AVOIDING COMMON PEDIATRIC ERRORS

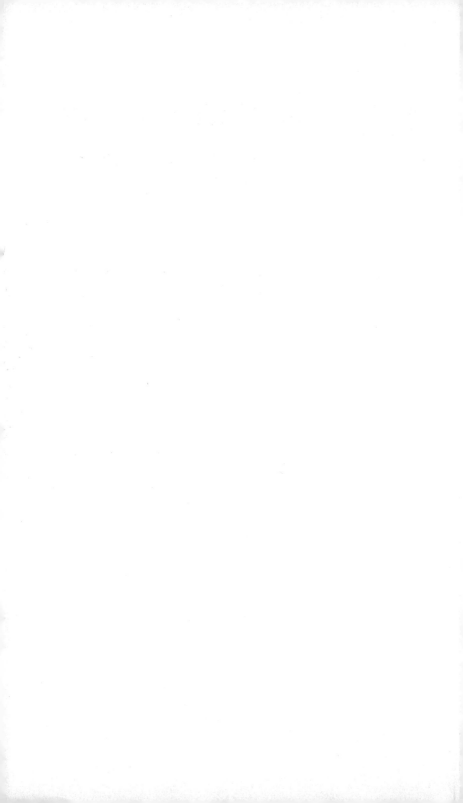

AVOIDING COMMON PEDIATRIC ERRORS

EDITOR

ANTHONY D. SLONIM, MD, DrPH
Vice President, Medical Affairs,
Carilion Medical Center

Senior Staff,
Carilion Clinic and Carilion Clinic Children's Hospital
Roanoke, Virginia

Professor, Medicine, Pediatrics, and Public Health
University of Virginia, School of Medicine and Public Health

Formerly
Executive Director, Center for Clinical Effectiveness
Attending Physician and Interim Chief, Critical Care Medicine
Children's National Medical Center
Washington, DC

SERIES EDITOR

LISA MARCUCCI, MD
Assistant Professor of Surgery
Division of Trauma and Critical Care
Department of Surgery
Thomas Jefferson University
Philadelphia, Pennsylvania

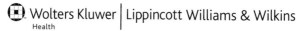
Wolters Kluwer | Lippincott Williams & Wilkins
Health
Philadelphia · Baltimore · New York · London
Buenos Aires · Hong Kong · Sydney · Tokyo

Acquisitions Editor: Sonya Seigafuse
Managing Editor: Ryan Shaw
Project Manager: Nicole Walz
Manufacturing Coordinator: Kathleen Brown
Marketing Manager: Kimberly Schonberger
Art Director: Risa Clow
Cover Designer: Marie Gardocky Clifton
Production Services: Aptara, Inc.

© 2008 by Lippincott Williams & Wilkins, a Wolters Kluwer business

All rights reserved. This book is protected by copyright. No part of this book may be reproduced in any form or by any means, including photocopying, or utilizing by any information storage and retrieval system without written permission from the copyright owner, except for brief quotations embodied in critical articles and reviews. To request permission, please contact Lippincott Williams & Wilkins at 530 Walnut Street, Philadelphia, PA 19016, via email at permissions@lww.com or via our website at lww.com (products and services.)

Printed in the United States

Library of Congress Cataloging-in-Publication Data

Avoiding common pediatric errors/editor, Anthony D. Slonim.
    p. ; cm.
Includes bibliographical references and index.
ISBN-13: 978-07817-7489-5
ISBN-10: 0-7817-7489-6
1. Pediatric errors—Prevention.   I. Slonim, Anthony D.
[DNLM: 1. Pediatrics—methods.   2. Child.   3. Diagnostic Techniques and Procedures.
4. Infant.   5. Medical Errors—prevention & control.   6. Therapeutics—methods.
WS 200 A961 2008]
RJ47.2.A96 2008
618.92—dc22

                                                                                2007051061

Care has been taken to confirm the accuracy of the information presented and to describe generally accepted practices. However, the authors, editors, and publisher are not responsible for errors or omissions or for any consequences from application of the information in this book and make no warranty, expressed or implied, with respect to the currency, completeness, or accuracy of the contents of the publication. Application of this information in a particular situation remains the professional responsibility of the practitioner; the clinical treatments described and recommended may not be considered absolute and universal recommendations.

The authors, editors, and publisher have exerted every effort to ensure that drug selection and dosage set forth in this text are in accordance with current recommendations and practice at the time of publication. However, in view of ongoing research, changes in government regulations, and the constant flow of information relating to drug therapy and drug reactions, the reader is urged to check the package insert for each drug for any change in indications and dosage and for added warnings and precautions. This is particularly important when the recommended agent is a new or infrequently employed drug.

Some drugs and medical devices presented in this publication have Food and Drug Administration (FDA) clearance for limited use in restricted research settings. It is the responsibility of health care providers to ascertain the FDA status of each drug or device planned for use in their clinical practice.

The publishers have made every effort to trace copyright holders for borrowed material. If they have inadvertently overlooked any, they will be pleased to make the necessary arrangements at the first opportunity.

To purchase additional copies of this book, call our customer service department at (800) 638-3030 or fax orders to (301) 223-2320. International customers should call (301) 223-2300. Visit Lippincott Williams & Wilkins on the Internet at: LWW.com. Lippincott Williams & Wilkins customer service representatives are available from 8:30 am to 6 pm, EST.

                                                      10 9 8 7 6 5 4 3 2 1

*Dedicated, as always, to my family.
Thank you for the reminders of what really
matters in life: love, health, and happiness.*

PREFACE

This book was developed to provide the pediatric component for the "Avoiding Common Errors" series. The content is focused on common pediatric medical problems that are associated with a patient safety component. These problems are relevant to the practicing pediatrician and pediatric trainees including medical students, residents, and fellows alike. The book's content of 250 concise "SNAFUs" is distributed proportionately across the core content areas for the American Board of Pediatrics' certification and recertification examinations.

The discussions presented here are not meant to be all encompassing, but rather draw attention to common "errors" in clinical practice. We have tried to keep the focus on important clinical topics that we have either experienced ourselves or learned from other colleagues. A guiding principle for the inclusion of scenarios was "if I only would have known that before it happened to me or my patients."

In addition, we are hopeful that this book will provide a practical guide for the care of patients. Medical decision making is based on incomplete information, considerable variability in presentation, and a need to recognize the emerging patterns of disease. When presented with a patient, our education allows physicians to progress stepwise, using a variety of tools to assist in delivering appropriate care. These areas are highlighted because they provide an opportunity for understanding where physician decision making may be flawed and thereby represent opportunities for patients to be harmed. Although each medical error is likely a combination of these physician processes, we tended to focus on the first breakdown point that needed to be kept in mind to avoid the error. We also recognize that medical decision making is more often an iterative "cycle" that begins with data gathering and ends up with additional data gathering after the first actions are taken (*Figure*). Nonetheless, we believe that this provided an important paradigm for combating medical errors occurring in the course of medical practice.

- **Data Gathering**: History and physical, laboratory, and radiographic testing, consultations, "workups," and knowledge of what the literature can offer.
- **Qualifying and Interpreting Data**: Assists in disease pattern recognition
- **Decision Making**: "What to do" and "What not to do"
- **Action Taking**: Operationalizing our decision for the patient's benefit

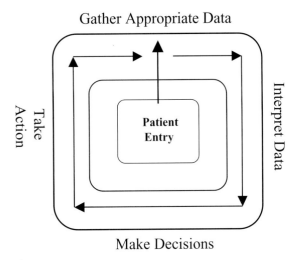

Gather Appropriate Data

Take Action

Interpret Data

Patient Entry

Make Decisions

Despite years of learning, I am humbled by how much is left to learn to effectively care for our patients. We must use every day to advance our own understanding of human disease, learn from the colleagues on our team, teach others about what we learn in our own practices and experiences, and enrich our lives by engaging with our patients and their families to provide the best care we know how, even when the outcomes for our most vulnerable patients may be less than optimal. These are the opportunities our profession provides us with and the true privilege that is ours, as physicians and pediatricians, to experience.

ANTHONY D. SLONIM, MD, DRPH

The editors welcome comments and suggestions at
sandson.marcucci@comcast.net

ACKNOWLEDGMENTS

AUTHORS:

Authorship can be a thankless job. You give all of your time, knowledge, and experience in writing a book chapter so that you can add a line to your CV and put a book on your shelf.

I would like to acknowledge and thank each one of the contributors for their efforts in turning this book into a product that we can all be proud of.

The greatest testament to our work would be that a child's life would be saved by someone who learned "What to do" or "What not to do" from our work.

ASSOCIATE EDITORS:

If you think authorship is thankless, try being an Associate Editor. More time, more energy, lots of editing, and a need to organize an entire book section and keep your contributors on task while meeting deadlines for the Editor—all of this with no special accolades.

I truly appreciate the work of this fine editorial group who met my demands, even when they were unreasonable. Importantly, this is their work. This group crafted the individual SNAFUS, guided their contributors through the process, and assured that the product that they gave to me was of the highest quality and on time. Thank you Jen, Jim, Sonya, David, John, Sophia, and Nailah.

SERIES EDITOR:

Dr. Lisa Marcucci, the Series Editor for the "Avoiding Common Errors" series has been a tremendous source of support and inspiration during this project. It is certainly difficult and often unnerving to rely upon others and allow them the autonomy and flexibility to get the job done. This is our second book together. In this effort, Lisa was consistent in providing amazing support by routinely checking in and making sure we were on task, but providing our editorial team with the latitude to be creative, work at our own pace, and create a product that we could "own." At particularly challenging times, I knew she was only a phone call or an e-mail away to discuss an idea or listen to me gripe about something that may not even be related to the project.

Lisa, I look forward to other opportunities to learn and collaborate with you.

SUPPORT:

Julie Owen, MHA

Thanks Jules for managing this project's details and alleviating the day-to-day disruptions that can be so distracting. I appreciate your special efforts at keeping me calm and providing support while we worked through this sometimes in pain-staking detail.

Robin Headley

Thank you Robin for all of the work you do make my life easier and more productive on a daily basis, and thanks for helping us to pull this together and meet our deadline.

CONTRIBUTORS

LINDSEY ALBRECHT, MD
Endocrinology Fellow
Department of Pediatrics
UC Davis Medical Center
Sacramento, California

JOHN T. BERGER, III, MD
Associate Professor
Department of Pediatrics
The George Washington University
Director of Cardiac Intensive Care
Divisions of Critical Care
    Medicine and Cardiology
Children's National Medical Center
Washington, DC

SONYA BURROUGHS, MD
Pediatrician
Physician Clinical Analyst, CTI Team
Children's National Medical Center
Washington, DC

DOROTHY Y. CHEN, MD, MPH
Physician
Department of Pediatrics
East Boston Neighborhood Health Center
East Boston, Massachusetts

MICHAEL R. CLEMMENS, MD
Director, Pediatric Hospitalist Program
Anne Arundel Medical Center
Annapolis, Maryland
Faculty, Children's National Medical
    Center
Assistant Professor of Pediatrics
George Washington University School of
    Medicine
Washington, DC

NAILAH COLEMAN, MD, FAAP
Pediatrician
Physician Clinical Analyst, CTI Team
Children's National Medical Center
Washington, DC

RUSSELL R. CROSS, MD
Medical Unit Director,
    Heart and Kidney Unit
Children's National Medical Center
Department of Cardiology
Assistant Professor of Pediatrics
The George Washington University
    Medical Center
Washington, DC

CRAIG C. DEWOLFE, MD
Assistant Professor of Pediatrics
Department of Pediatrics
The George Washington University
    School of Medicine
Pediatric Hospitalist
Children's Medical Center
Washington, DC

MADAN DHARMAR, MBBS
Graduate Researcher
Department of Pediatrics
University of California
    Davis Health System
Sacramento, California

MINDY DICKERMAN, MD
Pediatric Critical Care Fellow
Department of Critical Care
Children's National Medical Center
Washington, DC

MEGHA SHAH FITZPATRICK, MD
Fellow
Department of Critical Care Medicine
Children's National Medical Center
Washington, DC

ESTHER FORRESTER, MD
Pediatrician
Silver Spring, Maryland

WILLIAM GIASI, JR., MD
Pediatrician
Department of Pediatrics
Princeton Nassau Pediatrics
Pediatrician
Department of Pediatrics
University Medical Center at Princeton
Princeton, New Jersey

CYNTHIA GIBSON, MD
Division of Critical Care Medicine
Children's National Medical Center
Clinical Instructor, Pediatrics
The George Washington
    University School of Medicine
Washington, DC

ELLEN K. HAMBURGER, MD
Associate Clinical Professor of Pediatrics
Department of General Pediatrics
George Washington
    University School of Medicine
Associate Director of
    Graduate Medical Education
Department of Medical Education
Children's National Medical Center
Washington, DC

HEIDI HERRERA, MD
Division of Critical Care Medicine
Children's National Medical Center
Clinical Instructor, Pediatrics
The George Washington
    University School of Medicine
Washington, DC

LAURA HUFFORD, MD
Department of Pediatrics
Section of General Pediatrics
University of California,
    Davis School of Medicine
Sacramento, California

SARIKA JOSHI, MD
Fellow, Division of Pulmonary Medicine
Children's National Medica Center
Clinical Instructor, Pediatrics
The George Washington
    University School of Medicine
Washington, DC

BRIAN KIT, MD
Division of Hospital Medicine
Children's National Medical Center and
    Anne Arundel Medical Center
Annapolis, Maryland
Assistant Professor, Pediatrics
The George Washington University
    Medical Center
Washington, DC

YOLANDA LEWIS-RAGLAND, MD, FAAP
Community Pediatrician
Children's Health Project of DC
Children's National Medical
    Center
Washington, DC

JENNIFER MANISCALCO, MD, MPH
Assistant Professor
Department of Pediatrics
The George Washington School of
    Medicine and Health Sciences
Hospitalist
Department of Pediatrics
Children's National Medical Center
Washington, DC

EMILY RIEHM MEIER, MD
Fellow, Division of Hematology/Oncology
Children's National Medical Center
Washington, DC

NICKIE NIFORATOS, MD
Resident
General Pediatrics
Department of Graduate Medical
    Education
Children's National Medical Center
Washington, DC

JOHANN M. PETERSON, MD
Resident Physician
Department of Pediatrics
University of California,
    Davis, Medical Center
Sacramento, California

MICHAEL S. POTTER, BS
Graduate
Department of Computer Science
Virginia Polytechnic Institute and
    State University
Blacksburg, Virginia

CAROLINE E. RASSBACH, MD
Assistant Professor of Pediatrics
George Washington University
    School of Medicine and Health
    Sciences
Pediatric Hospitalist
Hospitalist Division
Children's National Medical Center
Washington, DC

RENÉE ROBERTS, MD
Assistant Professor of
    Anesthesiology and Pediatrics
Department of Anesthesiology
Children's National Medical Center
Washington, DC

**ANTHONY D. SLONIM,
    MD, DrPH**
Vice President, Medical Affairs
Carilion Medical Center
Senior Staff,
Carilion Clinic and Carilion Clinic
    Children's Hospital
Roanoke, Virginia
Professor, Medicine, Pediatrics, and Public
    Health
University of Virginia, School of Medicine
    and Public Health
Formerly:
Executive Director, Center for Clinical
    Effectiveness
Attending Physician and Interim Chief,
    Critical Care Medicine
Children's National Medical Center
Washington, DC

SOPHIA R. SMITH, MD
Division of Critical Care
    Medicine
Children's National Medical
    Center
Assistant Professor of Pediatrics
The George Washington
    University School of Medicine
Washington, DC

DAVID C. STOCKWELL, MD
Assistant Professor
Department of Pediatric Critical
    Care
George Washington University
    School of Medicine
Medical Director of Patient
    Safety
Department of Critical Care
Children's National Medical
    Center
Washington, DC

ANJALI SUBBASWAMY, MD
Division of Critical Care Medicine
Children's National Medical Center
Clinical Instructor, Pediatrics
The George Washington
    University School of Medicine
Washington, DC

**ELIZABETH M. WELLS,
    MD, MHS**
Resident
Department of Pediatrics
Children's National Medical Center
Washington, DC

CONTENTS

DEVELOPMENT AND ISSUES FOR SPECIFIC STAGES OF DEVELOPMENT

General Developmental Issues

Newborn and Infancy

Adolescence

HEALTH CARE GUIDANCE

Preventive Pediatrics

Psychosocial Issues

Nutrition

Substance Abuse

EMERGENCY MEDICINE AND CRITICAL CARE

ALLERGY, IMMUNOLOGY, INFECTIOUS DISEASE, AND RHEUMATOLOGY

Allergy

CONTENTS XXIII

92 Remember that erythema multiforme (EM) may be a sign of underlying hypersensitivity and may progress to Stevens-Johnson Syndrome (SJS), which can require aggressive fluid and skin care *Madan Dharmar, MD*.. 235

93 Provide supportive therapy for patients with Henoch-Schönlein purpura (HSP) *Emily Riehm Meier, MD*................................ 238

94 Patients who note a seafood or iodine allergy can safely receive intravenous (IV) contrast *Craig DeWolfe, MD*......................... 240

95 Many patients do not receive cephalosporins due to their penicillin allergy; most of these patients will not have an allergic response and can receive these drugs safely *Dorothy Chen, MD*............... 243

96 Proper vaccine administration is crucial to achieve the anticipated results. Know the methods for administering vaccines *Dorothy Chen, MD* 245

Infectious Diseases

97 Do not routinely test children for tuberculosis (TB) exposure *Yolanda Lewis-Ragland, MD*... 248

98 Do not avoid antibiotic use in patients with serious infections because of theoretical limitations *Yolanda Lewis-Ragland, MD*...... 250

99 Know that pinworms are a common cause of helminthic infection in the United States and may present with generic abdominal symptoms in children *Esther Forrester, MD* 252

100 Assure coverage for resistant *Streptococcus pneumoniae* with vancomycin if there is a concern for meningitis *Yolanda Lewis-Ragland, MD*... 254

101 Children who have suffered an infection for meningococcus should receive a work-up for an immunodeficiency (specifically a terminal complement disorder) *Lindsey Albrecht, MD*.......................... 257

102 Consider the diagnosis of Kawasaki disease in children with desquamation, fever, and rash *Lindsey Albrecht, MD* 259

103 Do not forget to use broad antimicrobial coverage for patients with osteomyelitis *Madan Dharmar, MD* 261

104 Know what to do for puncture wounds and the appropriate antibiotic therapy for pediatric patients *Laura Hufford, MD*.............. 264

Rheumatology

PEDIATRIC MEDICINE AND MEDICAL SUBSPECIALTIES

Cardiology

Endocrinology

Fluids, Electrolytes and Renal

Gastroenterology

Hematology

Pulmonology

PEDIATRIC SURGERY AND SURGICAL SUBSPECIALTIES

General Surgery

Trauma

NEUROMUSCULAR

Neurology

MISCELLANEOUS

Dermatology

Ethics

Genetic

Statistics

AVOIDING COMMON PEDIATRIC ERRORS

1

REMEMBER THAT THE PERSISTENCE OF PRIMITIVE REFLEXES IS A SIGN THAT THERE IS DAMAGE TO THE CENTRAL NERVOUS SYSTEM (CNS), SPECIFICALLY, A LACK OF HIGH-LEVEL CONTROL NECESSITATING A WORKUP FOR CEREBRAL PALSY (CP)

YOLANDA LEWIS-RAGLAND, MD

WHAT TO DO – INTERPRET THE DATA

The CNS is the control center for thinking, learning, and moving that develops in a highly organized and regulated sequence from conception. Movement patterns define this sequence at each developmental stage. These patterns are called primitive reflexes, which are important for survival. As the infant matures, the frontal lobes are responsible for suppressing primitive reflexes, but these may reappear during adulthood under certain conditions including dementia, traumatic lesions, and stroke. In infants who fail to suppress the primitive reflexes, CP must be entertained and currently, atypical primitive reflexes are also being investigated as potential early warning signs of Autism spectrum disorders.

PRIMITIVE REFLEXES ARE CHARACTERIZED BY:

- Automatic, stereotyped movements, directed by the brainstem
- Executed without involvement of higher levels of the brain (the cortex)
- Short-lived and replaced by more sophisticated structures (postural reflexes) controlled by the cortex once their function is no longer needed
- Retained if they do not fulfill their function or injury/insult occurs
- Considered aberrant and evidence of CNS immaturity if present beyond their usual time

WHAT IS CEREBRAL PALSY?

CP is a static encephalopathy caused by an insult to the brain during the prenatal, perinatal, or postnatal period. CP can lead to global dysfunction

ⓒ 2008 by Lippincott Williams & Wilkins, a Wolters Kluwer business

but always includes motor problems. CP is traditionally classified on the basis of the type of motor disorder. The revised classification now in use defines three main categories of motor disorders: (a) spastic (70%–80%), (b) dyskinetic (10%–15%), and (c) ataxic (<5%).

Spastic cases are further classified by involvement of the extremities. In quadriplegia (10%–15%), all four extremities are affected equally, and the trunk is involved. In diplegia (30%–40%), the lower extremities are affected more than the upper extremities. In hemiplegia (20%–30%), involvement is observed on one side of the body, including an arm and a leg. In monoplegia (rare), involvement is noted in one limb, either an arm or a leg; other causes should be ruled out.

CLINICAL PRESENTATIONS OF CEREBRAL PALSY

- Abnormal muscle tone is the most frequently observed symptom. The abnormalities may range from hypo- to hypertonic depending on the muscular resistance to passive movements.
- A definite hand preference before age 1 year is common (especially in patients with hemiplegia).
- An asymmetric crawl or failure to crawl
- Growth delay
- Joint contractures secondary to spastic muscles
- Persistent primitive reflexes: Examples such as Moro reflex, asymmetric tonic neck, symmetric tonic neck, palmar grasp, tonic labyrinthine, foot placement, are noted. A Moro reflex and a tonic labyrinthine should extinguish by the time the infant is aged 4 to 6 months; palmar grasp, by 5 to

---

TABLE 1.1	DIAGNOSTIC STUDIES FOR CEREBRAL PALSY

Laboratory Studies
- Thyroid studies
- Lactate level
- Pyruvate level
- Organic and amino acids
- Chromosomes
- Cerebrospinal protein: Levels may assist in determining asphyxia in the neonatal period. Protein levels can be elevated along with an elevated lactate to pyruvate ratio.

Imaging Studies
- CT provides diagnostic information for congenital malformations, intracranial hemorrhage, and periventricular leukomalacia.
- MRI is most useful after 2 to 3 weeks of life. MRI is the best study for assessing white matter disease in an older child.
- Evoked potentials are used to evaluate the anatomic pathways of the auditory and visual systems.

CT, computed tomography; MRI, magnetic resonance imaging.

6 months; asymmetric and symmetric tonic neck, by 6 to 7 months; and foot placement, before 12 months.

THE DIAGNOSTIC WORKUP FOR CEREBRAL PALSY

The diagnostic workup for CP included both laboratory and diagnostic radiologic studies, which are enumerated in *Table 1.1*. Neuroimaging studies can help to evaluate structural brain damage and to determine those at risk for CP. Data to support a definitive diagnosis of CP are lacking.

SUGGESTED READINGS

Cerebral Palsy Source. www.cerebralpalsysource.com. Accessed December 17, 2007.
National Institute of Neurological Disorders and Stroke. *Cerebral palsy: Hope through research:* Available at: www.ninds.nih.gov/disorders/cerebral_ palsy/detail_cerebral_palsy.htm. Accessed December 17, 2007.

REFER INFANTS DIAGNOSED WITH A SYNDROME KNOWN TO BE ASSOCIATED WITH MENTAL RETARDATION FOR EARLY INTERVENTION (EI) SERVICES AT THE TIME OF DIAGNOSIS EVEN THOUGH DEVELOPMENTAL DELAYS MAY NOT BE EVIDENT

ESTHER FORRESTER, MD

WHAT TO DO – TAKE ACTION

Early intervention (EI) applies to children of school age or younger who have or are at risk of developing a disability or other special need that may affect their development. The purpose of EI is to provide services to children and their families to lessen the effects of the condition. EI can be remedial or preventive in nature. Children are typically eligible for ongoing EI if they have at least one developmental delay with a 33% impact, or two delays of 25% impact as determined by professional testing. However, the criteria for qualifying for EI programs are established by state and local governments.

EI may focus on the child alone or on the child and the family together. An Individualized Family Service Plan (IFSP) is often formed based on the desired goals of the EIP. However, the EI official must also approve the final terms of each IFSP. Programs may be center-based, home-based, hospital-based, or a combination. Services range from identification (i.e., hospital or school screening and referral services) to diagnostic and direct intervention programs. EI may begin at any time between birth and school age. However, there are many reasons for it to begin as early as possible, principally to enhance the child's development, to provide support and assistance to the family, and to maximize the child's and family's benefit to society.

Child development research has established that the rate of human learning and development is most rapid in the preschool years. The timing of intervention becomes particularly important when a child runs the risk of missing an opportunity to learn during a state of maximum readiness. If the most teachable moments or stages of greatest readiness are not optimized, a child may have difficulty learning a particular skill at a later time.

EI services also have a significant impact on the parents and siblings of an exceptional infant or young child. The family of a young exceptional child often feels disappointment, social isolation, added stress, frustration, and helplessness. The compounded stress of the presence of an

© 2008 by Lippincott Williams & Wilkins, a Wolters Kluwer business

exceptional child may affect the family's well-being and interfere with the child's development. Families of children with a disability tend to experience increased instances of divorce and suicide, and the disabled child is more likely to be abused than the average child. EI can result in parents having improved attitudes about themselves and their child, improved information and skills for teaching their child, and more release time for leisure and employment. Parents of exceptional preschoolers also need early services to better provide the supportive and nourishing environment needed by the child.

A third reason for intervening early is that society will reap maximum benefits. The child's increased developmental and educational gains and decreased dependence on social institutions, the family's increased ability to cope with the presence of an exceptional child, and perhaps the child's increased eligibility for employment, provide economic and social benefits.

SUGGESTED READINGS

Kidsource Online. *What is early intervention?* http://www.kidsource.com/kidsource/content/early.intervention.html
Personal-Touch Early Intervention Program. *The EI process.* http://www.pthomecare.com/pdf/EI_process.pdf. Accessed March 2, 2007.

Additional Potential Sources

American Association on Intellectual and Developmental Disabilities. *Mental retardation: Definition, classification, and systems of supports.* 10th ed. Washington, DC: American Association on Intellectual and Developmental Disabilities; 2002.
Mental Retardation Management and Prognosis Pediatrics in Review http://pedsinreview.aappublications.org/cgi/content/extract/27/7/249 (subscription needed). Accessed December 17, 2007.

3

SEIZURE DISORDER SHOULD BE WORKED UP AGGRESSIVELY IN CHILDREN WITH MENTAL RETARDATION SINCE IT IS TEN TIMES MORE COMMON

ESTHER FORRESTER, MD

WHAT TO DO – GATHER APPROPRIATE DATA

Mental retardation (MR) or severe and profound intellectual disability generally occurs with other severe neurologic or psychiatric impairments, especially in individuals with acquired encephalopathy. Speech defects, epilepsy, and cerebral palsy (CP) are among the most common associated comorbid conditions. However, there are a number of syndromes associated with MR, all of which have their own associated features. Individuals with MR also have a significantly higher risk of sudden death than those without MR. The combination of MR with epilepsy or CP doubles the mortality compared to individuals with CP alone.

Epilepsy, which has a prevalence of <1% in the general population, has a prevalence of 20% to 30% in children with MR, independent of race. Notably, a diagnosis of epilepsy in this population can be difficult, given that patients with epilepsy commonly exhibit behaviors that resemble epilepsy. For example, generalized tonic extension crisis may occur in individuals with severe spasticity, resembling tonic–clonic seizures. Absence seizures may be mistaken for episodes of unresponsiveness that are frequently seen in patients with MR. Additionally, psychiatric disorders potentially responsible for self-destructive behavior in MR patients often need to be evaluated by neurologists to rule out frontal or temporal lobe seizures.

The prognosis of epilepsy in individuals with MR ultimately depends on the etiology of the MR. Some studies have shown a remission of seizures by the second decade of life, but the rate of remission is less than half that of children with normal intelligence—30% versus 70%. Generalizations in the prognosis of children with epilepsy and MR cannot be made, however, because MR is not uniform (*Tables 3.1* and *3.2*).

ⓒ 2008 by Lippincott Williams & Wilkins, a Wolters Kluwer business

TABLE 3.1	DEVELOPMENTAL CHARACTERISTICS RELATED TO LEVEL OF MENTAL RETARDATION (DSM-IV CRITERIA)*		
MILD RETARDATION	**MODERATE RETARDATION**	**SEVERE RETARDATION**	**PROFOUND RETARDATION**
75%–90% of all cases of retardation	~10%–25% of all cases of retardation	~10%–25% of all cases of retardation	~10%–25% of all cases of retardation
Function at 1/2–2/3 of CA (IQ: 50–70)	Function at 1/3–1/2 of CA (IQ: 35–49)	Function at 1/5–1/3 of CA (IQ: 20–34)	Function at <1/5 of CA (IQ: <20)
Slow in all areas	Noticeable delays, especially in speech	Marked and obvious delays; may walk late	Marked delays in all areas
May have no unusual physical signs	May have some unusual physical signs	Little or no communication skills but may have some understanding of speech and show some response	Congenital abnormalities often present
Can acquire practical skills	Can learn simple communication	May be taught daily routines and repetitive activities	Need close supervision
Useful reading and math skills up to grades 3–6 level	Can learn elementary health and safety habits	May be trained in simple self-care	Often need attendant care
Can conform socially	Can participate in simple activities and self-care	Need direction and supervision	May respond to regular physical activity and social stimulation
Can acquire vocational skills for self-maintenance	Can perform tasks in sheltered conditions	–	Not capable of self-care
Integrated into general society	Can travel alone to familiar places	–	–

NOTE: Additional problems with vision, hearing or speech, congenital abnormalities, seizures, emotional problems or cerebral palsy may be present.
DSM IV, *Diagnostic and Statistical Manual of Mental Disorders.* 4th ed.; CA, chronological age; IQ, intelligence quotient.
Adapted with permission from Pelegano JP, Healy A. Mental retardation. Part II. Seeing the child within. *Fam Pract Recertification.* 1992;14:63.

TABLE 3.2 COMMON SYNDROMES ASSOCIATED WITH MENTAL RETARDATION*

DIAGNOSIS	INCIDENCE	ETIOLOGY INCLUDING INHERITANCE	CLINICAL MANIFESTATIONS AND EARLY RECOGNITION	ASSOCIATED CONDITIONS	DIAGNOSTIC EVALUATION	PROGNOSIS	SPECIAL CONSIDERATIONS
Down syndrome	1 in 600–800 births	Results from extra copy of chromosome 21, usually a sporadic event; 2% of cases may be inherited from a balanced translocation carrier parent	Hypotonia; flat facial profile; upslanting palpebral fissures; small ears; in-curving fifth fingers; single transverse palmar creases	Slow growth; congenital heart defect; thyroid dysfunction; developmental delay, especially speech	Chromosome analysis in all patients; chromosome analysis of parents if translocation is found; pediatric cardiology evaluation with echocardiogram by 6 weeks of age	Cognitive limitations, with most in mild-to-moderate MR range; decreased life expectancy can be associated with congenital heart defect, especially if not recognized in early infancy	Except in cases where parent has a translocation, risk for recurrence is 1%
Fetal alcohol syndrome (FAS)	0.05–3 in 1,000 children diagnosed annually in United States	Alcohol consumption by mother during pregnancy	Diagnosis can be made at birth, based on history, baby's facial features (medial epicanthal folds, wide nasal bridge, small upturned nose, long philtrum, narrow or wide upper lip), low birth measurements	May include retardation, behavior problems, ADHD, seizures, autism	Good history and physical examination imperative; history of maternal drinking, pre- and postnatal growth retardation, dysmorphic facial features, CNS involvement; no laboratory tests available	Varies; growth may improve during adolescence and facial features may soften, but behaviors may cause serious problems	Many of these children are adopted; FAS and fetal alcohol effects (usually developmental and behavioral problems) are totally preventable

(Continued)

9

TABLE 3.2 (CONTINUED)

DIAGNOSIS	INCIDENCE	ETIOLOGY INCLUDING INHERITANCE	CLINICAL MANIFESTATIONS AND EARLY RECOGNITION	ASSOCIATED CONDITIONS	DIAGNOSTIC EVALUATION	PROGNOSIS	SPECIAL CONSIDERATIONS
Fragile X syndrome	1 in 2,000–3,000 male live births; females may also be affected	Abnormality in FMR-1 gene located on X chromosome; inherited in X-linked manner so males are more severely affected	Macrocephaly; large ears; enlarged testicles after puberty; hyperextensible fingers	Autism/autisticlike behaviors; developmental delay, especially speech; clumsiness; mitral valve prolapse	DNA testing for fragile X mutation (chromosome testing for fragile X misses up to 7% of cases); mothers of affected boys are obligate carriers of the gene	Normal life expectancy; mild-to-profound MR	Females usually less severely affected than males; up to 50% of females with mutation have MR or educational difficulties; risk for recurrence is 50%
Velocardiofacial syndrome	1 in 700 live births	Deletion of chromosome 22; usually de novo but may be inherited in an autosomal dominant manner	Cleft palate; congenital heart defect; speech delay; elongated face with almond-shaped eyes; wide nose with hypoplastic alae nasi; small ears; slender, hyperextensible fingers	Learning disabilities ± mild MR; psychiatric disorder in 10%	High-resolution chromosome analysis with chromosome painting (FISH) to detect chromosome 22 deletion; parents should also be tested	Normal life expectancy unless severe heart defect (e.g., truncus arteriosus, interrupted aortic arch) is present	Risk for recurrence as high as 50%, depending on family history

| Unknown cause of MR | 30%–50% of all cases of MR | Variable; diagnosis may evolve over time, so repeated evaluations may be helpful | Nonspecific cluster of minor malformations, delayed milestones, especially language development | Behavioral phenotype may also aid diagnosis as course evolves | Cytogenetic studies; brain imaging; metabolic studies | Will vary considerably based on etiology (if it can be established) and/or severity | Diagnostic techniques that may aid in diagnosis are constantly being refined |

DSM IV, *Diagnostic and Statistical Manual of Mental Disorders*, 4th ed.; CA, chronological age; IQ, intelligence quotient.

MR, mental retardation; ADHD, attention-deficit/hyperactivity disorder; CNS, central nervous system; FAS, fetal alcohol syndrome; FISH, fluorescence in situ hybridization.

Information from references 4, 5, 7 and 18.

*Tables 1 and 2 were copied directly from Daily DK, Ardinger HH, Holmes GE. Identification and evaluation of mental retardation." *Am Fam Physician.* 2000;61(4): 1059–1067, 1070.

SUGGESTED READINGS

Alvarez N. Epilepsy in children with mental retardation. http://www.emedicine.com/NEURO/topic550.htm. Accessed March 1, 2007.

Arvio M, Sillanpää, M. Prevalence, aetiology and comorbidity of severe and profound intellectual disability in Finland. *J Intellect Dis Res.* 2003;47(Pt 2):108–112.

Daily DK, Ardinger HH, Holmes GE. Identification and evaluation of mental retardation. *Am Fam Physician.* 2000;61(4):1059–1067, 1070.

4

REFER OLDER CHILDREN (OLDER THAN 3 YEARS) DIAGNOSED WITH MENTAL RETARDATION WHO ARE TOO OLD FOR EARLY INTERVENTION PROGRAM (EIP) TO PRESCHOOL PROGRAMS FOR CHILDREN WITH DISABILITIES (PPCD)

YOLANDA LEWIS-RAGLAND, MD

WHAT TO DO – TAKE ACTION

What Is Mental Retardation? Mental retardation (MR) is a term used to describe limitations in mental functioning and skills such as communicating, personal care, and social skills. These limitations will cause a child to learn and develop more slowly than a typical child. Children with MR may take longer to learn to speak, walk, and perform activities of daily living such as dressing or eating. They are likely to have trouble learning in school, having an inability to learn certain things and taking longer to learn things that they can learn.

HOW IS MENTAL RETARDATION DIAGNOSED?

To diagnose MR, professionals look at the person's intellectual functioning and adaptive skills. Intellectual functioning is usually measured by a test called an IQ (intelligence quotient) test. The average score is 100. People scoring <70 to 75 have MR. To measure adaptive behavior, professionals compare the child to other children of his or her age. Certain skills are important to adaptive behavior. These are:

- Daily living skills, such as getting dressed, going to the bathroom, and feeding one's self
- Communication skills, such as understanding what is said and being able to answer
- Social skills with peers, family members, adults, and others.

Approximately 87% of people with MR will have slower than average learning of new information and skills. When they are children, their limitations may not be obvious. They may not even be diagnosed with MR until they get to school. As adults, many people with mild MR can live independently. Others may not even be considered as having MR. The remaining 13% of people with MR score below 50 on IQ tests. These people experience difficulty in school, at home, and in the community. People with more severe

© 2008 by Lippincott Williams & Wilkins, a Wolters Kluwer business

MR will need intensive support for their entire life. Every child with MR is able to learn, develop, and grow. With help, all children with MR can live a satisfying life.

SIGNS OF MENTAL RETARDATION

There are many signs of MR including:

- Delayed sitting up, crawling, or walking than other children
- Learning to talk later, or have trouble speaking
- Difficulty with memory
- Lack of understanding for how to pay for things
- Difficulty understanding social rules
- Difficulty seeing the consequences of their actions
- Difficulty with solving problems
- Difficulty thinking logically

EARLY INTERVENTIONS FOR CHILDREN WITH MENTAL RETARDATION

A child with MR can do well in school but is likely to need individualized assistance. States are responsible for meeting the educational needs of children with disabilities. For children younger than 3 years, services are provided through an early intervention system. Staff work with the child's family to develop what is known as an Individualized Family Services Plan, or IFSP. The IFSP will describe the child's unique needs. It also describes the services the child will receive to address those needs. The IFSP will emphasize the unique needs of the family, so that parents and other family members will know how to help their young child with MR. For eligible school-aged children (including preschoolers), special education and related services are made available through the school system. School staff will work with the child's parents to develop an Individualized Education Program, or IEP. The IEP is similar to an IFSP. It describes the child's unique needs and the services that have been designed to meet those needs. Special education and related services are provided at no cost to parents.

TRANSITION FROM EARLY EDUCATION THROUGH HIGH SCHOOL

Many children with MR receive help with adaptive skills that enable them to transition into adolescence and early adulthood prepared for a level of self-sufficiency. These adaptive skills are needed to live, work, and participate in the community. Teachers and parents can help a child or adolescent work on these skills at both school and home. Some of these skills include:

- Clear communication with others
- Taking care of personal needs of daily living (dressing, bathing, going to the bathroom)

- Health and safety
- Home living (helping to set the table, cleaning the house, or cooking dinner)
- Social skills (manners, knowing the rules of conversation, getting along in a group, playing a game)
- Reading, writing, and basic math
- Travel (buses, subway, etc.)
- And as they get older, skills that will help them in the workplace.

Overall, there are a number of services available for children with MR. It is important to know what services are available to allow each child to optimize their developmental outcomes and participate in the world around them.

SUGGESTED READINGS

Mental Retardation: A Symptom and a Syndrome. www.uab.edu/cogdev/mentreta.htm

National Dissemination Center for Children with Disabilities. *Mental retardation fact sheet* (FS8). 2004. www.nichcy.org/pubs/factshe/fs8txt.htm. Accessed December 17, 2007.

U.S. Department of Education. *Guide to the individualized education program.* www.ed.gov/parents/needs/speced/iepguide/index.html. Accessed December 17, 2007.

5

KNOW THE DIFFERENT TYPES OF MENTAL RETARDATION (MR) AND DEVELOPMENTAL DELAY AS IT HAS IMPLICATIONS FOR TREATMENT AND COUNSELING

ELIZABETH WELLS, MD

WHAT TO DO – INTERPRET THE DATA

Three main types of developmental delay that pediatricians should know and understand are Aspberger syndrome, autism, and global developmental delay. Knowing the distinctions between the types of developmental delay and MR can lead to earlier diagnosis and referral for appropriate services and may have a positive effect on the long-term outcomes for affected children and their families.

According to the *Diagnostic and Statistical Manual of Mental Disorders,* 4th ed.; (DSM-IV) individuals with MR have an intelligence quotient (IQ) <70 and concurrent impairments in adaptive functioning in at least two of the following areas: communication, self-care, home living, social or interpersonal skills, use of community resources, self-direction, functional academic skills, work, leisure, health, and safety. MR must be diagnosed before age 18. The degree of MR is delineated by the IQ score, with an IQ of 55 to 69 signaling mild MR, an IQ of 40 to 54 signaling moderate MR, an IQ of 25 to 39 signaling severe MR, and an IQ of <24 signaling profound MR. The IQ level above which a child with MR is expected to benefit from a formal educational program is 50.

Although IQ testing is possible in the preschool years, the diagnosis of MR is usually not applied until the child reaches school age, when IQ testing is considered more reliable and reflective of the child's long-term abilities. Prior to that time, a diagnosis of "global developmental delay" is used and is sufficient to access appropriate support services within schools and public agencies.

Autism and Asperger syndrome are the two most common conditions classified as pervasive developmental disorders (PDDs). Often described as "autism spectrum disorders," these PDDs are marked by three central characteristics: impairments in social reciprocity, impairments in communication, and abnormalities of behavior.

Children with autism and Asperger syndrome both have impaired social learning. They often exhibit disabilities in initiating, responding to, and

---

ⓒ 2008 by Lippincott Williams & Wilkins, a Wolters Kluwer business

maintaining social interactions. They have particular difficulty with nonverbal communication, such as eye contact, gestures, and voice inflection. They have trouble integrating verbal and nonverbal components of communication. Most of these children have difficulty engaging in the "give–and-take" of social interactions.

Autism and Asperger syndrome are both characterized by communication impairments, and the degree of impairment helps define the differences between these syndromes. In children with autism, language is severely delayed and unusual or deviant, in both expressive and receptive areas. Cooing and babbling may develop in the first 6 months of life but then be lost, and speech develops late or not at all. In contrast, children with Asperger syndrome do not show delays in speech. When expressive language develops in children with PDD, it has impaired pragmatics. Early language often consists of echolalia and use of certain "stock phrases" or repetition of conversation from television. Other characteristics include confusion of personal pronouns, verbal perseveration (repeating something over and over or dwelling on a specific subject), and abnormalities of prosody (modulation of volume, pitch, rate of speaking). Although children with Asperger syndrome may have strong vocabularies, their language deficits include lack of "turn-taking" in conversations, preoccupation with their own areas of special interest, tangential or off-topic responses, and problems with abstract language.

The presence of repetitive and stereotypic behaviors is the third component in the diagnosis of an "autism spectrum disorder." Stereotypic motor behaviors include the flapping of hands, head banging, rocking, pacing, and twirling objects. These occur more frequently when the child is excited, stressed, or upset. During play, children with PDDs may prefer to line up cars or blocks in identical patterns rather than engage in imaginative or varied play. They also are often preoccupied with minor details or situations or objects. Older children show an all-consuming interest in certain topics or interests, such as maps or train schedules. Cognitive inflexibility is also reflected in the fact that these children have difficulty with transitions and do best with a predictable schedule and routine.

For a diagnosis of autism, a child must meet at least six of 12 DSM-IV criteria with at least two criteria relating to a disorder of social development, one relating to a disorder of communication, and one relating to a stereotypic behavior pattern. At least one of the above criteria must have an onset before 3 years of age, and the disturbance must not be better accounted for by another developmental disorder, such as Rett's disorder or childhood disintegrative disorder. Two thirds to three quarters of individuals with autistic disorder also have MR. Determining whether social communication lags behind other domains of development may aid in the classification of autism in patients with MR.

DSM-IV criteria for Asperger syndrome require qualitative impairment in social interaction and restricted repetitive and stereotyped patterns of behavior, interests and activities. The disturbance must cause clinically significant impairment in social, occupational, or other important areas of functioning. It is differentiated from autism by the fact that there is no clinically significant general language delay. In addition, there is no clinically significant delay in cognitive development or in the development of age-appropriate self-help skills, adaptive behavior, and curiosity about the environment.

All children should be monitored for developmental progress. Early identification of a developmental delay can help ensure access to resources and appropriate treatment and can enable a child to develop and use all of his or her capabilities.

SUGGESTED READINGS

American Association on Mental Retardation. *Mental Retardation: Definition, Classification, and Systems of Support,* 10th ed. Washington, DC: American Association on Mental Retardation, 2002.

American Psychiatric Association. *Diagnostic and Statistical Manual of Mental Disorders.* 4th ed. Washington, DC: American Psychiatric Association, 2000.

Batshaw ML, Shapiro BK. Mental retardation. In: Batshaw ML, ed. *Children with Disabilities, 5th ed.* Baltimore, MD: Paul H. Brookes; 2002:287–307.

Bauer, S. Autism and the pervasive developmental disorders: Part 1. *Pediatr Rev.* 1995;16(4):130–136.

Committee on Children with Disabilities. Technical report: The pediatrician's role in the diagnosis and management of autistic spectrum disorder in children. *Pediatrics.* 2001;107 (5):E85.

Towbin KE, Mauk JE, Batshaw ML. Pervasive developmental disorders. Batshaw ML, ed. *Children with Disabilities,* 5th ed. Baltimore, MD: Paul H. Brookes; 2002:365–388.

Walker WO Jr, Johnson CP. Mental retardation: Overview and diagnosis. *Pediatr Rev.* 2006;27(6);204–212.

6

WATCH FOR SIGNS OF MALNUTRITION EITHER UNDER- OR OVERNUTRITION, WHICH REPRESENT ADVERSE HEALTH CONSEQUENCES FOR CHILDREN

MICHAEL S. POTTER AND ANTHONY SLONIM, MD

WHAT TO DO – GATHER APPROPRIATE DATA

Although it less common in developed countries, malnutrition is still an important condition that can adversely affect pediatric health. The effects of malnutrition, depending on the extent of the condition, can persist into adulthood. Malnutrition is most often manifested as undernutrition; however, overnutrition, frequently resulting in obesity, has also become a major threat to children in the United States. Because childhood is largely a period of physical growth and development, an awareness of the common signs of malnutrition, including various anthropometric signs, is critical for quickly correcting dietary abnormalities. Vitamin deficiencies and surpluses also contribute to malnutrition and need to be considered when discussing problems with nutrition.

Undernutrition is a concept that conjures up different meanings for patients and providers based upon a number of societal factors. Depending on whether the deficiency is protein, energy, or micronutrients: the signs, symptoms, intervention, and treatment strategies will be different. Some of the presenting signs of undernutrition include growth failure, low birth weight, signs of specific vitamin and nutrient deficiencies (*Table 6.1*), and infectious diseases. A nutritional assessment is primarily based on the physical exam. There are three primary anthropometric indices that are used to determine the general cause or extent of undernutrition: height for age, weight for age, and weight for height. Although these metrics are good for an initial assessment, they are only one component of a more thorough assessment to determine the patient's nutritional status.

The deficiency of a single nutrient is often considered undernutrition. Typically, a deficiency in several nutrients leads to the term protein/energy malnutrition (PEM). Primary PEM, which is more prevalent in developing countries, is related to inadequate food intake. Secondary PEM, which is more prevalent in developed countries, is concerned with increased nutrient requirements, increased nutrient losses, and decreased nutrient absorption. The two most severe forms of PEM, marasmus and kwashiorkor,

© 2008 by Lippincott Williams & Wilkins, a Wolters Kluwer business

TABLE 6.1   PHYSICAL AND METABOLIC PROPERTIES AND FOOD SOURCES OF THE VITAMINS*

NAMES AND SYNONYMS	EFFECTS OF DEFICIENCY	EFFECTS OF EXCESS
Vitamin A: retinol (vitamin A₁) is an alcohol of high molecular weight; 1 μg of retinol = 3.3 IU vitamin A. Provitamin A: the plant pigments α-, β-, and γ-carotenes and cryptoxanthin; 1/6 activity of retinol	Nyctalopia, photophobia, xerophthalmia, conjunctivitis, keratomalacia leading to blindness; faulty epiphyseal bone formation; defective tooth enamel; keratinization of mucous membranes and skin; retarded growth; impaired resistance to infection	Anorexia, slow growth, drying and cracking of skin, enlargement of liver and spleen, swelling and pain of long bones, bone fragility, increased intracranial pressure, alopecia, carotenemia
Vitamin B Complex: thiamine: vitamin B₁; antiberiberi vitamin; aneurin	Beriberi, fatigue, irritability, anorexia, constipation, headache, insomnia, tachycardia, polyneuritis, cardiac failure, edema, elevated pyruvic acid in the blood, aphonia	None from oral intake
Riboflavin: vitamin B₂	Ariboflavinosis; photophobia, blurred vision, burning and itching of eyes, corneal vascularization, poor growth, cheilosis	Not harmful
Niacin: nicotinamide; nicotinic acid; antipellagra vitamin	Pellagra, multiple B-vitamin deficiency syndrome, diarrhea, dementia, dermatitis	Nicotinic acid (not the amide) is vasodilator; skin flushing and itching; hepatopathy
Folacin: group of related compounds containing pteridine ring, para-amino benzoic acid, and glutamic acid. Pteroylglutamic acid (PGA)	Megaloblastic anemia (infancy, pregnancy) usually is secondary to malabsorption disease, glossitis, pharyngeal ulcers, impaired immunity	Unknown
Cyanocobalamin: vitamin B₁₂	Juvenile pernicious anemia, due to defect in absorption rather than to dietary lack; also secondary to gastrectomy, celiac disease, inflammatory lesions of small bowel, long-term drug therapy (neomycin); methylmalonic aciduria; homocystinuria	Unknown

(continued)

TABLE 6.1   (CONTINUED)

NAMES AND SYNONYMS	EFFECTS OF DEFICIENCY	EFFECTS OF EXCESS
Biotin	Dermatitis, seborrhea; inactivated by avidin in raw egg white	None known
Vitamin B₆ active forms: pyridoxine, pyridoxal, pyridoxamine	Irritability, convulsions, hypochromic anemia; peripheral neuritis in patients receiving isoniazid; oxaluria	Sensory neuropathy
Vitamin C: ascorbic acid; vitamin C; antiscorbutic vitamin	Scurvy and poor wound healing	Oxaluria
Vitamin D: group of sterols having similar physiologic activity, D₂-calciferol is activated ergosterol. D₃ is activated 7-dehydrocholesterol in skin.1 µg = 40 IU vitamin D	Rickets (high serum phosphatase level appears before bone deformities); infantile tetany; poor growth; osteomalacia	Wide variation in tolerance; over 500 µg/24 hr toxic when continued for weeks; prolonged administration of 45 µg/24 hr may be toxic; nausea, diarrhea, weight loss, polyuria, nocturia, calcification of soft tissues, including heart, renal tubules, blood vessels, bronchi, stomach
Vitamin E: group of related chemical compounds—tocopherols with similar biologic activities	Requirements related to polyunsaturated fat intake; red blood cell hemolysis in premature infants; loss of neural integrity	Unknown
Vitamin K: group of aphthoquinones with similar biologic activities; K₁ is a phytoquinone	Hemorrhagic manifestations; bone metabolism	Not established; analogues may produce hyperbilirubinemia in premature infants

*Modified from Heird WC. Nutrition. In: Behrman RE, Kliegman RM, Jenson HB. *Nelson Textbook of Pediatrics,* 17th ed. Philadelphia: Saunders; 2004.

are typically considered as distinct disorders. Marasmus, also known as nonedematous PEM, is thought to result from inadequate energy intake, and it initially presents itself as a failure to gain weight, which is followed by weight loss. The skin then loses turgor and becomes loose as a result of the loss of subcutaneous fat. Muscle atrophy and hypotonia are also characteristic signs. Kwashiorkor, also known as edematous PEM, presents with indistinct symptoms such as lethargy and apathy. In its advanced stage, kwashiorkor results in a loss of stamina, inadequate growth, muscle loss, increased susceptibility to infection, vomiting, diarrhea, and edema. It is worth noting that edema can develop early and conceal weight loss. Other common signs in edematous PEM are dermatitis, depigmentation, hair thinning and loss.

Overnutrition, or obesity, is becoming an epidemic in developed countries. Children are experiencing the growing health risks that accompany obesity, and although genetic defects can rarely cause obesity in children, the most common cause relates to excess calorie consumption. The most common indicators include tall stature, slightly advanced bone age, and early puberty. In addition, many obese pediatric patients exhibit acanthosis nigricans, a hypertrophic hyperpigmentation of the skin. This condition puts children at a higher risk of developing type 2 diabetes and insulin resistance. Evaluation of body mass index and skinfold thickness may be helpful in determining overall body fat content.

Alhough nutritional issues are more commonly thought to plague impoverished nations, developed countries are not exempt from the effects of malnutrition. Being familiar with the signs of nutritional abnormalities in children is especially important to preventing future developmental issues.

SUGGESTED READINGS

Heird WC. Nutrition. In: Behrman RE, Kliegman RM, Jenson HB. *Nelson Textbook of Pediatrics*. 17th ed. Philadelphia: Saunders. 2004.

Speiser PW, Rudolf MCJ, Anhalt H, et al. Obesity Consensus Working Group. Childhood obesity. *J Clin Endocrinol Metabol*. 2005;90:1871–1887.

7

KNOW HOW TO SEQUENTIALLY EVALUATE NEONATAL CHOLESTASIS

ANJALI SUBBASWAMY, MD

WHAT TO DO – GATHER APPROPRIATE DATA, INTERPRET THE DATA

Neonatal cholestasis is a pathologic state of reduced bile formation or flow, where contents normally excreted into bile are retained and measurable in blood. The incidence is approximately one in 2,500 live births. It is a typical presenting feature of neonatal liver disease rather than a late manifestation. Mechanisms are hepatocellular (viral hepatitis, Dubin-Johnson syndrome) or obstructive (choledochal cyst, biliary atresia). There is an extensive differential diagnosis, including neonatal sclerosing cholangitis, cystic fibrosis, hypothyroidism, and tyrosinemia. When pathologic jaundice is noted, a workup should begin promptly and include:

- Fractionated bilirubin levels
- Blood type and Rh determination in mother and infant
- Direct Coombs testing in the infant
- Hemoglobin and hematocrit values
- Serum albumin levels: albumin binds bilirubin in a ratio of 1:1
- Ultrasound examination of the liver and bile ducts
- A radionuclide liver scan for uptake of hepatoiminodiacetic acid (HIDA) is indicated for suspected extrahepatic biliary atresia
- The only definitive diagnosis for biliary atresia is an intraoperative cholangiogram.

If the cause of the cholestasis is biliary atresia, expeditious surgical repair is necessary to avoid worsening cholestasis, hepatic fibrosis, and cirrhosis, which lead to portal hypertension, hepatic failure and death. Most infants present at 4 to 6 weeks of age, with a history of persistent jaundice and acholic stools. Operating before 60 days of age and having type 1 biliary atresia (obliteration of the common bile duct) are associated with favorable surgical

© 2008 by Lippincott Williams & Wilkins, a Wolters Kluwer business

outcomes. The aim of surgical repair, via the Kasai portoenterostomy, is to restore bile flow, alleviate jaundice, and abbreviate the cholangiodestructive process within the liver. Orthotopic liver transplantation is an option typically reserved for a failed Kasai procedure. Preoperative preparation for a Kasai procedure includes optimizing nutrition, administering 1 mg/day vitamin K by mouth/intramuscularly/intravenously to minimize perioperative coagulopathy. Some advocate preoperative antibiotics to minimize gut flora and postoperative trimethoprim-sulfa to minimize cholangitis. There are no studies proving the efficacy of any of these recommendations.

SUGGESTED READINGS

Bates MD, Bucuvalas JC, Alonso MH, et al. Biliary atresia: pathogenesis and treatment. *Semin Liv Dis.* 1998;18(3):281–293.
Middlesworth W, Altman RP. Biliary atresia. *Curr Opin Pediatr.* 1997;9(3):265–269.
Suchy FJ. Neonatal cholestasis. *Pediatr Rev.* 2004;25:388–396.

8

INFANTS WITH GREATER THAN 20% OF THEIR BILIRUBIN IN THE DIRECT FORM HAVE CHOLESTASIS OR OBSTRUCTION TO BILE FLOW. THE FIRST STEP IN EVALUATION OF PROLONGED JAUNDICE IS TO MEASURE TOTAL AND FRACTIONAL BILIRUBIN CONCENTRATIONS

YOLANDA LEWIS-RAGLAND, MD

WHAT TO DO – GATHER APPROPRIATE DATA

Jaundice is derived from the French word *jaune,* which means yellow, and is the term used to describe the yellowish discoloration caused by an excess amount of bilirubin in skin. Bilirubin is a yellowish-red pigment that is the result of red blood cell (RBC) breakdown in the natural RBC aging process, and is normally found in small amounts in the blood. Its appearance in newborns is primarily due to the immaturity of the newborn's liver, which cannot effectively metabolize the bilirubin and prepare it for excretion into the urine.

When too much bilirubin is made, the excess is dumped into the bloodstream and deposited in tissues for temporary storage. Most jaundice in newborn babies is a normal event and is not critical. In most cases, this jaundice appears between the second and fifth days of life and clears with time, often without treatment. Also, once this type of jaundice disappears, there is no evidence that it will appear again or that it has any lasting effects on the baby.

PHYSIOLOGIC JAUNDICE

Physiologic jaundice in healthy term newborns follows a typical pattern. The average total serum bilirubin level usually peaks at 5 to 6 mg/dL (86–103 μmol/L) on the third to fourth day of life and declines over the first week after birth. Bilirubin elevations of up to 12 mg/dL, with <2 mg/dL (34 μmol/L) of the conjugated form, can sometimes occur. Infants with multiple risk factors may develop an exaggerated form of physiologic jaundice in which the total serum bilirubin level may rise as high as 17 mg/dL (291 μmol/L) (Table 8.1).

Other factors that contribute to the development of physiologic hyperbilirubinemia in the neonate include an increased bilirubin load because of relative polycythemia, a shortened erythrocyte life span (80 days

© 2008 by Lippincott Williams & Wilkins, a Wolters Kluwer business

TABLE 8.1	RISK FACTORS FOR HYPERBILIRUBINEMIA IN NEWBORNS

Maternal factors
  Blood type ABO or Rh incompatibility
  Breastfeeding
  Drugs: diazepam (Valium), oxytocin (Pitocin)
  Ethnicity: Asian, Native American
  Maternal illness: gestational diabetes

Neonatal factors
  Birth trauma: cephalohematoma, cutaneous bruising, instrumented delivery
  Drugs: sulfisoxazole acetyl with erythromycin ethylsuccinate (Pediazole),
    chloramphenicol (Chloromycetin)
  Excessive weight loss after birth
  Infections: TORCH
  Infrequent feedings
  Male gender
  Polycythemia
  Prematurity
  Previous sibling with hyperbilirubinemia

TORCH, toxoplasmosis, other viruses, rubella, cytomegalovirus, herpes (simplex) viruses.

compared with the adult 120 days), immature hepatic uptake and conjugation processes, and decreased enterohepatic circulation.

BREAST MILK JAUNDICE

Breastfeeding jaundice is recognized in two phases: early-onset and late-onset.

Early Onset Breastfeeding Jaundice. Breastfed newborns may be at increased risk for early onset exaggerated physiologic jaundice because of relative caloric deprivation in the first few days of life. Decreased volume and frequency of feedings may result in mild dehydration and the delayed passage of meconium. Compared with formula-fed newborns, breastfed infants are 3 to 6 times more likely to experience moderate jaundice (total serum bilirubin level >12 mg/dL) or severe jaundice (total serum bilirubin level >15 mg/dL [257 μmol/L]).

Late-Onset Breast Milk Jaundice. Breast milk jaundice occurs later in the newborn period, with the bilirubin level usually peaking between days 6 and 14 of life. This late-onset jaundice may develop in up to one third of healthy breastfed infants. Total serum bilirubin levels vary from 12 to 20 mg/dL (340 μmol/L) and are nonpathologic. The underlying cause of breast milk jaundice is not entirely understood. Substances in maternal milk, such as ß-glucuronidases, and nonesterified fatty acids, may inhibit normal bilirubin metabolism. The bilirubin level usually falls continually after the infant is 2 weeks old, but it may remain persistently elevated for 1 to 3 months.

PATHOLOGIC JAUNDICE

All etiologies of jaundice beyond physiologic and breastfeeding or breast milk jaundice are considered pathologic. Features of pathologic jaundice include the appearance of jaundice within 24 hours after birth, a rapidly rising total serum bilirubin concentration (increase of more than 5 mg/dL/day), and a total serum bilirubin level >17 mg/dL in a full-term newborn. Other features of concern include prolonged jaundice, evidence

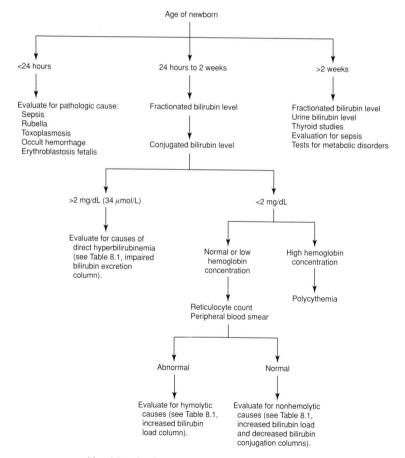

FIGURE 8.1. Algorithm for the suggested evaluation of a term newborn with hyperbilirubinemia.

of underlying illness, and elevation of the serum conjugated bilirubin level to >2 mg/dL or >20% of the total serum bilirubin concentration. Pathologic causes include disorders such as sepsis, rubella, toxoplasmosis, occult hemorrhage, and erythroblastosis fetalis.

LABORATORY EVALUATION

The initial evaluation of jaundice depends on the age of the newborn. If the serum conjugated bilirubin level is >2 mg/dL, the infant should be evaluated for possible hepatocellular disease or biliary obstruction. Using the following algorithm, clinicians are able to systematically evaluate the most likely cause of hyperbilirubinemia in a baby and initiate appropriate therapy (*Fig. 8.1*).

SUGGESTED READINGS

Hansen TWR. *Jaundice, neonatal.* 2006, eMedicine. www.emedicine.com/PED/topic1061.htm. Accessed December 17, 2007.

MedlinePlus Medical Encyclopedia: *Newborn jaundice.* 2007. www.nlm.nih.gov/medlineplus/ency/article/001559.htm. Accessed. *Newborn jaundice.* 2005. www.emedicinehealth.com/newborn_jaundice/article_em.htm. Accessed December 17, 2007.

9

BE CAREFUL WHEN EXAMINING THE NEWBORN INFANT. OFTEN A MULTITUDE OF RASHES, MORPHOLOGIC VARIATIONS AND UNUSUAL EYE FINDINGS CAN BE FOUND AND DO NOT REQUIRE A WORKUP, BUT OCCASIONALLY THE DIAGNOSTIC HALLMARKS OF A SERIOUS RASH ARE SUBTLE

LAURA HUFFORD, MD

WHAT TO DO – INTERPRET THE DATA

Erythema toxicum is a benign rash that usually presents in the first days of life and self resolves by 7 days. The rash varies in appearance from blotchy, erythematous macules to yellow pustules on an erythematous base. The lesions are most commonly located on the trunk and extremities but can be seen on the face. The lesions also may wax and wane and may change location within a few hours. If the diagnosis is in question, a pustule can be opened, and the cells treated with a Wright stain will reveal an eosinophilic predominance.

Unlike the benign nature of erythema toxicum, herpes simplex virus (HSV) causes a rash that is a warning sign to the examiner of serious infection. Infants usually acquire HSV when they pass through the birth canal and come into contact with the virus. Of note, HSV may be shed even if the mother is asymptomatic, so a negative history of maternal HSV does not rule out HSV infection in the newborn. Neonates may also become infected during pregnancy or postnatally when they come in contact with someone with herpes gingivostomatitis.

There are three classifications of neonatal infection: disease confined to the skin, eye, and mouth; confined to the central nervous system (CNS), such as encephalitis/meningitis; and disseminated disease which involves hepatitis, multiorgan failure, shock, and disseminated intravascular coagulation (DIC). CNS disease has an associated mortality of 50% and disseminated disease of at least 85% in the absence of appropriate antiviral therapy. Nearly 40% of patients with CNS or disseminated disease have skin lesions.

Typical lesions are clustered papules on an erythematous base that quickly evolve into thin walled vesicles which easily denude to reveal a shallow ulcer. Once skin lesions are discovered, they should be cultured for

---

© 2008 by Lippincott Williams & Wilkins, a Wolters Kluwer business

HSV and acyclovir therapy should be initiated immediately, and the patient should have further evaluation and assessment to determine the extent of the infection.

Ophthalmia neonatorum, or conjunctivitis within the first month of life, requires careful evaluation and appropriate treatment to prevent serious morbidity and mortality. By far, the most common form of neonatal conjunctivitis occurs within the first few days of life and is likely related to a chemical irritation from sliver nitrate administration shortly after birth. However, severe, purulent conjunctivitis within around the fifth day of life is a typical presentation of gonococcal conjunctivitis. The disease must be treated with multiple eye irrigations and intravenous administration of a third-generation cephalosporin to prevent local spread, perforation of the globe, and systemic disease. Silver nitrate and erythromycin are now routinely placed in newborn infants' eyes as prophylaxis against gonococcal conjunctivitis.

Chlamydia trachomatis conjunctivitis often presents with conjunctival erythema and a varying degree of discharge between weeks 1 and 2 of life. Pseudomembranous formation, scarring, and corneal infiltrates develop if left untreated. Other bacteria such as *Staphylococcus aureus* and *Pseudomonas* are relatively uncommon but important causes of ophthalmia neonatorum.

Viral pathogens, such as HSV, can also cause devastating damage to the neonatal eye. HSV conjunctivitis usually has a clear drainage with associated lymphadenopathy or clusters of vesicles. This infection warrants inpatient evaluation for additional organ involvement of HSV and treatment with acyclovir.

SUGGESTED READINGS

Kimberlin D. Herpes simplex virus, meningitis and encephalitis in neonates. *Herpes.* 2004; 11(Suppl 2):65A–76A.
O'Hara MA. Ophthalmia neonatorum. *Pediatr Clin North Am.* 1993;40:715–725.
Teoh DL, Reynolds S. Diagnosis and management of pediatric conjunctivitis. *Pediatr Emerg Care.* 2003;19(1):48–55.

10

KNOW THAT BLOODY STOOLS CAN BE AN ANXIETY-PROVOKING EVENT TO NEW PARENTS, BUT IS MOST OFTEN A BENIGN FINDING IN AN OTHERWISE WELL-APPEARING NEWBORN BABY. KNOW WHEN TO INTERVENE AND WHEN TO OBSERVE

LAURA HUFFORD, MD

WHAT TO DO – INTERPRET THE DATA

In newborns, one of the most common causes of blood in the stool is swallowed maternal blood. This occurs either during the delivery process or during breastfeeding if the mother's nipples are cracked and bleeding. If a maternal source is considered, then one can perform the Apt test to determine the origin of the blood. In this test, stool is mixed with water and centrifuged. Sodium hydroxide is added to the supernatant. If the blood is from the mother, the adult hemoglobin will denature and the sample will turn light brown. However, if the source of the blood is the infant, the sample remains pink because fetal hemoglobin is resistant to denaturation.

Anorectal fissures are another very common cause of rectal bleeding in children younger than 12 months. These fissures are usually seen upon close examination of the perineal skin and the anal canal. Often, they are small and caused by the passage of hard stool and resolve once the underlying constipation has been addressed.

Another common cause for blood in an infant's stool is food allergies. The top common allergens are cow's mild products and soy. Milk allergies occur in approximately 2% to 3% of infants, and it is typically outgrown by the age of 3 to 5 years. Symptoms include loose stools, vomiting, gagging, irritability or colic, and skin rashes. Avoiding milk-containing products is the treatment, and since January 2006, all U.S. food makers must clearly state on the package labels whether the foods contain milk or milk-based products. For infants, using a soy-based formula will sometimes work, but some infants may require using a hypoallergenic formula that contains pre-digested proteins.

Bloody stools in infants can also be the presenting sign of life-threatening conditions. One serious condition that should be considered in newborns is necrotizing enterocolitis (NEC). Associated symptoms can be apnea,

ⓒ 2008 by Lippincott Williams & Wilkins, a Wolters Kluwer business

abdominal distension, poor feeding or lethargy. Additionally pneumatosis intestinalis, air within the bowel wall, may be seen on radiographs. Although the etiology of NEC is unknown, it is likely multifactorial with bacterial overgrowth, enteral feeds, and hypoxia acting on immature intestinal mucosa to cause mucosal injury. The process continues, causing transmural and mucosal necrosis, and in severe cases, it causes perforation of the bowel wall. The incidence of NEC increases with lower gestational age; however, nearly 10% of cases occur in term infants. Treatment includes discontinuing all enteral feeds, intravenous antibiotics and supportive therapy. If perforation is suspected, then laparotomy and bowel resection may be indicated.

Another life-threatening cause of bloody stools in an infant is malrotation with midgut volvulus. Early in gestational development the gastrointestinal tract rapidly grows and protrudes into the yolk sac. The intestine then rotates 270 degrees in a counterclockwise fashion and returns into the abdominal cavity. Once inside the abdominal cavity, the bowel is fixed into place with the proximal portion of the bowel attached at the ligament of Treitz. If normal rotation fails to occur, a thin vascular stalk anchors the small bowel, which places the intestine at risk for midgut volvulus, torsion around this stalk, and subsequent bowel obstruction and ischemia. If torsion occurs, the patient may initially present with bilious emesis and abdominal distension. As the ischemic bowel begins to die, bloody stools, perforation, sepsis, and death can occur. Thus, early detection of malrotation with upper gastrointestinal contrast study is imperative. However, if an infant presents with bilious emesis and abdominal distension, they need no imaging and should undergo emergent operative management.

SUGGESTED READINGS

Fonkalsrud E. Rotational anomalies and volvulus. In: O'Neill JA, et al, eds. *Principles of Pediatric Surgery*. St. Louis: Mosby; 2003:477.

Gosche J, Vick L, Boulanger SC, et al. Midgut abnormalities. *Surg Clin North Am.* 2006;86: 285–299.

Liu N, Wu AH, Wong SS. Improved quantitative Apt test for detecting fetal hemoglobin in bloody stools of newborns. *Clin Chem.* 1993;11 (Pt 1):2326–2329.

Luig M, Lui K; NSW & ACT NICUS Group. Epidemiology of necrotizing enterocolitis–Part II: Risks and susceptibility of premature infants during the surfactant era: A regional study. *J Paediatr Child Health.* 2005;41(4):174–179.

Maayan-Metzger A, Itzchak A, Mazkereth R, et al. Necrotizing enterocolitis in full-term infants: Case-control study and review of the literature. *J Perinatol.* 2004;24(8):494–489.

11

NEONATAL CONJUNCTIVITIS SECONDARY TO *CHLAMYDIA TRACHOMATIS* SHOULD BE TREATED WITH ORAL ANTIBIOTICS TO PREVENT THE DEVELOPMENT OF ASSOCIATED PNEUMONIA

BRIAN KIT, MD

WHAT TO DO – TAKE ACTION

Chlamydia trachomatis is an obligate intracellular organism that may be transmitted to neonates from mothers who have cervical infections. This occurs primarily because of delivery through an infected vaginal canal, although documented cases of transmission following c-section are reported. For the neonate, Chlamydia infections are manifested as conjunctivitis, pneumonia, or both. Of neonates who are born to mothers with Chlamydia infections, 25% to 50% will develop conjunctivitis, and 5% to 20% will develop pneumonia. The time of onset for Chlamydia conjunctivitis is 5 to 14 days. The onset of pneumonia is typically 2 weeks to 3 months, with the majority of infants presenting by 2 months. Symptoms may appear earlier, particularly in infants born to mothers with premature rupture of membranes. Of infants who develop Chlamydia pneumonia, 50% had a history of conjunctivitis. Neonates who received prophylaxis with silver nitrate, erythromycin ointment, or tetracycline in the newborn period are still at risk for developing Chlamydia infections because these interventions are ineffective against Chlamydia; neonates receiving these interventions are protected against Neisseria conjunctivitis.

Physical findings of Chlamydia conjunctivitis include a watery discharge that progresses to a purulent discharge with associated eyelid swelling and erythema. The manifestations are generally unilateral but may be bilateral. Untreated Chlamydia infections may result in conjunctiva and corneal scarring over the course of months. The accurate diagnosis of chlamydial conjunctivitis is essential to ensure appropriate management. Because Chlamydia is an intracellular organism, a diagnosis requires obtaining cells by scraping the upper or lower conjunctiva rather than collection of the exudates. Culture is the gold standard for diagnosis, although polymerase chain reaction studies have excellent sensitivities and specificities.

Classically, patients with Chlamydia pneumonia present with a staccato cough, tachypnea, and are afebrile. Auscultation often reveals crackles, but

© 2008 by Lippincott Williams & Wilkins, a Wolters Kluwer business

no wheezing. The chest x-ray shows hyperinflation with bilateral interstitial infiltrates. Untreated Chlamydia pneumonia may lead to respiratory distress and apnea, particularly in younger infants.

Erythromycin at a dose of 50 mg/kg/day divided in four doses for 14 days is the recommended strategy for Chlamydia conjunctivitis. Treatment for Chlamydia conjunctivitis is more effective with oral erythromycin therapy when compared with topical treatment. Oral erythromycin therapy also results in greater eradication of nasopharyngeal colonization in comparison to topical treatment. Despite its advantages over topical therapy, oral erythromycin is effective in 80% of cases of conjunctivitis and requires close follow-up and a possible second dose of erythromycin for treatment failures. Eradication of nasopharyngeal colonization reduces the risk of developing Chlamydia pneumonia. The treatment for patients presenting with Chlamydia pneumonia is oral erythromycin 50 mg/kg/day divided in four doses for 14 days.

Because Chlamydia conjunctivitis precedes Chlamydia pneumonia in 50% of patients, appropriate management of patients with Chlamydia conjunctivitis is essential to prevent the development of pneumonia and its associated complications.

SUGGESTED READINGS

American Academy of Pediatrics. *Chlamydia trachomatis.* In: Pickering LK, Baker CJ, Long SS, et al, eds. *Red Book: 2006 Report of the Committee on Infectious Diseases.* 27th ed. Elk Grove Village, IL: American Academy of Pediatrics; 2006:253–257.

Hammerschlag MR, Cummings C, Roblin PM, et al. Efficacy of neonatal ocular prophylaxis for the prevention of chlamydial and gonococcal conjunctivitis. *N Engl J Med.* 1989;320(12):769–772.

Hammerschlag MR, Roblin PM, Gelling M, et al. Use of polymerase chain reaction for the detection of *Chlamydia trachomatis* in ocular and nasopharyngeal specimens from infants with conjunctivitis. *Pediatr Infect Dis J.* 1997;16(3):293–297.

Patamasucon P, Rettig PJ, Faust KL, et al. Oral vs topical erythromycin therapies for chlamydial conjunctivitis. *Am J Dis Child.* 1982;136:817–821.

12

VIGOROUS NEONATES BORN THROUGH MECONIUM-STAINED AMNIOTIC FLUID DO NOT REQUIRE ENDOTRACHEAL INTUBATION AND TRACHEAL SUCTIONING IMMEDIATELY AFTER DELIVERY. THIS PRACTICE SHOULD BE RESERVED FOR NEONATES WITH EVIDENCE OF FETAL DISTRESS AND PERINATAL DEPRESSION

JENNIFER MANISCALCO, MD

WHAT TO DO – TAKE ACTION

In utero passage of meconium occurs in up to 20% of births, usually in term or near-term neonates. There is a correlation between fetal distress or hypoxia and the passage of meconium prior to delivery. Aspiration of meconium-stained amniotic fluid (MSAF) occurs in up to 10% of such infants, either before delivery, during birth, or during resuscitation. Meconium aspiration can lead to proximal and peripheral airway obstruction, chemical pneumonitis, and persistent pulmonary hypertension. The clinical manifestations of meconium aspiration syndrome (MAS) are variable, ranging from mild tachypnea and hypoxia to fulminant respiratory failure.

As such, treatment of MAS can range from supportive care to full cardiopulmonary support. Infants with severe MAS may require conventional or high-frequency ventilation, surfactant therapy, inhaled nitric oxide, or extracorporeal membrane oxygenation. Mortality is typically <10%, but can be much higher in certain settings. In survivors, the most common sequelae are pulmonary, including prolonged oxygen requirement, exercise-induced bronchospasm, reactive airway disease, and chronic lung disease. Neurologic sequelae, including hypoxic ischemic encephalopathy, can occur but are more closely related to the occurrence of intrauterine asphyxia.

To prevent MAS, traditional teaching has encouraged two methods of suctioning for neonates born through MSAF. The first is intrapartum suctioning, which entails suctioning of the neonate's nasopharynx and oropharynx after the delivery of the head but prior to the delivery of the shoulders. The second is endotracheal intubation immediately following delivery, with application of suction as the tube is removed. Repeat intubation with tracheal suctioning until the secretions clear is often practiced. Early studies demonstrated a decline in the rate of MAS and a decline in the morbidity

ⓒ 2008 by Lippincott Williams & Wilkins, a Wolters Kluwer business

and mortality rate associated with MAS, with the implementation of endotracheal intubation and tracheal suctioning alone or in combination with intrapartum suctioning.

A recent randomized controlled trial assessed the efficacy of intrapartum suctioning for decreasing the risk of MAS. No such effect was noted. Further, randomized controlled trials have not demonstrated a reduction in the risk of developing MAS for vigorous term infants who undergo immediate endotracheal intubation and tracheal suctioning following birth. Although exact definitions vary, vigorous infants were generally defined as those with a heart rate >100 beats per minute, spontaneous respiratory effort, and reasonable tone. In one study, there was a 3.8% complication rate among neonates who underwent endotracheal intubation. Complications included bradycardia, laryngospasm, hoarseness or stridor, apnea, bleeding at the vocal cords, and cyanosis. In most cases, these complications were very brief and self-resolving.

Based on the results of these studies, the Neonatal Resuscitation Guidelines endorsed by the American Heart Association and the American Academy of Pediatrics do not recommend routine intrapartum suctioning for infants born through MSAF, or endotracheal intubation for vigorous term infants born through MSAF. Because infants born through MSAF with evidence of fetal distress and associated perinatal depression are at increased risk of developing MAS, immediate endotracheal intubation and tracheal suctioning is still recommended.

SUGGESTED READINGS

American Heart Association, American Academy of Pediatrics. 2005 American Heart Association (AHA) guidelines for cardiopulmonary resuscitation (CPR) and emergency cardiovascular care (ECC) of pediatric and neonatal patients: Neonatal resuscitation guidelines. *Pediatrics.* 2006:117(5):e1029–1038.

Dargaville PA, Copnell B; Australian and New Zealand Neonatal Network. The epidemiology of meconium aspiration syndrome: Incidence, risk factors, therapies, and outcome. *Pediatrics.* 2006;117:1712–1721.

Vain NE, Szyld EG, Prudent LM, et al. Oropharyngeal and nasopharyngeal suctioning of meconium-stained neonates before delivery of their shoulders: multicentre, randomised controlled trial. *Lancet* 2004;364:597–602.

Velaphi S, Vidyasagar D. Intrapartum and postdelivery management of infants born to mothers with meconium-stained amniotic fluid: evidence-based recommendations. *Clin Perinatol.* 2006;33:29–42.

Wiswell TE, Gannon CM, Jacob J, et al. Delivery room management of the apparently vigorous meconium-stained neonate: results of the multicenter, international collaborative trial. *Pediatrics* 2000;105(1 Pt 1):1–7.

13

INFANTS BORN TO MOTHERS POSITIVE FOR HEPATITIS B SURFACE ANTIGEN SHOULD RECEIVE BOTH HEPATITIS B VACCINE AND HEPATITIS B IMMUNE GLOBULIN (HBIG) WITHIN 12 HOURS OF BIRTH

BRIAN KIT, MD

WHAT TO DO – TAKE ACTION

Hepatitis B is caused by hepatitis B virus (HBV), a member of the Hepadnaviridae family. HBV is transmitted from person to person through exposure to infected blood or bodily fluids. Exposure may result from sexual contact with an infected person or perinatal transmission from an infected mother to her infant. Infection may also occur as a result of a needlestick injury from an infected person or from blood transfusions.

Perinatal exposure to hepatitis B results in a high rate of transmission of HBV, largely occurring during blood exposures during labor and delivery. The risk that an infant will acquire HBV from an infected mother is dependent on the mother's serologic status, with a 70% to 90% transmission for infant born to mothers who are hepatitis B surface antigen (HBsAg)-positive and hepatitis E antigen (HBeAg)-positive, and 5% to 20% transmission for infants born to mothers who are mothers who are HBsAg-positive but HBeAg-negative. In older children and adults, approximately 5% of persons who develop an acute hepatitis B infection will develop a chronic carrier state, while neonates acquiring hepatitis B from perinatal transmission have approximately 95% chance of becoming chronic carriers. A chronic carrier state increases the risk for hepatocellular carcinoma and liver cirrhosis.

Prevention has been a highly effective method of reducing hepatitis B transmission from mother to her baby. A regimen that includes active immunization with the hepatitis B vaccine and passive immunization with hepatitis B immune globulin (HBIG) results in a chronic carrier state in approximately 5% of infants. All pregnant women should be screened for hepatitis B in the first trimester, and again in the third trimester high-risk patients should be tested.

Infants born to mothers who are HBsAG-positive, including preterm babies who weigh <2 kg (4.4 lb) at birth, should receive the HBIG within 12 hours of birth and the first hepatitis B vaccine within 12 hours of birth. These babies will require laboratory evaluation of HBV serologies (HBsAg

© 2008 by Lippincott Williams & Wilkins, a Wolters Kluwer business

and anti-HBsAG) performed at 9 months of age to assess response to vaccination. Continuation of the three-dose vaccination regimen should begin at 1 to 2 months in accordance with the recommendations of the Center for Disease Control and Prevention's Recommendations of the Advisory Committee on Immunization Practices. The exceptions are infants who are <2 kg at birth. Because of concerns of lower immune response of infants <2 kg, those who receive the vaccine within the first 12 hours of life will require a total of four vaccinations to complete the HBV vaccine series. If the baby is preterm and weigh >2 kg the schedule for term babies should be followed.

Term or preterm infants >2 kg who are born to mothers with unknown hepatitis B status should receive the first dose of the hepatitis B vaccine within the first 12 hours of life. The mother should also be screened for hepatitis B. HBIG should be administered within the first week of the neonate's life if the results of testing indicate that the mother is positive. In the infant <2 kg at birth, regardless if they are term or preterm, the first hepatitis B vaccine should be administered within 12 hours of birth. These mothers should be tested immediately. If the serology results are not available by 12 hours or if the mother is HBsAG-positive, the babies should receive HBIG. Continuation of the vaccination regimen generally will begin at 1 to 2 months and should be performed in accordance with the Center for Disease Control and Prevention's Recommendations of the Advisory Committee on Immunization Practices. Of note, if the preterm infant weighs <2 kg at birth, they will need a fourth hepatitis B vaccine.

SUGGESTED READINGS

American Academy of Pediatrics. In: Pickering LK, ed. *Red Book: 2006 Report of the Committee on Infectious Diseases.* 27th ed. Elk Grove Village, IL; American Academy of Pediatrics; 2006:337.

Beasley RP, Hwang LY, Lee GC, et al. Prevention of perinatally transmitted hepatitis B virus infections with hepatitis B virus infections with hepatitis B immune globulin and hepatitis B vaccine. *Lancet.* 1983;2(8359):1099–1102.

14

MONITOR GLUCOSE LEVELS IN THE INFANT. HYPOGLYCEMIA IN THE NEWBORN IS IMPORTANT AND MAY GO UNDETECTED

HEIDI HERRERA, MD AND NICKIE NIFORATOS, MD

WHAT TO DO – GATHER APPROPRIATE DATA

Glucose is the major source of energy for tissue metabolism, particularly in the brain, where lack of alternate energy stores makes glucose an essential substrate. If there is a lower than normal glucose level in the blood, so that basic metabolic demands cannot be met, hypoglycemia results. A number of physiologic factors can leave the newborn particularly susceptible to hypoglycemia. Infants have an increased brain-to-body weight ratio, with a proportionately higher demand for glucose. In addition, newborns have an immature counter-regulatory response, which limits the use of alternate fuels, such as lactate and ketone bodies, in meeting basic metabolic requirements. Immediate consequences of hypoglycemia in the neonate include poor outcomes, worsening sepsis, and asphyxia. In the longterm, neonatal hypoglycemia may lead to impaired neurodevelopmental outcomes; some studies suggest that recurrent severe hypoglycemia may result in neuronal necrosis, contributing to impaired neurodevelopment.

Immediately after birth, the infant transitions from a maternal source of glucose to their own internal stores. Initially, the major source of neonatal glucose is from hepatic glycogen, via glycogenolysis. Within the first few hours of life, the neonate then develops the additional ability to maintain glucose levels via gluconeogenesis. Decreased stores, increased demands, or inadequate metabolic responses may disrupt the infant's transition to independent glycemic control. *Table 14.1* provides the common neonatal risk factors that may predispose the infant to hypoglycemia. Premature infants or small for gestational age (SGA) infants have decreased glycogen stores, putting them at risk for hypoglycemia. Septic infants, or infants with hypoxic-ischemic injuries, may have increased demands for glucose. If the infant is unable to meet these increased demands, hypoglycemia results. Infants of diabetic mothers (IDMs) frequently have islet-cell hypertrophy and higher than normal insulin levels. When transitioning from maternal glucose stores to their own stores, the insulin level may remain elevated, leading to hypoglycemia.

Infants with mild hypoglycemia may remain asymptomatic. When present, signs of hypoglycemia include jitteriness, poor suck, or unstable vital signs (*Table 14.2*). The spectrum of signs and symptoms of hypoglycemia

ⓒ 2008 by Lippincott Williams & Wilkins, a Wolters Kluwer business

---

TABLE 14.1   RISK FACTORS

Prematurity
Small for gestational age
Intrauterine growth retardation
Asphyxia
Hypothermia
Sepsis
Infant of diabetic mother
Erythroblastosis fetalis
Exposure to β-agonist tocolytics
Familial hyperinsulinism
Inborn errors of metabolism
Endocrine disorders (pan-hypopituitarism, adrenal
    insufficiency, hypothyroidism, etc.)

---

are variable and nonspecific, which is why the clinician must have a high index of suspicion for hypoglycemia to recognize, test, and treat it appropriately. Most nurseries have developed standard protocols to screen high-risk infants. Although each infant's threshold for adequate glucose levels varies, depending on their unique metabolic needs, commonly accepted values for hypoglycemia in a term infant include blood values <2.0 mmol/L (<35 mg/dL) or plasma values <2.2 mmol/L (<40 mg/dL).

What to watch out for: If the initial history and physical exam rule out common causes for hypoglycemia such as prematurity, SGA, or IDM, the clinician must suspect sepsis.

What to watch out for: If hypoglycemia persists for >1 week, the clinician must suspect more unusual but chronic causes, including hyperinsulinemia, endocrine disorders, and inborn errors of metabolism.

MANAGEMENT

For asymptomatic infants whose hypoglycemia has been noted on an initial screen, initial management is to provide enteral feeds (breastmilk or formula).

TABLE 14.2   CLINICAL SIGNS

Respiratory	Tachypnea
	Apnea
	Respiratory distress
Cardiovascular	Tachycardia
	Bradycardia
Neurologic	Jitteriness
	Lethargy
	Weak suck
	Temperature instability

These infants should continue to be monitored for 12 to 24 hours. If there is a second episode of preprandial hypoglycemia, intravenous (IV) therapy should be considered, even if the infant remains asymptomatic, recent literature suggests better neurodevelopment outcomes occur with better glycemic control. For symptomatic infants or high-risk infants, immediate IV therapy should be considered, as follows:

> Bolus: 200 mg/kg dextrose (or 20 mL/kg of D10W),
> THEN
> Continuous: 5 to 8 mg/kg/min of glucose
> If hypoglycemia recurs, repeat bolus and increase infusion by 15% to 20%

Once glucose levels have been stable for 12 to 24 hours, wean IV therapy (reduce the infusion rate by 10% to 20% each time blood glucose > 50 mg/dL (2.8 mmol/L))

What to watch out for: Dextrose concentrations > 12.5% should ONLY be administered via central catheter NOT by peripheral IV.

SUGGESTED READING

McGowan JE. Neonatal hypoglycemia. *Pediatr Rev.* 1999;20:e6–e15.

15

EMERGENTLY MANAGE THE ILL NEWBORN IN THE DELIVERY ROOM

SARIKA JOSHI, MD

WHAT TO DO – TAKE ACTION

Pediatricians should be familiar with the management of newborn infants in the delivery room. The International Guidelines 2000 Conference on Cardiopulmonary Resuscitation (CPR) and Emergency Cardiac Care (ECC) updated the prior 1992 recommendations established after the Fifth National Conference on CPR and ECC. The most important aspect of this management is the establishment of adequate ventilation.

At birth, the newborn must make the dramatic transition from placental gas exchange and fluid-filled lungs to pulmonary gas exchange with air-filled lungs. The lungs expand, pulmonary blood flow increases, and pulmonary vascular resistance decreases. Some antepartum factors associated with risk for the newborn's transition to be difficult include maternal diabetes, pregnancy-induced hypertension, poly- or oligohydramnios, and premature rupture of membranes. Some intrapartum risk factors for the newborn to have a difficult transition are breech presentation, premature labor, chorioamnionitis, or meconium-stained amniotic fluid.

It is recommended that at least one person skilled in neonatal resuscitation attend every delivery, and that another person, able to perform a complete resuscitation, should be immediately available. About 1% to 10% of newborns require some form of assisted ventilation. The need for intervention is based on evaluation of the newborn's respirations, heart rate, and color. Gasping and apnea indicate the need for assistance with ventilation. Heart rate, which is most easily assessed by feeling the pulsations at the base of the umbilical cord, should be greater than 100 beats per minute. The newborn should be pink, although acrocyanosis is a normal finding at birth. Neonatal resuscitation can be broken down into four categories of intervention: (a) basic steps, (b) ventilation, (c) chest compressions, and (d) administration of medications and fluids.

The basic steps of neonatal resuscitation include warming the infant, clearing the airway, stimulation, and oxygen administration. Heat loss increases the newborn's need for oxygen consumption. To prevent heat loss, the newborn should be rapidly dried under a radiant warmer, with continued

© 2008 by Lippincott Williams & Wilkins, a Wolters Kluwer business

removal of the wet linens. Airway clearance involves the appropriate positioning of the infant, with the newborn placed on its back or side with the head neutral or somewhat extended, and the removal of secretions, by wiping away from the nose and mouth. If suctioning is necessary, a bulb syringe is generally adequate, with the mouth being suctioned prior to the nose to minimize the risk of aspiration. If a suction catheter is required, care must be taken to avoid long or aggressive suctioning, as stimulation of the posterior pharynx can result in a vagal response and bradycardia. If the amniotic fluid is stained with meconium, the newborn's mouth and nose are suctioned on delivery of the head. In depressed infants (e.g., poor respirations, muscle tone, or heart rate), drying and suctioning are delayed, and the newborn is immediately intubated for tracheal suctioning, a process that is repeated until the airway is cleared of meconium or until further resuscitation is required.

The two remaining basic steps include stimulation and oxygen administration. The goal of stimulation is for the newborn to start and continue adequate respirations. Usually the drying and suctioning that accompanies each resuscitation is all that is required to stimulate the child. If these interventions are not adequate, then gentle rubbing of the newborn's back or flicking the soles of the feet can be employed. One hundred percent oxygen should be administered to all newborns requiring resuscitation to treat hypoxia.

If the infant's respiratory effort remains depressed, positive pressure ventilation should be initiated. Additional indications for positive pressure ventilation include gasping, apnea, heart rate <100 beats per minute, and central cyanosis. For the majority of newborns, a bag and mask provide satisfactory ventilation, which is best measured by watching for bilateral chest expansion. Forty to 60 breaths per minute, or 30 if the infant also requires chest compressions, should be provided. An orogastric tube should be placed to avoid gastric inflation. After 30 seconds, the infant should be reassessed. If spontaneous respirations are still inadequate, or the heart rate is <100 beats per minute, bag-mask ventilation should be continued. If a bag and mask cannot provide satisfactory ventilation, the newborn should be intubated. Chest compressions are indicated if, despite satisfactory ventilation with 100% oxygen for 30 seconds, heart rate is <60 beats per minute. Compressions are delivered on the lower third of the sternum with two thumbs on the sternum and fingers encircling the chest and back. The chest should be compressed to a third of its anteroposterior diameter. Chest compressions and breaths should be delivered in a 3:1 ratio with 90 compressions and 30 breaths per minute. After 30 seconds, the infant is reassessed. Compressions should continue until heart rate is >60 beats per minute.

Epinephrine is indicated if, despite satisfactory ventilation with 100% oxygen and chest compressions for 30 seconds, the heart rate remains <60 beats per minute. Intravenous or endotracheal epinephrine should be administered every 3 to 5 minutes as indicated, at a dose of 0.1 to 0.3 mL/kg of a 1 to 10,000 dilution. Volume expansion, with normal saline or Ringer's lactate, should be considered in any newborn who fails to respond to resuscitation, especially if blood loss or shock is suspected. The fluids should be given over 5 to 10 minutes with an initial dose of 10 mL/kg.

Although most newborns require nothing more than basic steps in the delivery room, pediatricians should be comfortable with more advanced neonatal resuscitation. Establishment of adequate ventilation is the key, because bradycardia is usually the result of poor lung inflation and hypoxia.

SUGGESTED READINGS

Kattwinkel J, Niermeyer S, Nadkarni V, et al. ILCOR advisory statement: resuscitation of the newly born infant. An advisory statement from the pediatric working group of the International Liaison Committee on Resuscitation. *Circulation.* 1999;99:1927–1938.

Niermeyer S, Kattwinkel J, Van Reempts P, et al. International Guidelines for Neonatal Resuscitation: An excerpt from the Guidelines 2000 for Cardiopulmonary Resuscitation and Emergency Cardiovascular Care: International Consensus on Science. Contributors and Reviewers for the Neonatal Resuscitation Guidelines. *Pediatrics.* 2000;103(3):E29.

16

KNOW HOW TO EVALUATE AND MANAGE AMBIGUOUS GENITALIA IN THE DELIVERY ROOM

HEIDI HERRERA, MD

WHAT TO DO – TAKE ACTION

Evaluation and management of the newborn with ambiguous genitalia should be immediately evaluated for potential life-threatening, salt-wasting form of congenital adrenal hyperplasia (CAH). Due to the complexity of the medical, emotional, and psychosocial dilemma, early intervention is essential.

Two main disorders are seen with ambiguous genitalia: disorders of gonadal differentiation (gonadal dysgenesis and true hermaphroditism) and disorders of steroidogenesis (CAH, 5α-reductase deficiency, and androgen insensitivity). Other causes include androgen insensitivity, maternal hyperandrogenism, and environmental or drug exposure.

The newborn with gonadal dysgenesis is a phenotypic male infant with a 46, XX karyotype who can present at birth with abnormal genitalia ranging from cryptorchidism to significant genital ambiguity, or a phenotypic female with 46, XY karyotype who may not be diagnosed at birth. The usual diagnosis is made when the patient presents with delayed puberty or primary amenorrhea. These patients usually have Müllerian structures due to the absence of anti-Müllerian hormone. Both of these diagnoses are usually associated with infertility. They may also have phenotypic characteristics of Turner syndrome (webbed neck, short stature, shield chest) due to the 45, X cell lines. Patients with streak gonads are at increase risk for neoplastic transformation.

True hermaphroditism may present with a spectrum of genital ambiguity. They have both ovarian tissue with mature Graafian follicles and testicular tissue with seminiferous tubules present on histologic evaluation. Both Müllerian and Wolffian ductal structures may be present. Fertility is variable.

Steroidogenesis begins with the conversion of cholesterol to pregnenolone. The adrenal gland produces enzymes related to the production of cortisol and aldosterone, and the gonads express enzymes related to the production of androgens and sex steroids. One of the most frequently encountered mutations is the 21-hydroxylase gene. The female infant will present

---

© 2008 by Lippincott Williams & Wilkins, a Wolters Kluwer business

with variable degrees of virilization. The male infant will be diagnosed when signs of mineralocorticoid insufficiency are observed (electrolyte disturbance, dehydration) as in the classical salt-losing CAH, or early pubic hair development as in nonclassical CAH. Other forms of CAH with ambiguous genitalia includes 11β-hydroxylase deficiency (female virilization, glucocorticoid insufficiency, and hypertension), 3β-hydroxysteroid dehydrogenase (HSD) deficiency (female virilization, male external undervirilization, with corticosteroid, and possibly mineralocorticoid, insufficiency), and more rare conditions include 17α-hydroxylase/17,20-lyase deficiency and 17β-HSD deficiency.

The 5α-reductase deficiency results in insufficient conversion of testosterone to dihydrotestosterone, resulting in variable degrees of undervirilization in the male infant.

Mutations in the genes related to androgen receptor production or function leads to inappropriate androgen action in sex-steroid responsive tissues. Individuals may present on a spectrum from complete testicular feminization—with normal female external genitalia and absent uterus—to partial forms of insensitivity, with various levels of virilization. Complete form of androgen insensitivity may be diagnosed early in life with a prenatal karyotype.

The initial step in the diagnostic process is the physical examination. Focusing on palpable gonads, symmetry of the external genitalia, and any additional congenital anomalies can help to determine the etiology. Ambiguous genitalia may present as clitoral enlargement with palpable labioscrotal mass, microphallus with hypospadias, and clitoromegaly with labial fusion. Additionally, if the male newborn has bilateral or unilateral unpalpable testes and hypospadias, he should be considered as having an intersex disorder until proven otherwise regardless of the appearance of the external genitalia.

A newborn should have an ultrasound of the abdomen and pelvis in the immediate perinatal period. An ultrasound can detect gonads in the inguinal region and the presence or absence of a uterus. A retrograde study can aid in outlining the anatomy of the internal genitalia. An abdominal and pelvic computed tomography scan can further visualize the location of gonadal tissue. Laparoscopy may be the definitive procedure to isolate and sample gonadal tissue to identify the gonadal dysgenesis. The newborn with ambiguous genitalia requires an evaluation of karyotype, serum electrolytes, 17-hydroxyprogesterone, testosterone, luteinizing hormone, and follicle-stimulating hormone levels immediately in the perinatal period. If the 17-hydroxyprogesterone level is elevated, then CAH exists. Abnormal electrolytes in salt-losing CAH do not usually occur in the first week but must be followed closely by the end of the first week of life if suspicious of CAH. If normal, further endocrine evaluation of androgen hormone axis is required. Determining the levels of 11-deoxycortisol and deoxycorticos-terone with help differentiate between 21-hydroxylase and 11β-hydroxylase deficiencies. Elevated levels indicate 11β-hydroxylase deficiency and low levels confirm 21-hydroxylase deficiency.

After the appropriate diagnosis is made, treatment should be started. In CAH, corticosteroid and mineralocorticoid replacement is started. Salt replacement is occasionally needed for salt-losers in the newborn period. Levels of 17-hydroxyprogesterone, androstenedione, and rennin are moni-tored to adjust dosing.

In summary, once a newborn is observed to have ambiguous genitalia, there should be immediate support to the family to provide basic information and education on sexual development and diagnostic steps to determine the etiology of the ambiguity while assuring that hemodynamic, fluid, and electrolyte status remains stable. The ultimate goal is to establish the most appropriate sex for rearing.

SUGGESTED READINGS

Hyun G, Kolon TF. A practical approach to intersex in the newborn period. *Urol Clin North Am.* 2004;31:435–443.

Leslie JA, Cain MP. Pediatric urologic emergencies and urgencies. *Pediatr Clin North Am.* 2006;53:513–527.

Palma Sisto PA. Endocrine disorders in the neonate. *Pediatr Clin North Am.* 2004;51:1141–1168.

17

IDENTIFY THE ETIOLOGY OF CYANOSIS IN THE NEWBORN

RUSSELL CROSS, MD

WHAT TO DO – INTERPRET THE DATA

The detection of persistent cyanosis in the neonate can be difficult because of the changing physiology in the first several hours following delivery, but it is an important marker for a number of pathologies. Cyanosis, a blue discoloration of the skin, results from an increased concentration of reduced (deoxygenated) hemoglobin, typically about 3 g/dL, in the capillary bed. The amount of reduced hemoglobin is a function of the S-shape of the hemoglobin-dissociation curve, which is in turn influenced by the concentration of hemoglobin, the amount fetal hemoglobin present, abnormalities in the hemoglobin itself, and other physiologic parameters such as temperature, pH, and pCo_2. The actual percent oxygen saturation at which cyanosis becomes clinically evident is widely variable, depending on the factors mentioned above, but on average cyanosis is evident when the oxygen saturation less than low 80s. From a clinical standpoint, cyanosis results from either a reduction of arterial oxygen saturation, an increased extraction of oxygen at the capillary level, or an abnormality in the hemoglobin itself.

Focusing on pathologies that result in a reduced arterial oxygen saturation, the causes are straight-forward; either there is diminished oxygen exchange at the alveolar level or desaturated blood is bypassing the alveolus altogether. Diminished oxygen exchange in the alveolus can result from inadequate ventilation, obstruction to airway flow, or abnormalities in the alveolar wall that result in poor exchange of gases. Examples of the latter include pneumonia, meconium pneumonitis, pulmonary edema, and cystic fibrosis. Abnormalities that result in desaturated blood bypassing the alveolus include an intracardiac right-to-left shunt or an intrapulmonary shunts. Intracardiac shunts may result from either from cyanotic congenital heart disease (CHD) or pulmonary hypertension resulting in a right-to-left shunt at the ductal or intracardiac level. Intrapulmonary shunts can arise from an arteriovenous malformation or fistula, for example. The clinician most frequently is faced with distinguishing whether cyanosis is a result of pulmonary or cardiac disease but should remember that other less causes of cyanosis also exist.

© 2008 by Lippincott Williams & Wilkins, a Wolters Kluwer business

As with any other diagnosis, details of the history may hold important clues as to the cause of cyanosis in the newborn. For instance, knowing whether there was meconium at delivery and the adequacy of airway suctioning in the delivery room can help to raise the suspicion of meconium aspiration syndrome and resulting pulmonary hypertension. Other perinatal history such as time of membrane rupture, presence of maternal fever, and maternal infectious disease history may increase the suspicion for neonatal pneumonia or sepsis. The onset of cyanosis may also be helpful. For instance, at 12 to 24 hours of life in the absence of other symptoms, cyanosis is may result from CHD that becomes evident when the patent ductus closes.

Thorough pulmonary and cardiovascular examinations are important in differentiating the causes of cyanosis. Patients who have signs of respiratory distress such as tachypnea, along with grunting, nasal flaring, or intercostal retractions are more likely to have a pulmonary cause for cyanosis. The respiratory distress in these patients is evidence of the body's attempt to increase alveolar ventilation. Patients with cyanotic CHD may be tachypneic, but they typically do not have other signs of respiratory distress. Patients with a pulmonary cause for cyanosis will also be more likely to have abnormal breath sounds. On cardiac auscultation, attention should be focused on evaluation of the second heart sound in addition to screening for the presence of a murmur. The second heart sound normally has splitting that varies with inspiration, and the presence of a single second heart sound may indicate severe stenosis or absence of either the aortic or pulmonary valve. A loud second heart sound is also evidence for pulmonary hypertension. Likewise, presence of a murmur may indicate CHD.

Evaluation of the distribution of the cyanosis is also important. Patients may have "differential cyanosis" as a result of pulmonary hypertension or certain cyanotic CHD. In the case of pulmonary hypertension with a patent ductus and a right-to-left shunt, there may be diminished oxygen saturation in the lower half of the body as a result of shunting of deoxygenated blood from the right ventricle being shunted through the ductus into the descending aorta. In contrast, patients with transposition of the great arteries may have "reverse differential cyanosis" with the upper half of the body having lower oxygen saturation. This is because the deoxygenated blood leaving the right ventricle passes into the ascending aorta, first reaching the upper body vessels. When the aortic blood flow passes the patent ductus, some mixing occurs with the more fully saturated blood in the pulmonary artery, increasing the oxygen saturation of the blood delivered to the lower half of the body.

In clinical practice, the differentiation between pulmonary and cardiac causes of cyanosis can be difficult. An easy test that can help to make the differentiation is the hyperoxia challenge. The hyperoxia challenge involves placing the patient on 100% oxygen for 20 minutes and observing the oxygen content (PaO_2) before and after. When cyanosis is caused by a fixed shunt outside the alveolar level of the lungs (e.g., cyanotic CHD), the arterial pO_2 will not increase significantly on 100% oxygen because the blood that is bypassing the lung has no opportunity for increased oxygen absorption. In contrast, when the cyanosis results from lung disease at the capillary level, an increased alveolar O_2 content will result in increased diffusion across the alveolar-capillary interface, thereby increasing arterial pO_2. Pulmonary hypertension with a patent ductus can complicate the test because the cyanosis in this setting is created by right-to-left shunt across the patent ductus arteriosus (external to the lung). With the application of 100% O_2, there can be some diminishment in the pulmonary hypertension, which both increases the amount of blood going to the lungs and diminishes the ductal right-to left shunt. The effect of both of these is to increase arterial oxygen content to a level intermediate to that typically seen with cardiac compared to lung disease.

Cyanotic CHD can be subdivided into two physiologic groups: those that have obstruction to pulmonary blood flow and those that have normal to increased pulmonary blood flow but with obligate mixing of venous and arterial blood. Examples of CHD with obstruction to pulmonary blood flow include tetralogy of Fallot, pulmonary stenosis or atresia, and certain forms of tricuspid atresia and Ebstein malformation. These types of cyanotic heart disease may be "ductal dependent" if they require ductal patency in order to provide adequate pulmonary blood flow. Ductal patency is ensured by the use of intravenous prostaglandins. Examples of CHD for which there is normal to increased pulmonary blood flow with obligate mixing are transposition of the great arteries and truncus arteriosus. In transposition of the great arteries, the aorta and pulmonary artery are switched and arise from the incorrect ventricle. The degree of cyanosis in this lesion is a function of the amount of mixing that occurs between the systemic and pulmonary circulation. Patients with transposition may also be "ductal dependent" in the sense that they require ductal patency to provide adequate mixing of venous and arterial blood. In truncus arteriosus, there is a single great vessel arising from the heart which becomes the aorta and from which the pulmonary arteries arise. This anatomy creates obligate mixing in the heart which results in cyanosis. Other examples of cyanotic CHD resulting from intracardiac mixing include total anomalous pulmonary venous return, hypoplastic left heart syndrome, and certain forms of double outlet right ventricle.

SUGGESTED READINGS

Kuehl KS, Loffredo CA, Ferencz C. Failure to diagnose congenital heart disease in infancy. *Pediatrics.* 1999;103(4 Pt 1):743–747.

Reich JD, Miller S, Brogdon B, et al. The use of pulse oximetry to detect congenital heart disease. *J Pediatr.* 2003;142:268–272.

Tingelstad J. Consultation with the specialist: nonrespiratory cyanosis. *Pediatr Rev.* 1999;20:350–352.

18

CHECK FOR FEMORAL PULSES
IN INFANTS AND NEWBORNS

RUSSELL CROSS, MD

WHAT TO DO – GATHER APPROPRIATE DATA

Coarctation of the aorta is a discrete narrowing of the aortic arch, typically located between the origin of the left subclavian artery and the more distal insertion of the ductus arteriosus. Coarctation accounts for 5% to 8% of patients with congenital heart disease (CHD) and is one of the most commonly missed forms of CHD. The acute physiologic effects of a significant coarctation or other aortic arch obstruction include progressive hypoperfusion of the lower body, with potential development of metabolic acidosis, tachycardia, tachypnea, diminished cardiac function, and, in severe cases, shock. The effects of a coarctation may not be evident early in life because the ductus is usually patent and provides flow to the descending aorta distal to the level of the obstruction. Once the ductus closes, all systemic flow must traverse the aortic arch. If there is a significant coarctation, the negative physiologic effects described above will ensue. In cases of milder coarctation, the patient may not develop acute symptoms, but early detection of coarctation of the aorta is vital in preventing premature cardiovascular disease and long-term systemic hypertension.

The timing of ductal closure can make early diagnosis of coarctation of the aorta difficult because lower body blood flow is adequately maintained as long as the ductus is patent. The patent ductus will typically begin closing in the first few hours to a couple of days of life. It is important that a thorough cardiac examination with emphasis on evaluation of potential coarctation be performed during this time frame, as well as into the first several well child visits. As the ductus closes, an increasing volume of blood will be forced through the narrowed coarctation area to provide lower body flow. This may create a murmur on auscultation, but the murmur can be difficult to differentiate from that of a closing ductus. Because the murmur is nonspecific, evaluation of central pulses and peripheral blood pressure in all four extremities is of the utmost importance in the newborn cardiac examination. When there is a significant coarctation of the aorta in the absence of adequate ductal flow, one can appreciate diminished pulse volume in the central pulses distal to the area of the coarctation. The blood pressure in these extremities will also

© 2008 by Lippincott Williams & Wilkins, a Wolters Kluwer business

be lower, and the examiner may appreciate a delay in the timing of the pulse in those extremities distal to the narrowing. It is important that the pulses and blood pressure be assessed in all four extremities, not just the right arm and a leg. The presence of an aberrant right subclavian artery could place the origin of that vessel distal to the level of the coarctation, which would make the blood pressure and pulses in the right arm lower than what would be expected, thus "masking" the coarctation. It is also important that the evaluation be performed in all extremities with the child quiet and at the same approximate time so as to minimize error created by changes in blood pressure secondary to agitation or other physiologic changes. An evaluation for coarctation should be performed in any patient with a blood pressure difference between extremities of >20 mm Hg, systemic hypertension, a palpable difference in pulse strength, or absent femoral pulses.

As mentioned earlier, an aortic coarctation may not be severe enough to cause significant symptoms early in life, but its presence does place the individual at increased risk for long-term hypertension and other problems. Therefore, the evaluation of any murmur or workup for systemic hypertension should include careful palpation of all four extremity central pulses and measurement of four extremity blood pressures. The examiner should ensure that there is no difference in intensity or delay in timing of pulse arrival from upper to lower extremities. A palpable central pulse delay or "lag" is a hallmark of a significant coarctation and usually corresponds to a demonstrable across the coarctation.

SUGGESTED READINGS

Brickner ME, Hillis LD, Lange RA. Congenital heart disease in adults. First of two parts. *New Engl J Med*. 2000;342(4):256–263.

Ing FF, Starc TJ, Griffiths SP, et al. Diagnosis of coarctation of the aorta in children: a continuing dilemma. *Pediatrics*. 1996;98(3 Pt 1):378–382.

Lu CW, Wang JK, Chang CI, et al. Noninvasive diagnosis of aortic coarctation in neonates with patent ductus arteriosus. *J Pediatr*. 2006;148:217–221.

19

CONSIDER THAT A NEWBORN WITH A SEPTIC PICTURE BUT NO FEVER MAY HAVE A DUCTAL-DEPENDENT HEART LESION, ESPECIALLY LEFT-SIDED DISEASE LIKE CRITICAL AORTIC STENOSIS, COARCTATION OF THE AORTA, OR HYPOPLASTIC LEFT HEART SYNDROME

RUSSELL CROSS, MD

WHAT TO DO – INTERPRET THE DATA

The differential diagnosis of the neonate presenting with nonspecific symptoms such as tachypnea, lethargy, poor feeding, poor perfusion, or hypothermia is broad. Neonatal sepsis is frequently considered as one of the top diagnoses in such cases, but it must also be remembered that certain forms of congenital heart disease (CHD) can present in a similar fashion. The absence of a fever in a newborn that otherwise has the presentation of sepsis should especially raise the suspicion for a ductal-dependent congenital cardiac lesion.

The ductal-dependent forms of CHD are those that depend on a patent ductus arteriosus to supply adequate systemic or pulmonary blood flow. These lesions can be confused with neonatal sepsis because the timing of onset of symptoms correlates with the natural history of ductal closure at several hours to several days of life. The neonates may initially appear well and have no significant clinical findings until the ductus closes. The onset of symptoms can then be abrupt and life-threatening, as flow to the systemic or pulmonary bed becomes limited. One category of ductal-dependent CHD is that of left-sided outflow obstruction, including severe aortic stenosis, coarctation of the aorta, interrupted aortic arch, and hypoplastic left heart syndrome. In all of these cases, the systemic blood flow is initially maintained by the presence of a patent ductus arteriosus, and the neonate continues to have a fetal circulation with the right ventricle providing systemic blood flow. The neonate with left-sided outflow obstruction is unable to transition to the normal postnatal left-dominant circulation when the ductus closes. The left-sided outflow obstruction results in decreased cardiac output with diminished systemic perfusion. The ultimate clinical picture is that of metabolic acidosis and shock associated with the nonspecific symptoms mentioned above. Likewise, patients with a right-sided ductal dependent

ⓒ 2008 by Lippincott Williams & Wilkins, a Wolters Kluwer business

lesion are those that rely on the patent ductus to maintain pulmonary perfusion. These lesions include severe pulmonary stenosis, tetralogy of Fallot, and various forms of pulmonary atresia. In these cases, transition to postnatal circulation creates a dramatic decrease in pulmonary blood flow, resulting in a similar septiclike picture along with significant cyanosis.

The initial treatment for all ductal dependent lesions is the rapid initiation of intravenous prostaglandin E_1 (PGE_1) which maintains patency of the ductus arteriosus and of the fetal-circulation. PGE_1 is typically started as a continuous infusion of $0.1\ \mu g/kg/min$, and then weaned as tolerated to a dose of 0.025 to $0.05\ \mu g/kg/min$ when hemodynamic stability is achieved. PGE_1 is lifesaving in patients with ductal-dependent lesions and should be started in any case with a significant suspicion of such CHD. The common side effects of PGE_1 include apnea, hyperpyrexia, flushing, and hypotension. The patient must be monitored closely for a need for ventilatory support and may benefit from fluid and inotropic drugs.

The use of prenatal diagnosis and screening programs to evaluate for ductal-dependent lesions has decreased the number of patients with congenital heart disease who present in this septiclike state. Prior knowledge of the ductal-dependent lesion allows for initiation of PGE_1 in the delivery room and minimizes the development of adverse clinical outcomes associated with ductal closure. Studies have demonstrated that prior knowledge of such lesions and the ability to intervene early has positive benefits as it relates to surgical outcome, hospital course, and mortality. It is also known that in the absence of prenatal diagnosis, early clinical diagnosis and intervention of ductal-dependent CHD also improves clinical outcome. This once again emphasizes the importance of a high clinical suspicion for the diagnosis of ductal-dependent CHD in the neonate with nonspecific septiclike symptoms.

SUGGESTED READINGS

Brown KL, Ridout DA, Hoskote A, et al. Delayed diagnosis of congenital heart disease worsens preoperative condition and outcome of surgery in neonates. *Heart*. 2006;92:1298–1302.
Colletti JE, Homme JL, Woodridge DP. Unsuspected neonatal killers in emergency medicine. *Emerg Med Clin North Am*. 2004;22:929–960.

20

CHILDREN WITH CONGENITAL DIAPHRAGMATIC HERNIA (CDH) MAY HAVE REDUCED OXYGEN SATURATIONS. WHEN THIS OCCURS, IT IS IMPORTANT TO NEEDLE THE "GOOD SIDE" WHEN A PROBABLE PNEUMOTHORAX IS SUSPECTED

RENÉE ROBERTS, MD

WHAT TO DO – TAKE ACTION

CDH is a condition in which a defect in the diaphragm allows abdominal viscera to herniate into the thorax. The incidence is estimated to be 1 in 2,000 to 5,000 births. Approximately 30% die before birth and 50% of newborns have other anomalies such as cardiac, genitourinary, gastrointestinal, and chromosomal defects. Eighty-five percent of the defects are left-sided, and all CDH infants have some component of pulmonary hypoplasia and pulmonary artery hypertension.

The cause of CDH is not known. The relationship between the developing diaphragm and the lung has been the subject of intense laboratory effort. The big question involves which comes first, the diaphragmatic defect or the lung hypoplasia. It is hypothesized that lung development proceeds normally until 9 to 10 weeks of development, but if the pleuroperitoneal folds fail to close or muscularize at 8 weeks, the intestine is able to pass into the thorax, causing mediastinal shift, compression of thoracic contents, and impairment of subsequent pulmonary growth on **both** lungs.

CDH has been associated with abnormalities on nearly every chromosome and more commonly with chromosomal duplications or deletions syndromes such as Turner (monosomy), as well as Down, Edward, and Patau (all trisomies). Most cases of CDH, however, occur as isolated nonsyndromic presentations. Associated anomalies are present in a high percentage of fetuses (approaching 40%).

Luckily, CDH is increasingly diagnosed not by neonatal symptoms of respiratory distress, but by prenatal imaging. The findings include polyhydramnios absence of the stomach in the abdomen and presence of abdominal contents in the chest. Newborns with CDH are usually in respiratory distress at the time of delivery. Physical findings include a scaphoid abdomen, displaced heart tones and absent breath sounds on the side of the hernia. Chest and abdominal radiographic findings consist of a bowel gas pattern

© 2008 by Lippincott Williams & Wilkins, a Wolters Kluwer business

in the chest with mediastinal shift. If not diagnosed prenatally, most infants present in the first day of life, but 10% may present later and usually do well because they have sufficient pulmonary function to survive.

In a CDH study group of 2,636 patients, overall survival rate for CDH was 67% but dropped to 41% in those with heart defects. The most common heart defect is ventricular septal defect (42%). Other numerous attempts have been made to correlate prenatal imaging with postnatal outcome, with mixed results. Things such as small lung volume, liver partially or fully intrathoracic, and right-sided heart defects have been found to correlate with poor outcome.

Over the years, CDH management has shifted from a surgical emergency to a physiologic emergency, which necessitates aggressive proactive and efficient management and stabilization of affected newborns. The physiologic emergency arises from the respiratory distress, which is caused by potentially reversible pulmonary hypertension and irreversible pulmonary hypoplasia. Efforts to improve survival have focused primarily on these aspects of hypoplasia and hypertension. Treatments include fetal interventions (tracheal clips), extracorporeal membrane oxygenation (ECMO), surgery, surfactant, nitric oxide, and pulmonary vasodilators (sildenafil). But there remains a paucity of randomized controlled clinical trials in the CDH literature, which makes it difficult to compare differences in therapy, and most of these therapies have not been supported by an evidence based Cochrane review. However, there is a database (the Congenital Diaphragmatic Hernia Study Group) of >2,500 patients providing important information about CDH care and outcome.

Initial management of congenital diaphragmatic hernia consists of endotracheal intubation to minimize distention of the abdominal viscera in the chest, continuous nasogastric tube decompression, and intravenous (IV) access for fluids and sedation, and inotropic support. Use of paralytic agents may be necessary, and ventilatory strategies to minimize hypoxia and give adequate ventilation should be done in consultation with a neonatologist. The effects of systemic hypotension and acidosis, which exacerbate pulmonary hypertension, may be minimized with use of IV fluids and vasopressors. The child may require high-frequency ventilation, inhaled nitric oxide, or ECMO before surgical repair.

Most institutions now agree that although once considered a surgical emergency, children with CDH should not undergo surgical repair for 24 hours and beyond for a number of reasons. Preoperative stabilization by waiting for the pulmonary gas exchange and respiratory compliance to improve during the first day of life is advantageous. And there is no convincing evidence that delayed repair is harmful, although this delay does not decrease risk of pulmonary hypertension or morbidity from the condition itself. Definitive surgery includes decompression of the lungs by reduction of the abdominal viscera and primary closure of the diaphragmatic defect. If the diaphragm is inadequate, reconstruction can be done with use of nearby musculature or prosthetic material.

The single most significant advance in treatment of CDH has been the development of a neonatal ventilation strategy that significantly limits inflation pressure, allows tolerance of hypercapnia and relative postductal hypoxemia, and eliminates hyperventilation. Survival rates improve dramatically with the introduction of these lung-protective strategies that avoid hyperventilation and limit inflation pressures to <25 cm of water. The prior ventilation mode of the 1980s and 1990s included hyperventilation and induced alkalosis to decrease pulmonary hypertension and control ductal shunting. However, these therapies never showed improved survival, and studies of CDH mortality showed that pulmonary barotrauma as evidenced by alveolar damage, pneumothorax, and pulmonary hemorrhage were dominant findings at postmortem examination. Iatrogenic barotrauma represented a potentially avoidable cause of mortality in CDH patients and was postulated to contribute to 25% of CDH deaths.

Even today, if respiratory status worsens in a child with CDH, pneumothorax on the side **opposite** the hernia must be suspected. It is clear that barotrauma, which most frequently present as a pneumothorax but manifest in other aspects of lung failure, is associated with decreased survival in CDH. Depending on the severity though, the baby may not even be symptomatic from a pneumothorax. On physical examination, breath sounds may be diminished on the affected side. A chest radiograph often diagnoses the presence of a pneumothorax; however, transillumination of the chest provides an immediate diagnosis. On transillumination, the entire affected hemithorax lights up, whereas the unaffected side does not light up as intensely. Rapid decompression of a symptomatic pneumothorax can be achieved by inserting an IV catheter into the second intercostal space along the mid-clavicular line, removing the stylet and aspirating while advancing the catheter. A more secure evacuation of the pneumothorax is accomplished by inserting a chest tube into the pleural space under sterile conditions.

Although most infants who have CDH survive without major neurologic sequelae, newborns who have more severe CDH have small lungs and are at risk for hypoxemia, acidosis, poor perfection, and ECMO, and thus are more at risk for hypoxic ischemic brain injury, affecting later life. Because CDH is increasingly diagnosed during fetal life and expanded use of three-dimensional ultrasound and fetal magnetic resonance imaging have improved diagnostic detail and accuracy. Although chromosomal abnormalities and severe congenital heart lesions negatively impact CDH outcome, survival at several centers that favor strict lung protective strategies exceeds 80% in patients who have isolated CDH.

SUGGESTED READINGS

Das UG, Leuthner SR. Preparing the neonate for transport. *Pediatr Clin North Am.* 2004;51(3):581–598.

Kays DW. Congenital diaphragmatic hernia and neonatal lung lesions. *Surg Clin North Am.* 2006;86(2):329–352.

Okada PJ, Hicks B: Neonatal surgical emergencies that present with respiratory distress. *Clin. Pediat. Emerg. Med.* 2002;3(1):.

21

HUMAN BOTULISM IMMUNOGLOBULIN INTRAVENOUS (BIG-IV) IS SAFE AND EFFECTIVE FOR INFANT BOTULISM, BUT THE EQUINE BOTULISM ANTITOXIN HAS NOT BEEN USED TO TREAT PATIENTS WITH INFANT BOTULISM IN THE UNITED STATES

CYNTHIA GIBSON, MD

WHAT TO DO – MAKE A DECISION, TAKE ACTION

Infant botulism causes acute bulbar dysfunction, weakness, and respiratory failure in infants infected with the neurotoxin-producing *Clostridium botulinum* spores. Common clinical presenting symptoms include constipation, weak cry, poor feeding, ptosis, inactivity, and respiratory distress. Physical findings consist of hypotonia, weakness, diminished or absent gag reflex, ptosis, mydriasis, weak suck, and weak cry. The diagnosis is made by a high clinical suspicion and detection of the botulinum toxin and isolation of the spores from stool samples.

Clinical management is primarily supportive. Historically, an equine antitoxin was used for therapy that neutralized toxin molecules not yet bound to nerve endings. However, side effects occurred in 20% of patients, including hypersensitivity reactions, anaphylaxis, and serum sickness. This was commonly used in adult patients but was never recommended for infant botulism because of the side effects seen in the adult population. The equine antitoxin is no longer considered beneficial, especially in the face of a self-limited disease.

A human-derived antitoxin, human botulism immunoglobulin (BIG) is now available for treatment of infant botulism, and has been shown to reduce length of stay and severity of illness, including the need for mechanical ventilation and tube feedings. BIG-IV was approved by the U.S. Food and Drug Administration in 2003. It consists of immunoglobulin prepared from the plasma of donors immunized with pentavalent botulinum toxoid. Side effects are usually minor (flushing during infusion) although hypotension and anaphylaxis can occur, as with any immunoglobulin product. Prompt treatment of infant botulism with BIG-IV is safe and effective, and reduces hospital stay.

ⓒ 2008 by Lippincott Williams & Wilkins, a Wolters Kluwer business

SUGGESTED READINGS

Arnon SS, Schechter R, Maslanka SE, et al. Human botulism immune globulin for the treatment of infant botulism. *N Engl J Med.* 2006;354:462–471.

Cox N, Hinkle R. Infant botulism. *Am Fam Physician.* 2002;65:1388–1392.

Shapiro RL, Hatheway C, Swerdlow DL. Botulism in the United States: a clinical and epidemiologic review. *Ann Internal Med.* 1998:129(3):221–228.

Thompson JA, Filloux FM, Van Orman CB, et al. Infant botulism in the age of botulism immune globulin. *Neurology.* 2005;64:2029–2032.

22

THE VOMITING OF BILE-STAINED FLUID IN THE FIRST FEW DAYS OF LIFE SHOULD BE CONSIDERED INTESTINAL OBSTRUCTION UNTIL PROVEN OTHERWISE

CYNTHIA GIBSON, MD

WHAT TO DO – INTERPRET THE DATA

Intestinal obstruction, often atresia, presents in the first few days of life as bilious vomiting sometimes accompanied by abdominal distention and failure to pass meconium. Infants are often premature and small for gestational age and a prenatal diagnosis may be made in babies with polyhydramnios. Intestinal obstruction with bilious vomiting in neonates is caused by duodenal atresia, malrotation, volvulus, jejunoileal atresia, meconium ileus, and necrotizing enterocolitis. Babies with stenosis present as newborns or later with recurrent vomiting and failure to thrive.

The diagnosis can be made on the presenting symptoms and plain abdominal x-rays. The presence of dilated bowel loops and air-fluid levels should prompt urgent consultation with a pediatric surgeon. The number of dilated loops usually indicates the level of obstruction and contrast studies are not required to make the diagnosis. Patients presenting with delayed symptoms may need an upper gastrointestinal study with small bowel follow through to assess for a midgut stenosis. Treatment of intestinal atresia is operative following adequate fluid resuscitation and electrolyte correction.

SUGGESTED READINGS

Gosche J, Vick L, Boulanger SC, et al. Midgut abnormalities. *Surg Clin North Am.* 2006;86:285–299.

Halter J, Basel T, Nicolette L, et al. Common gastrointestinal problems and emergencies in neonates and children. *Clin Fam Prac.* 2004;6:731–754.

Kimura K, Loening-Baucke V. Bilious vomiting in the newborn: rapid diagnosis of intestinal obstruction. *Am Fam Physician.* 2000;61:2791–2798.

© 2008 by Lippincott Williams & Wilkins, a Wolters Kluwer business

23

DON'T FORGET TO INQUIRE ABOUT SEXUAL ACTIVITY IN ADOLESCENT PATIENTS. MANY CONDITIONS, INCLUDING MONOARTICULAR ARTHRITIS, MAY REPRESENT AN UNDERLYING SEXUALLY TRANSMITTED DISEASE (STD)

ESTHER FORRESTER, MD

WHAT TO DO – GATHER APPROPRIATE DATA

Septic arthritis is usually caused by bacterial infection and results in inflammation of the synovial membrane with purulent effusion into the joint capsule. Gram-positive aerobes are the etiologic agent in 80% of cases, regardless of age group. However, practitioners need to be alert for *Neisseria gonorrhea* infections in sexually active adolescents who present with tenosynovitis, joint pain, fever, and skin lesions. Sixteen percent of the arthritis-dermatitis infections occur in individuals ages 10 to 19 years old and have a female predominance. Arthritis is the most common systemic complication of *N. gonorrhea,* usually occurring within 1 month of exposure. Up to two thirds of affected patients have migratory polyarthralgias, while one-quarter have pain in a single joint, with the knee being the most common site of purulent gonococcal arthritis.

Septic arthritis is the most destructive arthritis and empiric therapy is essential. Patients with suspected disseminated gonococcal infections (DGIs) should be hospitalized for initial therapy, particularly if concerns for compliance are raised (i.e., being adolescents), the diagnosis is uncertain (joint and blood cultures are rarely positive once arthritis is present), or if purulent synovial effusions or other complications (i.e., perihepatitis, endocarditis, or meningitis) are present. The Centers for Disease Control and Prevention (CDC) recommends ceftriaxone 1 g intramuscular or intravenous every 24 hours for DGI in patients weighing >45 kg (99 lb). This treatment should be continued for 24 to 48 hours. Once the patient improves, therapy can be switched to oral cefixime, ciprofloxacin, ofloxacin, or levofloxacin for at least

© 2008 by Lippincott Williams & Wilkins, a Wolters Kluwer business

TABLE 23.1	REGIMEN FOR TREATING SEPTIC ARTHRITIS	
REGIMEN	**DRUG**	**DOSE**
Recommended Parenteral Regimen	Ceftriaxone	>45 kg: 1 g IV or IM q24h <45 kg: 50 mg/kg (max dose: 1 g) IM or IV in a single dose daily for 7 days
Alternative Parenteral Regimen	Cefotaxime Ciprofloxacin* Levofloxacin* Ofloxacin* Spectinomycin	>45 kg: 1 g IV q8h hours >45 kg: 400 mg IV q12h >45 kg: 250 mg IV daily >45 kg: 400 mg IV q12h >45 kg: 2 g IM q12h
Oral Regimen	Cefixime Ciprofloxacin* Levofloxacin* Ofloxacin	>45 kg: 400 mg BID >45 kg: 500 mg BID >45 kg: 500 mg daily >45 kg: 400 mg BID

BID, twice daily; q, every; h, hour; IV, intravenous; IM, intramuscular.
*Quinolones are not recommended in patients <18 years old OR in MSM (see text) or patients with a history of recent foreign travel or partners' travel, infections acquired in California or Hawaii, or infections acquired in other areas with increase quinolone resistant *Neisseria gonorrhea* prevalence.

1 week (*Table 23.1*). Children weighing <45 kg should receive ceftriaxone 50 mg/kg in a single daily dose for 7 days. Parenteral cephalosporins are the only recommended therapy in children because of insufficient data on the efficacy of oral cephalosporins for gonococcal infections in this patient population. Quinolones are relatively contraindicated in children weighing <45 kg due to a theoretic risk of articular cartilage damage. Quinolones should not be used to treat men who have sex with men, or patients with a history of recent foreign travel or partners' travel, infections acquired in California or Hawaii, or infections acquired in other areas with a high quinolone-resistant *N. gonorrhea* prevalence. Patients with presumed DGI should also be treated for *Chlamydia trachomatis* infections. The CDC recommends azithromycin 1 g orally or doxycycline 100 mg twice a day for 7 days for patients with uncomplicated infections. Physicians should also test patients with confirmed gonococcal infections for other STDs, including human immunodeficiency virus.

SUGGESTED READINGS

Center for Disease Control and Prevention. Sexually Transmitted Disease Treatment Guidelines 2006. http://www.cdc.gov/std/treatment/2006/urethritis-and-cervicitis.htm#uc6. Accessed March 1, 2007.

Miller KE. Diagnosis and treatment of *Neisseria gonorrhea* infections. *Am Fam Phys.* 2006; 73:1779–1784.

Munos G. "Septic Arthritis" eMedicine. http://www.emedicine.com/orthoped/topic437.htm. Accessed March 1, 2007.

Neinstein L, ed. *Adolescent Health Care: A Practical Guide.* 4th ed. Philadelphia, PA: Lippincott Williams & Wilkins; 2002:1125–1133.

24

KNOW HOW TO APPROPRIATELY WORK UP A BREAST MASS IN ADOLESCENT FEMALES

LINDSEY ALBRECHT, MD

WHAT TO DO – GATHER APPROPRIATE DATA

The discovery of a breast mass in an adolescent female understandably awakens concern in both the patient and her family. Fortunately, the majority of breast masses in this age group are benign, with fibroadenoma being the most common lesion identified. However, malignant tumors may occur on rare occasions, making accurate diagnosis of the newly discovered breast mass critically important in the adolescent population.

A fibroadenoma is a benign estrogen sensitive tumor that is identified in 70% to 95% of breast biopsy specimens in adolescent females. Their peak incidence is in late adolescence until the early 20s, though premenarchal cases have been described. A fibroadenoma usually presents as a firm rubbery nontender mass, often noted to be slowly enlarging over weeks to months. At the time of diagnosis, most fibroadenomas are 3 to 4 cm in size. Fibroadenomas are most often found in the upper outer quadrants of the breast, though they can occur elsewhere. They are not associated with nipple discharge. Overlying skin changes may be noted in a minority of cases, usually when the lesions are quite large. Lesions are typically solitary but may be multiple or bilateral in 10% to 25% of cases, a condition referred to as fibroadenomatosis. Some fibroadenomas regress spontaneously, while others remain stable in size or enlarge over time.

A juvenile or giant fibroadenoma is a fibroadenoma that is >5 cm in size. These masses are often noted to grow rapidly and sometimes reach sizes of >15 to 20 cm. The giant variant is less common than the regular form, but makes up a higher percentage of cases in early adolescence. Because giant fibroadenomas may compress or replace normal breast tissue, their potential for leading to a poor cosmetic outcome is greater.

Cystosarcoma phyllodes is a breast tumor with peak incidence in the fourth decade of life, although it occasionally occurs in adolescence. It is usually painless and slow growing and is usually larger than a fibroadenoma when discovered. It may be associated with overlying skin changes, nipple discharge, and axillary lymphadenopathy (usually due to tumor necrosis or associated infection). Cystosarcoma phyllodes is most often benign, but borderline and malignant forms exist.

© 2008 by Lippincott Williams & Wilkins, a Wolters Kluwer business

Other than fibroadenoma and cystosarcoma phyllodes, additional etiologies of a breast mass in the adolescent patient include breast abscess, fibrocystic change or other varieties of breast cyst, intraductal papilloma, lipoma, and findings related to fat necrosis. Neurofibromatosis, hemangiomas, hematomas, and other causes have also been reported.

Malignant breast tumors, when they occur in the adolescent female, typically arise from nonbreast tissue. Lymphomas, leukemias, and sarcomas are the most common of these tumors. Only about one third of malignant breast masses arise from primary breast tissue, with highest risk seen in the older adolescent and in those with a family history of breast cancer or BRCA-1 or BRCA-2 gene mutations. Adenocarcinoma is usually hard with indistinct borders, and is usually fixed or nonmobile. Nipple retraction or discharge, skin edema, lymphadenopathy, and signs or symptoms of metastatic disease may be present in some cases.

The workup of a newly discovered breast mass may vary depending on the characteristics of the lesion and the particular patient. Small, slow-growing, rubbery lesions consistent with a fibroadenoma can be observed over a period of several months. Imaging by ultrasound may be helpful in differentiating solid lesions from cystic ones, though it is not usually helpful in distinguishing amongst solid lesions. Mammography is not encouraged in the adolescent population, because the density of the breast parenchyma is high in this age group, which may obscure the lesion. Of course, a tissue diagnosis is needed for suspicious lesions, such as fixed, irregular-feeling or rapidly enlarging masses. Tissue has traditionally been obtained through excisional biopsy or open surgery, though newer evidence has supported the role of fine-needle aspiration (FNA) as a diagnostic tool in adolescent girls. FNA may be preferable to other more invasive methods given the high incidence of benign disease in adolescents, as well as the decreased likelihood of causing a poor cosmetic result in the developing breast. FNA can additionally be used to drain cysts, which may be both diagnostic and therapeutic.

Thus, in most cases, breast masses in the adolescent female are benign. When they occur, they can usually be managed conservatively. Additional workup is needed for suspicious or questionable lesions, however, given the rare possibility of malignant disease in adolescents.

SUGGESTED READINGS

Greydanus DE, Matysina L, Gains M. Breast disorders in children and adolescents. *Prim Care.* 2006;33:455–502.

Pacinda SJ, Ramzy I. Fine-needle aspiration of breast masses. A review of its role in diagnosis and management of adolescent patients. *J Adolesc Health.* 1998;23:3–6.

25

Although chest pain in adolescents is often related to gastroesophageal reflux disease (GERD) or anxiety, it can occasionally be pathologic and more serious conditions should be considered

Johann Peterson, MD

What to Do – Gather Appropriate Data

Adolescents who present to the emergency department with chest pain are often frightened, as are their families. Typically, however, their pain is unlikely to be due to a pathologic or abnormal cardiac condition. As the treating provider, one should immediately assess the child for signs of serious disease—including respiratory distress, poor perfusion, altered mental status, asymmetric breath sounds, wheezing or poor air movement, and unhealthy vital signs—while remembering that tachypnea, tachycardia, and diaphoresis may be caused by anxiety. Early auscultation of the chest and palpation of pulses will most often reassure both you and the patient. When in doubt, give supplemental oxygen. Assuming that this rapid assessment does not reveal urgent respiratory or circulatory problems, attempting to calm your patient and his or her family is a good next step. Inquiring about their concerns and assuring them that cardiac disease, although rare in adolescents, will be considered by evaluating the patient's signs.

Keeping an extensive differential in mind will help you conduct a thorough evaluation. It can be helpful to recall thoracic and abdominal anatomy. Many adolescents with acute chest pain will be worried about heart disease, so start there. Coronary ischemia is rare (but possible, especially in cocaine abuse or children with anomalous coronary arteries). Consider myocarditis, pericarditis, aortic dissection or ruptured aneurysm, arrhythmias such as supraventricular tachycardias, mitral valve prolapse (which is, in some opinions, associated with chest pain), and pulmonary hypertension. Pulmonary causes may include asthma, pneumonia, pleuritis or pleural effusion (a parapneumonic effusion related to infection or other disease, such as lupus), spontaneous or posttraumatic pneumothorax, and pneumonitis from intentional or accidental inhalations. In the chest wall, consider muscle strains, fractured ribs, costochondritis (idiopathic or viral, also known as Tietze syndrome), breast pain (often due to normal breast bud development in boys or

ⓒ 2008 by Lippincott Williams & Wilkins, a Wolters Kluwer business

girls, or to benign cysts in pubertal girls). Precordial catch, also known as a Texidor twinge, is a recurrent, sharp chest or side pain, usually lasting several seconds to a few minutes, and made worse by deep breathing, without an identifiable cause. It is thought to be benign, and most adolescents outgrow it. Among gastrointestinal causes, consider GERD, esophagitis, ruptured esophagus (Boerhaave syndrome, generally caused by excessive vomiting in eating disorders such as bulimia), and gas. Depression and anxiety can manifest with a chief complaint of chest pain. Approach the history and physical with these in mind.

Establish in detail the history of the chest pain, including exactly what the patient was doing at its onset, its qualities and exacerbating or relieving factors; whether or not the patient has have ever had chest pain before; and if he or she has symptoms such as palpitations, lightheadedness, syncope, wheezing, chest tightness, or cough, especially if they occur with exertion. Ask early if the patient know what caused the pain. Make sure to note fevers and recent illnesses, exposure to smoke or vapors, and medications. Some commonly prescribed macrolide and quinolone antibiotics, antipsychotics, and selective serotonin reuptake inhibitors (SSRIs) can prolong the QT interval. In young or developmentally delayed children, the consideration of aspiration or an esophageal foreign body needs to be considered. The adolescent should be questioned alone about drug use, specifically cocaine and tobacco.

The medical and family histories should include any congenital heart disease, conduction abnormalities, asthma, spontaneous pneumothorax, thoracic surgery, Marfan disease, Ehlers-Danlos, early coronary artery disease, and whether or not the patient ever had Kawasaki disease (ask by name, and ask about a febrile illness with the signs and symptoms of Kawasaki). Other clues to possible undiagnosed arrhythmias include seizures, fainting (especially with emotional stress), sudden death, and drowning. A very detailed history is usually the most useful piece in the diagnostic puzzle and is more likely to assure patients that your evaluation is complete than it is to frighten them with ominous diagnoses and thoughts of death that had not crossed their mind.

The physical examination should include a thorough auscultation of the chest for heart and breath sounds. Palpate every costochondral joint for tenderness; identify the liver edge; palpate the abdominal aorta; and look for xanthomas, xanthelasmas, and corneal arcus (which would alert you to the possibility of familial hypercholesterolemia leading to early coronary artery disease). Check for clues to Marfan syndrome, including joint laxity, scoliosis, pes planus, and a history of dislocated lens. Loeys-Dietz syndrome is a related and recently described syndrome consisting of hypertelorism, cleft palate or bifid uvula, and the tendency to develop dilated and tortuous vessels, including the aorta. Suspicion of either disease should prompt you to consider aortic dissection. Rash, arthritis, or ulcers on the palate may lead you to suspect lupus, raising the probability of pericarditis or pleuritis.

In one study, the percentage of adolescent patients with a cardiac cause of their chest pain ranged from 0% to 4%. The most commonly identified causes were musculoskeletal pain, costochondritis, and pain due to cough. Pain without an identifiable cause was also common, with 20% to 40% of cases ultimately listed as idiopathic. These studies also found that many patients are frightened they are having a heart attack or that their pain is due to cancer, especially girls with breast pain, which emphasizes the need for education and reassurance. There do not seem to be well-validated criteria for when to perform diagnostic testing or referral in chest pain, but the consensus is that screening tests should be avoided. If the history and physical reveal a benign cause or none at all, reassurance is all that is indicated. As with other types of chronic pain, adolescents with chronic or recurrent chest pain may benefit from keeping a pain log and having regular follow-up. If trauma or significant pulmonary disease is suspected, obtain a chest x-ray. In the rare case you do have reason to suspect heart disease, start with a chest x-ray and eletrocardiogram and consider echocardiogram or referral.

SUGGESTED READINGS

De Paepe A, Devereux RB, Dietz HC, et al. Revised diagnostic criteria for the Marfan syndrome. *Am J Med Genet.* 1996;62:417–426.

Driscoll DJ, Glicklich LB, Gallen WJ. Chest pain in children: a prospective study. *Pediatrics.* 1976;57(5):648–651.

Pantell RH, Goodman BW Jr. Adolescent chest pain: a prospective study. *Pediatrics.* 1983;71(6):881–887.

Roden DM. Drug-induced prolongation of the QT interval. *N Engl J Med.* 2004;350(10):1013–1022.

Selbst SM, Ruddy RM, Clark BJ, et al. Pediatric chest pain: a prospective study. *Pediatrics.* 1988;82(3):319–323.

26

USE EVERY EPISODE OF CARE WITH ADOLESCENT PATIENTS TO ASSURE GENITAL HEALTH

MADAN DHARMAR, MD

WHAT TO DO – GATHER APPROPRIATE DATA

Adolescence is an important developmental period with regard to sexuality and sexual behavior. Adolescents are at increased risk for sexually transmitted diseases (STD) for a variety of several behavioral and biological factors. Age at first intercourse and time between menarche and first intercourse, number of sexual partners, partners with multiple other partners, inconsistent protected sex, and alcohol and drug abuse are some of the behavioral factors associated with increased STDs in adolescents. Cervical ectopy or cervical immaturity and low levels of secretary immunoglobulin A (IgA) in adolescent females make them more susceptible to STDs.

When addressing the issue of STDs in adolescents, unique factors such as consent for diagnosis and treatment, confidentiality, parental notification, and mandatory reporting of sexual activity need to be kept in mind. Several of these issues, including behavioral and biological factors, should be addressed by clinicians who provide services to adolescents. Clinicians can also address the lack of knowledge and awareness about the risks and consequences of STDs and offer guidance, constituting true primary prevention, to help adolescents develop healthy sexual behaviors and prevent patterns of behavior that can undermine sexual health.

Assessing Sexual Health in an Adolescent: Clinical preventive services provided during an office visit must include screening for sexual behavior that may result in unintended pregnancy and STD, and screening for STDs in a sexually active patient. A great proportion of adolescents are not evaluated for risk of acquiring STDs during their office visit. Owing to an increased incidence of some STDs in adolescents, it is important for clinicians to assess the individual's sexual activity. Presenting symptoms and signs in a patient can be useful for obtaining relevant history and appropriate examination and tests to diagnose STDs. Common presentations of STDs are vaginal/urethral discharge, skin lesions, genital ulcers, and pelvic inflammatory disease (PID).

ⓒ 2008 by Lippincott Williams & Wilkins, a Wolters Kluwer business

Chlamydia Infection in Adolescents: The incidence of Chlamydia is highest among adolescent females aged 15 to 19 years. Though the number of Chlamydia cases reported annually is increasing, most cases are undiagnosed. Chlamydia is a bacterial infection transmitted sexually. Chlamydia is more commonly found in women than men, and is highest among adolescent females aged 15 to 19 years. The two most important risk factors are the age of the woman (i.e., adolescent) and a risk of multiple sexual partners. Chlamydia infection is usually asymptomatic. Due to underdiagnosis and lack of treatment, chlamydial infections can cause severe health consequences for women, including PID, ectopic pregnancy, and infertility. Symptomatic patients present with vaginal discharge, poorly differentiated abdominal pain, and increased frequency of urine and dysuria. Screening for chlamydial infection requires a pelvic examination that is usually uncomfortable, and is considered a barrier for screening adolescents. Urine testing for Chlamydia infection is more acceptable to patients and because of its ease of implementation, is more likely to detect a greater number of cases of PID and infertility. Antibiotic therapy is curative for Chlamydia infection. Repeated acquisition of STDs is common, with up to 40% of the annual incidence of chlamydial or gonococcal disease occurring in adolescents previously infected with the causative organisms. Many adolescents are re-infected within a few months of an index infection. Annual screening for Chlamydia is recommended.

Vaginal discharge is the most common presenting symptom in STDs. It can be either physiological or pathologic in origin. Candidiasis, Trichomonas, and bacterial vaginosis are three most common pathologic causes for vaginal discharge in adolescents. *Trichomonas* infection is classically associated with a greenish-yellow purulent discharge; candidiasis with a thick, white, adherent, "cottage cheeselike" discharge; and bacterial vaginosis with a thin, homogeneous, "fishy smelling" gray discharge. Urethral mucopurulent discharge is a common presentation of gonorrhoeae. Skin lesions are commonly caused by human papillomavirus (genital warts). Genital herpes is the most common cause for genital ulcers in adolescents and are usually associated with other genital lesions. Primary syphilis should also be considered in adolescent patients involved in high-risk sexual behavior.

SUGGESTED READINGS

Anderson MR, Klink K, Cohrssen A. An evaluation of vaginal complaints. *JAMA.* 2004;291(11):1368–1379.

Centers for Disease Control and Prevention. *STD Surveillance 2005.* Centers for Disease Control and Prevention. www.cdc.gov/std/stats/. Accessed December 18, 2007.

Ford CA, Best D, Miller WC. The pediatric forum: confidentiality and adolescents' willingness to consent to sexually transmitted disease testing. *Arch Pediatr Adolesc Med.* 2001;155(9):1072–1073.

Fortenberry JD. Adolescent substance use and sexually transmitted diseases risk: a review. *J Adolesc Health.* 1995;16(4):304–308.

Halpern-Felsher BL, Ozer EM, Millstein SG, et al. Preventive services in a health maintenance organization: how well do pediatricians screen and educate adolescent patients? *Arch Pediatr Adolesc Med.* 2000;154(2):173–179.

McCormack WM, Rosner B, McComb DE, et al. Infection with *Chlamydia trachomatis* in female college students. *Am J Epidemiol.* 1985;121(1):107–115.

Shafer MA, Pantell RH, Schachter J. Is the routine pelvic examination needed with the advent of urine-based screening for sexually transmitted diseases? *Arch Pediatr Adolesc Med.* 1999;153(2):119–125.

Shew ML, Fortenberry JD, Miles P, et al. Interval between menarche and first sexual intercourse, related to risk of human papillomavirus infection. *J Pediatr.* 1994;125(4):661–666.

27

Do not miss the diagnosis of ovarian torsion. Ovarian torsion can present with nonspecific complaints of abdominal pain, nausea and vomiting, and variable physical findings. Early diagnosis and treatment is essential to reduce the likelihood of a negative outcome

Michael Clemmens, MD

What to Do – Interpret the Data

Ovarian torsion is an uncommon condition with potentially serious complications. Torsion occurs when the ovary twists on its ligamentous pedicle.
Venous and then arterial blood flow are compromised, and the ovary becomes nonviable if the condition is not diagnosed and surgically corrected
within a short time. Ovarian torsion can occur in utero, during infancy, and
throughout childhood. The incidence is highest in postmenarchal girls. The
presence of an ovarian cyst or tumor increases the risk of torsion, although
approximately 50% of cases occur in girls with normal ovaries. An ovarian
cyst on a prenatal sonogram places the newborn infant at increased risk for
torsion and should alert the clinician to pursue the diagnosis if abdominal
signs and symptoms arise.

The most common presenting symptom is abdominal pain that is usually severe in nature. Older girls may localize the pain to one of the lower
quadrants. Nausea and vomiting are also frequently present. Fever is unusual unless the presentation is late. The clinical history often raises concerns about the possibility of appendicitis or a renal stone. The absence of
hematuria makes the diagnosis of a stone less likely. The abrupt onset of severe pain should point the clinician away from the diagnosis of appendicitis,
which usually has a more insidious onset.

The abdominal examination is often nonspecific. The abdomen may
be soft, although voluntary guarding is common. Involuntary guarding and
rebound tenderness are present in advanced cases. Palpation of a mass is
quite helpful but often difficult in younger children. When the diagnosis of
ovarian torsion is suspected, the imaging test of choice is an ultrasound of
the abdomen and pelvis with Doppler flow evaluation of arterial and venous

© 2008 by Lippincott Williams & Wilkins, a Wolters Kluwer business

circulation to the ovaries. Enlargement of the ovary or the presence of a cyst or mass is supportive of the diagnosis. The key diagnostic finding is usually the absence of venous flow from one of the ovaries. Absence of arterial flow is also diagnostic, but it is a late finding and its presence does not rule out the diagnosis of torsion. It is important to note that a significant number of torsions occur with apparently normal arterial flow. In these cases, the venous stasis likely causes increased ovarian pressure, edema, and hemorrhage that ultimately compromise tissue viability.

Initial management includes intravenous hydration and analgesia. The pain from ovarian torsion usually requires the use of narcotics. If peritonitis is suspected, then broad-spectrum antibiotic coverage should be instituted. Immediate surgical correction provides the best chance to avoid loss of ovarian function. Detorsion with ovarian preservation is the most desirable course. Many ovaries with a dusky appearance are salvageable. Tissue that is clearly nonviable is removed to prevent the development of peritonitis. Maintaining a high index of suspicion for ovarian torsion in girls with the acute onset of abdominal pain is the key to establishing an early diagnosis. The abrupt onset of severe lower abdominal pain, the presence of a mass, and lack of venous flow on ultrasound are highly suggestive of torsion. Immediate surgical consultation improves the prognosis for preserving ovarian viability.

SUGGESTED READINGS

Ben-Ami M, Perlitz Y, Haddad S. The effectiveness of spectral and color Doppler in predicting ovarian torsion. A prospective study. *Eur J Obstet Gynecol Reprod Biol.* 2002;104:64–66.

Brown MF, Hebra A, McGeehin K, et al. Ovarian masses in children: a review of 91 cases of malignant and benign masses. *J Pediatr Surg.* 1993;28:930–933.

Houdry D, Abbott JT. Ovarian torsion: a fifteen-year review. *Ann Emerg Med.* 2001;38:156–159.

Piipo S, Mustaniemi L, Lenko H, et al. Surgery for ovarian masses during childhood and adolescence: a report of 79 cases. *J Pediatr Adolesc Gynecol.* 1999;12:223–227.

28

PROVIDE ADOLESCENTS WITH THE OPPORTUNITY TO RECEIVE CONFIDENTIAL CARE

BRIAN KIT, MD

WHAT TO DO – TAKE ACTION

The health needs of adolescents differ from those of younger children. The adolescent struggles with independence. With greater independence, adolescents have more opportunities to engage in behaviors that place them at risk for health problems, including drug use and sexual activity. A behavioral assessment is essential in caring for adolescent patients. Addressing adolescent behaviors is often difficult for the medical provider. Among the reasons for difficulties are the practical limitations of effectively communicating with the adolescent and also concerns regarding the legal and ethical dimensions for providing care for this age group. Providers of medical services to the adolescent patient must create a welcoming environment for the patient so that she or he feels comfortable discussing problems. A nonjudgmental approach will encourage adolescents to disclose information about their behavior. Although the goal of the provider may be to perform an assessment of the adolescent's risk-taking behaviors, this is best done after establishing a rapport and the patient feels like the provider cares about him or her as an individual.

Providers should routinely interview their adolescent patients both with their parents in the room and also after asking the parent to leave the room so that the patient has every opportunity to discuss sensitive issues. Talking individually with adolescents is important because many adolescents want to talk about sensitive health information but fail to do so because of the lack of opportunities for private discussion.

Many pediatricians find it awkward to ask parents to leave the room during part of the interview, but most families respect the adolescent's need for privacy. Adolescents and their parent(s) should be informed of the right of adolescents to confidentiality and to consent for their own medical care. By communicating clear guidelines, there will be less room for confusion and increased chances that adolescents will seek the advice of medical personnel regarding sensitive issue in the future.

State and federal laws have been developed to provide protection to adolescents who are concerned about health problems but do not want to

© 2008 by Lippincott Williams & Wilkins, a Wolters Kluwer business

disclose the information to their parents and who may forgo medical care as a result. It is important for practitioners to be familiar with the laws of consent and confidentiality in their own state, because variability between states exists.

Informed Consent: Parental consent generally is required for the medical treatment of minors. However, there are situations in which an adolescent can give informed consent without the consent of a parent. These situations include emergency care, care for emancipated minors, and state-mandated situations.

- **Emergency care:** Patients who present to the emergency room for medical services are required under the federally defined Emergency Medical Treatment and Active Labor Act (EMTALA) to receive an appropriate medical screening and necessary testing. EMTALA preempts conflicting or inconsistent state laws, essentially rendering the problem of obtaining consent for the emergency treatment of minors a nonissue.
- **Emancipated minors:** The definition of emancipated minor differs by state. For example, some states define the emancipated minor as someone who is older than 16 years, lives apart from his or her parents, and is economically independent.
- **State-mandated situations**: These might include abortion services, treatment for sexually transmitted infections, prenatal care and delivery services, treatment for drug abuse, and outpatient mental health care.

Confidentiality: Parents generally have the right to medical information and records of their children. However, many states have given adolescents the right to confidentiality in specific situations, including state-mandated situations, as discussed above. Exceptions to confidentiality include reporting of sexual abuse, alerting authorities in the case of homicidal intentions, and taking appropriate measures to protect a suicidal patient.

By effectively communicating with adolescents, including discussions with adolescents without a parent present, and equipping them with knowledge regarding the rights of adolescents in consent and confidentiality, health care professionals will be in a position to maximize the health status of their adolescent patients.

SUGGESTED READINGS

Bitterman RA. The medical screening examination requirement. In: Bitterman RA, ed. *EMTALA: Providing Emergency Care Under Federal Law.* Dallas, TX: American College of Emergency Physicians, 2000:23–65.

Cheng TL, Savageau JA, Sattler AL, et al. Confidentiality in health care. A survey of knowledge, perceptions, and attitudes among high school students. *JAMA.* 1993; 269(11);1404–1407.

Committee on Pediatric Emergency Medicine of the AAP. Consent for emergency medical services for children and adolescents. *Pediatrics.* 2003;111(3):703–706.

Ford CA, Millstein SG, Halpern-Felsher BL, et al. Influence of physician confidentiality assurances on adolescents' willingness to disclose information and seek future health care. A randomized control trail. *JAMA.* 1997;278:1029–1034.

King NM, Cross AW. Children as decision-makers: guidelines for pediatricians. *J Pediatr.* 1989;115:10–16.

Resnick M, Blum RW, Hedin D. The appropriateness of health services for adolescents: youth's opinions and attitudes. *J Adolesc Health Care.* 1980;1(2):137–141.

29

FOR ADOLESCENT GIRLS WHO PRESENT WITH ABDOMINAL PAIN, ORDER A PREGNANCY TEST

MICHAEL S. POTTER AND ANTHONY SLONIM, MD

WHAT TO DO – GATHER APPROPRIATE DATA

Teen pregnancy in the United States is disproportionately more frequent than it is in other industrialized nations, and although there has been a recent decline, the epidemiology of adolescent pregnancy still warrants careful observation for postmenarchal teenage girls who present with abdominal pain. Pediatricians should be aware of pregnancy as a potential cause for abdominal pain.

The symptoms associated with adolescent pregnancy include morning sickness, swollen tender breasts, weight gain, and amenorrhea. The presentation of these symptoms is often vague and presents like a flulike syndrome, including headache, fatigue, and pain in the abdominal region. Doctors should be aware that denial of sexual activity as a result of embarrassment or fear of negative parental reactions does not sufficiently exclude pregnancy. A complete examination and appropriate diagnostic testing may be necessary to identify pregnancy. On physical examination, an enlarged uterus, cervical cyanosis, a soft uterus, or a soft cervix are strong indicators of intrauterine pregnancy. Pregnancy testing is recommended to complement the physical exam. The most sensitive pregnancy test, a quantitative beta-human chorionic gonadotropin (β-hCG) radioimmunoassay, is less commonly used because of its expense, but it is useful in diagnosing an ectopic pregnancy, a retained placenta, or a molar pregnancy. Urine pregnancy tests have sufficient sensitivity to be used as a screening tool.

Teen pregnancy is an especially private issue and confidentiality is essential when dealing with its effects. As the age of the pregnant teen decreases, one should be more concerned that sexual coercion or abuse may have been involved. In the event that a negative pregnancy test occurs, the test should be performed again in 2 weeks. Repeated negative test results may warrant additional counseling and intervention by family or other trusted individuals. The adverse affects of teen pregnancy are significantly reduced by prenatal care. Teen mothers are more at risk of not completing high school or maintaining a steady job. Children of teen mothers are at a greater risk of low birth weight and exhibit difficulties with cognitive functions.

© 2008 by Lippincott Williams & Wilkins, a Wolters Kluwer business

Pregnancy almost always results in major life changes for those involved. Teenagers who are psychosocially unprepared for pregnancy must be handled with care to assure a proper diagnosis and follow-up. The complications that can arise from unprepared early pregnancies make timely, accurate diagnoses essential.

SUGGESTED READING

Jenkins RR. Pregnancy. In: Behrman RE, Kliegman RM, Jenson HB, eds. *Nelson Textbook of Pediatrics.* 17th ed. Philadelphia, PA: Saunders; 2004; pages 671–73.

30

SEXUAL ABUSE IS AN IMPORTANT DIAGNOSIS TO CONFIRM FOR BOTH THE CHILD AND FAMILY SO THAT APPROPRIATE TREATMENT CAN BEGIN. REMEMBER THOUGH THAT SOME PHYSICAL FINDINGS THAT MAY BE SUGGESTIVE OF ABUSE, MAY NOT BE DEFINITIVE

YOLANDA LEWIS-RAGLAND, MD

WHAT TO DO – INTERPRET THE DATA

There is a wide range of nonabusive causes of physical and behavioral symptoms that serve as presenting complaints of sexual abuse victims; likewise, the physical findings are often vague and nonspecific, with many having other likely causes. For example, although erythema of the vaginal vestibule could be a tell-tale sign of sexual abuse, it is seen commonly in asymptomatic, nonabused, prepubescent girls, and in girls with irritant vulvovaginitis.

NORMAL VARIANTS

After years of anatomical analysis of female genitalia, it is accepted that there is wide variation in normal hymenal configuration and of vaginal orifice shape. It is important, therefore, to keep in mind some of the following presentations as normal variants:

- Septal remnants, seen as tags near the midline on either the anterior or posterior portion of the hymenal membrane
- Anterolateral hymenal flaps
- Periurethral bands
- Intravaginal ridges
- Thin labial adhesions.

© 2008 by Lippincott Williams & Wilkins, a Wolters Kluwer business

NONABUSIVE CAUSES OF IRRITATION

- Vulvovaginitis (due to chemical irritation, poor perineal hygiene or aeration, nonabusive frictional trauma, and contact dermatitis or itching and scratching due to pinworms or fomites)
- Urethral prolapse
- Lichen sclerosus et atrophicus
- Straddle injuries
- Foreign bodies
- Anal fissures/anal tags (often associated with constipation).

WHEN TO SUSPECT ABUSE

The diagnosis of child sexual abuse can often be made on the basis of a child's history. Sexual abuse is rarely diagnosed on the basis solely on physical examination or laboratory findings. As stated previously, physical findings are often absent even when the perpetrator admits to penetration of the child's genitalia. Many types of abuse leave no physical evidence, and mucosal injuries often heal rapidly and completely. In a recent study of pregnant adolescents, only two of 36 had evidence of penetration. Occasionally, a child presents with clear evidence of anogenital trauma without an adequate history. The difficulty of diagnosis is further complicated, since children may deny abuse.

SUSPICIOUS PHYSICAL FINDINGS

Findings that are concerning include:

- Abrasions or bruising of the genitalia
- An acute or healed tear in the posterior aspect of the hymen extending to the hymen's base
- A markedly decreased or absent hymenal tissue posteriorly
- Injury to or scarring of the posterior fourchette, fossa navicularis, or hymen
- Anal bruising or lacerations.

The interpretation of physical findings continues to evolve as evidence-based research becomes available. Certain positive findings, however, serve as very likely if not definitive indications of abuse. For example, the presence of semen, sperm, or acid phosphatase; a positive culture for *Neisseria gonorrhoeae* or *Chlamydia trachomatis*; or a positive serologic test for syphilis or human immunodeficiency virus infection make the diagnosis of sexual abuse a near certainty even in the absence of a positive history, if perinatal transmission of the sexually transmitted diseases has been excluded. However, it is important to recognize that because of its prolonged incubation period, the human papillomavirus may not produce lesions until several months to years after delivery, despite transmission at birth and, therefore, may need further investigation of the unsuspecting mother who often is unaware of her own infection.

REPORTING A CRIME

The medical evaluation is first and foremost an examination by a medical professional with the primary aim of diagnosing and determining treatment for a patient's complaint. When the complaint involves the possible commission of a crime, however, the physician must recognize legal concerns. The legal issues confronting pediatricians in evaluating sexually abused children include mandatory reporting of suspected abuse, with penalties for failure to report; involvement in the civil, juvenile, or family court systems; involvement in divorce or custody proceedings; and involvement in criminal prosecution of defendants in criminal court.

The fact remains that whatever the associated family dynamics, the situation of sexual abuse is always a delicate one and must be handled with the least inflammatory words and actions as possible. It is essential that the physician's role be clearly defined as an advocate for the child and that the physician remains nonaccusatory of parents or guardians until the facts have been obtained and other likely causes have been ruled out.

SUGGESTED READINGS

Kellogg N, and the Committee on Child Abuse and Neglect. The evaluation of sexual abuse in children. *Pediatrics.* 2005;116:506–512. (doi:10.1542/peds.2005-1336). www.pediatrics. aappublications.org/cgi/content/full/116/2/506. Accessed December 28, 2007.

Lahoti SL, McClain N, Girardet R, et al. Evaluating the child for sexual abuse. *Am Fam Physician.* 2001;63(5):889–892. Published March 1, 2001. www.aafp.org/afp/20010301/883.html. Accessed December 28, 2007.

Sexual Assault in Children and Adolescents. www.respyn.uanl.mx/especiales/2005/ee-11-2005/documentos/73.pdf

Topics in Emergency Medicine- Full text: Volume 24 (4) Dec. www.pt.wkhealth.com/pt/re/tme/fulltext.00007815-200212000-00007.htm

31

Remember the Contraindications to Diphtheria, Pertussis, and Tetanus (DPT) Immunizations and Use Alternatives Recommended by the American Academy of Pediatrics (AAP) and the U.S. Public Health Service

Esther Forrester, MD

What to Do – Make a Decision, Take Action

The overall goal of immunizations is to prevent disease. This revolution in science began with the invention of the smallpox vaccine by Jenner in 1796 and has evolved to include prevention of more than 12 diseases. The use of vaccines has actually led to the eradication of diseases (smallpox, wild-type poliomyelitis). Following the AAP and Centers for Disease Control and Prevention (CDC)–recommended immunization guidelines, however, is difficult. The CDC currently estimates that only two thirds of all 2-year-old children in the United States have received all appropriate immunizations. This can be further complicated when dealing with preterm (PT) and low-birth-weight (LBW) infants. There are many challenges to successful immunization. In fact, the increase in vaccine-preventable illnesses presents a challenge in and of itself.

Vaccine shortages pose another problem. From 2000 to 2005, there were shortages for nine of 12 of the recommended childhood immunizations. Millions of people were affected by prolonged shortages. The low supply resulted partly from a reduction in the number of manufacturers. The rising cost and financial barriers are additional challenges. Despite the increase in cost, vaccination is a cost-effective public health intervention. Unfortunately, children with fragmented health care often have incomplete immunizations.

There is also increasing public concern regarding adverse events occurring secondary to vaccination. Two of the most common public fears are: (a) the association between the measles, mumps, and rubella (MMR) vaccine and autism, and (b) thimerosal-containing vaccines and autism. In addition, the Vaccine Adverse Event Reporting System was established to scrutinize vaccine safety after U.S. Food and Drug Administration licensure. Clinicians may present a challenge when coupling medical liability concerns with vaccine administration. Public and professional lack of knowledge (schedule,

© 2008 by Lippincott Williams & Wilkins, a Wolters Kluwer business

necessity) also expounds the problem. As mentioned earlier, special populations may cause increasing concerns and intensified challenges.

Due to the many complications faced by PT and LBW infants, they are at greater risk for amplified morbidity from diseases that can be prevented by vaccine administration. Despite this fact, they are less likely to receive timely immunizations. This is due to clinician's concern for the patient to develop protective immunity after routine administration, and the patient's overall fragile state. The safety, immunogenicity, and durability of immune response have been extensively studied for hepatitis B vaccine (HBV), inactivated poliovirus (IPV), *Haemophilus influenza* type b (Hib), and pneumococcal and influenza viruses. PT and LBW infants should receive full doses of all routinely recommended childhood vaccines at a chronological age consistent with the schedule for full-term (FT) infants, with the exception of Hepatitis B.

The AAP recommends that the first dose of HBV be delayed in infants weighing <2,000 g and born to hepatitis B surface antigen (HBsAg)-negative mothers until the infant achieves a weight of 2,000 g or is 2 months of age. The recommendation results from studies that showed lower seroconversion rates and antibody levels in very LBW (<1,500 g) and extremely LBW (<1,000 g) infants immunized with HBV shortly after birth, when compared to FT infants and PT infants immunized at a later age. Chronological age of the medically stable PT infant at first dose administration is the best predictor of successful seroconversion regardless of birthweight or gestational age at birth. It is very important to remember that all PT and LBW infants born to HBsAg-positive mothers must receive hepatitis immune globulin (HBIG) within 12 hours of birth as well as HBV at different sites. If maternal status is unknown, PT and LBW infants should follow the same guidelines as infants born to HBsAg-positive mothers (HBV and HBIG at birth).

The safety and immunogenicity of DTP, diphtheria and tetanus toxoids and whole-cell pertussis (DTwP), Hib, and IPV has been proven by several studies and they are recommended to be given to PT and LBW infants beginning at a chronological age of 2 months. Despite this fact, significant delays persist. There is no increase in adverse events when the before-mentioned vaccines are given to PT and LBW infants, with one exception. There have been reports of cardiorespiratory events occurring within 72 hours of DTwP administration in extremely LBW infants younger than 31 weeks gestation, but not after the administration of DTP. The episodes were not found to have detrimental effects on the patient's medical course.

PT and LBW infants are at increased risk for morbidity associated with influenza and respiratory syncytial virus (RSV). Because of this, it is recommended that this population receives 2 doses of the inactivated influenza vaccine, given 1 month apart, beginning at 6 months' chronological age.

Household contacts, child care providers, and hospital nursery personnel of PT infants younger than 6 months and those with complications of prematurity (i.e., chronic lung disease), should receive the vaccine yearly. Palivizumab (respiratory syncytial virus monoclonal antibody) should be given to all PT infants younger than 32 weeks gestational age, and/or with chronic lung disease, and/or specific cardiac conditions. This is a monthly vaccination given during RSV season.

Anatomic limitations of PT and LBW infants should be taken into consideration when administering vaccines in this population. The anterolateral thigh is the site of choice, and muscle mass, or the lack thereof, should guide the choice of needle length. The appropriate size may be less than the standard needle length (7/8 to 1 inch) used in FT infants.

SUGGESTED READINGS

Abramson J, Baker C. Immunization of preterm and low birth weight infants. *Pediatrics.* 2003;112(1):193–198.

Cohn AC, Broder KR, Pickering LK. Immunizations in the United States: a rite of passage. *Pediatr Clin North Am.* 2005;52:669–693.

Pfister RE, Aeschbach V, Niksic-Stuber V, et al. Safety of DTaP-based combined immunization in very-low-birth-weight premature infants: frequent but mostly benign cardiorespiratory events. *J Pediatrs.* 2004;145:58–66.

32

DO NOT USE ORAL POLIO VACCINE (OPV) IN PATIENTS OR PATIENTS WHOSE CONTACTS HAVE IMMUNOSUPPRESSION

ANJALI SUBBASWAMY, MD

WHAT TO DO – MAKE A DECISION, TAKE ACTION

Live vaccines are composed of viral or bacterial strains that are deprived of their pathogenicity but can still replicate in the organism into which it is injected. These vaccines can provoke a nonpathogenic infection in vaccinated subjects, both inducing an antibody and a cellular immune response. Live attenuated vaccines, such as measles, mumps, and rubella (MMR) or yellow fever vaccine, have been widely used with proven efficacy. The oral poliomyelitis vaccine is composed of three attenuated strains prepared from the three wild virus types and is efficacious but mutations of the virus (in particular for type 3) can induce polio-associated paralysis by giving it back its original neurovirulence (number of cases 2:1,000,000). The emergence of circulating vaccine-derived poliovirus (cVDPV) strains is a real risk associated with the use of OPV. The cVDPV strains result form point mutations that occur in the Sabin (developer of oral vaccine) OPV strains. There may or may not be an exchange of parts of the viral genome with related nonpolio enteroviruses. This exchange typically occurs in areas where the live OPV is used and immunization rates are low. The oral polio vaccine is still used in most parts of the world to prevent transmission (cheaper than injected form). Since the World Health Assembly launched its polio eradication goal, outbreaks caused by cVDPV have been seen in the Amish populations in the United States.

Live bacterial vaccines can be classified as a self-limiting asymptomatic organism that stimulates an immune response to one or more expressed antigens. A nonvirulent or attenuated derivative of the pathogen is used to induce a response to the bacterium itself.

The OPV contains a live virus that is capable of provoking an immune response but not capable of causing disease. Unfortunately, it very infrequently changes to a more virulent form, and some people may maintain the living virus in their bodies, excreting it constantly. The injectable vaccine contains killed virus and is more expensive. The oral vaccine is easier to administer, but at some point, to eradicate all sources of the live virus, its

© 2008 by Lippincott Williams & Wilkins, a Wolters Kluwer business

use will have to end. Continuing to use OPV while immunization coverage is not appropriate or optimal and is like playing Russian roulette.

Paralytic poliomyelitis has been a reportable disease since the early part of the century. Since the advent of immunization, the Centers for Disease Control and Prevention has issued surveillance reports approximately once per decade. By the 1970s, the principal focus of these reports became vaccine-associated paralytic poliomyelitis (VAPP), which affected both OPV recipients, mostly young infants receiving their first OPV dose, and close contacts of OPV recipients, mostly nonimmune adolescents and young adults who were caregivers to recently immunized infants. Recipients of OPV and contacts of OPV recipients with primary B-cell immunodeficiency had more than a 3,000-fold increased risk of VAPP compared with those with no known immune disorders. Over the years, the proportion of contact cases decreased as polio vaccination rates improved, and the proportion of cases observed among immunodeficient persons increased; perhaps, because of increased awareness of their risk. Nonetheless, immunosuppression or contact with immunosuppressed persons remains an absolute contraindication to the OPV.

SUGGESTED READINGS

Gomber S, Agarwal KN. Polio eradication–target 2000. *Indian J Pediatr.* 1996;63(4):477–483.

Kimman TG, Boot H. The polio eradication effort has been a great success–let's finish it and replace it with something even better. *Lancet Infectious Dis.* 2006;6(10):675–678.

Molrine DH, Hibberd PL. Vaccines for transplant recipients. *Infect Dis Clin North Am.* 2001;15(1):273–305.

Saliou P. [Live vaccines.] [French] *Rev Prat.* 1995;45(12):1492–1496.

33

Do not prescribe oral over-the-counter (OTC) decongestants for children with colds

Laura Hufford, MD

What to Do – Take Action

OTC cough and cold medications are widely recommended and used throughout the United States by clinicians and patients, respectively. These medications often contain a combination of drugs, depending on the preparation. Pseudoephedrine, a decongestant, is a sympathomimetic agent, thought to reduce nasal congestion by causing vasoconstriction and, thus, decrease nasal and sinus edema. Antihistamines, such as diphenhydramine and brompheniramine, block histamine at the H1 receptor and reduce smooth muscle contraction. An antitussive, dextromethorphan, is an opioid narcotic and acts centrally to raise the threshold for coughing. An expectorant, guaifenesin, reduces stickiness of phlegm and should make secretions easier to cough up. Antipyretics, including acetaminophen and ibuprofen, are often added for fever and pain. Because each OTC preparation includes many of these medications, the parent is at greater risk for giving an overdose if they combine these medications.

In a recent study, 1,519 children were treated at emergency departments for adverse events related to cough and cold medications during 2004. Serious acute reactions included seizures, dysrhythmias, and ischemic cardiac and bowel events. Additionally, a review of coroner reports from two states in children younger than 12 months in 2005 revealed three deaths caused by these medications. The infants were age 1 to 6 months and had pseudoephedrine levels nine to 14 times the levels expected from administering recommended doses to children younger than age 2 years. Additionally, dextromethorphan was detected in the blood of two children and doxylamine in one child. It is unknown if the death was caused by an overdose, interaction of several medications, or related to underlying medical conditions not noted by the coroner.

OTC decongestants have not been well studied in children younger than age 2 years. Little data exist in the adult or pediatric population showing clinical symptomatic relief from these multidrug preparations. In a review of the pediatric literature, cough and cold medications did not show a significant change in symptoms when compared with placebo. Because dosing of cough

© 2008 by Lippincott Williams & Wilkins, a Wolters Kluwer business

and cold medications has not been studied in children younger than age 2 years, health providers often calculate a dose based on weight comparisons. This method of dosing medication in milligram per kilogram assumes that drug metabolism and drug effect are equal in children of all weights.

Using cough and cold medications in children should be questioned, given the lack of data showing beneficial effects in children. Great caution should be used in children younger than age 2 years, given the reported adverse events and absence of information regarding dosing regimens and safety profiles. Although the American Academy of Pediatrics guidelines do not specifically state that physicians should not prescribe or recommend OTC cough and cold preparations, they do state that physicians have the responsibility of educating parents about the lack of benefit and known risks of OTC cough and cold preparations. It is the belief of many that for those families who insist on using these medications, physicians should negotiate to discontinue use in 2 days if there is no appreciated benefit.

SUGGESTED READINGS

Centers for Disease Control and Prevention. Infant deaths associated with cough and cold medications–two states, 2005. *MMWR Morb Mortal Wkly Rep.* 2007;56(1):1–4.

National Electronic Injury Surveillance System–Cooperative Adverse Drug Events Surveillance Project. Conducted by the Center for Disease Control, Food and Drug Administration and the Consumer Product Safety Commission. http://www.cdc.gov/mmwr/preview/mmwrhtml/mm5415a2.htm CDC MMWR Weekly April 22, 2005 / 54(15);380–383 Assessing the National Electronic Injury Surveillance System–Cooperative Adverse Drug Event Surveillance Project–Six Sites, United States, January 1–June 15, 2004. (Date last reviewed: 4/21/2005)

Gunn VL, Taha SH, Liebelt EL, et al. Toxicity of over-the-counter cough and old medications. *Pediatrics.* 2001;108(3):e52.

Schroeder K, Fahey T. Over-the-counter cold medications for acute cough in children and adults in ambulatory settings. *Cochrane Database Syst Rev.* 2004;(4):CD001831.

34

To Help Prevent Vertical Transmission of Human Immunodeficiency Virus (HIV), Infants Born to Seropositive Mothers Should Receive Zidovudine (ZVT) for the First 6 Weeks of Life

BRIAN KIT, MD

What to Do – Take Action
Epidemiology

Perinatal transmission is the most common source of HIV infection among infants and children in the United States, accounting for >90% of children with acquired immunodeficiency syndrome (AIDS) <13 years. In the United States, the number of infants born with HIV in 2001 was between 280 and 370, compared with approximately 1,000 to 2,000 neonates with HIV born in 1991. During the same period, the number of mothers with HIV in the United States also increased. Much of the success of the declining transmission rates, despite rising number of pregnant women with HIV, is the result of increased HIV screening of pregnant women and the use of antiretroviral drugs for both mother and baby.

Human Immunodeficiency Virus Testing in Pregnancy

The American Academy of Pediatrics (AAP) and the American College of Obstetricians and Gynecologists issued a joint statement supporting universal testing with patient notification as a routine component of prenatal care. Optimally, results of HIV should be known prior to labor and delivery to facilitate antepartum and intrapartum treatment. If the mother's HIV status was not determined during pregnancy, the AAP encourages pediatricians to discuss with the mother benefits of early identification of HIV and recommends testing at that time.

Medication Strategy to Prevent Perinatal Transmission of Human Immunodeficiency Virus

In 1994, the results of Pediatric AIDS Clinical Trials Group (PACTG) Protocol 076 documented that a three-part zidovudine (ZDV) chemoprophylaxis regimen could reduce the risk of perinatal HIV transmission by approximately two-thirds. The regimen includes oral ZDV initiated at 14 to

© 2008 by Lippincott Williams & Wilkins, a Wolters Kluwer business

34 weeks' gestation and continued throughout pregnancy, followed by intra-venous ZDV during labor and oral administration of ZDV to the infant for 6 weeks after delivery. Oral administration of ZDV to the newborn is dosed as ZDZ, 2 mg/kg/dose every 6 hours.

Since 1994, several new therapies and treatment approaches for HIV and AIDS have evolved. Up-to-date information is available through many sources, including online at http://hivatis.org, which is a service of the U.S. Department of Health and Human Services. Despite the evolving man-agement strategies, it generally remains true that any prenatal treatment regimen should include ZDV whenever possible. In addition, regardless of antepartum treatment, all women should receive intrapartum ZDV and their newborns should receive a full 6 weeks of ZDV.

NEWBORN CARE

In addition to ZDV for 6 weeks to prevent the transmission of HIV, chil-dren should receive Bactrim chemoprophylaxis to prevent the development of *Pneumocystis carinii* pneumonia (PCP). PCP is a rapidly progressing and often fatal opportunistic infection that can be prevented with Bactrim chemo-prophylaxis. The greatest risk for PCP in children with perinatal acquired HIV occurs between 3 to 6 months of age. Bactrim prophylaxis is discon-tinued when HIV infection has been reasonably excluded, usually after two negative virology studies, with one of the tests performed before 4 months of age.

HUMAN IMMUNODEFICIENCY VIRUS
TESTING OF HUMAN IMMUNODEFICIENCY
VIRUS-EXPOSED INFANTS

Following recommended HIV screening strategies is important because HIV-exposed neonates are usually asymptomatic and have normal physi-cal exam findings during the neonatal period. Confusion about the appro-priate laboratory evaluation of HIV-exposed neonates among providers can result in unnecessary costs and emotional burdens to the family. Because of transplacental transfer of maternal antibodies, tests for antibodies (i.e., enzyme-linked immunoabsorbent assay [ELISA] and Western Blot) should not be used to make a diagnosis of HIV infection in children younger than 18 months of age. Virologic testing (i.e., HIV DNA polymerase chain reaction [PCR]) should be performed at birth, at 1 to 2 months of age, and at 3 to 4 months of age. A positive result at any point should be immediately repeated for confirmation. Babies who have three negative virologic tests should un-dergo antibody testing at 12 months of age. If this test is negative, screening should be repeated at 18 months of age with an antibody test. A positive HIV antibody test after 18 months indicates HIV infection. A negative test indicates no infection.

Early screening for HIV in pregnant women provides an opportunity for reducing the perinatal transmission of HIV. In the setting of HIV exposure during pregnancy, the pediatrician can ensure appropriate follow-up testing with virologic studies and treatment with ZDV for 6 weeks for the prevention of transmission of HIV. Prophylaxis with Bactrim to prevent PCP will reduce mortality of infants who are born with HIV.

SUGGESTED READINGS

American Academy of Pediatrics, American College of Obstetrics and Gynecology. Human immunodeficiency virus screening. Joint statement of the American Academy of Pediatrics and the American College of Obstetricians and Gynecologists. *Pediatrics.* 1999;104(1 Pt 1): 128–135.

Considerations for antiretroviral therapy in the HIV-infected pregnant woman. Available at: http://www.ncbi.nlm.nih.gov/books/bv.fcgi?rid=hstat2.section.10362. Accessed June 24, 2007.

U.S. Department of Health and Human Services. AIDSinfo. Available at: http://hivatis.org. Accessed June 24, 2007.

35

KNOW THAT ANTIBIOTIC PROPHYLAXIS OF DEER TICK BITES IS NOT RECOMMENDED. BE AWARE OF THE CLINICAL STAGES OF LYME DISEASE (LD) AND THE APPROPRIATE LABORATORY EVALUATION AND TREATMENT ASSOCIATED WITH EACH STAGE

MICHAEL CLEMMENS, MD

WHAT TO DO – GATHER APPROPRIATE DATA, INTERPRET THE DATA, MAKE A DECISION

LD is caused by the spirochete *Borrelia burgdorferi,* which is transmitted by the bite of the deer tick. It is endemic in the Northeast, the mid-Atlantic states, the upper Midwest, and in parts of southern California. Because interstate travel is so common, however, LD can be seen in any state. Not all deer tick bites lead to LD. The deer tick must remain attached for at least 48 hours and become engorged before it can transmit the spirochete. Because the tick falls off of its host when fully engorged, transmission of the spirochete may not occur and the tick bite often goes undetected.

The clinical course of LD is divided into three stages: early localized, early disseminated, and late. The cardinal manifestation of early localized disease is an erythema migrans (EM) rash, which classically looks like a target with concentric erythematous rings. Although constitutional symptoms occasionally occur, the presence of an EM rash is all that is required to make a diagnosis of early localized LD. Early disseminated disease manifests as multiple EM lesions, meningitis, facial nerve palsy, or heart block. Acute and chronic arthritis are the major manifestations of late disease in children. Of note, both early disseminated and late disease may occur without an antecedent history of erythema migrans.

Serologic testing is not helpful in early localized LD because a detectable immune response has not yet occurred. In the early disseminated and late stages of the disease, testing is useful and is performed in a two-stage process. The first test is a screening test, usually an enzyme-linked assay to detect serum immunoglobulin (Ig)M and IgG to the spirochete. The assay has a high specificity unless it is performed too early in the disease process. False positives, however, are common. Therefore, if the screening test is positive or equivocal, a Western Blot is performed. The test results need to be interpreted in light of the clinical picture.

© 2008 by Lippincott Williams & Wilkins, a Wolters Kluwer business

The treatment of LD varies with the stage and clinical manifestations. In early localized disease, oral antibiotics are appropriate. Amoxicillin is recommended for children younger than 8 years of age, and doxycycline is used for older patients. Most cases of early disseminated disease can also be treated with oral antibiotics. However, patients with meningitis or heart block require a course of intravenous ceftriaxone. Patients with late-stage LD can be treated with either an oral or intravenous course of antibiotics, depending on the clinical situation.

Antibiotic prophylaxis following a tick bite in a child is not generally recommended because the subsequent risk of developing LD is very low. In fact, the risk of developing LD is <1.5% when a nonengorged tick is detected within 48 hours of the bite. Furthermore, the majority of those who do develop the disease will have an EM rash at the site of the bite, which can be easily recognized by the patient or family. Early treatment can then be instituted. Taking the time to explain the low likelihood of disease development and provide reassurance to the child and family is very important.

LD may present without a history of tick bite. As a result, the provider must consider the diagnosis in any child with an EM rash, arthritis, meningitis, facial palsy, or heart block. Laboratory testing is not indicated in the early localized stage but is indicated for early disseminated and late-stage disease. When the Lyme screen is positive, a Western Blot must be done to confirm the diagnosis. Results should be related to the clinical findings. Antibiotic treatment is very effective and prophylaxis rarely indicated.

SUGGESTED READINGS

American Academy of Pediatrics. Lyme disease. In: Pickering LK, Baker CJ, Long SS, et al, eds. *Red Book: 2006 Report of the Committee on Infectious Diseases.* 27th ed. Elk Grove, IL: American Academy of Pediatrics; 2006:428–433.
Medical Letter. Treatment of Lyme disease. *Med Lett Drugs Ther.* 2005;47:41–43.
Steere AC. Lyme disease. *N Engl J Med.* 2001;345:115–125.

36

EDUCATE PARENTS ON THE APPROPRIATE PLACEMENT OF INFANTS DURING SLEEP TO PREVENT SUDDEN INFANT DEATH SYNDROME (SIDS)

BRIAN KIT, MD

WHAT TO DO – TAKE ACTION

SIDS is the sudden death of an infant younger than 1 year of age, which remains unexplained after a thorough case investigation, including performance of a complete autopsy, examination of the death scene, and review of the clinical history. SIDS is considered a diagnosis of exclusion. The etiology of SIDS is unknown. A popular hypothesis is the triple risk model, which suggests that SIDS occurs in infants with predisposing factors (i.e., genetic pattern) who experience a trigger (i.e., maternal smoking), at a vulnerable developmental stage of the central nervous or immune system.

Deaths from SIDS have been declining since 1992, the year a major intervention was sponsored by the American Academy of Pediatrics (AAP) to encourage parents to place their babies in nonprone positions when putting them in a crib to sleep. In 1991, according to the National Center for Health Statistics (NCHS), the SIDS death rate was 1.3 deaths per 1,000 live births. By 2004, the rate had fallen to 0.55 deaths per 1,000 live births. According to the NCHS, the total number of deaths from SIDS in 2004 was 2,246. The occurrence of SIDS is rare during the first month of life, increases to a peak between 2 and 3 months of age, and then becomes rare after 6 months. Despite reductions in SIDS deaths, it remains the number one cause of death for infants between ages of 1 month and 1 year.

Risk factors for SIDS include the following:

- Male gender
- Prematurity
- Low birth weight
- Maternal smoking during and after pregnancy
- Seasonal distribution with a peak in winter months
- Lower socioeconomic status
- Lower level of maternal education
- Little or no prenatal care
- Young maternal age

ⓒ 2008 by Lippincott Williams & Wilkins, a Wolters Kluwer business

- Higher parity
- Single parenthood
- Multiple gestation
- Prone sleeping
- Soft bedding
- Sleeping with potentially obstructive materials (stuffed toys, pillows, quilts, comforters).

The pediatrician and other providers of medical services should employ the AAP's most recent guidelines from the Task Force on Sudden Infant Death Syndrome when counseling parents and families about SIDS risks. Current evidence supports the following recommendations, although this list is not exhaustive:

- Place babies supine or on the back for every sleep.
- Ensure a safe sleeping environment, including a firm crib mattress covered by a sheet. Soft objects, including pillows, comforters, and stuffed toys, should be kept out of the sleeping environment.
- Smoking cessation for all caregivers should be encouraged.
- Encourage a sleep arrangement that includes babies sleeping in the same room as their parent, in their own crib or bassinet. Ideally, infants should not share a bed during sleep. Many people recommend this arrangement for the first 6 months to reduce the risks of SIDS.

Despite many comprehensive studies on the epidemiology of SIDS, the causative factors have yet to be determined. It remains the number one cause of death in children ages 1 month to 1 year. By counseling families on the benefits of supine sleeping, ensuring a safe sleep environment, and encouraging smoking cessation, pediatricians can help reduce the incidence of SIDS.

SUGGESTED READINGS

American Academy of Pediatrics Task Force on Sudden Infant Death Syndrome. The changing concept of sudden infant death syndrome: diagnostic coding shifts, controversies regarding the sleeping environment, and new variables to consider in reducing risk. *Pediatrics.* 2003;116:1245–1255.

Filiano JJ, Kinney HC. A perspective on neuropathologic findings in victims of the sudden infant death syndrome: the triple-risk model. *Biol Neonate.* 1994;65:194–197.

Guntheroth WG, Spiers PS. The triple risk hypotheses in sudden infant death syndrome. *Pediatrics.* 2002;110:e64.

National Center for Health Statistics (NCHS). National Vital Statistics Reports. Available at: www.cdc.gov/SIDS/SUID.htm Accessed December 28, 2007.

Willinger M, James LS, Catz C. Defining the sudden infant death syndrome (SIDS): deliberations of an expert panel convened by the National Institute of Child Health and Human Development. *Pediatr Pathol.* 1991;11:677–684.

37

KNOW THE RISK FACTORS FOR THE DIFFERENT TYPES OF ACNE, HOW TO MANAGE, DIAGNOSE, AND TREAT

ELIZABETH WELLS, MD

WHAT TO DO – GATHER APPROPRIATE DATA, INTERPRET THE DATA, MAKE A DECISION, TAKE ACTION

Acne vulgaris the most common dermatologic disorder treated by physicians, affecting 80% of persons aged 11 to 30 years old. Because acne usually presents in early adolescence, pediatricians must be familiar with current recommendations about acne management. Appropriate management depends on a number of factors, including the types and numbers of lesions present, the patient's experiences with medications, and personal preferences. Growing knowledge about the multifactorial etiology of acne has led to new recommendations in favor of combination therapy and against monotherapy with antibiotics.

The microcomedo is now known to be the precursor of all acne lesions, inflammatory and noninflammatory. It develops from the pilosebaceous unit, which consists of the hair follicle, the hair shaft, and the sebaceous gland. The four primary factors contributing to the development of acne lesions are abnormal desquamation of keratinocytes within the pilosebaceous unit, increased sebum production, proliferation of *Propionibacterium acnes* (a gram-positive anaerobe that resides in the pilosebaceous unit), and inflammation.

The two main types of acne lesions are comedonal and inflammatory, and their etiology depends on the relative contribution of the preceding factors. Noninflammatory acne lesions are comedones. They may be open (i.e., blackheads) or closed (i.e., whiteheads). Closed comedones are small white papules with no surrounding erythema, containing only a microscopic opening to the skin surface. *P. acnes* is associated with inflammatory lesions (i.e., pimples). Inflammatory lesions are characterized by erythema. They may be papules and pustules (<5 mm in diameter) or nodules, which measure >5 mm and involve more than one follicle. The severity of inflammatory/pustular acne depends on the level of antibody, complement, and cell-mediated immune responses to the bacterium, rather than an infectious etiology. Large deep lesions that coalesce may form cysts. Scars may develop as inflammatory lesions resolve. Facial scars may appear as small pits,

---

© 2008 by Lippincott Williams & Wilkins, a Wolters Kluwer business

whereas truncal scars tend to be small hypopigmented spots. Scars may be irreversible and their presence may lead clinicians to be more aggressive in selecting anti-inflammatory therapeutic agents.

When evaluating a patient with acne, a pediatrician should record the number of open comedones, closed comedones, and inflammatory lesions in each region of the face. A rating of mild means that about one fourth of the face is involved, and there may be few-to-several papules or pustules but no nodules or scarring. In moderate acne, about one half of the face is involved, and there are several-to-many papules or pustules and a few-to-several nodules and a few scars. Severe acne involves three quarters of the face and is characterized by many papules, pustules, and nodules, with scarring often present.

The distribution and severity of acne lesions correlates with pubertal/hormonal stage. Blackheads and whiteheads distributed in the midface occur early in puberty, while inflammatory lesions are more prevalent later, affecting the lateral cheeks, lower jaw, back, and chest. Premenstrual acne in girls is thought to be due to the effects of progesterone, which is dominant during the second half of the menstrual cycle and leads to increased production of sebum. Some birth control hormones improve acne, whereas others with a higher level of progesterone, such as Depo-Provera, worsen acne.

There is no evidence that chocolate or other foods cause acne, nor is most acne caused by dirt or poor hygiene. Acne may be worsened, however, by certain behaviors, such as wearing tight-fitting sports protection (e.g., chin straps, shoulder pads), touching the face a lot, or using skin and hair products that contain oily and harsh substances. Certain medications, such as lithium, rifampin, or corticosteroids, can also worsen acne. Familial tendency seems to play a role, although no one has quantified the genetic contribution.

The American Academy of Pediatrics Expert Committee for Acne Management and the Global Alliance to Improve Outcomes in Acne recommends combination therapy to target as many pathogenic factors as possible. Topical retinoids (e.g., tretinoin, adapalene, tazarotene) are now recommended as the foundation for most acne treatment. Retinoids target the microcomedo, are comedolytic, and have anti-inflammatory effects. Oral antibiotics, no longer recommended as single-drug therapy for acne, should be used only in moderate-to-severe acne, in combination with another agent, and for a maximum length of treatment of 8 to 12 weeks.

Algorithms for treating acne are available in the literature (see citations). They break down the treatment of acne by severity and type of lesion. For mild comedonal acne, a topical retinoid alone is recommended, with salicylic acid as an alternative. For mild inflammatory acne, a topical retinoid and a benzoyl peroxide (BPO), or a BPO and a topical antibiotic, is recommended. Moderate acne requires a topical retinoid, an oral antibiotic (such as doxycycline or tetracycline), and a BPO or a BPO with a topical antibiotic. If the moderate acne is also nodular, the addition of oral isotretinoin is recommended. The recommendation for severe nodular acne is similar to that for moderate nodular acne. Female patients have the added option of trying hormonal therapy. Maintenance therapy is recommended for all types of acne and includes a topical retinoid with or without BPO and a topical antibiotic.

Oral isotretinoin (Accutane) is a powerful medication sometimes indicated for patients with severe acne or acne that has not responded to conventional therapy with a topical retinoid, benzoyl peroxide, and oral antibiotic. The U.S. Food and Drug Administration warns that isotretinoin may also cause depression, psychosis, and rarely suicidal thoughts or suicide. There is not enough scientific evidence to prove or disprove a causal link between psychiatric morbidity and the use of retinoids. Patients should be warned about these side effects, along with the more common side effects of dry mucous membranes and increased sensitivity to light, as well as an increase in cholesterol, and muscle or joint pain.

Pediatricians should prepare patients for the fact that acne treatment takes 6 to 8 weeks to cause significant results. Follow-up visits are important for addressing compliance, treatment response, adverse effects, and the effectiveness of therapy. Physicians should also be aware that in some states prescription topical acne medications are not approved for Medicaid reimbursement. Although acne cannot be cured, proper management can impact the emotional well-being of the adolescent and limit the potential for physical scarring.

SUGGESTED READINGS

Krowchuk DP. Managing adolescent acne: a guide for pediatricians. *Pediatr Rev.* 2005;26(7): 250–261.
Strahan JE, Raimer S. Isotretinoin and the controversy of psychiatric adverse effects. *Int J Dermatol.* 2006;45(7):789–799.
Zaenglein AL, Thiboutot DM. Expert committee recommendations for acne management. *Pediatrics.* 2006;118(3):1188–1199.

38

PROVIDE ANTICIPATORY GUIDANCE AT WELL-CHILD VISITS

ELIZABETH WELLS, MD

WHAT TO DO – TAKE ACTION

The term anticipatory guidance refers to the practice in which pediatricians provide information and counsel parents about child development and behavior. It helps families understand what to expect during their child's, or adolescent's, current and approaching stage of development. Studies show parents value these interactions and, in general, view them favorably. Pediatricians should take steps to learn what families are doing and target the discussion to the particular needs of each family.

Guidelines published by the American Academy of Pediatrics (AAP) and by others through the Bright Futures collaborative focus on health behaviors that have profound effects on childhood health and well-being. Topics to be discussed with patients of all ages include healthy habits, prevention of illness, nutrition, oral health, sexuality, social development, family relationships, parental health, community interactions, self-responsibility, and school/vocational achievement. Certain safety topics are appropriate to raise at any age such as motor vehicle safety, sun protection, a tobaccofree home, and smoke detectors. The AAP urges pediatricians to provide counseling for violence prevention, including discussing firearms in the home, physical and sexual abuse, and media exposure. Below is a summary of particular topics that may be raised, according to patient age.

INFANTS (BIRTH TO 1 YEAR)

Nutrition discussions with parents of infants should cover breast milk and formula, food preparation, transitioning to solid food, preventing choking and avoiding honey, which, if it contains the spores of *Clostridium botulinum*, could cause botulism. Elimination is an important issue, particularly as an increase in the diversity of the diet can lead to changes in stooling patterns. Additionally, supplementation with iron and vitamin D should be discussed. Oral health topics include preventing bottle caries and fluoride supplements. Safety discussions should cover safe sleep environment, car seats, burn prevention, fall prevention, choking prevention, drowning prevention, and cardiopulmonary resuscitation. Discussions about development and behavior should involve milestones in motor abilities and language. Reading aloud

© 2008 by Lippincott Williams & Wilkins, a Wolters Kluwer business

should be introduced early on. Guidance about family relationships may include childcare and postpartum depression.

TODDLERS AND PRESCHOOL AGE (1–5 YEARS)

In the toddler/preschool age group, providers should check that patients are visiting the dentist and brushing habits should be discussed. Elimination (bowel and bladder) training is an important topic at this age. Injury prevention should cover traffic safety, burn prevention, fall prevention, drowning prevention, and dealing with strangers. Poison prevention includes keeping medicines and household products locked up and the poison control telephone number (1-800-222-1222) readily available. Behavior guidance may focus on discipline and temper tantrums.

SCHOOL AGE (6–11 YEARS)

Discussions with parents of school-age children about eating may focus on healthy food choices; nutritious breakfasts, lunches, and dinners; and pleasant family meal times. Injury prevention should include talks about sports and protective gear, the neighborhood and neighbors, and emergency plans. Water safety guidance includes talking about and teaching children to swim. Limiting television time and video games should be recommended, as these activities are associated with an increased risk of obesity and problematic behaviors. Pubertal development may be discussed during this time.

YOUNGER ADOLESCENTS (11–15 YEARS)

Body image and weight management should be incorporated in discussions about balanced diet and physical activity with adolescents. Avoidance of alcohol, cigarettes, and illicit drugs should be emphasized. Pediatricians should recommend sexual abstinence at this age and encourage teenagers to make healthy lifestyle choices for themselves. Parents should be asked about house rules and be reminded to provide for adequate supervision while away. Adolescents should be reminded not to ride in cars with drunk and/or distracted drivers. Resolving conflicts without violence should be discussed. Safe dating and parties may be discussed. Adolescents often forget or ignore safety practices and should be reminded about seat belts, bike helmets, and other measures for injury prevention. In-home firearms are particularly dangerous during adolescence, because of the potential for their impulsive use by teenagers.

OLDER ADOLESCENTS (16–21 YEARS)

In older adolescents, doctors should recommend managing weight through healthy eating and regular exercise of at least three times per week. The adolescent should also be encouraged to get adequate sleep. It is important to discuss avoiding anabolic steroids, cigarettes, and illicit drugs and to provide resources for those who do report substance abuse. Responsible driving should be addressed. In addition to sexual activity, adolescents should be educated on creating healthy relationships and on avoiding or removing themselves from relationships involving physical violence or emotional abuse. Additional guidance about social relationships may cover changing communication patterns within the family and handling separation from home. Future plans for education, work, sports, and general health should be discussed.

Outcomes research is still emerging about the best way for clinicians to provide anticipatory guidance. New research is focusing on challenges such as overcoming cultural barriers, reimbursement issues, and time-limitations. Anticipatory guidance is most effective when it is responsive to the individual needs of the children and the parents. Additionally, limiting the number of topics discussed at each visit might lead to increased retention, and five to eight topics may be the most appropriate number to address in one visit. The use of supplementary handouts is also encouraged. Current research suggests that effective anticipatory guidance consists of authoritative, useful information offered in a supportive manner, respectful of parental decision making. Intervening early and promoting positive approaches in a developmental context may provide a more comfortable forum for discussing these issues.

SUGGESTED READINGS

American Academy of Pediatrics. *Guidelines for Health Supervision III*. Elk Grove Village, IL: American Academy of Pediatrics; 2002.

Barkin AL, Scheindlin B, Brown C, et al. Anticipatory guidance topics: are more better? *Ambulatory Pediatrics*. 2005;5(6):372–376.

Bethell C, Reuland CH, Halfon N, et al. Measuring the quality of preventive and developmental services for young children: national estimates and patterns of clinicians' performance. *Pediatrics*. 2004;113(6 Suppl):1973–1983.

Committee on Psychosocial Aspects of Child and Family Health. American Academy of Pediatrics. The new morbidity revisited: a renewed commitment to the psychosocial aspects of pediatric care. Committee on Psychosocial Aspects of Child and Family Health. *Pediatrics*. 2001;108:1227–1230.

Gardner HG; American Academy of Pediatrics Committee on Injury, Violence, and Poison Prevention. Office-based counseling for unintentional injury prevention. *Pediatrics*. 2007;119(1):202–206.

Green M, Palfrey JS, eds. *Bright Futures: Guidelines for Health Supervision of Infants, Children, and Adolescents*. 2nd ed. Arlington, VA: National Center for Education in Maternal and Child Health; 2002.

Schmidt ME, Rich M. Media and child health: pediatric care and anticipatory guidance for the information age. *Pediatr Rev*. 2006;27(8):289–298.

Schuster MA, Duan N, Regalado M, et al. Anticipatory guidance: what information do parents receive? What information do they want? *Arch Pediatr Adolesc Med*. 2000;154:1191–1198.

39

KNOW THE APPROPRIATE PROCEDURES FOR LEAD SCREENING, DIAGNOSIS, TREATMENT, AND ABATEMENT

ELLEN HAMBURGER, MD

WHAT TO DO – GATHER APPROPRIATE DATA, INTERPRET THE DATA, MAKE A DECISION, TAKE ACTION

The prevalence of elevated blood lead levels (BLLs) among U.S. children has declined sharply in the last decade primarily because of marked reductions of lead in residential paint, gasoline, and dietary sources. The prevalence of BLLs $> 10 \, \mu g/dL$ among children 1 to 5 years old declined from 9% to 1.6% between 1991 and 2002, but there remain communities and populations that bear a disproportionate burden of plumbism, with over 300,000 children remaining at risk for exposure to harmful levels of lead.

The ingestion of lead-containing dust is the primary source of lead exposure in children. The major sources of lead dust are disruption of lead-containing paint and soil. Other sources of lead exposure include water and contaminated clothing of adults who have occupational exposure to lead. Although lead-based paint has not been in use for decades in the United States, it is estimated that more than 20 million housing units still contain lead-based paint or lead-soldered pipes, units more likely to be in poor condition and occupied by low-income families. Risk factors for increased lead burden include:

- Minority race/ethnicity (African American highest risk)
- Urban residence
- Low educational attainment
- Older (pre-1950) housing
- Recent immigration (including international adoption).

Screening efforts focus on high-risk children from 1 to 5 years of age because they are most likely to ingest lead in their environment from increased hand-to-mouth activity. Furthermore, once ingested, lead is more easily absorbed in young children and their central nervous system is more vulnerable to its effects, as compared to adults. Neurotoxicity of lead includes acute encephalopathy as well as long-term impairment. Population-based studies consistently demonstrate impaired neurocognitive development in

© 2008 by Lippincott Williams & Wilkins, a Wolters Kluwer business

children with a BLL >10 μg/dL even in the asymptomatic child. Further, a clear negative effect on cognition has been demonstrated with BLLs <10 μg/dL, previously thought to have little to no effect. Although intelligence is the primary outcome in most studies, there is evidence that lead is implicated in attention deficit and learning disorders as well.

Older recommendations called for universal screening of children between 1 and 2 years of age. Targeted screening of high-risk populations is the current guideline because of the reduced prevalence of elevated BLL. Current recommendations for screening are based on community prevalence figures to avoid unnecessary costs and false-positive diagnosis in low-risk areas and populations. All children receiving Medicaid; Supplemental Food Program for Women, Infants and Children, as well as those living in communities where more than 27% of housing was built before 1950, should have BLL determined at least once, starting when they are 1 year old. For children not eligible for Medicaid, screening guidance should be sought from state or local health agencies. Screening can include the use of questionnaires that have been locally validated and that have acceptable sensitivity and specificity. A risk questionnaire developed by the Centers for Disease Control and Prevention has been shown to correctly identify 64% to 87% of urban and suburban children who had BLLs >10 μg/dL.

A progressive series of recommendations exist for children who have positive blood lead screens. Those with levels >10 μg/dL should have the blood test repeated and followed closely. Children with levels from 20 to 44 μg/dL warrant having environmental evaluation, including abatement of housing if warranted. Abatement can increase BLLs if children live in the housing while walls are scraped and repainted. Thus, families must relocate during abatement. Chelation and evaluation for iron deficiency is recommended for children whose levels are >44 μg/dL, with hospitalization for those whose neurologic status is concerning because of levels $\geq$70 μg/dL. Detailed management recommendations can be found in the American Academy of Pediatrics statement referenced below.

SUGGESTED READINGS

American Academy of Pediatrics, Committee on Environmental Health. Lead exposure in children: prevention, detection, and management. *Pediatrics.* 2005;116:1036–1046.

Centers for Disease Control and Prevention. *Preventing Lead Poisoning in Young Children: A Statement by the Centers for Disease Control—October 1991.* Atlanta, GA: Department of Health and Human Services; 1991.

Rischitelli G, Nygren P, Bougatsos C, et al. Screening for elevated lead levels in childhood and pregnancy: an updated summary of evidence for the US Preventive Services Task Force. *Pediatrics.* 2006;118:e1867–e1895.

40

BE SURE TO ADDRESS FAMILY DISCORD DURING ANTICIPATORY GUIDANCE BECAUSE BOTH ADOLESCENT SUICIDE AND RUNAWAYS OCCUR MORE OFTEN WHEN ADOLESCENTS FEEL MARGINALIZED

SONYA BURROUGHS, MD

WHAT TO DO – GATHER APPROPRIATE DATA

Providing anticipatory guidance and/or counseling to adolescent patients is often a challenge, but it is an essential part of the adolescent exam and must be performed to encourage healthy living and choices. Oftentimes, opportunities for prevention are missed during routine visits. This may be due to the fact that screening guidelines are less clear for this age group. Regardless of the reason why prevention strategies are missed, it is detrimental to the patient because the incidence of the leading causes of adolescent morbidity and mortality could be decreased if proper anticipatory guidance is provided. Several tools have been developed to help ensure proper screening of adolescents, including *h*ome/health, *e*ducation/employment, *a*ctivities, *d*rugs, *d*epression, *s*afety, *s*exuality (HEADSS). The first step in providing anticipatory guidance to this age group is to provide a comfortable and confidential environment for the patient. To successfully communicate with the adolescent, the following strategies should be implemented:

- Address the patient directly and ask open-ended questions
- Listen attentively without interrupting
- Observe nonverbal communication
- Avoid making judgments based on a patient's appearance
- Ask for an explanation regarding unfamiliar slang terms that the patient uses.

The Federal Healthy People 2010 Initiative has identified several critical objectives pertinent to adolescent health care (*Table 40.1*).

© 2008 by Lippincott Williams & Wilkins, a Wolters Kluwer business

TABLE 40.1	ADOLESCENT HEALTH OBJECTIVES IDENTIFIED BY THE HEALTHY PEOPLE 2010 INITIATIVE

ENVIRONMENTAL FACTORS

Reduce the rate of death from motor vehicle crashes, increase seat belt use, and reduce the number of **adolescents** who ride with drunk drivers.
Reduce the homicide rate.
Reduce the number of **adolescents** who participate in physical fighting.
Reduce the number of students who carry weapons to school.

Mental health
Reduce the rates of suicide and attempted suicide.
Increase the number of **adolescents** who get adequate physical activity.

Physical activity
Reduce the number of **adolescents** who are overweight or at risk of becoming overweight.

Physical activity
Increase the number of **adolescents** who get adequate physical activity.

Sexual activity
Reduce the pregnancy rate.
Reduce the incidence of HIV, *Chlamydia,* and other sexually transmitted diseases.
Increase the number of **adolescents** who practice abstinence.

Substance abuse
Reduce death and injury from alcohol- and drug-related motor vehicle crashes.
Reduce the prevalence of drug and tobacco use and binge-drinking behaviors.

HIV, human immunodeficiency virus.

Accidents, suicide, and homicide are the leading causes of death in American adolescents. Other causes of morbidity in this population include drug and tobacco use, being runaways, poor nutrition, risky sexual behaviors, and inadequate physical activity. By providing appropriate anticipatory guidance, health outcomes can be improved.

Suicide is a major public health concern, and the adolescent population is greatly affected. In fact, approximately 2,000 adolescents per year die of suicide. The number is probably higher because some accidents are most likely suicide, but are not classified as such. Approximately 2 million adolescents aged 13 to 19 years *attempt* suicide each year. The number of adolescents reporting suicidal thoughts has decreased over the last decade. However, the number of attempts has remained constant. Suicidal ideation and attempts are higher in females. Completed suicide is higher in males than females (5.5:1) due to the more fatal methods used by males (i.e., firearms, hanging). In fact, firearms are the most common method of completed suicide for all age, sex, and ethnic groups. Ninety percent of adolescents who commit suicide have a coexisting psychiatric disorder. The "cluster" phenomenon has its greatest impact on this population and refers to suicide attempts that are preceded by exposure to another real or fictitious suicide attempt. The period of increased risk usually lasts for 1 to 2 weeks.

Approximately one third of patients who complete suicide had made a previous attempt. Risk factors associated with adolescent suicide include male sex, age older than 16 years, previous suicide attempt, mood disorder, substance abuse, poor social support, and access to firearms. Risk factors are similar for male and female adolescents, but the weight of the factors differs. For boys, the most important risk factor is a previous suicide attempt. This factor increases the risk 30-fold. For girls, major depression is the most important risk factor and increases the risk 12-fold.

With the use of proper screening tools, providing a comfortable, confidential environment, and improving communication with adolescent patients, preventative health counseling can make a difference in morbidity and mortality. One must be aware of age-related issues and risk factors. In providing proper anticipatory guidance, overall quality of life is enhanced.

SUGGESTED READINGS

Edelsohn GA, Gomez JP. Psychiatric emergencies in adolescents. *Adolesc Med Clin.* 2006;17:183–204.

Kennedy SP, Baraff LJ, Suddath RL, et al. Emergency department management of suicidal adolescents. *Ann Emerg Med.* 2004;43:452–460.

Stephens MB. Preventative health counseling for adolescents. *Am Fam Physician.* 2006;74:1151–1156.

41

BE SURE TO APPROPRIATELY ASSESS THE FINANCIAL STATUS OF FAMILIES THAT PRESENT FOR CARE SINCE ECONOMIC CHALLENGES ARE A RISK FOR CERTAIN DISEASES AND NONCOMPLIANCE WITH THE TREATMENT PLAN

JOHANN PETERSON, MD

WHAT TO DO – GATHER APPROPRIATE DATA

Understanding the social situation and environment of your patients helps in tailoring the counseling, screening, and preventive services you provide. Economic status is an important part of this information. Economic status has been well established as a risk factor for many health conditions. Over-all childhood mortality increases with lower incomes, especially mortality related to trauma (motor vehicle accidents and homicide) and fire. Many specific sources of morbidity and mortality are also inversely related to family income, and knowing your patient's financial status will allow you to focus on these known risks with support from clinical evidence.

Poor children are at greater risk for elevated blood lead levels, especially in the "high-normal" range of 5 to 10 μg/dL. Recall that children with these blood levels, although below the usual cut-off of 10 μg/dL, still have an increased risk of worse developmental outcomes. These children also have a higher risk of iron deficiency, so screening for anemia is especially important. There is some evidence that anemia per se is not sensitive enough as a screen for iron deficiency, which by itself seems to be related to impaired cognitive development even in the absence of anemia. Therefore, consider taking a more careful dietary history with such patients and consider obtaining protoporphyrin levels as a more sensitive screen for iron deficiency.

Poor children also tend to have more emergency department (ED) visits for asthma and are more likely to be admitted to the hospital when they do present to the ED, which suggests that their increased use of the ED results at least partly from more severe disease than children who are not poor. Children from lower-income homes are also more likely to die from respiratory disease. This understanding of the social elements of health care should motivate you to be especially thorough in your asthma care. Assure that your poor patients have backup inhalers and inhalers at school. Consider how much albuterol they are using and their degree of control. To some patients, using albuterol

© 2008 by Lippincott Williams & Wilkins, a Wolters Kluwer business

a few times per week is "not that much." You may take it for granted that inhaled steroids offer improved asthma control with minimal and acceptable adverse effects; however, many families are very reluctant to use inhaled steroids.

Neuropsychiatric disorders are another area in which poor children are at an increased risk. For example, a lower-income status confers an increased risk of anxiety disorders among adolescents. Poor children with autism and related disorders are diagnosed on average almost a year later than are children from wealthier families. Whether this is because of limited or unstable access to primary care or because they are referred to subspecialists later and present in ways that are more difficult to diagnose is unclear. Whatever the reason, your extra vigilance may help narrow the gap in autism diagnosis. Choose a brief, validated screening questionnaire such as the Childhood Autism Test (CHAT) and use it liberally. The school psychiatry Web site at Massachusetts General Hospital lists other options (http://www.massgeneral.org/schoolpsychiatry/screening_pdd.asp).

Finally, remember that once a diagnosis is made and a treatment plan is established, families need to purchase the medication and administer it correctly. Refractory conditions that would be expected to resolve or conditions that occur with frequent recurrences should be considered as noncompliance until proven otherwise. Treatment escalation will not benefit these patients if they are unable to afford the medications that you prescribe to treat their underlying problem.

SUGGESTED READINGS

Babin SM, Burkom HS, Holtry RS, et al. Pediatric patient asthma-related emergency department visits and admissions in Washington, DC, from 2001–2004, and associations with air quality, socio-economic status and age group. *Environ Health.* 2007;6:9.

Centers for Disease Control and Prevention (CDC). Blood lead levels–United States, 1999–2002. *MMWR Morb Mortal Wkly Rep.* 2005;54(20):513–516.

Crowell R, Ferris AM, Wood RJ, et al. Comparative effectiveness of zinc protoporphyrin and hemoglobin concentrations in identifying iron deficiency in a group of low-income, preschool-aged children: practical implications of recent illness. *Pediatrics.* 2006;118(1):224–232.

Mandell DS, Novak MM, Zubritsky CD. Factors associated with age of diagnosis among children with autism spectrum disorders. *Pediatrics.* 2005;116(6):1480–1286.

Schneider JM, Fujii ML, Lamp CL, et al. Anemia, iron deficiency, and iron deficiency anemia in 12-36-mo-old children from low-income families. *Am J Clin Nutr.* 2005;82(6):1269–1275.

Téllez-Rojo MM, Bellinger DC, Arroyo-Quiroz C, et al. Longitudinal associations between blood lead concentrations lower than 10 microg/dL and neurobehavioral development in environmentally exposed children in Mexico City. *Pediatrics.* 2006;118(2):e323–e330.

Roberts RE, Roberts CR, Xing Y. Rates of DSM-IV psychiatric disorders among adolescents in a large metropolitan area. *J Psychiatr Res.* 2006;41(11):959–967.

Wise PH, Kotelchuck M, Wilson ML, et al. Racial and socioeconomic disparities in childhood mortality in Boston. *N Engl J Med.* 1985 8;313(6):360–366.

42

REFER CHILDREN FOR SUPPORTIVE SERVICES WHEN RECOVERING FROM SEVERE ILLNESSES SUCH AS TRAUMATIC BRAIN INJURY (TBI) AND BURNS. THESE CONDITIONS REQUIRE MULTIMODALITY SUPPORT FOR THE CHILDREN TO REACCOMMODATE INTO THEIR SOCIAL POSITION

ELLEN HAMBURGER, MD

WHAT TO DO – TAKE ACTION

Children recovering from severe injuries, such as TBI and burns, are very likely to experience a range of neuropsychiatric and behavioral responses that require a multidisciplinary approach to assessment and treatment. Post-traumatic stress disorder (PTSD) is the psychiatric disorder that has been most clearly established as a sequela to these injuries, affecting as many as one third of patients. TBI patients are also at high risk for attention deficit disorder and cognitive impairment, as well as the mood, anxiety, and conduct disorders known to affect all patients who suffer severe illness. Intervention with appropriate therapy has improved long-term outcome and function.

The age of the child and the extent and nature of the injury will determine the modalities required to provide support for the child and his or her family in recovery and return to school and home. In most cases, emotional recovery is successful but slower than physical recovery after severe injury. An understanding of the range of sequelae and risk factors for adverse long-term outcome is important in coordinating the necessary multimodal rehabilitative approach. The following are factors are associated with children having a more difficult recovery:

- Prior history of trauma, particularly head injury
- Pre-existing mental health disorder, especially anxiety or depression
- Parental history of trauma
- Serious family problems such as history of abuse or neglect, parental mental illness, or substance abuse
- Chaotic social environment, including extreme poverty or community violence.

ⓒ 2008 by Lippincott Williams & Wilkins, a Wolters Kluwer business

Psychological evaluation is warranted for severely injured patients. Children may experience acute stress disorder (ASD) or PTSD. The diagnosis of PTSD is made after a child experiences an injury that causes him or her to react with intense fear, helplessness, or horror and meets symptom criteria in three primary clusters (re-experience of the event, avoidance or numbing, hyperarousal). Children with ASD (which occurs within the month after trauma) have similar symptoms but also experience dissociative symptoms (feelings that they are detached from their bodies, or that their surroundings are unreal or dreamlike). Children with ASD are at high risk for PTSD.

A large percentage of children develop conduct, sleep, mood, or anxiety disorders that require psychiatric intervention through medication and/or cognitive therapy. Child life staff can address the internalizing behaviors that are common in young injured children. Social withdrawal and depressive behaviors are often successfully addressed through play. Physical therapy to address physical limitations is important for physical as well as psychological recovery from injury. Children often avoid activities that they fear will produce pain, but exercise has been shown to improve long-term outcome in lung function, avoidance of contractures after burns, and overall exercise tolerance. Palliative care is also an important part of rehabilitation. TBI and burn patients often suffer pain long after the injury, which can contribute to depression and inability to return to normal activity.

Social work involvement is critical in the recovery phase. Parents may have difficulties coping with the injury and its aftermath and even suffer PTSD themselves. Understanding the nature of the home environment as well as anticipating challenges in planning for return to school are both important in guiding a successful adaptation to postinjury life for the child and family. Families will likely need help identifying community resources and anticipating the long adjustment period that awaits them on return home with their child.

SUGGESTED READINGS

Stoddard FJ, Ronefeldt H, Kagan J, et al. Young burned children: the course of acute stress and physiological and behavioral responses. *Am J Psychiatry.* 2006;163:1084–1090.

Stoddard FJ, Saxe G. Ten-year research review of physical injuries. *J Am Acad Child Adolesc Psychiatry.* 2001;40(10):1128–1145.

Zatzick DF, Grossman DC, Russo J, et al. Predicting posttraumatic stress symptoms longitudinally in a representative sample of hospitalized injured adolescents. *J Am Acad Child Adolesc Psychiatry.* 2006;45(10):1188–1195.

43

DO NOT IGNORE CHILDREN WHO ARTICULATE THAT THEY WANT TO KILL THEMSELVES OR HURT OTHERS

ELLEN HAMBURGER, MD

WHAT TO DO – TAKE ACTION

The child who expresses a desire to hurt himself or herself poses a serious concern that must be addressed. Suicide is the third leading cause of death among children 10 to 19 years old. There were close to 2,000 reported cases of suicide among children in 2004, accounting for 12.5% of all deaths among adolescents. The magnitude of the problem is probably even greater, given that underreporting is a known phenomenon. Depression leading to suicide is often unrecognized and, frequently, goes untreated due to poor access to health care and reticence to access mental health services.

When surveyed, nearly 25% of students in grades 9 to 12 reported that they seriously considered attempting suicide during the preceding 12 months. Almost 1 in 10 (8.7%) high school students has made an attempt. Among those who attempt suicide, 1% to 2% succeeds, with the incidence of completed suicide higher among boys than girls. Suicide attempts using guns are very concerning, as 90% of attempts with guns are fatal, making firearms the leading cause of death in youths who commit suicide.

Clearly, it is incumbent on the pediatrician to know risk factors associated with suicide as well as signs and symptoms of depression. Factors associated with a higher risk of suicide include:

- Homosexuality
- Interpersonal violence (victims and/or perpetrators)
- Alcohol or illicit drug use
- Access to guns in the home or at school
- Suicide of friend or family member
- Somatic complaints
- History of mental health treatment

Although suicide affects children from all racial, ethnic, and socioeconomic groups, certain groups have higher rates than others. Native American boys have the highest suicide rate, whereas African American girls have the lowest.

© 2008 by Lippincott Williams & Wilkins, a Wolters Kluwer business

Several factors reduce the risk of suicide attempt even in at risk adolescents. Adolescents who are connected to family and school, who do well in school, and who do not suffer mental illness are less likely to commit suicide. The presence of these protective factors can reduce the risk of a suicide attempt by as much as 70% to 85%. Clinicians should educate parents about the importance of nurturing children and adolescents.

Because depression is clearly a strong risk factor for pediatric suicide, the pediatrician should be alert to its signs and symptoms. Depression in children and adolescents can be similar to those in adults with signs such as anhedonia, feelings of sadness, helplessness, and hopelessness, changes in eating behavior, insomnia or hypersomnia, extreme fatigue, and inability to concentrate. Even more common, depressed children and teens present with somatic complaints and/or behavioral problems. Somatic complaints are often serial and nonspecific, including headache, abdominal pain, chest pain, dizziness, and fatigue. Behavior problems can include deterioration in school work, truancy, sexual acting out, substance abuse, vandalism, or running away.

All children 10 years of age or older, particularly those in the high-risk groups noted above, should be asked about their mood and sense of well-being at regular check ups. Reliable depression screens have been developed for regular office use. Patients who have a history of emotional problems, have access to firearms, are disconnected from school, have troubled relationships with parents and family, and who are recurrently involved in violence are at high risk.

Patients at high risk and those with symptoms of depression should be asked about suicidal thoughts with a question, such as "Have you ever felt so unhappy or depressed that you thought about killing yourself or wished you were dead?" When the answer is affirmative, the physician should ask specifically about previous attempts and the response to them and whether they have a clear plan (method, time, place) and access to guns. Such inquiry has not been shown to precipitate the behavior; in fact, the child often perceives it as a welcome answer to a cry for help. All families should be warned about the extreme danger of having guns in the home and advised to remove them immediately.

Management of patients who express a desire to hurt themselves must be tailored to individual circumstances and needs with appropriate engagement of psychiatric, school, and social service supports.

SUGGESTED READINGS

American Academy of Pediatrics. Committee on Adolescents. Suicide and suicide attempts in adolescents. *Pediatrics.* 2000;105(4 PT 1):871–874.

Borowsky IW, Ireland M, Resnick M. Adolescent suicide attempts: risks and protectors. *Pediatrics.* 2001;107:485–493.

Brent DA, Perper JA, Moritz G, et al. Firearms and adolescent suicide. A community case-control study. *Am J Dis Child.* 1993;1247(10):1066–1071.

Stein RE, Zitner LE, Jensen PS. Interventions for adolescent depression in primary care. *Pediatrics.* 2006;118:669–682.

44

DO NOT RECOMMEND BLADDER TRAINING EXERCISES FOR CHILDREN WITH ENURESIS

WILLIAM GIASI, JR., MD

WHAT TO DO – TAKE ACTION

Enuresis is a common urinary problem that occurs in childhood and encountered by primary care physicians. Enuresis is defined as the involuntary discharge of urine. Enuresis can be further classified as being primary versus secondary, as well as nocturnal versus diurnal. Primary enuresis is the diagnosis for the patient with nocturnal enuresis who has never been dry for extended periods. In secondary enuresis, the patient has onset of urinary incontinence after a continuous period of at least 6 months of bladder control. Nocturnal enuresis is involuntary and undesirable discharge of urine during the night or sleep beyond the age of anticipated bladder control. Diurnal enuresis in contrast is involuntary discharge of urine while the child is awake.

The true incidence of enuresis is unknown because of underreporting. The timing of when a patient presents to the pediatrician with enuresis is variable and is dependent on that family's concept of what is normal. It is estimated that 15% of 5-year-old children have primary nocturnal enuresis, never having achieved continence. Primary enuresis is twice as common as secondary enuresis; approximately 25% to 30% of children with enuresis have secondary enuresis. The incidence is increased in males 2:1 as compared to females. The rate of resolution amongst enuretics is approximately 10% to 15% per year, such that 5% of 10-year-old children and 1% of adolescents will remain incontinent. The view is the enuresis can be considered a clinical problem after the age of 4 or 5 years.

The typical sequence of developing continence in a child is to achieve nocturnal bowel control, daytime bowel control, daytime bladder control, and finally nocturnal bladder control. Urinary continence is developed through the enlargement of the child's bladder capacity, voluntary control of the sphincter muscles, and finally voluntary control of micturition.

The assessment of enuresis requires knowledge of the differential diagnosis and a thorough history, physical exam, and screening urinalysis. A thorough evaluation may identify a specific etiology or disorder with a specific and definitive treatment. Most patients, however, will not have an identifiable etiology for their enuresis. Generic treatments, conditioning,

© 2008 by Lippincott Williams & Wilkins, a Wolters Kluwer business

or pharmacologic interventions are available, depending on the child's and family's concern, motivation, and intelligence.

Generic interventions include responsibility reinforcement, voiding programs, fluid-intake programs, and arousal systems. These approaches are commonsense and have evolved over time. They are considered supportive but unproven. Bladder training exercises in which the child is asked to ingest large quantities of fluid and to hold the urine in the bladder without voiding until uncomfortable are not recommended. Teaching a child not to respond normally to the sensation of a full bladder and prescribing a therapy that is inherently painful is without merit. Furthermore, the results of studies that report on this therapy are either methodologically flawed or show no improvement.

Conditioning night awakening, utilizing portable alarms that alert the enuretic child to the sensation of a full bladder, are the most benign and successful of the nonpharmacologic treatments. Initial success rates are approximately 66%, with >50% experiencing long-term success. Conditioning, however, requires support on behalf of the physician to provide clear instructions and monitoring, as well as parental help to awaken the child to finish voiding. If the home environment is unable to support the patient, this will often lead to frustration and failure.

Retention-control training, also known as bladder training exercises, focuses on the observation that many children with enuresis have decreased functional bladder capacity. Bladder retention training proposes to increase bladder capacity by asking the child to hold urine at increasing intervals of time after sensing an urge to void. It has been reported to be effective in the literature. Nevertheless, the effort not to void despite urgency may be uncomfortable for the patient as well as the family. Furthermore, a Cochrane database review found that there was not enough evidence to evaluate retention-control training whether compared with controls, used as supplement to alarms, or versus desmopressin.

Enuresis is a common primary care problem. Knowledge of normal voiding dynamics, differential diagnosis, and systematic protocols allow the primary care provider to treat most children. Simple behavioral methods may be effective for some children; however, physicians should be aware that many are unproven and further trials are needed particularly in comparison to treatments known to be effective such as desmopressin, tricyclic antidepressants, and alarms.

SUGGESTED READINGS

Herndon CD, Joseph DB. Urinary incontinence. *Ped Clin North Am.* 2006;53:363–377.
Schulman SL. Voiding dysfunction in children. *Urol Clinic North Am.* 2004;31:481–490.

45

ENCOURAGE BREASTFEEDING FOR INFANTS

ESTHER FORRESTER, MD

WHAT TO DO – MAKE A DECISION, TAKE ACTION

It is widely accepted that human breast milk is the optimum food for infants. Not only does it provide essential nutrients for the developing infant, it changes in composition both during the lactation period and the lactation session to supply ideal nutrition according to the respective stages of development and hourly demand. For example, the fat content of breast milk is lowest early in the morning and highest in the afternoon. The amount of fat in breast milk also increases substantially towards the end of a session. The vitamin and mineral content of breast milk varies during the postpartum period, throughout nursing, and during weaning.

The mineral content of breast milk is highest immediately postpartum and decreases over time. During the first few days postpartum, colostrum is high in vitamin E, protein, zinc, magnesium, and antibodies. From day 3 to day 6 postpartum, colostrum enters a transitional form with increasing amounts of fat, lactose, and calories, while protein and immune factors gradually decrease. Magnesium levels begin to decrease after 18 months of lactation. Unlike other minerals, magnesium secretion is unaffected by constitutional variables such as adolescent motherhood, maternal malnutrition, smoking, gestation length, environment or stage of lactation.

The vitamin content transitions according to the fat- and water-solubility of vitamins and may vary according to the mother's diet and genetic makeup. However, if a mother is deficient, the volume of milk produced varies more than the vitamin composition. Generally, water-soluble vitamins (e.g., B, C, B_6) increase over time except for vitamins C and B_6. Fat-soluble vitamins (e.g., A, D, E, K) generally decrease over time.

There is a strong correlation between vitamin D content in breast milk and the 25-hydroxycalciferol (25-OH-D) concentration in serum of exclusively breastfed infants. However, there is no correlation between the

© 2008 by Lippincott Williams & Wilkins, a Wolters Kluwer business

concentration of vitamin D in mothers' serum and breast milk. Exclusively breastfed infants 0 to 12 months of age should receive at least 200 IU (5 μg) of vitamin D to prevent rickets. For infants not exposed to sunlight, up to 400 IU (10 μg) may be required.

Although the amounts of calcium and iron in breast milk are less than those found in cows' milk, the bioavailability is greater. Fifty percent of iron in human breast milk is absorbed, whereas only 4% to 10 % is absorbed from cows' milk or commercial infant formulas. The large amount of lactose in breast milk is believed to help absorb calcium, phosphorus, and magnesium. Lactose also nourishes intestinal bacteria, which in turn produce B vitamins for the infant.

These natural variations in breast milk represent a few of the reasons the American Academy of Pediatrics and the American Dietetic Association's recommend breast feeding for the first 4 to 6 months of life. As the nutritional and dietary demands of the infant increase, breastfeeding should be supplemented with solid foods for at least 12 months. Considering the impact that maternal nutrition status has on the quality and quantity of breast milk, breastfeeding mothers must also make conscious efforts to supplement their diets with vitamins and minerals and increase their caloric intake to adequately provide for breastfeeding infants.

SUGGESTED READINGS

Dórea JG. Magnesium in human milk. *J Am Coll Nutr.* 2000;19:210–219.

Cancela L, Le Boulch N, Miravet L. Relationship between the vitamin D content of maternal milk and the vitamin D status of nursing women and breastfed infants. *J Endocrinol.* 1986;110:43–50.

Karra MV, Udipi SA, Kirksey A, et al. Changes in specific nutrients in breast milk during extended lactation. *Am J Clin Nutr.* 1986;43:495–503.

Meyer L. *Breast Milk.* CD written February 21, 2000. Available at: http://uimc.discoveryhospital.com/main.php?id=1875. Accessed March 1, 2007.

Schuster E. Oregon State University Extension Family and Community Development. *Breast Milk Changes.* Available at: http://72.14.209.104/search?q=cache:f5-6HRiU0GsJ:extension.oregonstate.edu/fcd/nutrition/publications/nutrifocus/breastmilkchanges.pdf+vitamins+in+breast+milk&hl=en&ct=clnk&cd=35&gl=us. Accessed March 1, 2007.

Vitamin D Supplementation for Breastfed Infants—2004 Health Canada Recommendation. Available at: http://www.hc-sc.gc.ca/fn-an/nutrition/child-enfant/infant-nourisson/vita_d_supp_e.html. Accessed March 1, 2007.

46

KNOW WHEN TO TELL MOTHERS TO STOP BREASTFEEDING

YOLANDA LEWIS-RAGLAND, MD

WHAT TO DO – TAKE ACTION

Breastfeeding provides "human milk for human babies" for optimal brain development, immune system protection, and digestive compatibility. Research shows that breastfed babies have slightly higher intelligence quotients (IQs) than babies fed infant formula. They have fewer infections and the onset of allergies is delayed. Breastfed babies may have a reduced risk of obesity and chronic diseases, such as diabetes. Mothers who breastfeed may have a decreased risk of breast and ovarian cancers, and possibly a decreased risk of osteoporosis and hip fractures. Although any amount of breastfeeding is beneficial, exclusive breastfeeding for the first 6 months is associated with greater health benefits.

TRUE BREASTFEEDING CONTRAINDICATIONS

Despite the many benefits of breastfeeding, there are incidences and conditions in which breastfeeding is contraindicated. For example, galactosemia is a hereditary disease that is caused by the lack of a liver enzyme required to digest galactose. Galactose is a breakdown product of lactose, which is most commonly found in milk products. Because galactose cannot be broken down, it accumulates in the cells and becomes toxic. The body then produces abnormal chemicals, which causes the symptoms seen in infants with untreated galactosemia.

Galactosemia usually causes no symptoms at birth, but jaundice, diarrhea, and vomiting soon develop and the baby fails to gain weight. If not detected immediately, it results in liver disease, cataracts, mental retardation, and possibly death. Death can occur as early as 1 to 2 weeks of age from severe *Escherichia coli* bacteria infections. *E. coli* infections are common in untreated galactosemic infants. The American Liver Foundation recommends that all infants who develop jaundice be considered for galactosemia.

Other contradictions to breastfeeding include:

- Women actively using street drugs or heavily abusing alcohol
- Women infected with human immunodeficiency virus (HIV)—transmission to infants

© 2008 by Lippincott Williams & Wilkins, a Wolters Kluwer business

- Women with active untreated tuberculosis—infants may contract tuberculosis (TB) from close respiratory exposure associated with breastfeeding—after 14 days of treatment breastfeeding can be resumed
- Women undergoing chemotherapy for breast cancer
- Women taking certain medications should not breastfeed

Medications contradicted in breastfeeding mothers include:

1. Bromocriptine (Parlodel) (it suppresses prolactin)—milk letdown hormone
2. Lithium (used to treat manic–depressive disorder)—blood levels get too high in infants
3. Methotrexate (used to treat lupus and arthritis)—hinders the immune system
4. Ergotamine (used for migraine headaches)—causes vomiting, diarrhea, seizures
5. Several cancer therapy medications—too toxic for infant exposure.

TEMPORARY INTERRUPTION OF BREASTFEEDING

Other infectious conditions require temporary cessation of breastfeeding:

Chicken pox: Women with open chicken pox lesions that are weeping should not breastfeed until the lesions are completely healed; breastfeeding may resume after the infant has been administered immunoglobulin providing temporary protection against chicken pox.

Shingles: Women with shingles, another presentation of the varicella virus, can breastfeed if there are no lesions on the breast or if breast lesions are covered. This is possible because these women have antibodies to chicken pox virus that are passed through the breast milk to the infant, conferring additional protection against the disease.

Women with active herpes lesions on the breast should not breastfeed until the lesions have completely healed and symptoms have cleared.

CONDITIONS COMPATIBLE WITH BREASTFEEDING

Hepatitis B: Infected mothers may breastfeed their infants; infants treated with hepatitis immunoglobulin and hepatitis vaccine can be breastfed without increased risk of transmission.

Hepatitis A: Infants can be breastfed by their actively infected mothers once the infants have been given immune serum globulin and hepatitis A vaccine.

Hepatitis C: Infants can breastfeed since the transmission rate of hepatitis C is 4% regardless of whether they are breastfed or not.

Mastitis: One to 2% of women will develop mastitis, a breast infection. This usually occurs 1 to 5 weeks after delivery. The breast becomes tender, firm, and reddened; fever is common. Women with mastitis need antibiotic therapy. If a breast abscess develops, surgical drainage may be needed. These infections are caused by bacteria normally found in the infant's mouth. Breastfeeding can continue because it helps to resolve the mastitis more quickly and continues to benefit the infant.

Breastfeeding is an important nutritive and emotional link for mothers and babies. However, knowledge of the contraindications to breastfeeding can help prevent transmission of infectious agents to infants during this important activity.

SUGGESTED READINGS

Centers for Disease Control and Prevention. Breastfeeding: diseases and conditions: contraindicators. Available at: www.cdc.gov/breastfeeding/disease/contraindicators.htm. Accessed December 28, 2007.

Continuity Clinic Notebook. Breastfeeding-Advantages and Disadvantages. Available at: www.mcg.edu/pediatrics/CCNotebook/chapter1/breastfeedingfaqs.htm. Accessed on December 28, 2007.

MedlinePlus. Medical Encyclopedia: Galactosemia. Available at: www.nlm.nih.gov/medlineplus/ency/article/000366.htm. Accessed December 28, 2007.

47

INFANTS WHO ARE EXCLUSIVELY BREASTFED ARE AT INCREASED RISK FOR VITAMIN D DEFICIENCY AND ASSOCIATED RICKETS. ASSESS THESE INFANTS FOR ADDITIONAL RISK FACTORS SUCH AS DARK SKIN AND LIMITED SUN EXPOSURE AND CONSIDER VITAMIN SUPPLEMENTATION

JOHANN PETERSON, MD

WHAT TO DO – GATHER APPROPRIATE DATA

Vitamin D is a fat-soluble vitamin that is either produced in the skin with ultraviolet (UV) light exposure, or absorbed from the intestine in chylomicrons. Dietary vitamin D is available in two forms: D2 (ergocalciferol, derived from plants or yeast) or D3 (cholecalciferol, derived from animals or produced in human skin exposed to sunlight). D3 is the more physiologic and potent form, but D2 is historically the predominant form found in vitamin D supplements and fortified foods. Vitamin D is hydroxylated to 25-hydroxycalciferol (25-OH-D) in the liver, and hydroxylated again to calcitriol, or 1, 25-(OH)2-D in the kidney. The 25-OH-D form is measured in blood to assess vitamin D stores, and it has a half-life of about 2 weeks. The 1,25-(OH)2-D form is the most biologically active. Vitamin D is measured in international units (IU), where 1 IU is defined as 0.025 μg D3, which is 65 pmol D3. Units of other forms of vitamin D, (25-OH-D and 1,25-(OH)2-D) are defined as molar equivalents to D3 (i.e., 65 pmol = 1 IU).

The 1,25-(OH)2-D form is a hormone acting via a nuclear receptor (VDR), which in the presence of vitamin D binds the retinoic acid receptor (RXR). The RXR-VRD-vitamin D complex binds so-called vitamin D responsive elements in nuclear DNA and alters gene expression. In both renal tubular cells and in the intestinal epithelium, vitamin D increases absorption of calcium and phosphate. In bone, it stimulates both osteoblastic and osteoclastic activity. Recall that parathyroid hormone (PTH) is predominantly regulated by the plasma calcium level. PTH stimulates osteoclast activity and bone resorption, stimulates calcium resorption and phosphate loss in the renal tubule, and promotes hydroxylation of 25-OH-D to 1,25-(OH)2-D by the kidney. In vitamin D deficiency, poor calcium absorption stimulates PTH release, and renal calcium absorption and osteoclast activity are increased. Increased renal hydroxylation of 25-OH-D can often compensate

© 2008 by Lippincott Williams & Wilkins, a Wolters Kluwer business

for decreased levels of precursor to maintain normal or high levels of 1,25-(OH)-D with low levels of 25-OH-D. Decreased renal absorption results in low phosphate levels. Alkaline phosphatase is high, reflecting increased bone turnover.

Vitamin D deficiency is usually diagnosed by a serum vitamin D level <20 ng/mL, and levels <15 ng/mL represent severe deficiency. In children with growing bones, severe chronic vitamin D deficiency results in rickets, a disorder of bone development characterized by poor mineralization throughout the skeleton. This results in a tendency of the long bones to bend under the stress of walking (or muscle contraction in perambulatory children), and can produce varus or valgus deformities of the legs. The skull may be affected, with palpable softening (rachitic craniotabes), delayed closure of the fontanelles, frontal bossing, and exaggerated positional flattening of the occiput. Hypertrophy of the costochondral junctions produces the "rachitic rosary," which can progress to a Harrison groove when the ribs begin to contract. Epiphyses of the long bones widen, producing a characteristic appearance on x-ray. Tooth development is also delayed. Muscle weakness and hypotonia are common, and the hypocalcemia can be so severe as to cause tetany, seizures, laryngospasm, and dilated cardiomyopathy. Hypochromic anemia can be a feature of rickets. In older patients, vitamin D deficiency results in osteomalacia without the other characteristic skeletal changes of rickets.

Adequate vitamin D can be produced in the skin if there is sufficient sunlight exposure; however, the actual and required amount of sun exposure are difficult to determine in any given person. Vitamin D levels in healthy people vary with the season and persons living at high latitudes or in cities (where there is more shade) are less likely to receive adequate sunlight. Skin pigmentation and sunblock affect the amount of UV-B radiation available for vitamin D synthesis, and African Americans are more prone to vitamin D deficiency. In the United States, the recommended dietary intake of vitamin D in children is 200 IU/day, although this is the subject of some controversy. In Canada the recommendation is 400 IU/day, as it was in the United States previously. Human and unfortified cows milk usually provide around 20 to 25 IU/L vitamin D, although the level can be much higher in nursing mothers taking large doses of vitamin D or exposed to lots of sunlight. All infant formulas sold in the United States contain more than 400 IU/L, so an infant consuming 500 mL/day of formula is meeting the recommended intake. The American Academy of Pediatrics (AAP) recommends that vitamin D supplementation, in the form of a multivitamin, be provided to any infant who is exclusively breastfed or is taking in <500 mL/day of formula, beginning in the first 2 months of life, and to older children who do not "get regular sunlight exposure." Fortified cow's milk and orange juice should contain 100 IU/8 oz of vitamin D. Salmon and other salt-water fish are good sources of vitamin D, and shiitake mushrooms are a good source for vegans.

In cases of rickets or severe vitamin D deficiency, much higher doses must be administered. Several regimens have been used, including single oral doses of 150,000 to 600,000 IU, a single intramuscular dose of 600,000 IU, and daily oral doses of 2,000 IU for 4 weeks. Comparative trials are limited, but one study found a higher incidence of hypercalcemia after doses of 600,000 IU, and another reported a lower rate of adequate clinical response in children receiving the lower daily dose regimen. Therefore if there is no suspicion of malabsorption, a single oral dose of 300,000 IU is probably reasonable. Patients with malabsorption due to inflammatory bowel disease, cystic fibrosis, cholestasis, or chronic diarrhea are at risk for vitamin D deficiency and deficiency of the other fat-soluble vitamins (A, E, and K).

SUGGESTED READINGS

Cesur Y, Caksen H, Gündem A, et al. Comparison of low and high dose of vitamin D treatment in nutritional vitamin D deficiency rickets. *J Pediatr Endocrinol Metab.* 2003;16(8):1105–1109.

Gartner LM, Greer FR, Section on Breastfeeding and Committee on Nutrition. American Academy of Pediatrics. Prevention of rickets and vitamin D deficiency: new guidelines for vitamin D intake. *Pediatrics.* 2003;111(4 Pt 1):908–910.

Holick MF. Resurrection of vitamin D deficiency and rickets. *J Clin Invest.* 2006;116(8):2062–2072.

Houghton LA, Vieth R. The case against ergocalciferol (vitamin D$_2$) as a vitamin supplement. *Am J Clin Nutr.* 2006;84(4):694–697.

Lubani MM, al-Shab TS, al-Saleh QA, et al. Vitamin-D-deficiency rickets in Kuwait: the prevalence of a preventable disease. *Ann Trop Paediatr.* 1989;9(3):134–139.

Shah BR, Finberg L. Single-day therapy for nutritional vitamin D-deficiency rickets: a preferred method. *J Pediatr.* 1994;125(3):487–490.

48

MONITOR PATIENT'S WEIGHT AND PROVIDE APPROPRIATE GUIDANCE REGARDING NUTRITION AND PHYSICAL ACTIVITY TO PREVENT ADULT DISEASES

BRIAN KIT, MD

WHAT TO DO – GATHER APPROPRIATE DATA

Scope of the Problem. According to the Centers for Disease Control and Prevention (CDC), the prevalence of obese children in the United Sates tripled to 16% from 1980 to 2002. Despite this, pediatricians often both overlook and fail to disclose the diagnosis in affected children and teens. The increased prevalence of obesity has resulted in an increase in associated medical problems, including diabetes, hypertension, and dyslipidemia. These conditions are beginning to present during childhood. The focus on childhood obesity is based on evidence that obese children become obese adults and will be at risk for significant and lifelong comorbidity.

DEFINITIONS

To thwart the rise in childhood obesity and to avoid its associated complications, pediatricians and other providers must have an understanding of the definition of obesity and related terms. The key definitions are listed below.

- **Body Mass Index (BMI):** BMI, defined as weight in kilograms divided by height in meters squared (kg/m^2), is an indirect measurement of adiposity. Although there are limitations of its ability to measure adiposity, it is the most acceptable screen for obesity in children ages 2 to 18 years.
- **Underweight:** BMI <10th percentile for age.
- **Normal Weight:** BMI between the 10th and 85th percentile for age.
- **Overweight:** BMI >85th percentile for age.
- **Obese:** BMI >95th percentile for age.

HEALTH SUPERVISION FOR OVERWEIGHT AND OBESE CHILDREN

All patients should have a BMI calculated at least annually during a well-child visit and charted on the CDC's National Center for Health Statistics charts for BMI. The charts are available online at http://www.cdc.gov/

© 2008 by Lippincott Williams & Wilkins, a Wolters Kluwer business

growthcharts. If the child is overweight or obese, the practitioner should take into consideration the following points:

- Discuss with the family the clinical definition of obesity and the importance of early identification. Focus the discussion on the health benefits of addressing obesity and the child's positive qualities.

- A full history, including dietary history and activity history, should be taken from both the child and the parent. Questions regarding eating patterns and food choices may provide the clinician with opportunities to address areas of concerns, including consumption of foods with high calories but low nutritional value. Encourage the child and family to maintain a food journal, detailing the foods consumed during the day. Time spent in physical education and playing outdoors should be determined. Availability of community resources that promote exercise should be explored.

- Family history of obesity, hypertension, diabetes, and heart disease should be ascertained to identify the child's risks factors.

- Physical examination should be complete, with particular emphasis on items that may indicate complications of obesity, including hypertension, hirsutism, and acanthosis nigricans.

- Although there are no standards for laboratory evaluation, many clinicians will screen for diabetes (using a fasting glucose), insulin resistance (measuring an insulin level), and hyperlipidemia (measuring total cholesterol, triglycerides, and high-density lipoprotein [HDL]-cholesterol) in children who are obese.

- Develop a plan with the family that employs dietary and activity modifications. Evidence from the medical literature has confirmed the advantages of a combined dietary and exercise approach. Individual exercise routines will vary depending on needs and available resources. Ensure that the child is part of the process of developing the goals and meet with the family regularly to monitor progress.

- Psychosocial support, particularly for those children who are depressed, is a vital component of the treatment of obesity.

- Recognize that management of obesity is best done using a multidisciplinary approach, whenever possible, involving trained nurses, nurse practitioners, nutritionists, physicians, psychologists, and social workers. All these professionals can effectively help patients and their families monitor and change behavior.

CONCLUSION

The pediatrician and other providers of services for children are in a position to alter the course of obesity and its complications. Identifying the problem and developing an action plan that includes exercise and dietary modifications will have positive outcomes. Attention to the child's psychosocial needs is another key element of treatment.

SUGGESTED READINGS

Barlow SE, Dietz WH. Obesity evaluation and treatment: expert committee recommendations. The Maternal and Child Health Bureau, Health Resources and Services Administration and the Department of Health and Human Services. *Pediatrics.* 1998;102(3):e29.

Centers for Disease Control and Prevention. Children and teens told by doctors that they were overweight–United States, 1999–2002. *MMWR Morb Mortal Wkly Rev.* 2005;54(34):848–849.

Centers for Disease Control and Prevention. Prevalence of overweight among children and adolescents: United States, 1999–2002. National Health and Nutrition Examination Survey. Hyattsville, MD: U.S. Department of Health and Human Services, CDC, National Center for Health Statistics. Available at: www.cdc.gov/nchs/products/pubs/pubd/hestats/overwght99.htm. Accessed on December 28, 2007.

Cook S, Weitzman M, Auinger P, Barlow SE. Screening and counseling associated with obesity diagnosis in a national survey of ambulatory pediatric visits. *Pediatrics.* 2005;116(1):112–116.

Dietz WH, Robinson TN. Clinical practice. Overweight children and adolescents. *N Engl J Med.* 2005;352:2100–2109.

Dietz WH. Health consequences of obesity in youth: childhood predictors of adult disease. *Pediatrics.* 1998;101(3 Pt 2):518–525.

Hill JO, Trowbridge FL. Childhood obesity: future directions and research priorities. *Pediatrics.* 1998;101(3 Pt 2):570–574.

Hills AP, Parker AW. Obesity management via diet and exercise intervention. *Child Care Health Dev.* 1988;14:409–416.

Whitaker RC, Wright JA, Pepe MS, et al. Predicting obesity in young adulthood from childhood and parental obesity. *N Engl J Med.* 1997;337:869–873.

49

PROVIDE ADEQUATE CALCIUM AND PHOSPHORUS IN THE DIET OF A PREMATURE INFANT, USING A FORMULA DESIGNED FOR THIS AGE GROUP OR FORTIFIED HUMAN BREAST MILK, AND MONITOR FOR THE DEVELOPMENT OF METABOLIC BONE DISEASE OF PREMATURITY (MBDP)

BRIAN KIT, MD

WHAT TO DO – TAKE ACTION

Meeting the calcium and phosphorus demands of the premature infant represents a challenge for pediatricians from the early days in the neonatal intensive care unit (NICU) and continuing beyond discharge. The problem is a direct result of a shortened gestational period. The fetus acquires two thirds of its calcium and phosphorus stores during the third trimester. Infants born <30 weeks' gestation are particularly at-risk for calcium and phosphorus abnormalities, including MBDP. Other risk factors include a birth weight <1,500 g, prolonged immobilization, systemic illness, and chronic exposure to medications that negatively impact bone mineralization, such as furosemide (Lasix), steroids, and phenobarbital.

MDBP describes a constellation of abnormalities in premature infants that results in rickets, osteomalacia, and osteoporosis. The etiology of MBDP is a deficiency of calcium and phosphorus. Classic radiographic abnormalities associated with MBDP include fractures, osteopenia as demonstrated by a "washed out" appearance of the bones, and radiographic evidence of rickets with the classic metaphyseal changes. However, a loss of <40% of bone mineralization can occur without the radiographic changes suggestive of MBDP. Early identification of MBDP is better achieved with biochemical markers, including alkaline phosphatase and phosphorus. Classically, the practitioner will see low levels of phosphorus and elevated alkaline phosphatase. However, even with normal biochemical markers and normal radiologic findings, an infant may still be at risk for MBDP.

To prevent the development of MBDP, supplementation of calcium and phosphorus begins almost at the time of birth, initially parentally and then enterally. Babies are generally transitioned from total parental nutrition (TPN) when they are able to tolerate the change. The choice of nutrition for the enterally fed baby requires careful attention. *Table 49.1* reviews the

ⓒ 2008 by Lippincott Williams & Wilkins, a Wolters Kluwer business

TABLE 49.1	COMPARISON OF CALORIE, CALCIUM, AND PHOSPHORUS COMPOSITIONS OF DIFFERENT TYPES OF INFANT FORMULA			
CATEGORY	CALORIES (KCAL/OZ)	CALCIUM (MG/KG)	PHOSPHORUS (MG/KG)	EXAMPLE
Term Formula[a]	20	80	45	Enfamil, Similac
Transitional Formula[a]	22	120	70	Enfamil 22, Neosure 22
Preterm Formula[a]	24	200	105	Enfamil Premature 24, Similac Special 24
Breast Milk with Human Milk Fortifier[b]	24	150	80	Enfamil Human Milk Fortifier, Similac Human Milk Fortifier

[a] Calcium and phosphorus values reported are based on provision of 150 mL/kg/day.
[b] Calcium and phosphorus values reported are per 100 mL of breast milk with human milk fortifier.

different types of infant formula. Although breast milk has many advantages over other forms of nutrition, breast milk alone provides preterm infants with insufficient calcium and phosphorus for adequate bone mineralization and eventual growth. To circumvent this problem, expressed breast milk is supplemented with human milk fortifiers (HMF) or infants are given preterm formulas to reflect the intrauterine calcium accretion needs of 105 mg/kg/day, taking into consideration variances in absorption and losses. The appropriate duration of feeds with HMF and preterm formulas has not yet been determined, but most babies receive these interventions until they weigh approximately 2 kg or until discharge from the NICU, whichever is first.

Increasingly, the increased metabolic demands of infants born preterm have been shown to persist outside of the NICU. Graduates of the NICU, when compared with term infants, have decreased bone mineralization and are at increased risk of metabolic bone disease. The use of transitional formulas, which have a greater caloric density and more calcium and phosphorus compared to term formulas, has become fairly common for the premature infant who has achieved 2 kg or who is prepared for discharge from the NICU. There is no consensus regarding the duration of transitional formula, but some practitioners provide enriched formulas for infants born <1,500 g until 9 months corrected age. This is partially based on evidence that preterm infants taking formula with calcium concentrations of 700 mg/L have greater bone mineral content than those taking formula with calcium concentrations of 350 mg/L. For infants receiving primarily human breast milk, there is insufficient evidence to support the use of transitional formulas over breast milk once HMF is no longer necessary. Despite this, many experts will recommend two feedings per day with transitional formulas.

MBDP is a common problem in preterm infants. Prevention and early identification plays an important role in addressing the disease process. It is a difficult diagnosis to make, requiring a high index of suspicion. There are many questions in the scientific literature regarding interventions that should be taken to prevent the development of MBDP. The recommendations below should be used as guidelines to assist with the management, recognizing individual practices will vary depending on available resources and specific risk factors.

- **Prevention.** Calcium and phosphorus supplementation must begin in the NICU, with the use of breast milk with HMF or preterm formulas until approximately 2 kg. Depending on the clinical scenario, transitional formulas may be used to achieve higher calcium and phosphorus intake. The duration of supplementation may vary but should be considered until 9 months corrected age for those born <1,500 g.
- **Early Identification.** Measure alkaline phosphatase and phosphorus levels 4 weeks following discharge from the NICU for babies with risk factors. Correlate the results with the clinical picture because infants with MBDP may have normal biochemical markers. Frequent growth assessments are essential for early identification of infants who may not be meeting their nutritional needs, including calcium and phosphorus.

SUGGESTED READINGS

Bishop NJ, King FJ, Lucas A. Increased bone mineral content of preterm infants fed with a nutrient enriched formula after discharge from hospital. *Arch Dis Child.* 1993;68(5 Spec No):573–578.

Carver JD, Wu PY, Hall RT, et al. Growth of preterm infants fed nutrient-enriched or term formula after hospital discharge. *Pediatrics.* 2001;107:683–689.

Kuzma-O'Reilly B, Duenas ML, Greecher C, et al. Evaluation, development, and implementation of potentially better practices in neonatal intensive care nutrition. *Pediatrics.* 2003;111(4 Pt 2):e461–e470.

Lucas A, Fewtrell MS, Morley R, et al. Randomized trial of nutrient-enriched formula versus standard formula for discharged preterm infants. *Pediatrics.* 2001;108:703–711.

Morely R, Lucas A. Randomized diet in the neonatal period and growth performance until 7.5-8 years of age in preterm children. *Am J Clin Nutri.* 2000;71:822–888.

Rigo J, De Curtis M, Pieltain C, et al. Bone mineral metabolism in the micropremie. *Clin Perinatol.* 2000;27:147–170.

50

DO NOT PERFORM AN EXTENSIVE LABORATORY OR RADIOGRAPHIC EVALUATION FOR FAILURE TO THRIVE (FTT)

MICHAEL CLEMMENS, MD

WHAT TO DO – GATHER APPROPRIATE DATA

FTT is a common pediatric problem, especially during infancy. The diagnosis of FTT is made when a child's weight is less than the fifth percentile for weight-for-age or crosses two major percentile lines. Identifying the underlying cause of FTT is usually straightforward, but occasionally it requires an inpatient evaluation. The most important tools for determining the underlying cause of poor growth are a thorough history, complete physical exam, and a staged laboratory workup. There are few other areas in pediatrics where the history is so vitally important. Less often, the exam will hold a clue to the etiology. When the history and physical do not reveal the diagnosis, the laboratory evaluation is not likely to prove helpful. In some cases, carefully selected testing is still in order.

Traditionally, FTT has been classified as organic or nonorganic, although there is often considerable overlap. Many children will have mixed etiologies for their poor growth. Organic FTT reflects an underlying pathophysiologic abnormality, resulting in an inability to ingest, absorb, or utilize adequate nutrition to sustain normal growth. Conditions associated with increased metabolic demands may make the standard caloric intake inadequate. Examples of organic FTT include swallowing disorders, malabsorption, metabolic disorders, and congestive heart failure.

The great majority of FTT is nonorganic and occurs when an otherwise healthy child does not get enough nutrition to sustain normal growth. Difficulties with breastfeeding, caregiver misunderstanding about infant nutritional needs, and improper mixing of formula are three common examples of nonorganic FTT. Often, there are psychosocial factors, such as financial stress or caregiver mental illness, influencing the situation. Most patients with nonorganic FTT are treated successfully as outpatients.

A detailed history is the most powerful diagnostic tool for determining the cause of a child's FTT. Special attention to the nutritional and psychosocial history is paramount. The provider must take the time to learn about the child's diet and feeding behaviors, the caregiver's understanding of the

© 2008 by Lippincott Williams & Wilkins, a Wolters Kluwer business

child's nutritional needs, and the entire family's social situation. A skilled social worker may be able to contribute significantly to this process.

In addition, because abnormalities in any organ system can lead to FTT, a thorough physical exam should be performed. All growth parameters should be measured, plotted, and compared to prior data points. Other key elements of the exam include identification of dysmorphic features, signs of physical abuse or neglect, and possible effects of malnutrition. Observing the interaction between the child and caregiver may provide important clues to the psychosocial factors influencing the situation.

If the cause of FTT is not clear after a thorough history and physical exam, a 3-day diet diary and calorie count can provide critical information. Inadequate caloric intake is the most common cause of FTT. Screening laboratory and radiographic tests are helpful in only approximately 5% of cases. A directed laboratory or radiographic evaluation, guided by the findings on the history or physical exam, is more likely to be useful.

The major pitfall in the evaluation of a child with FTT is performing an inadequate history and physical examination. Most cases of FTT can be treated successfully as an outpatient. Often, a multidisciplinary approach, including social services and referral to a nutritionist, is useful. However, hospitalization is indicated if an accurate dietary history cannot be determined, if a trial of increased caloric intake in the home environment fails, if there are concerns about the safety of the home environment, or if an underlying pathologic process is identified.

SUGGESTED READINGS

Berwick DM. Nonorganic failure to thrive. *Pediatr Rev.* 1980;1:265–279.
Bithoney WG, Dubowitz H, Egan H. Failure to thrive/growth deficiency. *Pediatr Rev.* 1992; 13:453–460.
Krugman SD, Dubowitz H. Failure to thrive. *Am Fam Physician.* 2003;68:879–884.
Sills RH. Failure to thrive. The role of clinical and laboratory evaluation. *Am J Dis Child.* 1978; 132:967–969.

51

IF PATIENTS CANNOT MEET THEIR NUTRITIONAL NEEDS ORALLY, CONSIDER AUGMENTING WITH ADDITIONAL FEEDING BY TUBE RATHER THAN PARENTERALLY

CRAIG DEWOLFE, MD

WHAT TO DO – TAKE ACTION

Appropriate nutrition is vital to maintaining health and recovering from disease and injury. Research in this field has offered the practitioner many choices in nutritional formulation and delivery. Yet, when patients are unable to effectively meet their needs by mouth, enteral nutrition should be considered the next best choice. It is more physiologic, less costly, and associated with fewer complications than parenteral nutrition. Some studies suggest that it is underutilized in up to 60% of cases. Practitioners should familiarize themselves with the risks and benefits of enteral and parenteral nutrition while reconsidering the contraindications to gastrointestinal feeds. The use of a validated algorithm may offer additional assistance when maximizing nutritional delivery.

Patients are regularly placed on intravenous fluids or total parenteral nutrition (TPN) at the expense of oral or enteral feeds. However, research in areas as diverse as dehydration to respiratory failure suggests that oral hydration and enteral feeds are generally the preferred route of providing nutrition. Enteral feeds maintain the gastrointestinal lining, limit the translocation of enteric bacteria, provide enhanced utilization of nutrients, are easier to administer at a lower cost, and are associated with fewer infectious, metabolic and hepatobiliary risks than TPN.

Special formulas have been developed for patients of all ages and according to disease process. Some studies suggest that enteral nutrition for critically ill children should start with hypo- or isotonic lactose-free or elemental formulas advancing to a standard formula over 3 to 4 days. Additionally, rates in critically ill children can begin a 1 mL/kg/hr with stepwise increases every 4 to 6 hours to the goal calories. Alternative formulas or additives can be provided for children with fat malabsorption or azotemia/hyperammonemia. Practitioners should acquaint themselves with these formulations or regularly enlist the help of a nutritionist when offering the best substrate for the patient. The clinician should also consider the optimal route of enteral feeds, as each may carry their own set of risks and benefits. For example,

© 2008 by Lippincott Williams & Wilkins, a Wolters Kluwer business

flexible polyurethane or Silastic oral or nasogastric tubing may be the easiest access and promote gastric pH balance while limiting the risks of sinus disease or mucosal irritation from the larger tubing of the past. But they may place a patient with slow gastric empty or other risk factors associated with aspiration at greater risk for pneumonia than a fluoroscopic, endoscopic, or surgical transpyloric placement of the same tube. In patients who require prolonged enteral nutrition, tube enterostomies may minimize the risk of tube displacement and resolve concerns related to the physical appearance of the tube on the face.

Health care providers should ensure the safety of enteral nutrition by limiting the aspiration risk, preventing mechanical problems, and ensuring metabolic balance. First, to prevent aspiration, the practitioner should ensure correct placement of the tube, elevate the upper part of the body 30 degrees while infusing the formula, and check residuals. If problems persist, they should consider starting continuous feeds or placing a transpyloric tube. Other mechanical problems include tube migration into the esophagus or rarely into the trachea, local irritation and infection, or partial intestinal obstruction. Taking care to prevent these complications include proper tube measurement, placement, and stabilization. Thereafter, caretakers should recheck the tube placement regularly, clean the ostomy site daily, and limit leakage. Finally, to ensure metabolic balance, the practitioner should regularly assess the patient's nutritional status and fluid and electrolyte balance.

One should use the parenteral route only when the patient is at risk for malnutrition from not eating, has failed an enteral trial, or has severely diminished intestinal function. The practitioner may need to use parenteral nutrition in very low-birth-weight infants who are building up on enteral feeds, or in other patients with ischemic injury to the bowel, significant bowel resection, fistula, obstruction, malabsorption, or bleeding. When using parenteral nutrition, the possible complications include infection or thrombosis related to the intravenous catheter or metabolic disturbances. After parenteral nutrition has begun, the patient should be regularly monitored for complications and transitioned quickly to oral or enteral feeds.

Timely transition to enteral feeds is better assured by the use of a validated algorithm that regularly assesses the nutritional needs of every patient with the ultimate goal of providing enteral feeds as soon as possible. Such a protocol works by encouraging the initiation of enteral feeds, assessing and troubleshooting gastrointestinal tolerance, and advancing to goal feeds in a safe but efficient manner. One such algorithm in a multicenter randomized clinical trial in an intensive care unit was shown to improve the nutritional support to patients while hospital lengths of stay and mortality rates decreased.

In summary, enteral nutrition should be considered in patients who cannot effectively meet their nutritional needs by mouth. A greater appreciation of the benefits of enteral nutrition, contraindications, and the ways to manage risks will result in better patient outcomes.

SUGGESTED READINGS

American Society for Parenteral and Enteral Nutrition. Guidelines for the use of parenteral and enteral nutrition in adult and pediatric patients. *JPEN J Parenter Enteral Nutr.* 1993;17(4 Suppl):1SA–52SA.

Chellis MJ, Sanders SV, Webster H, et al. Early enteral feeding in the pediatric intensive care unit. *JPEN J Parenter Enteral Nutr.* 1996;20:71–73.

Martin CM, Doig GS, Heyland DK, et al. Multicentre, cluster-randomized clinical trial of algorithms for critical-care enteral and parenteral therapy (ACCEPT). *CMAJ.* 2004;170:197–204.

52

ENTERAL NUTRITION IS THE PREFERRED FEEDING MODALITY

NAILAH COLEMAN, MD

WHAT TO DO – MAKE A DECISION, TAKE ACTION

Nutrition provides adequate substrates, vitamins, minerals, and antioxidants for cell and organ metabolism. The maintenance of adequate nutrition is critical for preventing disease, and augmenting disease resolution. Unfortunately, there are times during a patient's disease course when enteral nutrition cannot be used or is ineffective. At this time, parenteral nutrition may be implemented to provide enough macro- and micronutrients to sustain life and aid in disease recovery.

Multiple reviews and meta-analyses demonstrate the benefits of enteral nutrition, when compared to parenteral nutrition. Patients receiving enteral nutrition have decreased infectious and noninfectious complications. Their cell-mediated immunity is improved and they experience less organ failure, improved wound healing, and nitrogen balance. Active use of the intestinal mucosa helps to preserve its integrity. With the early use of enteral nutrition, these patients have a reduced need for ventilatory support, decreased intensive care unit (ICU) and hospital lengths of stay.

Enteral nutrition also has complications associated with its use. Mechanical complications are the most common. The feeding tube can become obstructed, inhibiting the flow of nutrition. Infection, at the site of tube entry is a persistent risk. The patient can also have difficulties with electrolyte balance and adequate hydration. Patients receiving enteral nutrition may also experience gastroesophageal reflux, aspiration, refeeding syndrome, and diarrhea.

Despite these complications, enteral nutrition remains the nutritional method of choice. An absolute contraindication to enteral nutrition is mechanical obstruction. Relative contraindications include a the gastrointestinal tract unable to be used or inadequate for absorption. Additionally, clinicians may decide to use parenteral nutrition for convenience, ease of delivery, and perceived patient comfort. Common diseases that often require parenteral nutrition include cerebral palsy, multiple sclerosis, Crohn disease, congenital disorders, failure to thrive, and pancreatitis.

Once the decision is made to use parenteral nutrition, clinicians must continually review the patient's nutrition, infectious, and immune status, because complications are common. Infectious complications occur frequently

ⓒ 2008 by Lippincott Williams & Wilkins, a Wolters Kluwer business

and include catheter-related bloodstream infections and bacterial translocation of the nonfunctioning gut wall. In addition to becoming infected, the patient's catheter may become occluded due to a thrombus, a kink, or a precipitate. Patients may also exhibit metabolic disturbances, including elevated blood glucose levels and liver disease—mainly steatosis, steatohepatitis, cholestasis, and cirrhosis, the latter two of which are more common in children. Immune compromise and metabolic bone disease have also been seen in patients receiving parenteral nutrition. These complications contribute to an increased hospital length of stay.

Maintaining patients' nutritional status is critical to their overall health and to their disease process. The choice of enteral or parenteral nutrition should be carefully considered, taking into account the indications, benefits, and complications of both therapies. Parenteral nutrition is the preferred method to provide patient's with necessary substrate to meet metabolic needs during the course of illness and beyond.

SUGGESTED READINGS

DiBaise JK, Scolapio JS. Home parenteral and enteral nutrition. *Gastroenterol Clin North Am.* 2007:36:123–144.

Marik PE, Zaloga GP. Early enteral nutrition in acutely ill patients: a systematic review. *Crit Care Med.* 2001;29:2264–2270.

Peter JV, Moran JL, Phillips-Hughes J. A meta-analysis of treatment outcomes of early enteral versus early parenteral nutrition in hospitalized patients. *Crit Care Med.* 2005;33:213–220; discussion 260–261.

53

DO NOT MINIMIZE THE EFFECTS THAT DIET HAS ON METABOLISM

NICKIE NIFORATOS, MD

WHAT TO DO – INTERPRET THE DATA

Some diets are medications, too.

A clinician should never underestimate the role of diet in a child's health. A child's diet must meet basic metabolic functions but also provide adequate nutrition to allow for appropriate growth and development. A pediatrician's role is to ensure that the child's diet meets all metabolic and nutritional requirements in the prevention and management of disease, such as iron and vitamin D deficiencies. Diet, as source of treatment, is particularly important for a number of diseases, including phenylketonuria (PKU), epilepsy, diabetes, and renal disease.

Children with inborn errors of metabolism have unique metabolic and dietary requirements. A commonly screened inborn error of metabolism includes PKU. Patients with PKU lack the enzyme used to convert phenylalanine to tyrosine. As serum levels of phenylalanine rise, excessive levels of phenylalanine are transmitted across the blood–brain barrier, leading to deficiencies in the transfer of other essential amino acids. The resultant amino acid deficiencies lead to reduced neuronal protein and neurotransmitter synthesis, impaired brain development, and mental retardation. The mainstay of treatment for patients with PKU is diet; phenylalanine intake is limited with a low-protein diet, and a specific amino acid "cocktail" to provide sufficient amounts essential amino acids. In addition, patients with a metabolic disorder must be monitored for signs catabolism (e.g., intercurrent illness, overexertion, anorexia), as they promote the breakdown of internal protein stores, lead to toxic amounts of a specific substrate, like phenylalanine in PKU. Even a simple viral infection in patients with inborn errors of metabolism can lead to severe acidosis or hyperammonemia, which, in turn, can lead to coma or death. These patients should be treated aggressively at the first sign of illness to avoid (or treat) a metabolic crisis.

On the other end of the dietary protein-intake spectrum is the ketogenic diet, which encourages protein intake and limits carbohydrates. Ketogenic diets benefit patients with severe, refractory epilepsy, infantile spasms, or certain neurodegenerative disorders. Patients on ketogenic diets often require vitamin and mineral supplements, especially iron, calcium, and folic

ⓒ 2008 by Lippincott Williams & Wilkins, a Wolters Kluwer business

acid; however, vitamin supplements and medications cannot be placed in typical suspensions, which often contain a carbohydrate base. Be sure to prescribe all medications and supplements in the form of sugarfree drops or tabs.

Patients with diabetes mellitus must also pay close attention to their diet, in maintaining glycemic control. Using an insulin sliding scale in conjunction with carbohydrate counting leads to better glycemic control and the avoidance of both hypo- and hyperglycemia.

Renal disease is another condition that requires dietary modification. A high-protein diet can exacerbate uremia, a salt-losing nephropathy may require sodium supplementation, whereas comorbid hypertension may require sodium restriction. Vitamin D deficiency, due to renal disease, often leads to hyperphosphatemia and hypocalcemia and the need for dietary adjustments. Severe hyperkalemia may lead to fatal cardiac arrhythmias. Fluid retention may lead to ascites, pulmonary edema, or impaired cardiopulmonary function. Depending on the patient's unique fluid and electrolyte status, a renal diet must be individualized to each patient.

An inadequate diet may contribute to various diseases, as well. A low-iron diet in infancy may impair brain development. Anemia can result from a variety of dietary deficiencies, including iron deficiency, vitamin B_{12} deficiency, or folate deficiency. Infants who are exclusively breastfed, especially infants with darker skin and limited exposure to sunlight, may have inadequate vitamin D intake that can result in rickets.

Because of its importance in the maintenance of health and in the treatment of disease, a patient's diet should be monitored regularly to maximize health and to allow for early intervention should disease occur.

SUGGESTED READINGS

Goodman SI, Greene CL. Metabolic disorders of the newborn. *Pediatri Rev.* 1994;15(9): 359–365.

Haslam RH. Nonfebrile seizures. *Pediatr Rev.* 1997;18(2):39–49.

Kossof EH, Pyzik PL, McGrogan JR, et al. Efficacy of the ketogenic diet for infantile spasms. *Pediatrics.* 2002;109(5):780–783.

Weiss RA, Edelmann CM Jr. End-stage renal disease in children. *Pediatr Rev.* 1984;5(10):295–304.

54

ASSURE ADEQUATE PHOSPHATE LEVELS IN EXTREMELY MALNOURISHED PATIENTS BECAUSE THEY MAY EXHIBIT REFEEDING SYNDROME

CAROLINE RASSBACH, MD

WHAT TO DO – GATHER APPROPRIATE DATA

Patients with severe malnutrition may have a deficit of total body phosphate. Introduction of feeds can result in refeeding syndrome, characterized by life-threatening hypophosphatemia. Phosphate levels should be closely monitored and maintained during initial phases of refeeding.

The majority of the body's phosphate is stored in the form of adenosine triphosphate (ATP). Because phosphates are ubiquitous in foods, total body phosphate depletion occurs only in cases of severe malnutrition. Patients with severe malnutrition are more than 30% to 35% less than ideal body weight. In the pediatric population in the United States, anorexia nervosa and bulimia nervosa represent a large percentage of these cases. Children with chronic disease and those who are neglected or abused may also be affected.

Refeeding syndrome occurs because of rapid refeeding in a severely malnourished patient. Intravenous or enteral administration of carbohydrate stimulates insulin release by the pancreas, resulting in increased cellular uptake of glucose and phosphate, particularly in the liver and skeletal muscle. This acute shift of phosphate from the extracellular to the intracellular compartment in a patient with total body phosphate depletion results in acute hypophosphatemia. Refeeding syndrome can also cause hypoglycemia, hypokalemia, and hypomagnesemia by a similar mechanism. Fluid overload, edema, and gastrointestinal dysmotility also occur.

Clinical manifestations of hypophosphatemia include cardiac failure, neurologic abnormalities, and hemolytic anemia. Myocardial dysfunction has been attributed to impaired contractility from deficiency of ATP in myocardial cells. Hypophosphatemia may also cause arrhythmias, muscle weakness, rhabdomyolysis, and respiratory failure. Neurologic symptoms including encephalopathy, paresthesias, seizures, and coma can also occur.

Prevention of refeeding syndrome is extremely important. Feeds should be initiated slowly, with 1,000 to 1,600 kcal/day, and should be increased by 200 to 400 kcal/day. Phosphorus levels should be monitored daily for several

ⓒ 2008 by Lippincott Williams & Wilkins, a Wolters Kluwer business

days as feeds are advanced, and phosphorus supplements may be used either prophylactically or at the first sign of decreasing serum phosphorus levels. Oral supplements are generally safer than intravenous supplements; however, the latter are used for severe or clinically significant hypophosphatemia or in patients unable to take enteral supplements.

In patients with extreme malnutrition, phosphate levels should be monitored closely to prevent the life-threatening complications of refeeding syndrome. Feeds should be advanced slowly, and phosphorus supplements should be considered in patients at risk for the syndrome.

SUGGESTED READINGS

Fisher M. Treatment of eating disorders in children, adolescents, and young adults. *Pediatr Rev.* 2006;27(1):5–16.

Gaasbeek A, Meinders E. Hypophosphatemia: an update on its etiology and treatment. *Am J Med.* 2005;118(10):1094–1101.

Kellogg ND, Lukefahr JL. Criminally prosecuted cases of child starvation. *Pediatrics.* 2005;116(6):1309–1316.

55

AUSCULTATE THE CHEST WITH PATIENTS IN THE STANDING POSITION DURING PREPARTICIPATION EXAMINATIONS (PPES)

SONYA BURROUGHS, MD

WHAT TO DO – GATHER APPROPRIATE DATA

Preparticipation sports screening is an essential yet difficult tool used for athletic clearance. This purpose of the screening is to identify those at risk for sudden cardiac death and to enlist restrictions for those with known factors that predispose the athlete to sudden death. Despite its importance, the ability of this screening to identify those at risk varies and is questionable. The thoroughness and expertise of clinicians vary, and this factor understandably affects the screening process and overall findings. Only 3% of trained athletes who experienced sudden cardiac death were previously suspected of having a cardiovascular abnormality during the preparticipation sports exam. Thankfully, sudden cardiovascular death is a rare phenomenon, affecting 1 in 200,000 to 300,000 individual student athletes per academic year. The risk for sudden death in young athletes with cardiovascular disease is 2.5 times higher than in nonathletes. In the United States, sudden cardiac death most commonly occurs with basketball and football. Males account for 90% of the cases.

The medical history is the most important aspect of the cardiovascular PPE. It should focus on the presence of symptoms such as: near-syncope, syncope, dizziness, chest pain, chest tightness, and fatigue. Medication history, including questions regarding illicit and performance-enhancing drug use, is extremely important. The history should also elicit information concerning Kawasaki disease, rheumatic fever, myocarditis, arrhythmias, hypertension, congenital heart disease, and heart murmurs. A history of seizures or near-drowning may indicate long QT syndrome. Pertinent findings in the family history include: congenital heart disease, long QT syndrome, Marfan syndrome, and cardiomyopathy.

© 2008 by Lippincott Williams & Wilkins, a Wolters Kluwer business

> **TABLE 55.1 RED FLAGS IN THE HISTORY OR PHYSICAL EXAMINATION**
>
> - Syncope or near-syncope on exertion
> - Chest pain/discomfort on exertion
> - Palpitations at rest
> - Excessive shortness of breath or fatigue with activities
> - Family history of Marfan syndrome, cardiomyopathy, long QT syndrome, or clinically significant arrhythmias
> - Family history of premature, sudden death
> - Irregular heart rhythm
> - Weak or delayed femoral pulses
> - Fixed, split second heart sound
> - Any systolic murmur graded 3/6 or greater
> - Any diastolic murmur
> - Stigmata of Marfan syndrome
> - Chest pain in Turner syndrome

The physical exam of the PPE begins with the vital signs. Blood pressure and pulse must be compared with age-specific norms. If hypertension is present (blood pressure >90th percentile for age, height, and sex), a four-extremity blood pressure is warranted. The general examination should focus on looking for features suggestive of Marfan syndrome (pectus deformity, arm span greater than height, kyphoscoliosis, and arachnodactyly). When examining the heart, one should focus on heart sounds, and the presence of clicks and murmurs. The chest should be auscultated while the patient is standing and supine. The standing position accentuates the dynamic obstruction murmur of HCM. The abdominal exam should focus on detecting organomegaly, and femoral pulses must be assessed as a screening tool for aortic coarctation. *Table 55.1* provides several "red flags" for the preparticipation history and physical exam.

These flags should prompt a pediatric cardiology consultation. Approximately 75% of all sudden deaths are due to cardiovascular disease; HCM is the most common cause.

HCM has an autosomal dominant inheritance pattern, with a prevalence of approximately 0.2% of the general population. It is characterized by an asymmetrically thickened left ventricular wall (≥12 mm). It leads to impaired perfusion of the myocardium because of the thickened wall. Perfusion is worst with elevated heart rates. It is often clinically silent and presents with sudden cardiac death. Features that may raise suspicion for this condition include heart murmur, family history, abnormal electrocardiogram (ECG) tracing, or symptoms of left ventricular outflow obstruction. Other cardiac conditions leading to sudden death include congenital coronary artery anomalies, congenital long QT syndrome, Marfan syndrome,

TABLE 55.2	ABSOLUTE CONTRAINDICATIONS TO SPORTS PARTICIPATION

- Pulmonary vascular disease with cyanosis and large right-to-left shunt
- Severe pulmonary hypertension
- Severe aortic stenosis or regurgitation
- Severe mitral stenosis or regurgitation
- Cardiomyopathies
- Vascular form of Ehlers-Danlos syndrome
- Coronary anomalies of wrong sinus origin
- Catecholaminergic polymorphic ventricular tachycardia
- Acute phase of pericarditis
- Acute phase of myocarditis (at least 6 mo)
- Acute phase of Kawasaki disease (at least 8 wk)

mo, month; wk, week.

and commotio cordis. *Table 55.2* provides several absolute contraindications for sports participation.

SUGGESTED READINGS

Cava JR, Danduran MJ, Fedderly RT, et al. Exercise recommendations and risk factors for sudden cardiac death. *Pediatr Clin North Am.* 2004;51:1401–1420.

Singh A, Silberbach M. Consultation with the specialist: cardiovascular preparticipation sports screening. *Pediatr Rev.* 2006;27:418–424.

56

KNOW WHEN TO RESTRICT SPORTS PARTICIPATION FOR CHILDREN WITH CARDIAC DISEASE DUE TO AN INCREASED RISK OF SUDDEN DEATH

NAILAH COLEMAN, MD

WHAT TO DO – TAKE ACTION

Although rare, sudden cardiac death in children does occur, increasing in prevalence with age through adolescence. The risk of sudden cardiac death in children may be increased in those participating in strenuous activity due to an increase in the dynamic and static demands made on the cardiovascular system. Thus, it is important for pediatricians to recognize those children at risk for sudden cardiac death and to restrict potentially their sports activities.

Sudden cardiac arrest is defined as "the sudden cessation of cardiac activity so that the victim becomes unresponsive with no normal breathing and no signs of circulation." When it occurs in children, sudden cardiac arrest is usually caused by an inherited or congenital cardiac malformation (e.g., tetralogy of Fallot, transposition of the great arteries), an arrhythmia (e.g., Wolf-Parkinson-White [WPW] syndrome, long QT syndrome), an acute medical condition leading to inflammation of the heart (e.g., myocarditis), or to commotio cordis, a sudden impact to the chest that causes ventricular fibrillation or ventricular tachycardia. Regardless of the cause, sudden cardiac arrest should be treated with prompt cardiopulmonary resuscitation and activation of the emergency response system.

The initial determination of an athlete's cardiovascular readiness for sports play should occur with the preparticipation exam. A detailed history, including family history of cardiac events and early cardiac death; a review of systems, including a history of dizziness, chest pain, or other symptoms with exertion; vital signs, which may show hypertension or tachycardia; and a cardiac exam, which may demonstrate a heart murmur, can alert pediatricians to the presence of a cardiac abnormality that needs further analysis and complete or partial restriction from sporting activities. Should any concerns for cardiac disease be found in the preparticipation physical, the athlete should be referred to a cardiologist for a more thorough analysis.

Athletes with structural heart disease may be at increased risk of sudden cardiac death, depending on their primary cardiac lesion and on the success

© 2008 by Lippincott Williams & Wilkins, a Wolters Kluwer business

of their repair. Often these athletes, especially when unrepaired or with a suboptimal repair, are restricted to low-intensity activities that limit the dynamic and static stresses put on the cardiovascular system.

Cardiomyopathies, including restrictive, dilated, and hypertrophic cardiomyopathy, can lead to sudden cardiac death in the athlete, with hypertrophic cardiomyopathy leading the group. A family history of sudden death is extremely important to elicit in this group of patients. One also might find signs of left-sided ventricular hypertrophy with ST-T changes on the athlete's electrocardiogram. An echocardiogram should confirm the diagnosis and, depending on the patient's cardiac function, the athlete may be limited to low intensity activities or may be excluded from sports participation completely.

Myocarditis, acute or chronic, and often associated with a viral infection, can also lead to sudden cardiac death in athletes. These athletes may present with a fever due to the viral infection, persistent tachycardia, mild ventricular ectopy, decreased exercise tolerance, or congestive heart failure. Athletes with myocarditis should not participate in sports activities.

Coronary artery disease in children can also lead to sudden cardiac death. The most common congenital coronary artery anomaly leading to sudden cardiac death in children is anomalous left coronary artery (ALCA). Often, children with ALCA are asymptomatic until they participate in activities of exertion. Strenuous activity in these children can cause syncope, palpitations, or chest pain, secondary to decreased blood supply to the heart muscle itself and acute ischemia. The most common acquired coronary artery anomaly in children is coronary artery aneurysm from Kawasaki disease. The pediatric athlete with coronary artery disease may be limited to low intensity activities or may be excluded from sports participation completely.

Pediatric valvular heart disease (e.g., aortic stenosis and mitral valve prolapse) may also lead to sudden cardiac death. Early symptoms may include syncope, arrhythmia, dyspnea, and chest pain with exertion. An echocardiogram can determine the degree of cardiac deficiency related to the valvular problem. The restriction in sports activities in valvular heart disease depends on the severity of the aortic stenosis or mitral valve prolapse. Of note, mitral valve prolapse may be associated with Marfan syndrome or other connective tissue diseases, so athletes with these conditions should be given additional attention.

Primary arrhythmias that are not associated with a congenital cardiac malformation, including WPW, sick sinus syndrome, and complete atrioventricular block, rarely lead to sudden cardiac death. Should sudden cardiac death occur in these patients, it is usually due to ventricular fibrillation from an accessory pathway for WPW or to extreme bradycardia or atrial fibrillation for sick sinus syndrome. Presenting with syncope, patients with long

QT syndrome, however, are at increased risk of sudden cardiac death. Beta-blockers have been shown to decrease the risk of sudden cardiac death in patients with long QT syndrome. Patients with arrhythmias and without symptoms (e.g., chest pain, syncope) may participate fully in sporting activities; however, those with symptoms should be referred to a cardiologist for a more thorough analysis.

SUGGESTED READINGS

Batra AS, Hohn AR. Consultation with a specialist: palpitations, syncope, and sudden cardiac death in children: who's at risk? *Pediatr Rev.* 2003;24:269–275.

Committee on Sports Medicine and Fitness. American Academy of Pediatrics: Medical conditions affecting sports participation. *Pediatrics.* 2001;107:1205–1209.

Hazinski MF, Markenson D, Neish S, et al. and the American Heart Association Emergency Cardiovascular Care Committee. Response to cardiac arrest and selected life-threatening medical emergencies: the medical emergency response plan for schools. A statement for healthcare providers, policymakers, school administrators, and community leaders. *Pediatrics.* 2004; 113(1 Pt 1):155–168.

Metzl JD. Preparticipation examination of the adolescent athlete: part 2. *Pediatr. Rev.* 2000;22: 227–239.

57

RECOGNIZE THE FEMALE ATHLETE TRIAD

NAILAH COLEMAN, MD

WHAT TO DO – GATHER APPROPRIATE DATA

In the athletic world, as in other parts of general society, there are certain sports (e.g., cheerleading, figure skating, and rowing) where a slim build is not only desirable but beneficial to an athlete's performance or placement in a certain sporting category. Unfortunately, the attainment of a slim build often results in a trio of signs and symptoms known as the female athlete triad, comprised of disordered eating, menstrual dysfunction, and osteoporosis.

Disordered eating can take many forms, ranging from restricting food intake (e.g., anorexia) to binging or purging (e.g., bulimia) to taking medications to promote weight loss (e.g., laxatives, diuretics). Athletes will also partake in excessive exercising or wear rubber suits while exercising to increase their weight loss. All of these disordered eating practices can help contribute to the two remaining parts of the triad.

In general, menstrual dysfunction more commonly exists among female athletes, as opposed to nonathletic females. This menstrual dysfunction can take various forms, including amenorrhea, both primary and secondary; oligomenorrhea; and luteal phase deficiency. Primary amenorrhea is diagnosed when a female has had no menses by the age of 16 or has had no menses within 4.5 years of breast development. After having begun to menstruate, a female that has 3 to 6 consecutive months without a menses is said to have secondary amenorrhea. Oligomenorrhea denotes a cycle that exists >35 days in duration. Luteinizing hormone (LH) pulsatility is dependent on a female's energy reserve. If a female has increased expenditure with decreased energy intake, the energy deficiency causes abnormal LH pulsatility suppression and, menstrual irregularity.

Osteoporosis is defined as decreased bone mass due to premature bone loss or poor bone formation. In female athletes, this decreased bone mass is related to low estrogen levels. Ironically, certain sports that cause increased stress to certain bone groups may cause increased bone density in only those bone groups. For example, female gymnasts—at risk for the female athlete triad, due to the emphasis the sport puts on size and physique—may have increased lower extremity bone density, from the stress placed on the lower skeleton.

© 2008 by Lippincott Williams & Wilkins, a Wolters Kluwer business

Early recognition of the female athlete triad is critical to prevention of injury and short- and long-term sequelae. In the short term, using laxatives, diuretics, and rubber suits can result in dehydration and decreased performance. Long-term consequences of the female athlete triad can be functional, including decreased speed, endurance, and strength; and physiological, including electrolyte disturbances and end-organ dysfunction (e.g., cardiac and endocrine).

The preparticipation physical is the ideal time to probe for signs of the female athlete triad. In addition to obtaining a good history from the athlete, it is also important to listen to any concerns expressed by the athlete's parents, friends, and coaches. A thorough evaluation of the patient's menstrual dysfunction should include a pregnancy test and evaluation for other pathologic conditions, including hypothyroidism (thyroid-stimulating hormone), pituitary tumor (prolactin), or polycystic ovarian syndrome (pelvic exam, testosterone, LH, dehydroepiandrosterone sulfate [DHEA-S], and 17-hydroxyprogesterone). In addition, an evaluation of the patient's bone mineral density may be warranted.

After diagnosis, treatment of the female athlete triad often involves a multidisciplinary team of physicians, nutritionists, and mental health specialists. On occasion, however, an unaware female athlete may only need dietary education on her body's energy needs while playing her sport. Estrogen supplementation may be helpful for those with hypothalamic amenorrhea, restoring menstrual function and improving bone mineral density.

SUGGESTED READINGS

American Academy of Pediatrics. Committee on Sports Medicine and Fitness. Medical concerns in the female athlete. *Pediatrics.* 2000;106:610–613.

American Academy of Pediatrics. Committee on Sports Medicine and Fitness. Promotion of healthy weight-control practices in young athletes. *Pediatrics.* 1996;97:752–753.

58

KNOW HOW TO TREAT THE DIFFERENT TYPES OF LIGAMENTOUS INJURIES (SPRAINS, STRAINS, DISLOCATIONS, SUBLUXATIONS)

NAILAH COLEMAN, MD

WHAT TO DO – INTERPRET THE DATA

Over the past two decades, the rate of musculoskeletal sports injury, including soft tissue injury, in children has risen. This increase has also made it increasingly important that pediatricians be able to recognize and treat effectively soft tissue musculoskeletal injuries, including sprains, strains, subluxations, and dislocations.

To accurately diagnose a soft tissue musculoskeletal injury, one must be able to distinguish one injury type from another. Sprains are caused by the overstretching and partial tearing of a ligament. Excessive stretching of a muscle, resulting in pain and swelling, is a strain. A subluxation is the partial separation of a joint with some continued union between the two bones' articular cartilages. An example of a common subluxation in young children, often associated with a sudden pull to an outstretched arm, is the "nursemaid elbow." Complete separation of the articular cartilages of two bones in a joint is a dislocation, relatively uncommon in children and associated with major trauma and fractures.

In general, there are four phases of recovery for an athlete with soft tissue injury. The goal of the first phase is to limit additional injury and to control pain and swelling. The next phase begins the athlete's active rehabilitation with the gradual improvement in the strength and flexibility of the injured area. The third phase of rehabilitation progresses from the second, with the addition of proprioception and endurance training to the strength and flexibility work. This third phase will continue until the athlete has nearly regained his normal function. The fourth and last phase of rehabilitation begins at the athlete's return to his or her sport. Initial phases of rehabilitation should be supported with adequate analgesics, so as to avoid disuse during recovery. Attention should also be paid to the strength, flexibility, and fitness of noninjured areas during the athlete's rehabilitation, as well as to the athlete's general psyche. To avoid separation from his team, the athlete should be encouraged to attend games and practices with teammates.

The first phase of rehabilitation is commonly referred to as "RICE therapy": rest, ice, compression, and elevation. The "rest" for an athlete is

© 2008 by Lippincott Williams & Wilkins, a Wolters Kluwer business

the limitation of activity—to avoid any pain during or within 24 hours of the activity. Ice, placed in a plastic bag and applied directly to the skin for 20 minutes, comprises the next part of RICE therapy and will help not only to control the pain but to also control the swelling associated with the injury. Ice should be applied three to four times a day for the first 48 hours after injury and, at a minimum, daily afterwards, while swelling and/or pain persist. The next part of RICE therapy is compression, which involves the application of an elastic bandage—above and below the injury—to promote resorption of injury-related edema. If the compression bandage is applied too tightly, venous drainage may be impaired, so this should be avoided. For the last part of RICE therapy, the injured area should be kept elevated as much as possible, which will also help to decrease swelling.

Pediatric soft tissue musculoskeletal injury usually heals quickly, requiring little additional therapy and minimal immobilization. Often, soft tissue injuries in children require only the first phase of rehabilitation (i.e., RICE therapy), after which they can make a fairly rapid (within weeks) return to play.

SUGGESTED READINGS

Hergenroeder AC. Prevention of sports injuries. *Pediatrics.* 1998;101:1057–1063.
Huurman WW, Ginsburg GM. Musculoskeletal injury in children. *Pediatr Rev.* 1997;18:429–440.
Sachs HC. Dislocations. *Pediatr Rev.* 2000;21:433–434.

59

BE AWARE OF SUBSTANCE USE IN THE ATHLETE WHO IS ATTEMPTING TO ENHANCE PERFORMANCE

NAILAH COLEMAN, MD

WHAT TO DO – GATHER APPROPRIATE DATA

Athletes have been using performance-enhancing substances for as long as there has been athletic competition. In fact, the prevalence of the use of performance-enhancing substances has increased over time. Classified as supplements, prescriptions medications and banned/illicit substances, performance-enhancing substances have found their uses in the world of sports, for both theoretical and proven reasons.

Supplements can be packaged as such when sold as a beneficial supplement and not defined as a drug or proclaimed to treat a medical condition. Adolescent athletes most commonly utilize supplement performance-enhancing substances. Currently used supplements include creatine, androstenedione, antioxidants, and amino acids. Creatine, naturally found in the body and utilized for energy production via its conversion to phosphocreatine, has been used in the sporting world since 1992. The use of creatine in the adolescent population is increasing due to several potential reasons, including its claim as a "natural" supplement, its easy access on the Internet, and its routine use by collegiate and professional athletes. The premise behind its use is that the added creatine allows for more readily available aerobic energy and decreased use of anaerobic metabolism, as increased levels of phosphocreatine lead to increased conversion of adenosine diphosphate (ADP) to adenosine triphosphate ATP. Creatine, however, does not work without strength training, and its side-effect profile is still unknown at this time. Recent reports suggest a reversible renal dysfunction related to decreased glomerular filtration rate. Androstenedione, also available for use for some time, is believed to work as a precursor to testosterone; however, it remains on the supplement list due to lack of efficacy in clinical trials. Androstenedione use in a prepubertal athlete could, in theory, cause premature puberty or premature closure of the growth plates. Amino acid supplements are often used to achieve a positive nitrogen balance; antioxidants are used for their immunity-promoting properties.

© 2008 by Lippincott Williams & Wilkins, a Wolters Kluwer business

Prescription medications are obtained by a physician for a specific medical purpose but may also have beneficial effects with regards to sports participation when used at supratherapeutic doses or in healthy athletes. Beta-agonists, such as albuterol, have both anabolic and stimulating effects, and because of this, they have been banned from use by the International Olympic Committee, if used without a medical indication (e.g., bronchospasm). Other prescription medications that may have additional benefits in healthy athletes include narcotics, which, by decreasing pain, can increase an athlete's stamina and ability; beta-blockers, which, when used in sports that require accuracy (e.g., archery), can decrease anxiety; and diuretics, which can be used to alter one's form (e.g., in body-building) and to dilute one's urine (e.g., for drug testing).

Banned/illicit substances are those that are either banned by athletic competition governing boards or declared illegal by law. Some banned/illicit substances may also be supplements and/or prescription medications. Most of the banned/illicit substances are anabolic steroids and their derivatives or other hormones and hormone analogs. Steroids, increasingly used by adolescent athletes, are used for their anabolic and/or anticatabolic effects. Anabolic steroids are purported to increase muscle mass and strength and to decrease recovery time. Unlike many supplements, steroids have a well-defined side-effect profile, including acne, hirsutism, hypertension, psychosis, premature closure of the growth plates, and decreased sexual function. In addition, anabolic steroid use in adolescents had been linked to other illicit substance abuse in adolescents. Commonly used androgenic compounds include anti-estrogens, which inhibit the conversion of androgens to estrogen, and dehydroepiandrosterone (DHEA), a precursor to androgens and utilized for their androgenic effect. Additional banned/illicit substances include stimulants, such as caffeine and ephedra, which are used to increase one's endurance and to increase fatty acid breakdown, and "blood doping," such as nontherapeutic transfusions or erythropoietin, which is also used to improve one's endurance. The ideal time to screen for the use of performance enhancing substances is at the preparticipation exam. A detailed history with pointed, but nonjudgmental, questions should be used to elicit an athlete's use of performance enhancing substances. Questions should focus on the use of any substance, including vitamins, herbs, and minerals, to help with sports competitions, workouts, or one's general appearance. Appropriate screening and diagnosis could then help to keep our young athletes safe and competing well into the future.

SUGGESTED READINGS

American Academy of Pediatrics. Committee on Sports Medicine and Fitness. Adolescents and anabolic steroids: a subject review. *Pediatrics.* 1997;99:904–908.

Koch JJ. Performance-enhancing: substances and their use among adolescent athletes. *Pediatr Rev.* 2002;23(9):310–317.

Metzl JD, Small E, Levine SR, et al. Creatinine use among young athletes. *Pediatrics.* 2001;108: 421–425.

60

AVOID BETA BLOCKERS FOR PATIENTS WITH ASTHMA OR OTHER OBSTRUCTIVE AIRWAY DISEASE

LINDSEY ALBRECHT, MD

WHAT TO DO – INTERPRET THE DATA, MAKE A DECISION, TAKE ACTION

Hypertension in childhood is defined as a systolic blood pressure and/or diastolic blood pressure greater than the 95th percentile for age, gender, and height on multiple occasions. In the past decade, the detection and management of pediatric hypertension has evolved, partly because normative data has become available and the long-term consequences have been more clearly elucidated. Additionally, given the increasing incidence of childhood obesity and the association with elevated blood pressure, hypertension is being recognized as a major health issue in the pediatric population. Although lifestyle modification plays an important role in pediatric hypertension, medical management is often required.

Pharmacologic therapy should be initiated when lifestyle modification fails or in the presence of secondary hypertension, symptomatic hypertension, or end organ damage (often left ventricular hypertrophy). To begin, single drug therapy is recommended. When initiated, treatment may be with angiotensin-converting enzyme (ACE) inhibitors, angiotensin receptor blockers, calcium channel blockers, beta blockers, or diuretics. Specific classes of medication are used preferentially in certain disease states; for example, ACE inhibitors have been shown to be efficacious in preventing disease progression in children with proteinuric renal disease.

Beta-receptor antagonist drugs, or beta blockers, work by competitively reducing receptor occupancy by catecholamines and other beta agonists. Because catecholamines have positive inotropic and chronotropic effects on the heart, beta blockade leads to a reduction in heart rate and a reduction in myocardial contractility. Beta-2 receptor blockade leads initially to increased peripheral vascular resistance, but with chronic use, the resistance returns

© 2008 by Lippincott Williams & Wilkins, a Wolters Kluwer business

to normal. Beta blockers do not reduce blood pressure in normotensive individuals but do reduce blood pressure in hypertensive ones. In children, they are safe and effective.

Patients with asthma or underlying airway disease may suffer an increase in airway resistance or bronchoconstriction following treatment with beta blockers. Bronchoconstriction occurs because beta-2 receptor blockade in bronchial smooth muscle leads to smooth muscle contraction. This affect may be subtle, with mild symptoms including wheezing or dyspnea on exertion, but may be life-threatening. More severe bronchoconstriction does not seem to occur in individuals without underlying pulmonary disease. Because of this, nonselective beta blockers (those with no preference for the cardiac or beta-1 subtype of beta receptors), such as propranolol, are contraindicated in children with asthma. Some beta receptor antagonists, such as metoprolol and atenolol, are designed to selectively work on beta-1 receptors, and these medications are considered to be less likely to cause pulmonary side effects. However, because even the selective forms have some affinity for the beta-2 receptors, they should be used with caution in asthmatics and others with obstructive airway disease.

Hypertension in the pediatric population is an increasingly recognized problem. Pharmacologic therapy is often required, and when needed, the patient's underlying health should be taken into consideration. In particular, beta blocker use in asthmatics and others with pulmonary disease may have severe consequences related to a potential for bronchoconstriction.

SUGGESTED READINGS

Flynn JT, Daniels SR. Pharmacologic treatment of hypertension in children and adolescents. *J Pediatr.* 2006;149(6):746–754.

National High Blood Pressure Education Program Working Group on High Blood Pressure in Children and Adolescents. The fourth report on the diagnosis, evaluation, and treatment of high blood pressure in children and adolescents. *Pediatrics.* 2004;114(2 Suppl 4th Report):555–576.

61

ALWAYS CALCULATE THE DOSE OF
MEDICATIONS YOURSELF

MICHAEL S. POTTER, NICKIE NIFORATOS, MD,
HEIDI HERRERA, MD AND ANTHONY SLONIM, MD

WHAT TO DO – TAKE ACTION

Medication errors are a major patient safety problem for children and physicians have a role in their prevention.

Medical errors represent a major public health problem in the United States, and medication errors represent an important subset with specific challenges for providing safe care for children. Medication errors lead to prolonged hospitalizations, unnecessary evaluations and treatments, and occasionally death. Pediatric patients are particularly vulnerable to these errors since dosages are prescribed based upon the child's weight or body surface area (*Fig. 61.1*). Children also cannot intercept errors like adults can, and the pharmacokinetics of certain drugs are age-dependent and require alterations in prescribing (*Fig. 61.1*).

To combat these sources of prescribing error, physicians should always make a point of performing medication calculations themselves, making use of computerized calculations and other decision support tools, such as reference texts and ordering outlines, that help to provide appropriate reference material at the point of calculating and prescribing.

Documentation of the formula used and the actual calculations is helpful, because calculation errors can be detected more effectively.

Wt: 13 kg
Allergies: none
Erythromycin 150 mg (12 mg/kg/dose) PO every 6 hours

In addition to recognizing calculation errors with this type of documentation, dosage errors can also be identified. In the example above, a therapeutic dose of erythromycin to treat an acute infection is 50 mg/kg/day; however, the use of erythromycin as a prokinetic agent is dosed at 20 mg/kg/day. A number of sources are available to help the physician confirm the dose of a medication, including *The Harriet Lane Handbook* and personal digital assistant (PDA) programs, such as Epocrates.

© 2008 by Lippincott Williams & Wilkins, a Wolters Kluwer business

- Different and changing pharmacokinetic parameters between patients at various ages and stages of maturational development.
- Need for calculation of individualized doses based on the patient's age, weight (mg/kg), body surface area (mg/m^2), and clinical condition.
- Lack of available dosage forms and concentrations appropriate for administration to neonates, infants, and children. Frequently, dosage formulations are extemporaneously compounded and lack stability, compatibility, or bioavailability data.
- Need of precise dose measurement and appropriate drug delivery systems.
- Lack of published information or Food and Drug Administration-approved labeling regarding dosing, pharmacokinetics, safety, efficacy, and clinical use of drugs in the pediatric population.

FIGURE 61.1. Factors Placing Pediatric Patients at Increased Risk for Adverse Drug Reactions (From Levine SR, Cohen MR, Blanchard NR, et al. Guidelines for preventing medication errors in pediatrics. *J Pediatr Pharmacol Ther*. 2001;6: 426–442).

Many hospitals have initiated computerized provider order entry programs (CPOE) to help standardize medication prescribing. These systems allow the medications to be ordered with a weight-based dose (i.e., mg/kg) and also allow the program to perform the appropriate calculation. Although these systems provide important safety nets, particularly in preventing errors caused by difficult-to-read penmanship, these programs are not foolproof and require a number of precautions. If the CPOE system prompts the user with common doses, the physician must select the appropriate dose for the desired effect. For example, in ordering ceftriaxone, there may be an automatic prompt for 50 mg/kg intravenous (IV) daily; however, if treating a patient for meningitis, the physician must recognize that the meningitic doses of the antibiotic is 50 mg/kg/dose IV twice a day (BID).

Whether a physician is using a CPOE system or paper-and-pen prescriptions, a number of additional safety measures should be considered for calculating medication doses. A physician must recognize if the per-kilogram dosage, when calculated, exceeds the total daily dose. Adult medication doses have been calculated on the average ideal body weight of 60 to 75 kg. Generally, a pediatric patient weighing >60 kg is prescribed medications on adult-dose regimens, rather than a per-kilogram regimen; however, almost all medications have a recommended total daily dose, which may be reached even in children weighing <60 kg. To illustrate this point, consider the treatment of meningitis in a 45-kg patient. The maximum dose of ceftriaxone is 4 g per 24 hours, so this child should be given the antibiotic according to the total daily dose (2,000 mg BID) rather than the calculated dose (50 mg/kg BID, which would be 2,250 mg BID).

The route of administration and the route of excretion also play significant roles in determining medication doses. Generally speaking, the bioavailability of a medication is greater when administered parenterally (i.e., IV) than enterally (i.e., by mouth [PO]). Often, the difference is small and PO/IV doses are the same; however, in cases where there is a significant difference in bioavailability, the doses differ based on route of administration. For example, an initial dose of labetalol is 2 mg/kg/dose when given orally, but only 0.2 mg/kg/dose, when given intravenously, a 10-fold difference in dosage. The route of excretion is most pertinent to patients with impaired renal or hepatic function. In patients with renal failure, medications can be adjusted by either increasing the interval of administration (i.e., from every 4 hours to every 8 hours) or by decreasing the dose amount (i.e., from 4 mg/kg to 2 mg/kg). Dose adjustments are less common in liver failure. Rather than changing the drug dose, the drug choice is given greater attention to preserve function; for example, using nonsteroidal anti-inflammatory drugs rather than acetaminophen to pain or fever.

Drug form (tab vs. suspension) is also pertinent in medication orders. In these instances, the conversion from drug dose (i.e., mg) to drug volume (i.e., mL) must also be considered and calculated correctly. For example, amoxicillin suspensions can be made in the following concentrations: 200 mg/5 mL or 400 mg/5 mL. A patient prescribed 400 mg of amoxicillin will be instructed to take 10 mL of the first suspension but only 5 mL of the second.

Many mistakes can be made in calculating doses in routine medication orders. To minimize mistakes, the provider should always have access to a drug reference guide, calculate doses themselves, and consider the treatment strategy, including what is being treated and what is the therapeutic goal.

SUGGESTED READINGS

Kumm S. University of Kansas School of Nursing. *Basic Drug Calculations Review.* Available at: http://classes.kumc.edu/son/nurs420/clinical/basic_review.htm. Accessed July 27, 2007.
Levine SR, Cohen MR, Blanchard NR, et al. Guidelines for preventing medication errors in pediatrics. *J Pediatr Pharmacol Ther.* 2001;6:426–442.

62

AVOID PHENYTOIN SUSPENSION IN PATIENTS WITH FEEDING TUBES

JOHN T. BERGER, III, MD

WHAT TO DO – MAKE A DECISION, TAKE ACTION

Phenytoin is an important medication for the treatment of primary and secondary generalized tonic–clonic seizures, partial seizures, and status epilepticus. Consistent serum concentrations of phenytoin are essential for maintaining effective seizure control. Phenytoin, however, has several properties including nonlinear pharmacokinetics, a narrow therapeutic window, and uneven absorption that pose challenges for maintaining steady serum concentrations. Consistent administration and formulation will reduce the variability.

Phenytoin's metabolism has nonlinear (Michaelis-Menten) kinetics. At low serum concentrations, a fixed percentage of drug is metabolized in a given time (first-order kinetics). At higher serum levels (at the high end of the normal therapeutic range), a fixed amount of drug is metabolized per unit time (zero-order kinetics), because the metabolic pathways are saturated. Consequently, when serum levels are high, even a small dose increase may produce a very big increase in serum levels. Additionally, factors such as hepatic dysfunction and fever can alter phenytoin clearance. Phenytoin interacts with many drugs, which may increase or decrease concentrations of it or other concomitantly used anticonvulsants.

The administration of phenytoin suspension in conjunction with enteral nutrition through nasogastric (NG) feeding tubes has been associated with erratic phenytoin absorption, subtherapeutic concentrations, and breakthrough seizures. Postulated mechanisms include chelation to proteins and electrolytes in the enteral feeding, binding to NG tubing, and alterations in gastrointestinal pH, resulting in precipitation of phenytoin. If possible, continuous NG feeds should be held for 2 hours before and 2 hours after phenytoin administration to avoid decreased serum levels. The suspension should be diluted and the nasogastric tube should be thoroughly irrigated after administration.

Phenytoin suspension is reported to settle and result in uneven drug distribution and subsequently variability in drug delivery. The only study to address the question showed that even poorly shaken suspensions maintained uniform concentrations for up to 4 weeks. More important to variable

© 2008 by Lippincott Williams & Wilkins, a Wolters Kluwer business

dosing may be inaccurate measuring of the concentrated suspension, as small variations in volume may produce a large change given phenytoin's pharmacokinetics. Parents should be instructed not only to shake the suspension prior to each dose but also to measure carefully. Commercially available brand and generic phenytoin products may differ in phenytoin content and other formulation characteristics that can affect bioavailability. These differences may occasionally result in an increase or decrease in serum phenytoin levels, which in turn might adversely affect seizure control or cause toxicity when patients are switched from one preparation to another. Additional serum monitoring is warranted when substituting new formulations of phenytoin.

SUGGESTED READINGS

Bader MK. Case study of two methods for enteral phenytoin administration. *J NeurosciNurs.* 1993;25(4):233–242.

Sarkar MA, Garnett WR, Karnes HT. The effects of storage and shaking on the settling properties of phenytoin suspension. *Neurology.* 1989;39(2 Pt 1):207–209.

Soryal I, Richens A. Bioavailability and dissolution of proprietary and generic formulations of phenytoin. *J Neurol Neurosurg Psychiatry.* 1992;55(8):688–691.

63

GIVE KETAMINE IN PATIENTS WITH SIGNIFICANT CARDIAC DISEASE OR SEPSIS

RUSSELL CROSS, MD

WHAT TO DO – MAKE A DECISION, TAKE ACTION

Ketamine is a direct-acting anesthetic that is widely used in pediatric practice because of its dissociative properties and perceived beneficial cardiovascular effects. It is frequently used in the emergency department setting for minor procedures and is used in other areas for induction of anesthesia. Most other sedative and anesthetic agents result in some degree of cardiovascular depression in the form of hypotension, bradycardia, or direct negative inotropic effects. Ketamine, in contrast, typically causes an increase in heart rate, systemic blood pressure, and systemic vascular resistance. These effects result partially from inhibition of catecholamine reuptake, but also from direct sympathetic stimulation, resulting in increased release of catecholamines. Various studies have shown that ketamine can have either a negative or positive inotropic effect on cardiac function, with the overall effect being dosage dependent but generally negative. Because of these somewhat unpredictable cardiovascular effects, ketamine must be used with caution in certain situations, especially when patients are catecholamine depleted.

Ketamine should be used cautiously in patients who are critically ill or who are acutely traumatized. In these clinical settings, the patient may be effectively catecholamine depleted and unable to mount a sympathetic response to counteract the negative inotropic effect of ketamine. This combination could result in cardiovascular collapse in patients who are septic or otherwise critically ill. Similarly, ketamine should be avoided in patients with limited myocardial reserve or congestive heart failure. These patients may similarly be catecholamine depleted and unable to increase sympathetic tone. Alternatively, those patients who can mount a sympathetic response may have a reduced cardiac output resulting from increased afterload in the setting of a failing myocardium with limited reserve.

Ketamine should, likewise, be avoided in patients who cannot otherwise tolerate an increased afterload, such as those patients with significant pre-existing hypertension or those at risk for myocardial ischemia. Ketamine has also been shown to increase both intracranial and intraocular pressure, so it should be used cautiously in patients who have a space-occupying central

© 2008 by Lippincott Williams & Wilkins, a Wolters Kluwer business

nervous system lesion or who are at risk for increased intracranial or intraocular pressures.

SUGGESTED READINGS

Bovill JG. Intravenous anesthesia for the patient with left ventricular dysfunction. *Semin Cardiothorac Vascu Anesth.* 2006;10(1):43–48.

Sprung J, Schuetz SM, Stewart RW, et al. Effects of ketamine on the contractility of failing and nonfailing human heart muscles in vitro. *Anesthesiology.* 1998;88(5):1202–1210.

Waxman K, Shoemaker WC, Lippmann M. Cardiovascular effects of anesthetic induction with ketamine. *Anesthes Analg.* 1980;59(5):355–358.

64

PHENYTOIN GIVEN PERIPHERALLY IS CAUSTIC AND CAN DAMAGE PERIPHERAL VEINS, IT IS ALSO ARRHYTHMOGENIC. FOSPHENYTOIN IS A VERY SAFE ALTERNATIVE

DAVID STOCKWELL, MD

WHAT TO DO — MAKE A DECISION

Phenytoin is one of the most useful anticonvulsant medications available for the pediatric practitioner. Although benzodiazepines are typically the first-line therapy in an emergent situation, use of phenytoin or fosphenytoin is valuable for treating most types of seizure disorders and status epilepticus, with the exception of absence seizures.

Phenytoin's mechanism of action is by blocking voltage-sensitive sodium channels in neurons, leading to decreased neuronal electrical recovery. Its administration can cause occasional serious adverse effects, including impairment of myocardial contractility, dysrhythmias, hypotension, and cardiac arrest, as well as the less serious but concerning adverse local effects, including phlebitis, purple glove syndrome, and tissue necrosis.

The parenteral form of phenytoin is dissolved in 40% propylene glycol and 10% ethanol and adjusted to a pH of 12; sodium hydroxide is added to maintain solubility. Extravasation of the solution may cause skin irritation or phlebitis. Therefore, it is recommended that intravenous (IV) phenytoin be given via central venous access. Phenytoin administered intravenously at a rate >50 mg/min may cause hypotension and arrhythmias. These complications are believed to be secondary to the diluent, propylene glycol.

Historically, this preparation was the only form of phenytoin available. The pro-drug fosphenytoin was approved by the U.S. Food and Drug Administration (FDA) as an alternative IV as well as intramuscular (IM) preparation. The advantages are that this preparation can be given peripherally and has a smaller side effect profile than the standard form of phenytoin.

Fosphenytoin, the disodium phosphate ester of phenytoin, is a parenteral phenytoin pro-drug that is rapidly converted to phenytoin by blood and tissue phosphatases after IV and IM injection. Many of the adverse local and systemic effects with IV administration of phenytoin occur much less frequently with administration of fosphenytoin. Fosphenytoin, which is more water soluble, does not contain the same diluents and its pH is more neutral. Although fosphenytoin appears to have a better safety profile than

© 2008 by Lippincott Williams & Wilkins, a Wolters Kluwer business

IV-administered phenytoin, it costs considerably more than either IV or oral phenytoin preparations.

Dosing of fosphenytoin is performed by using "phenytoin equivalents." Therefore, the dosing is identical to phenytoin.

SUGGESTED READINGS

ACEP Clinical Policies Committee; Clinical Policies Subcommittee on Seizures. Clinical policy: Critical issues in the evaluation and management of adult patients presenting to the emergency department with seizures. *Ann Emerg Med.* 2004;43(5):605–625.

Browne TR, Kugler AR, Eldon MA. Pharmacology and pharmacokinetics of fosphenytoin. *Neurology.* 1996;46(Suppl 1):S3–7.

Leppik IE, Boucher BA, Wilder BJ, et al. Pharmacokinetics and safety of a phenytoin prodrug given i.v. or i.m. in patients. *Neurology.* 1990;40:456–460.

65

BE SELECTIVE IN YOUR CHOICE OF NEUROMUSCULAR BLOCKER, DEPENDING ON THE PATIENT'S UNDERLYING ORGAN FUNCTION

RENÉE ROBERTS, MD

WHAT TO DO – INTERPRET THE DATA

When choosing a neuromuscular blocker for intubation, one should take into account how long the procedure will be, how long the patient is expected to remain intubated in the recovery room or intensive care unit, and the patient's underlying physiologic status. The presence of underlying organ dysfunction, particularly hepatic and renal systems, can affect the metabolism and excretion of these drugs and lead to a longer half-life and duration of action.

In patients with hepatic failure, depending on the nondepolarizing neuromuscular blocker used, the initial dose required may be larger due to an increase in the volume of distribution but the amount used to redose will be lower due to a reduction in plasma clearance. Pancuronium is metabolized to a limited degree by the liver and its effects will be moderately prolonged in liver failure. Vecuronium is excreted by the biliary system but its duration of action is modestly prolonged by liver failure when used in standard doses. Similarly, rocuronium's duration of action is modestly prolonged in severe liver disease. Cisatracurium is a good choice is liver failure because its metabolism and elimination are *independent* of liver dysfunction. However, do not limit yourself to cisatracurium when choosing a neuromuscular blocker (NMB) for patients with liver failure. Cisatracurium's duration of action may be least affected by liver failure but takes 2 minutes to provide good intubation conditions, which is longer than rocuronium, so consider both the onset and duration of action when choosing a nondepolarizing NMB.

When choosing a NMB for patients with chronic renal failure, one must consider when the last dialysis was performed to ascertain volume status. In addition, a serum potassium level, preferably within the past 24 hours, is an essential laboratory value to determine prior to surgery to determine if anesthesia can be safely induced and if succinylcholine is an option during intubation. An intubation dose of succinylcholine will raise the serum potassium by 0.5 mEq/L. Other electrolyte abnormalities are also important. For example, magnesium prolongs the duration of nondepolarizing NMB by

© 2008 by Lippincott Williams & Wilkins, a Wolters Kluwer business

competing with calcium at the prejunctional sites. Although some studies have shown it can reduce the onset of action of pancuronium, magnesium is not used in standard practice as an adjunct to NMB. Pancuronium's long duration of action will increase in patients with renal failure, because pancuronium is primarily excreted by the kidneys. Vecuronium's duration of action will also be prolonged; however, it depends only secondarily on renal excretion, which makes it an acceptable choice but a rarely used alternative. Rocuronium is eliminated slightly by the kidneys, so its duration of action will not be significantly prolonged by renal dysfunction. Of the nondepolarizing NMB, cisatracurium will provide the most predictable neuromuscular blockade because its metabolism is least dependent on renal function. In fact, cisatracurium undergoes degradation in the plasma by organ-independent Hoffman elimination. However, as in patients with liver dysfunction, if a rapid sequence intubation is required, succinylcholine or rocuronium are more appropriate choices.

The studies on the affect of acid–base balance and NMB have primarily investigated pancuronium and vecuronium because these are some of the oldest and most widely established nondepolarizing NMBs. Acidemia prolongs the duration of a nondepolarizing NMB, whereas alkalemia will shorten it. Some explanations include the effect of pH on the binding of vecuronium on acetylcholine receptors, the effect of intracellular Ca^{2+} on the neuromuscular junction, and the effect of pH on blood flow to the muscle. For practical purposes, however, the intubation and maintenance doses will remain the same.

When in doubt, before redosing a NMB, monitor the neuromuscular function with a peripheral nerve stimulator. Common sites to test include the ulnar nerve and the facial nerve. If there are no twitches on the Train-of-four, do not redose. Also, if you suspect that the NMB is lasting longer than predicted, be sure that the patient is receiving adequate sedation and analgesia to cover the period of neuromuscular blockade.

SUGGESTED READINGS

Fawcett WJ, Haxby EJ, Male DA. Magnesium: physiology and pharmacology. *Br J Anaesth.* 1999;83:302–320.

Khuenl-Brady KS, Pomaroli A, Pühringer F, et al. The use of rocuronium (ORG 9426) in patients with chronic renal failure. *Anaesthesia.* 1993;48(10):873–875.

Morgan GE, Mikhail MS, Murray MJ, et al. *Clinical Anesthesiology.* 3rd ed. New York: McGraw-Hill; 2002:954–959.

Yamauchi M, Takahashi H, Iwasaki H, et al. Respiratory acidosis prolongs, while alkalosis shortens, the duration and recovery time of vecuronium in humans. *J Clinic Anesth.* 2002;14(2):98–101.

66

RECOGNIZE TRICYCLIC ANTIDEPRESSANT (TCA) TOXICITY AND MANAGE IT AGGRESSIVELY

HEIDI HERRERA, MD

WHAT TO DO – INTERPRET THE DATA

Although selective serotonin reuptake inhibitors are more popular, TCAs are still commonly prescribed in the treatment of enuresis, obsessive-compulsive disorder, and attention-deficit-hyperactivity disorders in children. These drugs are well-absorbed orally and are metabolized by the liver. TCA toxicity occurs by the following mechanisms: inhibiting norepinephrine and serotonin reuptake at the nerve terminals, creating anticholinergic blockade, directing α-adrenergic blockage, and blocking the cardiac myocytes fast sodium channels. The latter mechanism is a hallmark of TCA toxicity because it slows down phase zero of the action potential depolarization, and causes a widened QRS complex on the electrocardiogram (EKG).

Exposure to TCA dosages >5 mg/kg tend to be symptomatic and >15 mg/kg lethal. Early toxicity may present with signs and symptoms of anticholinergic toxidromes and central nervous system (CNS) involvement. The former include mydriasis, flushing, dry mouth, urinary incontinence, diminished bowel activity, hyperthermia, tachycardia; and the latter demonstrates mental status changes, confusion, hallucinations, and delirium. Mortality is attributed to cardiovascular collapse and CNS toxicity, including seizure and coma. CNS toxicity can be attributed partially to inhibition of the chloride ionophore on the γ-aminobutyric acid channel complex. In general, seizures are usually generalized and self-limited in nature. Signs of significant toxicity can be expected within 6 hours of ingestion.

EKG findings can help to confirm TCA toxicity in the pediatric population. Signs include sinus tachycardia, ventricular dysrhythmias, heart block, widening QRS and QTc intervals, and an R wave >3 mm in lead aVR. A

© 2008 by Lippincott Williams & Wilkins, a Wolters Kluwer business

QRS duration of >100 ms is a marker of toxicity, including hypotension, coma, and airway instability.

The management of TCA toxicity includes aggressive airway protection and hemodynamic support. Patients should be placed on a continuous cardiac monitor, with adequate intravenous access, and supplemental oxygen. For neurologic deterioration with mental status changes, patients should be intubated and mechanically ventilated. Seizures can be treated with benzodiazepines. Barbiturates should be avoided due to potential hypotension. Phenytoin is not recommended for seizure control because it induces ventricular dysrhythmias in animal models. For TCA-induced cardiotoxity, widening QRS complex >100 ms, ventricular dysrhythmias, and hypotension, the first line of therapy is alkalinization with sodium bicarbonate. Starting with an IV bolus dose of 1 to 2 mEq/kg in children is appropriate, with a goal of keeping serum pH >7.5. The patient should also be monitored for hypokalemia. Antidysrhythmic medications, classes IA and IC, are contraindicated for potential of TCA-induced cardiotoxicity. Dopamine and norepinephrine may be used to overcome the α-blockade-induced hypotension. Physostigmine is contraindicated because it leads to seizures and dysrhythmias.

In general, patients with accidental ingestion of TCAs who are asymptomatic may be observed in the emergency department for 6 hours after ingestion. If no evidence of toxicity is observed, the child may be discharged home. If symptomatic, the patient should be appropriately assessed and treated as discussed above.

SUGGESTED READINGS

Henry K, Harris CR. Deadly ingestions. *Pediatr Clin North Am.* 2006;53:293–315.
Michael JB, Sztajnkrycer MD. Deadly pediatric poisons: nine common agents that kill at low doses. *Emerg Med Clin North Am.* 2004;22:1019–1050.

67

Do not give charcoal for iron, alcohol, or lithium ingestions — it is ineffective

Craig DeWolfe, MD

What to Do — Interpret the Data, Make a Decision, Take Action

Activated charcoal is the best proven technique for eliminating most toxic ingestions. Charcoal's large surface area adsorbs poisons and reduces the amount of free agent available for absorption by means of van der Waals forces and covalent binding. Up to 75% of the toxin may be eliminated when a dose of 1 g of charcoal per kg is given in the first hour of ingestion and repeated every 4 hours as needed. It is especially effective in enhancing the elimination of theophylline, phenobarbital, and carbamazepine, as it can decrease the reabsorption of these drugs as they move through the gut during enterohepatic recirculation, but charcoal is not indicated in all ingestions. It should be used based only on its efficacy for a specific toxin, the toxicity of the ingestion, the elapsed time from ingestion, and individual patient characteristics such as their cooperation, level of consciousness, and presence of vomiting.

There are several significant risks associated with charcoal administration. If it is vomited, which occurs in 15% of treated patients, and then aspirated, it can result in pneumothorax, empyema, pulmonary parenchymal injury, or bronchiolitis obliterans. If charcoal is inadvertently instilled in the lungs through a misplaced orogastric or nasogastric tube, it can result in death.

Importantly, charcoal is ineffective in adsorbing or eliminating alcohols, hydrocarbons, metals, and minerals. Specifically, it should not be used to treat iron, alcohol, lithium, or magnesium ingestions, as the risk far exceeds any benefit. In fact, during the period of 1995 to 1998, more children died from the administration of activated charcoal than the ingestion of alcohol, lithium, or magnesium. Only iron was associated with more deaths.

Although the evidence is limited due to the lack of clinical trials and the limits of case reports and animal and human volunteer models, there are techniques available to reduce the toxicity of iron, alcohol, and lithium overdoses. Treatment may include any combination of supportive care, whole-bowel

© 2008 by Lippincott Williams & Wilkins, a Wolters Kluwer business

irrigation, chelation agents, and hemodialysis. In any ingestion, consult the poison control center for specific recommendations.

Lithium toxicity may occur with acute, acute on chronic, or chronic ingestions. The patient may present with gastrointestinal symptoms before tissue distribution causes other central nervous system symptoms. Manifestations include tremor, clonus, agitation, lethargy, delirium, seizures, coma, myocardial dysfunction, and arrhythmia. If ingestion is suspected, a blood lithium level should be assessed on presentation and 2 hours later to evaluate for increasing levels. Whole-bowel irrigation is the treatment of choice, as charcoal is ineffective. Large volumes of polyethylene glycol electrolyte solution should be administered until the rectal effluent is clear. Often a nasogastric tube needs to be placed, the head of bed positioned at 45 degrees to decrease the likelihood of vomiting and aspiration, and the airway protected in patients with a depressed level of consciousness. In patients who have renal dysfunction, severe neurologic dysfunction, and lithium concentrations ≥4 mEq/L in an acute ingestion or ≥2.5 mEq/L in a chronic ingestion, hemodialysis should be considered. Redistribution between intra- and extracellular compartments necessitates repeated and prolonged dialysis sessions.

Acute iron poisonings are one of the most common pediatric ingestions and are associated with the greatest risk of death. Throughout the 1980s and 1990s, iron ingestions accounted for 2% of the total number of poisonings in the United States. Toxic ingestions of 20 mg/kg of elemental iron are associated with direct corrosive injury to the gastrointestinal mucosa and are commonly associated with fluid and blood losses leading to shock. Ingestions >60 mg/kg of elemental iron often lead to hepatotoxicity, metabolic acidosis, coagulopathy, and cardiovascular collapse. If syrup of ipecac is available at home, the patient may benefit from its use on the way to the emergency department (ED). In the ED, the patient should be treated with fluids and cardiovascular care. To determine the extent of poisoning, the clinician should obtain iron levels in addition to blood gases, electrolytes, liver function tests, and coagulation studies. Plain abdominal films should be obtained to evaluate for radiopaque iron particles, which may be treated with cathartics and whole-bowel irrigation. Finally, for iron levels >500 μg/dL or for evidence of systemic toxicity with lower iron levels, deferoxamine is the iron-chelating agent of choice. The intravenous route of deferoxamine is preferred and is generally dosed at 15 mg/kg/hour over 8 to 24 hours, depending on the extent of toxicity.

Children can ingest excessive alcohol form beverages, elixirs, and personal care products, such as mouthwash and aftershave. Manifestations include hypoglycemia, central nervous system depression, respiratory depression, hypotension, and death. The health care provider should evaluate the patient with a measurement of serum electrolytes, glucose, and a blood ethanol level, in addition to a more broad-spectrum drug screen in appropriate circumstances. Management is primarily supportive. The clinician should provide parenteral fluids while correcting any hypoglycemia and electrolyte disruptions. Airway management is important in the obtunded patient with emesis or in a patient with respiratory depression.

In summary, activated charcoal is an important and useful agent in the treatment of most toxic ingestions. Alcohol, hydrocarbon, metal, and mineral ingestions are an important exception to this rule and will not benefit from charcoal administration. Rather, toxin-specific treatments are indicated with the guidance of a toxicologist or poison control center.

SUGGESTED READINGS

McGuigan MA. Acute iron poisoning. *Pediatr. Ann.* 1996;25:33–38.
McGuigan ME. Poisoning potpourri. *Pediatr Rev.* 2001;22:295–302.
Shannon M. Primary care: ingestion of toxic substances by children. *N Engl J Med.* 2000;342:186–191.
Zimmerman JL. Poisonings and overdoses in the intensive care unit: general and specific management issues. *Crit Care Med.* 2003;31:2794–2801.

68

KNOW THAT DIGOXIN HAS A NARROW THERAPEUTIC WINDOW WITH SEVERAL COMPLICATIONS AND TOXICITIES

MINDY DICKERMAN, MD

WHAT TO DO – INTERPRET THE DATA, TAKE ACTION

Obtaining digoxin levels in specific circumstances can be lifesaving.

Digoxin is the most widely used cardiac glycoside. These agents inhibit the sodium-potassium-adenosine triphosphate (Na^+-K^+ATPase) pump and, therefore, block active transport of Na^+ and K^+ across cell membranes. Increased intracellular Na^+ reduces the transmembrane Na^+ gradient and subsequently increases activity of the Na^+-Ca^+ exchanger, which causes intracellular calcium to rise. It is this increased intracellular Ca^+ that augments myofibril activity in cardiac myocytes, causing a positive inotropic action and therefore is used for treatment of congestive heart failure. Digoxin is also used to slow the ventricular rate in certain tachyarrhythmias.

Digoxin can cause toxicity by increasing vagal tone that may lead to direct atrioventricular depression and arrhythmias. Clinically, a patient may present with acute or chronic digoxin toxicity. There are several dysrhythmias that can result, most commonly frequent premature ventricular beats. Bidirectional ventricular tachycardia is specific for digoxin toxicity but is rarely seen. Noncardiac symptoms of toxicity may include anorexia, nausea, vomiting headache, fatigue, depression, dizziness, confusion, memory loss, delirium, and hallucinations. Visual disturbances, specifically xanthopsia, seeing yellow halos around objects, have been reported. Vague symptoms can lead to a misdiagnosis of viral syndrome, so a high degree of suspicion must be maintained. Chronic toxicity may lead to renal failure.

Digoxin toxicity can occur if a condition or medication changes the metabolism or excretion of the drug. This can happen if a patient is in renal failure. Some of the medications that can affect digoxin metabolism include quinidine, cyclosporine, verapamil, tetracycline, erythromycin, and rifampin.

If you suspect your patient has digoxin toxicity, immediately place the patient on a cardiac monitor. Bradycardia is the most common vital sign change. If stable, these patients should have an electrocardiogram performed and a chemistry and digoxin level drawn. Hyperkalemia will usually be seen

© 2008 by Lippincott Williams & Wilkins, a Wolters Kluwer business

in acute toxicity due to the inhibition of the Na^+-K^+-ATPase and a resultant rise in extracellular K^+. Hyperkalemia may not be seen in chronic digoxin toxicity because the kidneys had time to compensate or the patient is on diuretics that promote potassium excretion.

Serum digoxin levels need to be interpreted with caution. High levels do not always indicate toxicity. In the case of an acute exposure, digoxin will slowly redistribute into the tissues after it is absorbed in the plasma. False-positive results may occur in the presence of digoxin, such as immunoreactive substances, which can be seen in neonates, pregnancy, and other disease states. Therapeutic levels in children are reported between 0.5 and 2.0 ng/mL. Levels >10 ng/mL may be associated with significant toxicity and treatment with digoxin-specific Fab should be considered.

If a patient with digoxin toxicity has cardiac dysrhythmias with hemodynamic instability, Fab fragments are first-line therapy Digoxin-specific Fab fragments are antibody fragments produced by enzymatic cleavage of sheep immunoglobulin G antibodies to digoxin. Several antiarrhythmics have been used to treat digoxin toxicity associated dysrhythmias. Antiarrhythmics that depress atrioventricular nodal conduction are contraindicated because they can worsen cardiac toxicity. If there has been an acute ingestion within 6 to 8 hours, charcoal can be administered for gastrointestinal decontamination. Intravenous potassium and magnesium may be beneficial in patients with chronic digoxin toxicity. Calcium and beta blockers should be avoided. Electrical cardioversion should be performed with extreme caution and as a last resort.

SUGGESTED READINGS

Antman EM, Wenger TL, Butler VP Jr, et al. Treatment of 150 cases of life-threatening digitalis intoxication with digoxin-specific Fab antibody fragments. Final report of a multicenter study. *Circulation.* 1990;81:1744–1752.

Morris SA, Hatcher HF, Reddy DK. Digoxin therapy for heart failure: an update. *Am Fam Physician.* 2006;74:613–618.

69

THE MOST EFFICIENT PARENTERAL CHELATING AGENT FOR LEAD IS CALCIUM DISODIUM ETHYLENE DIAMINE TETRAACETIC ACID

MINDY DICKERMAN, MD

WHAT TO DO – GATHER APPROPRIATE DATA, INTERPRET THE DATA

Severe lead toxicity is defined as a venous blood lead level ≥ 70 μg/dL, or having symptoms of encephalopathy. It is a medical emergency even if the child is asymptomatic. Parenteral chelating agents are the mainstay of therapy for these children and can be lifesaving. In 1950, calcium disodium ethylene diamine tetraacetate (CaNa2EDTA) was found to be clinically useful as a chelating agent in the treatment of lead poisoning. Similar to dimercaprol, also known as British Anti-Lewisite or BAL, CaNa2EDTA increases the urinary excretion of lead through the formation of nonionizing soluble chelate. CaNa2EDTA has very low bioavailability orally and treatment necessitates hospitalization and parenteral administration.

The appropriate protocol for administration of CaNa2EDTA is controversial. Its use may cause increased lead concentration in the central nervous system and subsequent increased intracranial pressure. Therefore, CaNa2EDTA is recommended only after administered of dimercaprol. CaNa2 EDTA can be administered 4 hours after the first dose of dimercaprol and once urine output is established. CaNa2EDTA can be administered intravenously or intramuscularly. The intravenous route is usually preferred because it is less painful than the intramuscular route and it permits continuous chelation. However, the intramuscular route should be used in patients with acute encephalopathy. In addition to the possible elevation in intracranial pressure, the major side effects of CaNa2EDTA include local reactions at the injection site, fever, hypercalcemia, the excretion of other essential minerals, and renal dysfunction. The renal dysfunction can manifest as rising blood urea nitrogen, proteinuria, or hematuria. There has been a case report describing the effectiveness of intraperitoneal CaNa2EDTA therapy in patients with renal failure requiring chelation therapy. The use of disodium salt alone (Na2EDTA), as opposed to calcium disodium salt (CaNa2EDTA), is crucial because it may result in severe hypocalcemia and possible death.

© 2008 by Lippincott Williams & Wilkins, a Wolters Kluwer business

The hepatic and renal function of the patient must be observed during chelation therapy. This includes regular monitoring of transaminases, electrolytes, blood urea nitrogen, creatinine, and renal analyses. CaNa2EDTA should be temporarily discontinued if the patient becomes anuric although dimercaprol should be continued. It is also necessary during treatment to monitor for arrhythmias by continuous electrocardiogram monitoring and have frequent neurologic assessments.

These chelating agents are very effective at removing lead from the blood, soft tissues, and the brain and, therefore, can reverse acute encephalopathy, anemia, and renal insufficiency caused by lead intoxication. The effect of using dimercaprol and CaNa2EDTA together were found in the 1960s to reduce the mortality secondary to severe lead intoxication from 66% to about 2%. In contrast to the effects chelation has on mortality and acute symptoms, this therapy does not affect the neurologic sequelae of chronic lead toxicity.

SUGGESTED READINGS

Committee on Drugs. Treatment guidelines for lead exposure in children. *Pediatrics.* 1995;96 (1 Pt 1):155–160.

Dietrich KN, Ware JH, Salganik M, et al. Effect of chelation therapy on the neuropsychological and behavioral development of lead-exposed children after school entry. *Pediatrics.* 2004;114:19–26.

Markowitz ME, Bijur PE, Ruff H, et al. Effects of calcium disodium versenate (CaNa2EDTA) chelation on moderate childhood lead poisoning. *Pediatrics.* 1993;92:265–271.

70

KNOW WHAT TO DO FOR THE EMERGENT RECOGNITION AND TREATMENT OF DESIGNER DRUG OVERDOSE

NAILAH COLEMAN, MD

WHAT TO DO – INTERPRET THE DATA, MAKE A DECISION, TAKE ACTION

Although alcohol and marijuana are the most common drugs of abuse by adolescents, there is another class of drugs being used by this age group with increasing frequency, known as "club drugs." Named after the locations of their frequent use (night clubs and raves), club drugs range from stimulants to depressants to hallucinogens.

Commonly used club drug stimulants include 3, 4-methylenedioxy-methamphetamine (MDMA), also known as ecstasy, XTC, and X; and methamphetamine, also known as speed, crank, and crystal. MDMA, a selective serotonergic neurotoxin taken orally, also has hallucinogenic properties. Its effects can be felt within 30 minutes of ingestion and last for up to 8 hours. An overdose could result in sympathetic hyperactivity, abnormal behavior, and fever, which is the main source of the more serious complications, including acute renal failure, seizures, and coma. Management of MDMA overdose includes a cooling blanket for hyperthermia, adequate control of hypertension, and benzodiazepines for agitation and seizures.

Methamphetamine, the N-methyl homolog of amphetamine, acts by increasing the release of and inhibiting the breakdown of catecholamines. It can be smoked, snorted, injected, or taken orally, and its rate of effect is directly related to its method of intake. The side effects of methamphetamine relate to its stimulant effect on peripheral alpha- and beta-receptors and include fever, tachypnea, hypertension, insomnia, anorexia, paranoia, and psychosis. Management of amphetamine overdose includes a cooling blanket for hyperthermia, adequate control of hypertension, and haloperidol for the psychosis.

Ketamine, gamma-hydroxybutyrate (GHB), and flunitrazepam comprise the commonly used club drug depressants. Flunitrazepam—whose

© 2008 by Lippincott Williams & Wilkins, a Wolters Kluwer business

brand name is Rohypnol and whose street names include roofies, Mexican valium, and the forget-me-pill—has the same anxiolytic, sedative, and antiepileptic effects as other benzodiazepines. Because it is a depressant, its side effects include hypotension, drowsiness, confusion, and dizziness. Due to its disinhibitive and amnestic effects, flunitrazepam is also known as a "date rape" drug.

GHB, another central nervous system depressant, is also called liquid ecstasy, soap, and goop. Available in multiple forms, including liquid, powder, and tablet, it can be easily made at home with instructions from the Internet. With its effects of euphoria and intoxication, it has also gained the classification as a "date rape" drug. Adverse effects can range from drowsiness and nausea to respiratory depression, seizure, and coma. Fortunately, GHB has a short duration of effect, with an onset of action of 10 to 20 minutes and a total effect time of up to 4 hours.

With its induction of dreamlike states, ketamine also falls within the depressant and "date rape" drug category. Also known as special K, vitamin K, and cat valium, ketamine can cause amnesia at lower doses and depression, hypertension, and respiratory depression at higher doses.

Club drug hallucinogens, in addition to MDMA, include d-lysergic acid (or lysergic acid diethylamide, LSD) and phencyclidine (PCP). LSD, derived from morning glory seeds, may also be called acid, dotes, and sugar. In addition to the hallucinations for which it is known, LSD can also engender a feeling of euphoria. Management of a negative LSD reaction includes a calm interaction with the patient as well as haloperidol for extreme reactions and seizures.

Phencyclidine, also known as angel dust, supergrass, and wack, produces its hallucinogenic effects by inhibiting the reuptake of catecholamines. Severe adverse effects of PCP include hypertension, hypotension, hypothermia, seizures, and delirium. Management of a negative PCP reaction includes putting the patient in a calm, dark, padded room while the drug effects dissipate. Haloperidol and diazepam can be used to treat the seizures and the delirium.

SUGGESTED READINGS

Greydanus DE, Patel DR. Substance abuse in adolescents: a complex conundrum for the clinician. *Pediatr Clin North Am.* 2003;50:1179–1223.
Rimsza ME, Moses KS. Substance abuse on the college campus. *Pediatr Clin North Am.* 2005;52:307–319.

71

WHEN CHILDREN OR ADOLESCENTS PRESENT WITH A CHANGE IN MENTAL STATUS, RESPIRATORY DEPRESSION, GASTROINTESTINAL COMPLICATIONS, OR PANCREATITIS, CONSIDER ALCOHOL ABUSE AS AN UNDERLYING CAUSE

MICHAEL S. POTTER AND ANTHONY SLONIM, MD

WHAT TO DO - GATHER APPROPRIATE DATA, INTERPRET THE DATA

Alcohol abuse is becoming more and more prevalent in the pediatric population, and children are being introduced to alcohol at younger ages than before. Approximately 40% of nonautomotive accidental deaths are attributed to alcohol abuse, and alcohol, as a legal drug, contributes to more deaths in young people than all illegal drugs combined. Therefore, pediatricians need to be familiar with the effects of alcohol overdose syndrome and the complications of chronic exposure.

Because alcohol depresses the central nervous system, euphoria, grogginess, talkativeness, impaired short-term memory, and an increased pain threshold are commonly exhibited in patients suffering from alcohol overdoses. Respiratory depression can occur if serum levels are significant. Furthermore, alcohol inhibits the normal operation of the pituitary antidiuretic hormone. When alcohol is consumed in a large quantity at one time, gastrointestinal complications are not uncommon. Acute erosive gastritis is the most common of these complications, and it manifests itself as epigastric pain, anorexia, vomiting, and guaiac-positive stools. Be aware, however, that vomiting and midabdominal pain can also be the result of acute alcoholic pancreatitis. If elevated serum amylase and lipase levels are detected, then a diagnosis of acute alcoholic pancreatitis becomes more likely.

There are also social manifestations associated with alcohol overdose, and although it is not common for younger adolescents to become alcoholics, if the following social symptoms are observed, then the patient should be considered as having an impairment from alcohol: having been drunk several times in a single year, having problems with school authorities and the police, having problems with peers, having been criticized about drinking habits by members of the opposite sex, and having driven while drunk.

© 2008 by Lippincott Williams & Wilkins, a Wolters Kluwer business

Diagnostically, children are three to four times as likely to develop an alcohol-related disorder if their parents are alcoholics. If children present with disorientation, lethargy, or coma, then alcohol overdose syndrome should be suspected. The smell of alcohol can be helpful for making a positive diagnosis, but blood tests can confirm the diagnosis. Although in most jurisdictions a serum level >80 to 100 mg/dL corresponds to intoxication, serum levels >200 mg/dL pose a significant risk of death, and levels >500 mg/dL, are generally fatal.

The primary mechanism of death by alcohol overdose is respiratory depression. Therefore, ventilatory support is essential while the liver works to eliminate alcohol from the body. Approximately 20 hours is required to reduce the blood-alcohol level from 400 mg/dL to 0 mg/dL in nonalcoholic patients. If the patient has a blood level >400 mg/dL, dialysis may be warranted.

When consumed in moderation by adults, alcohol represents negligible health risks. However, children metabolize this drug differently than adults and may lack the appropriate social and developmental attributes to manage their behavioral changes, effectively leading to both physical and social complications or abuse.

SUGGESTED READING

Jenkins RR. Substance Abuse. In: Behrman RE, Kliegman RM, Jenson HB. *Nelson Textbook of Pediatrics*. 17th ed. Philadelphia: Saunders; 2004, pages 653–61.

72

BE AWARE OF THE POTENTIAL FOR OPIATE (HEROIN) DRUG ABUSE IN ADOLESCENTS

MICHAEL S. POTTER AND ANTHONY SLONIM, MD

WHAT TO DO - GATHER APPROPRIATE DATA

Heroin use in the United States has seen a steady decline since the 1980s and is less of a concern today than it has been in past decades. Unfortunately, it is important for pediatricians to be familiar with the manifestations and management of heroin abuse if it presents in their patients.

Depending on the route of delivery, heroin's affects on the body will be different. Heroin induces euphoria, blunts pain, and results in pinpoint pupils. A lowered body temperature is suggested as a sign of heroin's affect on the hypothalamus. Vasodilation is a major cardiovascular manifestation, and alveolar hypoventilation is a characteristic of respiratory depression. "Track marks," which are hypertrophic linear scars that follow the course of large veins, are a frequently occurring dermatologic lesion associated with chronic heroin use; however, more easily overlooked are the smaller peripheral scars that occur from injection into smaller veins. If injected subcutaneously, heroin causes fat necrosis, lipodystrophy, and atrophy. Not surprisingly, abscesses secondary to unsterile drug administration techniques are a common occurrence. In addition, endocarditis with *Staphylococcus aureus*, cerebral microabscesses, and viral infections with hepatitis B and human immunodeficiency virus can all result from unsterile drug administration. Although its cause is unknown, a loss of libido is also a characteristic of heroin use. Addicted children may often find themselves in difficult circumstances to support a drug habit and prostitution is not an uncommon means of supporting these addictions. Constipation results from decreased smooth muscle propulsive contractions and increased anal sphincter tone. Finally, abnormal serologic reactions are frequent with heroin abuse, which include false-positive Venereal Disease Research Laboratory (VDRL) and latex fixation tests.

After approximately 8 hours without the use of heroin, a withdrawal syndrome begins in chronic users, which is characterized by a period of physiologic disequilibrium for a period of 24 to 36 hours. Early signs of this syndrome include yawning, lacrimation, mydriasis, inability to sleep, voluntary muscle cramping, diarrhea, tachycardia, and systolic hypertension. In rare cases, the patient may experience seizures. Methadone and diazepam are both safe medications to assist with the detoxification from heroin.

© 2008 by Lippincott Williams & Wilkins, a Wolters Kluwer business

A heroin overdose is an acute reaction that may lead to death if not managed appropriately in drug users. Stupor, coma, seizures, respiratory distress, cyanosis, and pulmonary edema are common signs of overdose. Naloxone, an opiate antagonist, can be administered intravenously to assist with managing the heroin toxicity. Treatment for heroin overdose includes supporting the airway, breathing, and circulation. Naloxone can be administered by intravenous infusion.

The danger of heroin overdose, although considerably less frequent than 20 years ago, is still a threat to pediatric patients. Peer and social pressures can make illicit drug use seem more appealing to adolescents, and pediatricians should be adequately prepared to handle acute and chronic drug abuse problems in their patients.

SUGGESTED READING

Jenkins RR. Substance Abuse. In: Behrman RE, Kliegman RM, Jenson HB. *Nelson Textbook of Pediatrics.* 17th ed. Philadelphia: Saunders; 2004, pages 653–61.

73

BECAUSE THE CLASSIC SIGNS AND SYMPTOMS OF THE APPENDICITIS ARE NOT ALWAYS PRESENT IN CHILDREN, THE PROVIDER MUST HAVE A HIGH INDEX OF SUSPICION FOR THIS CONDITION

MICHAEL CLEMMENS, MD

WHAT TO DO – GATHER APPROPRIATE DATA

Ultrasound and computerized tomography (CT) may provide additional information.

Acute appendicitis is the most common cause of emergency abdominal surgery in children. It occurs throughout childhood but is most common during the second decade of life. Appendicitis occurs infrequently in children younger than 2 years of age. Diagnosis and surgical intervention before perforation is the most important determinant of a good clinical outcome.

Appendicitis develops when the lumen of the appendix is obstructed by a fecalith, food, lymphoid tissue, or tumor. Obstruction leads to bacterial overgrowth and inflammation of the appendiceal wall. Perforation is common after 48 hours and very common after 72 hours. Rupture of the appendix is followed in most instances by generalized peritonitis from contamination with fecal bacterial flora.

Presenting symptoms vary with age. Early diagnosis is especially difficult in children who are younger than 4 years of age. For many reasons, the appendix may already be ruptured at the time most infants and toddlers present for care. These young children may not be able to complain of pain and often present with symptoms suggestive of acute gastroenteritis, such as vomiting and irritability. In addition, the disease may evolve more quickly in this age group. Children of preschool and school age typically present with fever, abdominal pain, and vomiting. Anorexia is almost always present. Older school-aged children and teenagers are more likely to localize their pain to the right lower quadrant.

The examination of the abdomen in a child with symptoms of appendicitis is a challenge for even the experienced clinician. Care should be taken to make the child as calm and comfortable as possible. Warm hands and a slow, gentle approach are helpful. Flexing the child's knees to relax the abdominal muscles may aid the examination. Distracting the child with conversation or a story may serve to minimize voluntary guarding. The examiner

© 2008 by Lippincott Williams & Wilkins, a Wolters Kluwer business

should watch the child's face for signs of discomfort while gently palpating the abdomen.

Classic findings of right lower quadrant tenderness are difficult to elicit in the child younger than 2 years of age. More often, there is diffuse abdominal tenderness and distension. The child may appear systemically ill. The presence of fever is variable. Guarding, generalized or focal tenderness, and rebound may all be present. On occasion, a mass is felt. Older children are more likely to show findings localized to the right lower quadrant.

The triad of fever, vomiting, and abdominal tenderness should always raise the suspicion of appendicitis. Supportive lab findings include a leukocytosis with a left shift, and an elevated C-reactive protein. The presence of ketones and an elevated urine specific gravity are usually noted. Pyuria may be seen. Postmenarchal girls should have a pregnancy test to rule out potential complications from pregnancy and to guide further treatment if positive.

When the diagnosis of appendicitis is clear, immediate surgical consultation is in order. In other instances an ultrasound or CT scan of the abdomen and pelvis should be ordered. Ultrasound is sensitive and specific, but accuracy is dependent upon the skill of the technician and radiologist. CT with oral and intravenous contrast is very accurate. Radiation exposure, however, is significant. CT of the abdomen and pelvis exposes the child to the same amount of radiation as 100 to 250 chest x-rays. CT should, therefore, be used judiciously, and radiation doses should be reduced when scanning children when possible.

Preoperative care includes intravenous hydration and pain control. Appropriate doses of narcotic analgesics do not mask the significant physical findings of acute appendicitis. Antibiotics should be administered if perforation is likely or confirmed.

SUGGESTED READINGS

Alloo J, Gerstle T, Shilyansky J, et al. Appendicitis in children less than 3 years of age: a 28-year review. *Pediatr Surg Int.* 2004;19:777–779.

Kwok MY, Kim MK, Gorelick MH. Evidence-based approach to the diagnosis of appendicitis in children. *Pediatr Emerg Care.* 2004;20:690–698.

Paulson EK, Kalady MF, Pappas TN. Clinical practice. Suspected appendicitis. *N Engl J Med.* 2003;348:236–242.

Rothrock SG, Pagane J. Acute appendicitis in children: emergency department diagnosis and management. *Ann Emerg Med.* 2000;36:39–51.

74

DO NOT MISS THE DIAGNOSIS OF SEPSIS OR PNEUMONIA IN A PATIENT WITH SICKLE CELL DISEASE AND FEVER

EMILY RIEHM MEIER, MD

WHAT TO DO – INTERPRET THE DATA

Sickle cell anemia (SCD) is a chronic hemolytic anemia affecting 1 in 400 African Americans in the United States. End-organ damage from the persistent anemia and vaso-occlusion from irreversibly sickled cells has been well documented. One of the earliest organs affected is the spleen, placing children with SCD at increased risk for overwhelming bacterial sepsis. Patients with SCD also have poor opsonization of encapsulated organisms, related to decreased serum concentrations of opsonic antibodies. Asplenic patients require higher concentrations of antibody to effectively eliminate organisms, placing SCD patients at even higher risk for sepsis.

Streptococcus pneumoniae is the most common cause of sepsis in SCD patients. Early detection with newborn screening programs, allowing for early institution of penicillin prophylaxis, and widespread availability of immunizations against pneumococcus and *Haemophilus influenzae* type b have dramatically reduced the incidence of bacterial sepsis. Nonetheless, SCD patients with fever demand special consideration and treatment to prevent adverse clinical outcomes.

With the development of third-generation cephalosporins, most febrile SCD patients can now be managed as outpatients. However, certain patients are considered high risk and continue to require inpatient admission. The presenting signs and symptoms, coupled with diagnostic studies can help to determine if a patient is standard or high risk. Each febrile sickle cell patient should have a thorough history and physical examination performed. Blood cultures, urinalysis, complete blood count with white blood cell (WBC) differential and reticulocyte count should be obtained. All patients, even those without respiratory signs or symptoms, should have a chest radiograph (CXR). Patients are considered high risk if they are ill-appearing, had a fever $\geq 40^\circ$C, WBC >30,000/μL or <5,000/μL, a new pulmonary infiltrate on CXR, history of pneumococcal sepsis, penicillin noncompliant, platelet count <100,000/μL, rapidly enlarging spleen, or younger than age 1 year. High-risk patients need to be admitted to the hospital for intravenous antibiotics and observation for at least 48 hours. Standard-risk patients can

ⓒ 2008 by Lippincott Williams & Wilkins, a Wolters Kluwer business

safely receive 50 to 75 mg/kg of ceftriaxone and be discharged home. These patients need to return the next day to receive a second dose of ceftriaxone.

Pneumonia in a sickle cell patient can lead to acute chest syndrome (ACS), defined as a new pulmonary infiltrate on CXR accompanied by fever, chest pain, tachypnea, or hypoxia. ACS is the leading cause of death in sickle cell patients and requires aggressive treatment to prevent serious sequelae. One recent study found that 60% of pulmonary infiltrates found in febrile sickle cell patients were not suspected by the treating clinician. This study failed to demonstrate a constellation of symptoms to accurately predict new pulmonary infiltrates in febrile SCD patients. Therefore, all patients should have a CXR as part of the diagnostic workup.

SUGGESTED READINGS

Morris C, Vichinsky E, Styles L. Clinician assessment for acute chest syndrome in febrile patients with sickle cell disease: is it accurate enough? *Ann Emerg Med.* 1999;34:64–69.

West DC, Andrada E, Azari R, et al. Predictors of bacteremia in febrile children with sickle cell disease. *J Pediatr Hematol Oncol.* 2002;24:279–283.

Wilimas JA, Flynn PM, Harris S, et al. A randomized study of outpatient treatment with ceftriaxone for selected febrile children with sickle cell disease. *N Engl J Med.* 1993;329:472–476.

75

FEEL FOR LOWER EXTREMITY PULSES IN TRAUMA PATIENTS

RUSSELL CROSS, MD

WHAT TO DO – GATHER APPROPRIATE DATA

A trauma evaluation requires a complete and thorough examination beyond the ABCs of resuscitation. Secondary assessment includes careful examination of distal pulses. Absent lower extremity pulses could indicate aortic injury, vascular trauma from an adjacent fracture, or extremity compartment syndrome.

Patients with blunt aortic injury may show signs such as upper extremity hypertension, diminished femoral pulses ("pseudocoarctation"), and an intrascapular murmur. The presence of all three are distinctly uncommon, and diminished femoral pulses in a patient with history of blunt chest trauma or motor vehicle accident should always alert one to think of hidden aortic injury. Dissection should be suspected in any patient with a widened mediastinum on chest radiograph although a normal x-ray does not rule out an injury. Further imaging for dissection includes computed tomography scan or transesophageal echocardiogram.

Blunt aortic injury as part of blunt chest trauma, is responsible for 10% to 15% of motor vehicle-related deaths. It is a lethal injury that provides the surgeon with a small window of opportunity for effective surgical intervention. This window is often missed because the injury may be asymptomatic initially, followed later by catastrophic bleeding or other complications. In more than half the cases, the involved aortic segment is the proximal descending aorta just distal to the origin of the left subclavian artery. Less common is involvement of the aortic arch, the distal thoracic aorta at the diaphragm, or multiple sites.

The classic mechanism of blunt aortic injury is sudden deceleration during a frontal-impact motor vehicle collision or a fall from height; however, the possibility of blunt aortic injury should be considered in all victims of motor vehicle collision, regardless of the point of impact. The dominant pathophysiologic event in blunt aortic injury is sudden deceleration with creation of a shear force between a relatively mobile part of the thoracic aorta and an adjacent fixed segment. The three major points of fixation are the atrial attachments of the pulmonary veins and vena cava, the ligamentum arteriosum, and the diaphragm. The resulting tear may involve either part

© 2008 by Lippincott Williams & Wilkins, a Wolters Kluwer business

of the aortic wall or may be a full-thickness disruption that is contained by periadventitial and surrounding tissues.

Careful serial physical examination along with a high degree of clinical suspicion is needed to diagnose acute compartment syndrome. Absence of distal pulse along with pain out of proportion usually is diagnostic, although the presence of distal pulses cannot exclude the diagnosis of compartment syndrome.

Compartment syndromes in the lower extremity are often caused by open and closed fractures associated with arterial injury, gunshot wounds, extravasation at venous and arterial access sites, limb compression, burns, constrictive dressings, and tight casts. The rapid diagnosis and management of compartment syndrome is paramount to achieving a successful clinical outcome.

The common cause of compartment syndrome in an extremity is muscle edema, resulting from direct trauma to the extremity that causes an increase in compartment pressure, preventing venous outflow, causing backflow congestion, and worsening the cycle of increasing pressure and muscle ischemia. When there is a long bone fracture, the situation is exacerbated by fracture bleeding, which produces a space-occupying hematoma. Reducing the fracture increases the compartment pressures secondary to a decrease in the volume of the osseofascial space. External compressive casts or bandages further reduce the ability of the compartment to expand.

SUGGESTED READINGS

Fabian TC, Richardson JD, Croce MA, et al. Prospective study of blunt aortic injury: Multi-center Trial of the American Association for the Surgery of Trauma. *J Trauma.* 1997;42: 374–383.

Mattox KL. Red River anthology. *J Trauma.* 1997;42:353–368.

Whitesides TE, Heckman MM. Acute compartment syndrome: update on diagnosis and treatment. *J Am Acad Orthop Surg.* 1996;4:209–218.

76

DO NOT ASSUME THAT A NEGATIVE DRUG SCREEN MEANS THAT NO DRUGS OF ABUSE WERE USED. MANY DRUGS OF ABUSE ARE NOT IDENTIFIED ON STANDARD URINE DRUG SCREENING SAMPLES

MICHAEL S. POTTER AND ANTHONY SLONIM, MD

WHAT TO DO – INTERPRET THE DATA

Like all diagnostic tests, it should not be assumed that a negative drug screen indicates with perfect accuracy that no illicit drugs have been used by the patient. Although rapid urine drug tests allow the quick detection of a wide variety of drugs, there are other factors to consider when interpreting the results of these tests. General urine drug tests should only be used as an initial screening mechanism for determining whether a drug of abuse is present in a patient. More-specific drug tests should be considered after an initial screen is performed and analyzed. A urine drug screen is most valuable when the diagnosis is unknown, that is, when one is not certain whether symptoms are being caused by drugs or by disease.

There are several techniques used for drug detection, including chromatographic methods, immunoassays, and chemical and spectrometric techniques. Chromatography is used for broad-spectrum analysis, whereas immunoassays are used for specific analysis. Being aware of what drug coverage is available in particular toxicology screens is helpful. Most tests identify analgesics, amphetamines, antidepressants, barbiturates, cocaine, ethanol, and opiates. Drugs that are not commonly found in standard drug screens include bromide, carbon monoxide, chloral hydrate, clonidine, cyanide, organophosphates, tetrahydrozoline, colchicines, cyanide, iron, β-blockers, calcium-channel blockers, clonidine, and digitalis. Note that traces of many drugs persist for lengths of time that may not be clinically relevant depending on the situation. Realizing that false-positive and false-negative results are not uncommon is essential for making clinically sound decisions. As such, confirmation analyses may be required. In addition, inquiring about the patient's legal drug use can help to clarify toxicology screening results. Aspirin and acetaminophen, for example, are very common analgesic ingredients in many medications, so measuring their prevalence should be considered (*Table 76.1*).

ⓒ 2008 by Lippincott Williams & Wilkins, a Wolters Kluwer business

TABLE 76.1	QUALITATIVE URINE DRUG SCREENS:	
DRUG/TOXIN	INTERFERENTS/ IRRELEVANTS[a]	COMMENTS
Amphetamines	Chlorpromazine, ephedrine/pseudoephedrine, desoxyephedrine, *Ephedra* sp., mexiletine, phenylephrine, phenylpropanolamine, selegiline	Vicks nasal inhaler (desoxyephedrine) and selegiline also cause positive GC-MS; chiral confirmation is required. Interferents in older assays include labetalol and ranitidine
Benzodiazepines	Oxaprozin—false-negative result	Poor detection of parent drugs with absent or low concentration of oxazepam metabolite (e.g., alprazolam, lorazepam, triazolam)
Cocaine	Coca leaf teas	Most reliable urine screen
Opiates/opioids	Poppy seeds; ofloxacin; rifampin	Does not detect semisynthetic or designer opioids (e.g., fentanyls, meperidine, methadone, propoxyphene)
Phencyclidine	Dextromethorphan, diphenhydramine, ketamine; thioridazine	—
Tetrahydrocannabinol	Dronabinol, hemp consumables	Positive result is seldom clinically relevant
Tricyclic antidepressants	Cyclobenzaprine, diphenhydramine, phenothiazines	

CG-MS, gas chromatography-mass spectrometry.
Ford MD, Acute Poisoning. In: Cecil RL, Goldman L, Bennett JC, eds. *Cecil Textbook of Medicine*, 22nd ed. Philadelphia: WB Saunders; 2004. Chapter 106, pages 628–40. Modified from Table 106–4.
[a] Irrelevants are agents causing true positive but clinically irrelevant results.

When determining which specimen to collect for use in a drug screen, note that urine is the best specimen for producing the highest rate of positive findings among the greatest number of drugs when compared to gastric aspirates or serum. Obviously, the earlier the urine is collected, the more drugs can be detected because some drugs have short detection intervals. When extraordinary screening is available, adding a blood sample to the urine can produce a slightly higher yield of positives. Gastric aspirates frequently contain high concentrations of parent drugs, which is helpful when a drug is already metabolized to an appreciable extent and cannot be identified based on urinary metabolites.

Being conscious of what drug tests are available at one's medical institution can help to properly diagnose suspected drug abuse-related illnesses.

TABLE 76.2	URINE SCREENING FOR DRUGS COMMONLY ABUSED BY ADOLESCENTS				
DRUG	MAJOR METABOLITE	INITIAL	FIRST CONFIRMATION	SECOND CONFIRMATION	APPROXIMATE RETENTION TIME
Alcohol (blood)	Acetaldehyde	GC	IA		7–10 hr
Alcohol (urine)	Acetaldehyde	GC	IA		10–13 hr
Amphetamines	—	TLC	IA	GC, GC/MS	48 hr
Barbiturates	—	IA	TLC	GC, GC/MS	Short-acting (24 hr); long-acting (2–3 wk)
Benzodiazepines	—	IA	TLC	GC,GC/MS	3 days
Cannabinoids	Carboxy– and hydroxymetabolites	IA	TLC	GC/MS	3–10 days (occasional user; 1–2 mo (chronic user)
Cocaine	Benzoyl ecgonine	IA	TLC	GC/MS	2–4 days
Methaqualone	Hydroxylated metabolites	TLC	IA	GC/MS	2 wk
Heroin	Morphine Glucuronide	IA	TLC	GC, GC/MS	2 days
Morphine	Morphine Glucuronide	IA	TLC	GC, GC/MS	2 days
Codeine	Morphine Glucuronide	IA	TLC	GC, GC/MS	2 days
Phencyclidine		TLC	IA	GC, GC/MS	8 days

GC, gas chromatography; IA, immunoassay; TLC, thin-layer chromatography; MS, mass spectrometry. (Modified from Chapter 105, Table 105–3. Jenkins RR. In: Kliegman RM, ed. *Nelson Textbook of Pediatrics.* Philadelphia: WB Saunders, 2007).

Recognizing which drugs are commonly missed in routine drug screens and which drugs—illicit or otherwise—result in false positives can also prevent time-wasting, erroneous drug tests from being ordered (*Table 76.2*).

SUGGESTED READINGS

Ford MD. Acute poisoning. In: Goldman L, Ausiello D, eds. *Cecil Textbook of Medicine*. 22nd ed. Philadelphia: Saunders; 2004, pages 328–40.

Jenkins RR. Substance abuse. In: Behrman RE, Kliegman RM, Jenson HB, eds. *Nelson Textbook of Pediatrics*. 17th ed. Philadelphia: Saunders; 2004, pages 653–62.

Lee J. Poisonings. In: Robertson J, Shilkofski N, eds. *The Harriet Lane Handbook: A Manual for Pediatric House Officers*. 17th ed. Philadelphia: Elsevier Mosby, 2005, pages 17–71.

Osterloh JD. Laboratory testing in emergency toxicology. In: Ford MD, Delaney KA, Ling LJ, et al, eds. *Clinical Toxicology*. Philadelphia: WB Saunders Company; 2001.

77

AN ARTERIAL BLOOD GAS (ABG) IS NOT NEEDED TO DOCUMENT RESPIRATORY FAILURE. CARE FOR THE PATIENT FIRST AND INTUBATE WHEN NECESSARY

DOROTHY CHEN, MD

WHAT TO DO – TAKE ACTION

Respiratory failure is the inability of the respiratory system to facilitate adequate gas exchange and meet the metabolic needs of the body. Failure of the respiratory system can be caused by abnormalities in the respiratory, neuromuscular, or central nervous system. Respiratory distress is defined as signs of increased work of breathing, nasal flaring, use of accessory muscles, and inspiratory retractions. This does not always accompany respiratory failure, because respiratory failure can be due to lack of respiratory effort. Within the pulmonary system, there can be hypoventilation, diffusion impairment, intrapulmonary shunting or a ventilation-perfusion mismatch. Abnormal arterial pO_2 and pCO_2 is found in respiratory failure, but it is not necessary to measure and document these values prior to initiating care. Physical exam is the key to determining respiratory failure and treatment should not be delayed for blood gas analysis.

The ABCs of Pediatric Advanced Life Saving are vital to recognizing respiratory failure; patients should be assessed for *a*irway, *b*reathing, and *c*irculation. The airway should be examined to be clear and maintainable without intervention. For breathing, it is important to assess for signs of upper and lower airway obstruction, respiratory rate, respiratory effort, the adequacy of ventilation, use of accessory muscles, and signs of cyanosis. When assessing circulation, evaluate responsiveness, heart rate, blood pressure, and perfusion. If respiratory failure is identified, intubation should be initiated. Timely intervention and treatment of respiratory failure improves outcomes. The natural progression of respiratory failure will result in pulseless cardiac arrest, so intervention should not be delayed.

ABG analysis is useful in evaluating perfusion, ventilation, and respiratory versus metabolic acidosis. However, one ABG is only a single lab value and still needs to be considered in the context of the clinical scenario. It can be obtained as a component of the comprehensive evaluation and as confirmation of the clinical exam, but ABGs are not required before intervening

© 2008 by Lippincott Williams & Wilkins, a Wolters Kluwer business

and treating a patient for respiratory failure. The basics of Pediatric Advance Life Saving should always be initiated: access *a*irway, *b*reathing and *c*irculation.

SUGGESTED READING

American Academy of Pediatrics, American Heart Association. *PALS Provider Manual*. Dallas: American Academy of Pediatrics, American Heart Association; 2002.

78

INTRAVENOUS (IV) FLUID MANAGEMENT IS INDICATED AS THE FIRST THERAPEUTIC INTERVENTION FOR ALL TYPES OF SHOCK

CAROLINE RASSBACH, MD

WHAT TO DO – TAKE ACTION

Shock occurs when the oxygen and nutrient supply is insufficient to meet the metabolic demands of the body. Shock can be classified as hypovolemic, septic, distributive, and cardiogenic. Hypovolemic shock is the most common type of shock in children. It is usually the result of fluid-losing states such as diarrhea, blood loss, or burns. The effect is decreased intravascular volume, decreased preload, and decreased stroke volume. When hypovolemic shock occurs as a result of fluid and electrolyte losses, both intravascular and interstitial fluid volume is decreased. Physical signs are classic for dehydration, including sunken eyes, depressed fontanelle, dry mucous membranes, cool extremities, decreased peripheral pulses, and poor skin turgor. In contrast, patients with hypovolemic shock because of increased capillary permeability have intravascular hypovolemia with interstitial euvolemia. Such is the case with burns and nephrotic syndrome. Physical signs include mental status changes, increased capillary refill, decreased peripheral pulses, and decreased urine output without the classic signs of dehydration. Extremities may be edematous. Treatment of hypovolemic shock consists of replacement of fluids. When shock is secondary to blood loss, fluid replacement should include blood products.

Septic shock occurs as a consequence of bacterial, fungal, or viral infection. It is defined as hypotension despite adequate fluid resuscitation and inadequate perfusion. Signs of inadequate perfusion may include lactic acidosis, oliguria, or altered mental status. In children, septic shock can present as classic "warm shock," with high cardiac output and low systemic vascular resistance, or as "cold shock" with decreased cardiac output and elevated systemic vascular resistance. Septic shock should be treated with IV fluids and broad-spectrum antibiotics. Following resuscitation with at least 60 mL/kg of isotonic fluid, vasopressors may be required to maintain blood pressure. In addition, cortisol replacement may be indicated if adrenal insufficiency occurs.

Distributive shock, also known as vasodilatory shock, occurs because of abnormal regulation of blood flow, resulting in functional hypovolemia.

ⓒ 2008 by Lippincott Williams & Wilkins, a Wolters Kluwer business

One example of distributive shock is anaphylactic shock, a hypersensitivity reaction that occurs immediately after exposure to an allergen. The result is an immunoglobulin (Ig)E-mediated massive release of cytokines by mast cells and basophils. Angioedema, hypotension, and third-spacing ensue and can be life-threatening. Immediate treatment with subcutaneous epinephrine, as well as fluid resuscitation, is imperative. In addition, airway management and treatment with antihistamines and steroids are required.

Another example of distributive shock is neurogenic shock, which results from injury to the central nervous system (CNS). Neurogenic shock is usually transient and occurs after an acute injury to the CNS. There is generalized loss of sympathetic vascular and anatomic tone. Cardiac contractility is preserved and can usually increase to maintain cardiac output without raising the heart rate. Eventually, however, cardiac output may be compromised by lack of venous return. As a result, neurogenic shock may demonstrate hypotension in the absence of tachycardia. Treatment includes volume resuscitation and vasopressors.

Cardiogenic shock is the last major category of shock and results from cardiac abnormalities that cause decreased myocardial contractility, arrhythmias, left ventricular outflow tract obstruction, and large left-to-right shunts. With cardiogenic shock, fluid resuscitation should be judicious, as the patient may present in fluid overload or in volume depletion. Vasopressors and inotropes may be beneficial.

In both septic shock and distributive shock, a low systemic vascular resistance is the primary problem. In contrast, in hypovolemic shock and cardiogenic shock, the primary problem is a reduced cardiac output. The earliest physical sign of all types of shock is tachycardia. The heart rate and stroke volume increase to sustain cardiac output. Systemic vascular resistance is also maximized to maintain blood pressure. This is accomplished by diverting blood from less essential organs, such as the skin, kidneys, and skeletal muscles, to essential organs, such as the brain, heart, lungs, and adrenal glands. In the early stages of shock, also known as compensated shock, blood pressure is maintained as a result of this diversion, but blood flow to the less essential organs is compromised. Physical signs to evaluate for shock should include heart rate and end-organ perfusion, such as capillary refill, urine output, mentation, and peripheral pulses.

With all types of shock, the blood pressure drops only after the body maximizes heart rate and systemic vascular resistance. At this point, the patient may rapidly decompensate, as vital organs no longer receive the oxygen and nutrients they need. Hypotension represents an advanced stage of shock, known as decompensated shock, and has a high mortality rate. Multisystem organ failure and death may result.

Practitioners must recognize early signs of shock to initiate treatment and prevent morbidity and mortality. Patients should be treated initially according to the ABCs: airway stabilization, oxygen therapy, and establishment of vascular access. Large-bore peripheral IV lines, intraosseous lines, or central venous catheters are required. Fluid resuscitation should begin with a 20 mL/kg bolus of isotonic crystalloid. Fluid status should be reassessed and the need for subsequent therapy considered, including further IV fluids, pressors, or antibiotics. If the patient does not have cardiogenic shock, boluses may be repeated up to 60 to 80 mL/kg in the first 1 to 2 hours. The patient should be closely monitored for signs of fluid overload. In the absence of renal disease, urine output of 1 to 2 mL/kg/hr is a useful indicator of adequate organ perfusion.

In summary, all categories of shock have similar physical manifestations and a common endpoint. Physical signs present in all types of shock include tachycardia and poor perfusion to end organs. In addition, the initial treatment for all types of shock is also the same and includes resuscitation with intravenous fluids.

SUGGESTED READINGS

Frankel LR and Mathers LH. Shock Chapter 57.2. In: Behrman RE. *Nelson Textbook of Pediatrics*, 17th ed. Philadelphia: WB Saunders; 2004.

McKiernan CA, Lieberman SA. Circulatory shock in children: an overview. *Pediatr Rev.* 2005;26(12):451–460.

79

DO NOT WASTE TIME TRYING TO GET AN INTRAVENOUS (IV) LINE ON AN INFANT IN SHOCK WHEN AN INTRAOSSEOUS (IO) LINE WILL DO JUST AS WELL

WILLIAM GIASI, JR., MD

WHAT TO DO – TAKE ACTION

There are thousands of emergencies every year that require the resuscitation of infants and children. These emergencies can occur in almost any setting and providers need to be prepared to intervene. The goal in any resuscitation is to maintain adequate oxygenation and perfusion while interventions are taken to stabilize the child. Resuscitation should proceed in an orderly fashion beginning with the ABCs: *a*irway, *b*reathing, and *c*irculation.

As part of the circulation sequence during advanced life support, it is necessary for the provider to establish venous access as a route to administer medications, fluids, and blood products, and to obtain blood for analysis. Nevertheless, even in the hands of experienced providers, obtaining IV access in pediatric patients can be difficult. The preferred site for access is the one that is readily accessible and will not interfere with the resuscitation. There are several peripheral sites that providers should familiarize themselves with where IV access can be obtained. Central venous access is another option in the event that the proper equipment and trained personnel are available. An attempt to establish peripheral and central venous access can be approached simultaneously.

If peripheral or central venous access is unattainable in <1 minute during resuscitation, current recommendations urge the use of IO cannulation. The administration of potentially lifesaving drugs and interventions should not be delayed while attempting venous access. IO access provides access to a noncollapsable venous network, which can serve as a rapid, safe, and reliable route via which drugs, fluids, and blood products may be administered. Following the establishment of IO access, providers can continue to explore other peripheral and/or central routes of access to support the patient's ongoing care.

In the infant and child, the anteromedial surface of tibia is the preferred site for insertion of the IO needle because it is a large bone with a thin layer of subcutaneous tissue. The location and anatomy of this region allows for

© 2008 by Lippincott Williams & Wilkins, a Wolters Kluwer business

landmarks to be readily palpated, access obtained, and does not interfere with airway management or cardiopulmonary resuscitation.

SUGGESTED READINGS

Mathers LH and Frankel LR. Chapter 57.1 Pediatric Emergencies and Resuscitations. In: Behrman RE, Kliegman RM, Jenson HB, eds. *Nelson Textbook of Pediatrics.* 17th ed. Philadelphia: Saunders; 2004, pages 291–95.

Stanley R. Intraosseous infusion. In: Roberts JR, Hedges JR, eds. *Roberts: Clinical Procedures in Emergency Medicine,* 4th ed. Philadelphia: Saunders; 2004, pages 475–85.

Zaritsky A. Vascular access. In: American Heart Association. *PALS Provider Manual.* Dallas, TX: American Heart Association; 2002:155–172.

80

Assure that Patients with Severe Asthma and Status Asthmaticus Receive Adequate Intravascular Volume Expansion

David Stockwell, MD

What to Do – Take Action

Asthma is one of the most common illnesses in pediatrics, with considerable variation in presentation. Patients can have an asthma attack with mild respiratory difficulties and not require more than an intermittent inhaled β-agonist. Alternatively, a severe asthmatic patient may require mechanical ventilation or even extracorporeal life support. Although an asthma attack that requires endotracheal intubation is rare, it is important to identify the risk factors for intubation. These include low socioeconomic status, active tobacco smoking or second-hand smoke exposure, parenteral history of allergy or asthma, prior intubation, intercurrent respiratory infection, prior asthma emergency room visit in past year, prior asthma hospitalization in past year, and steroid dependence.

Children require mechanical ventilation for asthma when they have profound hypoxemia, life-threatening respiratory muscle fatigue, or altered mental status. However, high airway pressures, barotrauma, and patient-ventilator dyssynchrony complicate mechanical ventilation in patients with asthma. Although potentially lifesaving, use of mechanical ventilation during an asthma exacerbation is associated with an increased risk of death from asthma. Therefore, the decision to intubate an asthmatic should not be made lightly. These patients are at high risk for cardiac dysfunction. A particularly difficult combination of factors merges to impact the asthmatic patient's cardiac preload. Namely, dehydration, increased pulmonary vascular resistance due to bronchospasm, and the addition of positive pressure to the thoracic cavity will also decrease venous return to the heart and increase resistance to pulmonary blood flow. All of these factors combine to dramatically lower preload for the left ventricle.

Typically people with severe enough asthma to consider intubation have dehydration owing to the extreme work of breathing and lack of fluid intake. These patients have often been sick for a number of hours and have extreme respiratory difficulty. Their insensible losses due to their respiratory distress are high.

© 2008 by Lippincott Williams & Wilkins, a Wolters Kluwer business

Bronchospasm severe enough to cause the typical hyperexpanded lung findings on chest x-ray limits left ventricular preload. While the chest is hyperexpanded, the resistance to pulmonary blood flow increases due to the over filled alveoli increasing pulmonary vascular resistance. In addition, hyperexpanded chests can decrease systemic venous return to the heart by increasing the resistance in the vena cava.

Finally, by adding positive pressure ventilation to a hyperexpanded chest there is typically an exacerbated reduction in cardiac preload. Similar to the mechanism of action for the hyperexpanded chest, the systemic venous return is limited due to increased resistance in both vena cava. Additionally, positive pressure ventilation will increase intrathoracic pressures because there is a chance from negative pressure ventilation to positive pressure ventilation. The combination of all of these factors can lead to severe cardiac depression and hypotension. It is important to understand that the increased positive pressure from bag-mask ventilation is the initial period that cardiac dysfunction is observed. If unrecognized as decreased preload, it will progress as a patient is placed on a ventilator. Providing the patient with isotonic intravenous solution as a bolus prior to intubation is sound practice. This will augment venous return to the heart and decrease the likelihood of cardiac depression.

SUGGESTED READINGS

LeSon S, Gershwin ME. Risk factors for asthmatic patients requiring intubation. I. Observations in children. *J Asthma*. 1995;32(4):285–294.

Roberts JS, Bratton SL, Brogan TV. Acute severe asthma: differences in therapies and outcomes among pediatric intensive care units. *Crit Care Med*. 2002;30:581–585.

81

REMEMBER THAT A COMES BEFORE B AND C. IF YOU HAVEN'T PROTECTED THE AIRWAY, YOU HAVEN'T EFFECTIVELY CARED FOR THE PATIENT

RENÉE ROBERTS, MD

WHAT TO DO – TAKE ACTION

The guidelines for cardiopulmonary resuscitation (CPR) and emergency cardiovascular care for pediatric and neonatal patients contains recommendations designed to improve survival from sudden cardiac arrest and acute life-threatening cardiopulmonary problems. They have recently been revised, but this does not imply that the use of earlier guidelines is outdated. It is important that pediatric caregivers be familiar with these guidelines and the changes. In particular, the guidelines continue to emphasize that *cardiac* arrest in children is most often the *end result of respiratory arrest.* Thus a lone rescuer for an unresponsive child should begin with 30 compressions and two breaths, then activate the emergency medical services system. This approach is thought to optimize the chances for quick resuscitation of children with primary respiratory arrest, before complete cardiopulmonary arrest occurs. Two-rescuer CPR in children is the only situation that deviates from the 30:2 ratio recommended for compressions and breaths; for two-rescuer CPR in children, two breaths should be given after every 15 compressions. Otherwise, CPR recommendations for children closely parallel those for adults where basic life support should always be remembered as an "ABCD" approach to cardiopulmonary arrest: *a*irway, *b*reathing, *c*irculation, *d*efibrillation. Guidelines for advanced life support for children also are similar to those for adults, with a few notable exceptions: vasopressin and atropine not recommended for pulseless electrical activity; defibrillation should be dosed on weight (4 joules per kg); and the use of intraosseous (IO) access is permissible if intravenous (IV) access is not established quickly.

Changes in the guidelines include caution about use of endotracheal tubes. Confirmation of tube placement requires exhaled carbon dioxide detection and is recommended especially when a prompt increase in heart rate does not occur after intubation. Furthermore, all rescue breaths given over 1 second with sufficient volume need to produce a visible chest rise. Lastly, correct placement must be verified when the tube is inserted, during transport, and whenever the patient is moved. With an advanced airway in place,

© 2008 by Lippincott Williams & Wilkins, a Wolters Kluwer business

CPR is not done in cycles but rather chest compressions are performed continuously at a rate of 100 per minute without pauses for ventilation, which should be 8 to 10 breaths per minute. Remember an increase in heart rate is the primary sign of improved ventilation during resuscitation.

   The unexpected difficult pediatric airway that may be encountered during resuscitation is subdivided into the nonemergency (can ventilate but cannot intubate) and emergency pathways (cannot ventilate and cannot intubate). Management for the unexpected difficult pediatric airway involves maintaining adequate oxygenation while a definitive course of action is pursued. Unfortunately, infants have an increased metabolic rate and decreased functional residual capacity, which makes the time between the loss

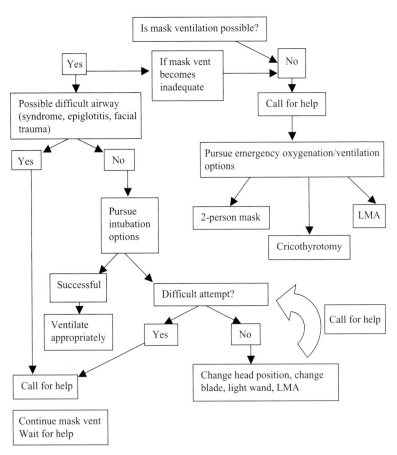

FIGURE 81.1. Algorithm for management of an unexpected difficult airway. LMA, laryngeal mask airway.

of the airway and resultant hypoxemia with secondary neurologic injury significantly diminished compared with adults. Approximate time to zero oxygen saturation from an inspired oxygen concentration of 90% is 4 minutes in a 10-kg child, whereas the same event in a healthy adult takes 10 minutes. If there is any question of a possibility of difficulty with ventilation or intubation due to airway, face, or neck abnormalities, appropriate personnel (anesthesia) should be notified immediately. This can include facial and neck trauma, craniofacial syndromes, infectious causes (e.g., epiglottitis, large abscesses deforming the mouth head or neck), and masses encroaching on the trachea or mediastinum. A timely call for experienced airway assistance will result in the best possible outcome. *Figure 81.1* is an algorithm for management of an unexpected difficult airway.

The laryngeal mask airway has proven to be an extremely useful device in the emergency pathway when used by health care providers. It is an effective device for ventilation and an effective conduit for intubation. It is easily inserted blindly and requires a relatively low level of skill. However, caution must be used because this is a supraglottic device, so if glottic or subglottic obstruction to ventilation is present it will be ineffective, and transtracheal jet ventilation via percutaneous needle cricothyrotomy must be pursued. In addition, protection against aspiration is not assured.

In the new guidelines, induced hypothermia ($32-34°C$ for 12–24 hours) may be considered if a child remains comatose after resuscitation. Studies show that infants without signs of life after 10 minutes of resuscitation show either a high mortality rate or severe neurodevelopmental disability, thus in the child who already has conditions with unacceptable high morbidity and congenital anomalies associated with certain early death, discontinuation of resuscitation is justified.

SUGGESTED READINGS

American Heart Association. 2005 American Heart Association (AHA) guidelines for cardiopulmonary resuscitation (CPR) and emergency cardiovascular care (ECC) of pediatric and neonatal patients: pediatric basic life support. *Pediatrics.* 2006;117(5):e989–e1004.

Cayley WE. Understanding 2005 AHA Guidelines for CPR and emergency care. *Am Fam Physician.* 2006;73(9):1644.

Wheeler M. The difficult pediatric airway. *Anesthesiol Clin North Am.* 1998;16(4):743–761.

82

REMEMBER THAT THE TREATMENT OF PATIENTS WITH DIABETIC KETOACIDOSIS (DKA) IS DEPENDENT UPON THE PROVISION OF INSULIN

RENÉE ROBERTS, MD

WHAT TO DO – MAKE A DECISION

The insulin infusion should never be discontinued until the acidosis is corrected. Rather, use additional sources of dextrose containing intravenous (IV) fluids if hypoglycemia develops.

DKA is the presenting symptom in approximately 40% of children and teenagers at the time of diagnosis and the most frequent diabetes-related cause of death in children, teenagers, and young adults. Most DKA-related morbidity and mortality can be avoided via early recognition and early intervention.

The underlying pathophysiologic cause of DKA is an absolute or relative deficiency of insulin. Declining insulin production lowers the ratio of insulin to glucagon, which leads to excess hepatic glucose production stimulating glycogenolysis and gluconeogenesis. When the serum glucose rises above 200 mg/dL, the renal threshold for glucose reabsorption is exceeded, causing osmotic diuresis with increased urine output. Physiologic stress from acidosis and progressive dehydration stimulates release of the counterregulatory hormones, cortisol, catecholamines (epinephrine and norepinephrine), and growth hormone. These hormones shift the metabolism of carbohydrate, protein, and lipids; and further increase hepatic glucose production, ketogenesis, and peripheral insulin resistance, thereby worsening acidosis and dehydration. The acidosis and dehydration in turn accelerate the development of DKA by further stimulating increase in the counterregulatory hormones. This cycle is responsible for the development of severe ketoacidosis.

The classic triad of DKA is hyperglycemia, ketosis, and acidosis. Presenting symptoms include polyuria polydipsia, weight loss, abdominal pain, nausea, vomiting, tachycardia, and hypoperfusion (cool extremities, decreased capillary refill, dry mucous membranes, poor skin turgor). The following lab criteria are used to diagnose DKA: blood glucose >250 to 300 mg/dL, pH <7.3, serum bicarbonate <15mEq/L, urinary ketones >3+, serum ketones positive. Furthermore, there is a high anion gap metabolic

© 2008 by Lippincott Williams & Wilkins, a Wolters Kluwer business

acidosis due to the ketoacids. Severe DKA should be treated as a potentially life-threatening condition, thus frequent monitoring of patient status, and accurate intake and output, electrolytes, and blood pH is crucial.

The initial interventions should be

1. To ensure adequate ventilation and cardiovascular function and satisfactory mental status. If there is hemodynamic instability, inability to protect the airway, and obtundation, this is severely decompensated diabetes should be managed in the intensive care unit (ICU).
2. Correct fluid deficits and electrolyte disturbances with fluid therapy. This includes frequent monitoring and blood work every 1 to 2 hours.
3. Continuous low-dose insulin to interrupt ketoacidosis and minimize osmotic diuresis.
4. Correct metabolic acidosis with fluids and insulin.
5. Treat any underlying cause (infection).
6. Monitor for complications.

Volume expansion should be initiated immediately (usually 10–20 mL/kg) with isotonic saline over 30 to 60 minutes. A recent study in 2004 showed most clinician's assessment of children with DKA often underestimate the severity of dehydration. If the child is obviously in shock or very hypotensive or has poor perfusion (cap refill <3 seconds) then an extra 10 mL/kg should be bolused. The deficit (plus maintenance) should be corrected evenly over 24 to 48 hours and include losses from diarrhea, vomiting, and osmotic diuresis. Potassium should be added to the rehydration fluid, usually by adding 30 to 40 mEq/L. The goal is to maintain potassium levels in the range of 4 to 5 mEq/L To prevent hypokalemia both from fluid administration and insulin, the potassium level should be checked to prevent cardiac arrhythmias. Kidney function should also be checked before administering any exogenous potassium.

Blood glucose will decline quickly during the early treatment of DKA as a result of volume expansion and insulin action. The same amount of glucose in a larger extracellular volume allows the blood glucose to fall rapidly by 200 to 400 mg/dL/hr, or about 23%. This reduction is *not* dependent on insulin administration or action. After the initial drop, a decline in blood glucose level >100 mg/dL/hr should not be exceeded in the treatment of DKA because more rapid correction of serum glucose concentration increases the risk of cerebral edema. The optimal rate of decrease of serum glucose is 50 to 70 mg/dL/hr.

Because all patients are in a state of absolute or relative insulin deficiency, exogenous insulin must be provided during therapy. The insulin reverses protein breakdown and lipolysis, and suppresses ketone body and ketoacid formation, thus interrupting the excess production of acid. Insulin will also lower blood glucose by inhibiting glycogenolysis and gluconeogenesis and stimulating glucose uptake. IV insulin is clearly the route of choice for initial therapy because the absorption of subcutaneous or intramuscular insulin may be reduced or delayed.

The most effective means of insulin replacement is a continuous infusion of "low-dose" regular insulin (0.1 U/kg) followed by a continuous infusion of 0.1 U/kg/hr (not to exceed 5–7 U/hr). This allows a steady state of circulating insulin concentration. The insulin should be infused separately so the rate can be maintained separate from the rehydration fluid, which then can be changed independently. It is wise to flush the tubing with the insulin solution as some will adhere to the infusion tubing and bag.

The rate of insulin infusion should not be reduced because of falling blood glucose in the absence of significant correction of the ketoacidotic state. Instead dextrose should be added to the IV solution to maintain the desired blood glucose level. A solution of 5% dextrose is added to the IV fluids when plasma glucose level falls to ≤ 250 mg/dL. This addition allows continued administration of insulin until the acidosis and ketonemia have resolved, and prevents iatrogenic hypoglycemia. One method to allow good glycemic control is to have two glucose concentrations (0% and 10%), then the rate of infusion of both bags can be adjusted to administer between 0% and 10% glucose.

The insulin infusion should not be discontinued until the acidoses and ketonemia have improved significantly and the anion gap is normal or near normal. Resolution of ketosis and the attainment of a serum bicarbonate level ≥ 18 mEq/L indicate that the IV insulin may be stopped. However when converting to subcutaneous insulin, time must be allowed for steady state. It is vital then to continue the IV insulin (half-life of 7 minutes) to prevent rapid onset of hyperglycemia.

Complications of DKA include hypoglycemia, fluid overload causing congestive heart failure and aspiration of gastric contents in those with altered mental status. The most morbid complication, however, is cerebral edema (1%–2% of children). Although subclinical cases of cerebral edema are evident on a computed tomography scan for many children in DKA, the progression to fulminant cerebral edema is dire. Even with accurate and careful management, symptomatic cerebral edema occasionally occurs in children with severe DKA within 24 hours after therapy initiation without any apparent cause. Although many mechanisms have been proffered, the only correlating symptoms include high blood urea nitrogen concentrations at presentation and more profound hypocapnia. The best treatment of cerebral edema is early mannitol (0.2–1 g/kg over 30 minutes) and decrease in fluid administration rate with an immediate neurology consult and transfer to the ICU. The signs and symptoms include headache, deteriorating level of consciousness, development of seizures, recurrence of vomiting, and signs of increasing intracranial pressure (hypertension, bradycardia, papilledema). About one third of children with cerebral edema die, and one third are neurologically impaired.

SUGGESTED READINGS

Glaser N. Pediatric diabetic ketoacidosis and hyperglycemic hyperosmolar state. *Pediatr Clin North Am.* 2005;52(6):1611–1635.

Magee MF, Bhatt BA. Endocrine and metabolic dysfunction syndromes in the critically ill. *Crit Care Clin.* 2001;17(1):75–106.

White NH. Diabetic ketoacidosis in children. *Endocrinol Metab Clin North Am.* 2000;29(4):657–682.

83

KNOW HOW TO TREAT ACUTE SEIZURES IN CHILDREN AND HOW TO AGGRESSIVELY MANAGE STATUS EPILEPTICUS

CYNTHIA GIBSON, MD

WHAT TO DO – TAKE ACTION

A common definition of a seizure is a transient, involuntary alteration of consciousness, behavior, motor activity, sensation, or autonomic function. A postictal period, often described as decreased responsiveness, usually follows most seizures. Epilepsy is a condition of recurrent seizures. Status epilepticus refers to continuous or recurrent seizure activity lasting >30 minutes without recovery of consciousness.

A seizure can have many possible causes, often due to an underlying pathologic process. Determining the cause will assist with making treatment decisions. Categories of diagnoses include infectious, neurologic, metabolic including electrolyte or glucose disturbances, traumatic, toxicologic, oncologic, or idiopathic. Obtaining a detailed history, including a description of the seizure will assist with making the diagnosis. Precipitating factors such as trauma, ingestion, fever, or signs of systemic illness should also be elucidated.

Regardless of a seizure's cause, the acute management remains the same. Initial management should always include assessment of the ABCs: stabilization of the airway, breathing, and circulation, and then stopping the seizure. Most patients do require some type of pharmacologic intervention to stop the seizure.

Benzodiazepines are the initial drugs of choice for the acute management. Lorazepam is preferred due to its rapid onset and long half-life and can be given intramuscularly if intravenous access has not been obtained. Diazepam is another choice with a rapid onset, but has a shorter duration and patients often need a long-term agent to prevent recurrence. Diazepam can be administered rectally. If, the seizures continue despite multiple benzodiazepine doses, then phenytoin or fosphenytoin is often the next choice and is given initially as a loading dose. Careful monitoring must follow because cardiovascular side effects can occur. Persistent seizures and neonatal seizures are often treated with phenobarbital, but monitoring for respiratory depression and hypotension are necessary.

Status epilepticus requires aggressive management, which may include continuous infusions of midazolam or phenobarbital with continuous

© 2008 by Lippincott Williams & Wilkins, a Wolters Kluwer business

electroencephalograph monitoring and mechanical ventilation. If the seizure activity still persists despite the above therapeutic interventions, then the determination of a specific cause requiring other therapies may be necessary; these include treatment of infection, correction of increased intracranial pressure, and correction of electrolyte disturbances or hypoglycemia.

Brief seizures rarely have lasting effects on the brain. However, prolonged seizures can lead to lactic acidosis, rhabdomyolysis, hyperkalemia, hyperthermia, and hypoglycemia, which can all be associated with permanent neurologic injury. For this reason, aggressive intervention to stop the seizure activity is critical.

SUGGESTED READINGS

Appleton R, Choonara I, Martland T, et al. The treatment of convulsive status epilepticus in children. The Status Epilepticus Working Party, Members of the Status Epilepticus Working Party. *Arch Dis Child.* 2000;83(5):415–419.

Friedman MJ, Sharieff GQ. Seizures in children. *Pediatr Clin North Am.* 2006;52:257–277.

Hirtz D, Berg A, Bettis D, et al. Practice parameter: treatment of the child with a first unprovoked seizure: Report of the Quality Standards Subcommittee of the American Academy of Neurology and the Practice Committee of the Child Neurology Society. *Neurology.* 2003;60:166–175.

84

CONSIDER THE BROAD-DIFFERENTIAL DIAGNOSIS FOR RESPIRATORY DISTRESS IN CHILDREN

SARIKA JOSHI, MD

WHAT TO DO – GATHER APPROPRIATE DATA

It is important for pediatricians to recognize the signs and symptoms of respiratory distress, as it is a common presenting complaint for children. With a careful history and physical exam, it is possible to narrow down the broad differential for respiratory distress so that appropriate treatment may be started. Respiratory distress is characterized by increased work of breathing (i.e., tachypnea, flaring, retractions) often in association with pulmonary exam findings such as stridor, wheezing, and rales.

Important elements of the history for a child with respiratory distress include trauma, voice changes (i.e., muffled, hoarse), and associated symptoms, such as fever. Prior episodes of respiratory distress or any chronic medical conditions are also significant parts of the history. Physical exam should start with vital signs, especially respiratory rate and oxygen saturation. The World Health Organization defines tachypnea (in breaths per minute) based on age: >60 for age <2 months, >50 for ages 2 months to 1 year, >40 for ages 1 to 5 years, >20 for age >5 years. Remember that for febrile children, each degree Celsius increase may cause an increase of up to 10 breaths per minute. In addition to the respiratory rate, pay attention to the respiratory pattern. For instance, Kussmaul breathing and Cheyne-Stokes breathing occur with metabolic acidosis and central nervous system (CNS) processes, respectively.

Prior to auscultation, careful observation of the child in respiratory distress may provide important clues to the diagnosis. Mental status changes, such as combativeness or somnolence, may indicate severe hypoxia or hypercarbia. Cyanosis is a late sign in the hypoxic child. The child will assume a position that decreases work of breathing. For example, a child with upper airway obstruction may assume the "sniffing position." Observe whether there is nasal flaring, head bobbing, retractions (supraclavicular, intercostal, substernal), or grunting, all of which signify respiratory distress. If there is cough, listen to the quality: hoarse or barky (suggests upper airway problem), tight and persistent (suggests lower airway obstruction), or loose and productive (suggests infection). On auscultation, particularly note stridor,

© 2008 by Lippincott Williams & Wilkins, a Wolters Kluwer business

wheezing, rales, and decreased breath sounds. Stridor is generally an inspiratory noise from upper airway obstruction. Wheezing is usually an expiratory noise from lower airway obstruction. Rales are typically an inspiratory noise from lower airway reinflation, which occurs in pneumonia and pulmonary edema. Decreased breath sounds may indicate local areas of collapse, consolidation, or fluid.

Armed with your history and physical exam findings, it is then conceptually helpful to categorize the child with respiratory distress as follows: (a) upper airway obstruction; (b) asymmetric breath sounds, no upper airway obstruction; (c) symmetric breath sounds, no upper airway obstruction. Children with upper airway obstruction will have symptoms such as stridor, voice changes, and dysphagia. Some causes of afebrile upper airway obstruction in children are foreign body, neck trauma, and upper airway burns. Causes of febrile upper airway obstruction include croup, retropharyngeal abscess, and epiglottitis. Asymmetric breath sounds indicate a focal pulmonary process. An important cause of afebrile asymmetric breath sounds, often with a history of trauma, is pneumothorax. Atelectasis can produce this picture, with or without fever. Lobar pneumonia is a cause of febrile asymmetric breath sounds, typically associated with rales. Symmetric breath sounds suggest a diffuse pulmonary process or a nonpulmonary process. Pulmonary processes that present in this manner include viral or atypical pneumonia (usually with fever and rales), asthma (generally with wheezing), and bronchiolitis (typically with fever, rales, and wheezing). Significant nonpulmonary etiologies to consider are myocarditis, metabolic acidosis, and CNS processes.

In summary, the differential diagnosis of respiratory distress in children is broad and necessitates a careful history and physical exam. Important features include recognition of the signs of increased work of breathing and auscultation of symptoms such as stridor, rales, wheezing, and differential breath sounds.

SUGGESTED READINGS

Margolis P, Gadomski A. The rational clinical examination. Does this infant have pneumonia? *JAMA.* 1998;279:308–313.

Zaritsky AL, Nadkarni VM, Hickey RW, et al., eds. *Pediatric Advanced Life Support Provider Manual.* Dallas, TX: American Heart Association; 2002.

85

KNOW HOW TO AGGRESSIVELY WORK UP ALTERATIONS IN CONSCIOUSNESS IN CHILDREN

CYNTHIA GIBSON, MD

WHAT TO DO – GATHER APPROPRIATE DATA

Alteration of consciousness involves reduced awareness initially of self, then of environment, and then the inability to be aroused. Different terms are used to describe alterations in consciousness. Confusion represents a loss of clear thinking and impaired cognition and decision making. Disorientation accompanies confusion. Delirium is a disturbed ability to focus, sustain, or shift attention, and children often have extreme mental or motor excitement. Lethargy resembles slumber with some arousal with moderate stimulation but also with quick return to the sleep state. Stupor is a condition of deep sleep or unresponsiveness except to repetitive vigorous stimuli. A coma is a state in which a person is unresponsive to all stimuli, including pain, and is the most profound degree of altered consciousness.

Arousal depends on intact communication between the reticular activating system (RAS) and its targets in the hypothalamus, thalamus, and cerebral cortex. The RAS is located within the brainstem and functions to regulate arousal in response to signals from the environment. Consciousness can be altered by dysfunction within the brainstem, impairment of both cerebral hemispheres, or by insults that globally depress neuronal activity. In children, there are many causes of altered consciousness, with the differentiation being between structural and nonstructural or medical conditions. A mnemonic exists that is helpful for remembering general categories: AEIOU TIPS. A- alcohol, abuse of substance; E-epilepsy, encephalopathy, electrolyte abnormalities, endocrine; I-insulin, intussusception; O-overdose, oxygen deficiency; U-uremia; T-trauma, temperature abnormality, tumor; I-infection; P-poisoning, psychiatric condition; S-shock, stroke. *Table 85.1* provides a list of differential diagnoses.

Coma is a medical emergency and the evaluation of coma and other altered states requires a rapid, comprehensive, systematic approach. A thorough history is critical, and the etiology may be apparent from the symptoms present leading up to coma. Information about the onset of the neurologic symptoms is very important. An abrupt change often indicates an acute event, such as a central nervous system hemorrhage or obstructive hydrocephalus.

© 2008 by Lippincott Williams & Wilkins, a Wolters Kluwer business

TABLE 85.1	DIFFERENTIAL DIAGNOSIS OF ALTERED LEVEL OF CONSCIOUSNESS

STRUCTURAL CAUSES

Cerebral vascular accident
Cerebral vein thrombosis
Hydrocephalus
Intracerebral tumor
Subdural empyema
Trauma

MEDICAL CAUSES

Anoxia
Diabetic ketoacidosis
Electrolyte abnormalities
Encephalopathy
Hypoglycemia
Hypothermia/hyperthermia
Infection/sepsis
Inborn errors of metabolism
Intussusception
Meningitis/encephalitis
Psychogenic
Postictal state
Toxins
Uremia

A gradual onset over days or hours suggests a metabolic, infectious, or toxic cause. A history of trauma, even minor, will help direct the workup. Evidence of ingestion or availability of prescription or nonprescription drugs should also be determined.

The physical examination can help differentiate structural from medical causes. Assessment of vital signs is important, with specific alterations in blood pressure, heart rate, and respirations being key evidence. The Cushing triad—systemic hypertension, bradycardia, and abnormal respirations—is a late sign of increased intracranial pressure. The neurologic examination is initially brief and should be directed at determining if the pathology is structural or medical in nature. Assessment of the level of consciousness, motor responses, and brainstem reflexes may indicate dysfunction in specific regions of the brain. A funduscopic examination should always be included in the physical examination, and the presence of retinal hemorrhages in a baby or young child should raise concern for shaken baby syndrome.

Workup should include early imaging of the brain with a computed tomography or magnetic resonance imaging scan, which can provide a rapid and accurate diagnosis and possible need for surgical intervention. Laboratory assessment should include blood glucose, serum electrolytes, arterial blood gas, liver function tests, as well as ammonia, complete blood count, blood urea nitrogen, creatinine, urine drug screen, and blood culture. If a metabolic disorder is considered, then urine organic acids and serum amino acids should be obtained. Suspected central nervous system infection warrants a lumbar puncture as soon as the child is stable enough for it to be performed and a mass lesion has been ruled out.

An altered level of consciousness in a child has many possible etiologies, but with proper and rapid assessment an accurate diagnosis can be made and proper therapies provided.

SUGGESTED READINGS

Avner JR. Altered states of consciousness. *Pediatr Rev.* 2006;27(9):331–338.

Farrell K, Selby K. Neurologic disorders, "Coma." In: Baldwin GA, ed. *Handbook of Pediatric Emergencies.* 2nd ed. Philadelphia: Little, Brown, and Company; 1994.

Kirkham FJ. Non-traumatic coma in children. *Arch Child Dis.* 2001;85(4):303–312.

Michelson D, Thompson L, Williams E. Evaluation of Stupor and Coma in Children. Up to Date, version 15.1, May 2006. http://patients.uptodate.com/topic.asp?file=ped_neur/6748. Accessed December 20, 2007.

86

AFTER CONSIDERATION OF THE ABCs IN AN ACUTELY BURNED PEDIATRIC PATIENT, MANAGEMENT SHOULD BE DIRECTED AT FLUID MANAGEMENT, PREVENTION OF INFECTION, AND PAIN CONTROL

CYNTHIA GIBSON, MD

WHAT TO DO – TAKE ACTION

Children with burn injuries require complex care, involving medical, surgical, critical care, and rehabilitation services. Assessment always initially involves evaluation of the ABCs. Most severely burned patients are intubated for airway protection and respiratory support. There may be presence of direct injury due to inhalation injury or secondary injury due to activation of systemic inflammatory response. Proper fluid management, prevention of infection, and adequate pain control are important factors for the continued care of burn patients.

Burn trauma leads to hypovolemic and distributive shock, due to generalized microvascular injury and interstitial third spacing. There are ongoing fluid shifts throughout resuscitation and recovery. Fluid resuscitation formulas have been developed based on the percentage of body surface area (BSA) burned and weight of the patient. The Parkland formula is the most widely used formula. The formula provides resuscitation with isotonic crystalloid solution at 4 mL/kg per percentage of BSA burned plus the maintenance intravenous fluid (IVF) rate; the first half of fluid resuscitation is provided over the first 8 hours and the second half over the next 16 hours. This formula provides an estimate of fluid requirements and continual clinical parameters must be assessed to adjustment the fluid resuscitation to meet the patient's physiologic demands. The most common parameter to monitor is urine output. If the urine output is 1 to 2 mL/kg/hr, then fluid management is appropriate. If the output is <1 mL/kg/hr, an increase in fluid resuscitation, such as a fluid bolus may be necessary. When the output is >3 mL/kg/hr, the fluid rate should be decreased to two-thirds the calculated Parkland formula recommendation. Judicious use of fluid may avert such complications as pulmonary edema, cerebral edema, or acute electrolyte fluctuations.

A significant burn compromises the integrity of the skin, therefore, compromising the immune function locally and systemically, as well as the

© 2008 by Lippincott Williams & Wilkins, a Wolters Kluwer business

ability of the body to regulate temperature and fluids. Infection of burn wounds accompanied with local and systemic immune dysfunction is a serious life-threatening complication. Use of topical antimicrobial agents in the care of burn wounds is standard once the wounds have been débrided. These help limit the colonization and prevent infection within the wound. Superficial burns do not require treatment with antimicrobial ointments. These ointments are best utilized in the care of superficial partial thickness burns. Deep partial thickness or full-thickness burns often require skin grafts and use of topical antimicrobials help prevent infection in anticipation of grafting. Common agents used include bacitracin (which is especially useful for facial burns), silver sulfadiazine (Silvadene) and mafenide acetate (Sulfamylon). There is currently no role for prophylactic intravenous antibiotics in the management of children with burn injuries.

Children with inhalation injuries pose a special circumstance for emergency and critical care physicians. Clinical evidence of inhalation injury includes respiratory distress, hypoxemia, hoarseness, stridor, wheezing, oropharyngeal blistering, tongue swelling, carbonaceous sputum, and singed eyebrows and nasal hairs. A high index of suspicion must be maintained in the care of the burned child. Early intubation is recommended if inhalation injury is suspected because of the anatomy of the pediatric airway and its susceptibility to rapid occlusion by edema. Monitoring of carboxyhemoglobin levels can help determine the degree of carbon monoxide poisoning and the need for high concentration of oxygen to displace carbon monoxide from hemoglobin. A prolonged high-oxygen requirement may be an indication of the severity of the acute lung injury. The lung injury may not manifest until 24 to 48 hours after the initial burn injury. Management is supportive, with mechanical ventilation and lung protective strategies and aggressive pulmonary toilet. There is no defined role for the use of systemic steroids in the treatment of burn patients, even with acute lung injury.

Pain control is another important component in the management of pediatric burn patients. Inadequately treated pain has important physiologic and emotional complications. Adequate analgesia, usually with a narcotic analgesic and continued reassessment, is an important accompaniment to fluid and infection prevention.

Children with burn injuries pose special challenges to physicians. Appropriate fluid management, prevention of infection, and wound care that promotes wound healing have improved the survival in these patients. Pain control reduces the emotional scars associated with these injuries.

SUGGESTED READINGS

Duffy BJ, McLaughlin PM, Eichelberger MR. Assessment, triage, and early management of burns in children. *Clin Ped Emerg Med*. 2006;7(2):82–93.

Ipaktchi K, Arbabi S. Advances in burn critical care. *Crit Care Med*. 2006;34(9 Suppl):S239–S244.

87

DO NOT MISS SEPSIS IN BABIES THAT PRESENT WITH FEVER

CYNTHIA GIBSON, MD

WHAT TO DO – INTERPRET THE DATA

Evaluation and treatment of a neonate for possible bacterial infection and sepsis is one of the most common pediatric practices. Signs and symptoms of sepsis in a neonate are quite broad and include respiratory distress, lethargy or irritability, fever or hypothermia, hypo- or hyperglycemia, acidosis, hypotonia, poor feeding apnea, cyanosis, seizures, poor perfusion, shock, unexplained jaundice, or simply "not looking well." Ten percent of full-term babies with fever not due to environmental causes may have bacterial sepsis.

Because the neonate's response to sepsis is generic and often confusing, a systematic approach that does not vary is important for assuring that all infants with potential sepsis are identified. Evaluation of a neonate with fever should include a complete history and physical. Laboratory investigations include a complete blood cell count with a white blood cell differential, blood culture, urine culture, and lumbar puncture. Other potentially useful tests may include a chest x-ray, C-reactive protein, erythrocyte sedimentation rate, and a bacterial antigen profile. Although the large proportion of septic workups in infants are negative, the method exists to assure that those babies with potentially devastating meningitis are identified and treated early. Treatment should begin as soon as possible and include antibiotics that cover organisms commonly found in the neonatal period, including group B streptococci and *Escherichia coli*.

SUGGESTED READINGS

Bergman DA, Mayer ML, Pantell RH, et al. Does clinical presentation explain practice variability in the treatment of febrile infants? *Pediatrics.* 2006;117:787–795.

Gerdes JS. Diagnosis and management of bacterial infections in the neonate. *Pediatr Clin North Am.* 2004;51:939–959.

Van den Bruel A, Bruyninckx R, Vermeire E, et al. Signs and symptoms in children with a serious infection: a qualitative study. *BMC Fam Pract.* 2005;6:36.

© 2008 by Lippincott Williams & Wilkins, a Wolters Kluwer business

88

SEVERE CLINICAL PRESENTATIONS OF DISEASES USUALLY HIGHLIGHT IMPORTANT OPPORTUNITIES FOR AGGRESSIVE DIAGNOSTIC TESTING AND TREATMENT

ANJALI SUBBASWAMY, MD

WHAT TO DO – GATHER APPROPRIATE DATA

Consider a diagnosis of Langerhans cell histiocytosis (LCH) as a possibility in cases of severe seborrheic dermatitis, especially if atrophy, ulceration, or purpura is present.

Seborrheic dermatitis, commonly known as cradle cap, is frequently seen in infants and children. Typical lesions are scaly, oily, and located on the scalp and sometimes behind the ears. A papulosquamous disorder patterned on the sebum-rich areas of the scalp, face, and trunk, it is commonly aggravated by changes in humidity or seasons, scratching, or emotional stress. It can present in combination with atopic dermatitis. Seborrheic dermatitis is uncommon in children after infancy and before puberty. In this older age group, scalp scaling is likely to be due to other causes such as tinea capitis, atopic dermatitis, or psoriasis. For severe lesions, refractory to the usual therapies, an expanded differential diagnosis must be entertained. This includes disorders with potential for organ involvement, such as LCH.

LCH is a group of idiopathic disorders characterized by the proliferation of specialized bone marrow-derived Langerhans cells (LCs) and mature eosinophils. The Birbeck granule is the histopathological hallmark. The term LCH is generally preferred to the older term, histiocytosis X. The Histiocyte Society has divided histocytic disorders into three different groups: (a) dendritic cell histiocytosis, (b) erythrophagocytic macrophage disorders, (c) malignant histiocytosis. LCH belongs in group 1. The clinical spectrum ranges from an acute fulminant, disseminated disease (Letterer Siwe) to a few indolent, chronic lesions of bone or other organs called eosinophilic granulomas. Hand-Schüller-Christian disease is an intermediate form that classically presents as the triad of diabetes insipidus, proptosis, and lytic bone

ⓒ 2008 by Lippincott Williams & Wilkins, a Wolters Kluwer business

lesions. Disseminated disease appears more commonly in children younger than 2 years of age, whereas the chronic and acute disseminated forms are most common in children ages 2 to 15 years.

An ongoing debate exists over whether this is a reactive or neoplastic process. The exact pathogenesis is still unclear. Although the disease is rare, with an annual incidence of 0.5 to 5 cases per million per year, it can be serious. More than one half of patients younger than 2 years with disseminated LCH and organ dysfunction die of the disease, whereas unifocal LCH and most cases of congenital self-healing histiocytosis are self-limited. Patients of all ages are affected. Establishing the diagnosis and extent of disease will facilitate the prompt initiation of appropriate therapy, which ranges from excision of solitary lesions to steroids or chemotherapy for disseminated disease.

Signs of LCH depend on the localization and extent of the disease. The clinical spectrum of LCH is broad. Cutaneous manifestations occur in up to 80% of patients with disseminated disease. These lesions may be noduloulcerative in the oral, axillary, perineal, perivulvar, or retroauricular regions. Extensive coalescence, scaling, or crusting may occur. Lesions consist of closely set petechiae and yellow-brown papules topped with scales and crust. The papules may coalesce to form an erythematous, weeping eruption, mimicking seborrheic dermatitis. Intertriginous lesions are often exudative, and secondary infection and ulceration may occur.

The differential diagnosis includes seborrheic dermatitis, Wiskott-Aldrich syndrome, acrodermatitis enteropathica, erythema toxicum, neonatorum, incontinentia pigmenti, mastocytosis, and acropustulosis of infancy. The diagnostic workup should include histologic examination of skin lesions, appropriate radiographs, hematologic and chemistry profiles, and looking for bone and organ involvement when indicated.

SUGGESTED READINGS

Braier J, Chantada G, Rosso D, et al. Langerhans cell histiocytosis: retrospective evaluation of 123 patients at a single institution. *Pediatr Hematol Oncol.* 1999;16(5):377–385.

McDonald LL, Smith ML. Diagnostic dilemmas in pediatric/adolescent dermatology: scaly scalp. *J Pediatr Health Care.* 1998;12(2):80–84.

Williams M. Differential diagnosis of seborrheic dermatitis. *Pediatr Rev.* 1986;7:204–211.

89

DO NOT ADMINISTER IMMUNOGLOBULINS (IGS) FOR LOW IGA LEVELS

ESTHER FORRESTER, MD

WHAT TO DO – INTERPRET THE DATA

IgA deficiency is the most common primary immunodeficiency, with an occurrence ranging from 1/400 to 2,000 individuals. The frequency of IgA deficiency is greater in people of European descent and may be as high as 1 in 500. In the United States, whites are affected more than blacks by a ratio of 20:1. Asian Americans have an even lower incidence, with the occurrence in Japanese descendents being 1 in 18,500 persons.

IgA deficiency may be primary or secondary (acquired), sporadic, or familial. Both serum and secretory IgA are lacking in most patients and, rarely, one or the other is lacking. Inheritance is either autosomal recessive or dominant. The primary defect in selective IgA deficiency is related to a failure of B cells to differentiate in response to appropriate stimuli to mature isotype-switched surface IgA-positive B cells and IgA-secreting plasma cells. The basis for the defect is not known. Certain drugs, such as phenytoin, D-penicillamine, sulfasalazine, and hydroxychloroquine, have been associated with this entity. Congenital cases of noninherited IgA deficiency in association with rubella, cytomegalovirus, and *Toxoplasma gondii* have been reported.

Although some studies have reported recurrent infections in as many as 50% of IgA-deficient patients, most of these individuals are healthy. Some patients develop symptoms after an uneventful childhood and early adulthood. Recurrent or chronic upper and lower respiratory tract infections result in bronchiectasis or cor pulmonale in insufficiently treated patients. Gastrointestinal infection with *Giardia lamblia* infection is common as are a spruelike syndrome, ulcerative colitis, and Crohn disease.

The incidence of autoimmune and collagen vascular diseases, including rheumatoid arthritis, systemic lupus erythematosus, autoimmune hepatitis, hemolytic anemia, and endocrinopathies, is also increased, with reports of up to 25% of patients being affected.

Patients with undetectable levels of IgA antibodies may develop anti-IgA antibodies after the administration of blood products. Once sensitized, these patients are at risk for anaphylactic reactions if they receive blood products

© 2008 by Lippincott Williams & Wilkins, a Wolters Kluwer business

containing even small amounts of IgA. An antibody response to cow's milk protein is also common.

The variability in clinical expression is explained by several factors. Symptoms may be attenuated by an increased excretion of monomeric IgM in these patients' secretions, which helps to compensate for the lack of IgA. Symptoms may be worsened by the association of an IgG subclass deficiency.

Intravenous Ig (IVIG) replacement therapy is the treatment of choice for most primary B-cell disorders with hypogammaglobulinemia, including x-linked agammaglobulinemia, common variable immunodeficiency, immunodeficiency with thymoma, and most of the combined immunodeficiencies. However, selective IgA deficiency has no treatment. Therapy should be directed toward the specific disease. Administration of IVIG to patients with IgG subclass deficiency is not recommended unless antibodies are absent or there is no response to prophylactic antibiotics. Gammaglobulin is not used in selective IgA deficiency unless IgG2 subclass deficiency or antibody deficiency is also present. The prognosis is the same as the associated disorder.

SUGGESTED READINGS

Cooper MA, Pommering TL, Korányi K. Primary immunodeficiencies. *Am Fam Physician.* 2003;68:2001–2008.

Makhoul I, Claxton D, Rybka W. Pure B-cell Disorders. Available at: www.emedicine.com/med/topic216.htm. Accessed March 2, 2007.

National Primary Immunodeficiency Resource Center. Selective IgA Deficiency. Available at: http://www.info4pi.org/faq/index.cfm?Section=faq&CFID=24824785&CFTOKEN=51564784#24. Accessed March 1, 2007.

90

RECOGNIZE THE SIGNS OF ANAPHYLAXIS (TYPE I HYPERSENSITIVITY) AND KNOW HOW TO TREAT IT AGGRESSIVELY

YOLANDA LEWIS-RAGLAND, MD

WHAT TO DO – INTERPRET THE DATA, MAKE A DECISION, TAKE ACTION

Anaphylaxis is an acute, multisystem, and severe allergic reaction, known also as type I hypersensitivity reaction. The term comes from the Greek words *ana* (again) and *phylaxis* (protection). Anaphylaxis occurs when a person is exposed to a trigger substance, called an allergen, to which they are sensitized. Re-exposure to the trigger substance intensifies what is normally a protective immune response and it become detrimental.

CLASSIFICATION

Gell and Coombs classified hypersensitivity reactions into four types:

- **Type I reactions** (i.e., immediate hypersensitivity reactions) involve immunoglobulin (Ig) E-mediated release of histamine and other mediators from mast cells and basophils.
- **Type II reactions** (i.e., cytotoxic hypersensitivity reactions) involve IgG or IgM antibodies bound to cell surface antigens, with subsequent complement fixation.
- **Type III reactions** (i.e., immune-complex reactions) involve circulating antigen–antibody immune complexes that deposit in postcapillary venules, with subsequent complement fixation.
- **Type IV reactions** (i.e., delayed hypersensitivity reactions, cell-mediated immunity) are mediated by T cells rather than by antibodies.

TYPE I HYPERSENSITIVITY

Type I hypersensitivity reactions are extremely important to recognize and treat because their reactions are immediate; abrupt in onset, usually occurring within 15 to 30 minutes from the time of exposure; and potentially life threatening. This "immediate" reaction assists with the identification of the triggering antigen. Anaphylaxis is related to the action of IgE and other anaphylatoxins, which act to release histamine and other mediators from mast cells during degranulation. Histamine has a number of effects, including the vasodilation of arterioles and constriction of bronchioles in the lungs.

© 2008 by Lippincott Williams & Wilkins, a Wolters Kluwer business

Signs and Symptoms. Patients with anaphylaxis may report or experience the following signs and symptoms:

- Respiratory distress
- Hypotension
- Fainting
- Unconsciousness
- Urticaria
- Flushed appearance
- Angioedema (swelling of face, neck and throat)
- Tears (due to angioedema and stress)
- Vomiting
- Pruritus (itching)
- Diarrhea
- Abdominal pain
- Anxiety

Treatment. The first thing to consider in a patient experiencing anaphylaxis is the cause of the reaction, if it can be identified, and the withdrawal of the offending agent (i.e., stop drug infusion, remove bee stinger). This point is often overlooked but is an essential part of practice. Next, the patient needs to be assessed for airway involvement because a rapid constriction of the airway can lead to respiratory failure and respiratory arrest. Patients with respiratory compromise may require intubation. Occasionally, laryngeal edema will be so severe that oral intubation is difficult and a tracheostomy needs to be performed. The level of consciousness and vital signs can assist in directing interventions.

Interventions.

- Epinephrine should be administered immediately. Epinephrine prevents worsening of airway constriction, stimulates the heart to continue beating, and may be lifesaving. It acts on β_2-adrenergic receptors in the lung as a powerful bronchodilator. Tachycardia results from stimulation of β_1-adrenergic receptors of the heart. Repetitive administration of epinephrine can cause tachycardia and arrhythmias. The administration of 0.3 to 0.5 mL of a 1:1,000 dilution is often prescribed.
- The rapid administration of isotonic intravenous fluids should be administered to restore blood pressure.
- Vasoactive agents (i.e., dopamine) may be prescribed if hypotension persists and is unresponsive to fluids.
- H1- and H2-receptor blockers can alleviate pruritus and urticaria. Cimetidine, when combined with any of several H1 antihistamines, blocks histamine-induced hypotension.

- Albuterol nebulizers can be used to treat bronchospasm.
- Corticosteroids help to prevent or control the latent phase of the reaction.

Patients are often observed in the hospital because of biphasic reactions with recurrent symptoms even after the patients condition has stabilized. Usually, patients do well with acute management after the offending agent is removed and the patient's condition stabilized.

SUGGESTED READINGS

Anand MK, Routes JM. eMedicine—Hypersensitivity Reactions, Immediate. Available at: www.emedicine.com/med/topic1101.htm. Accessed December 20, 2007.

Hypersensitivity—Global Advanced Trait Descriptions. Available at: www.similarminds.com/types/hypersensitivity.html. Accessed December 20, 2007.

Hypersensitivity Reactions. Available at: www.pathmicro.med.sc.edu/ghaffar/hyper00.htm. Accessed December 20, 2007.

91

PATIENTS WITH T LYMPHOCYTE DEFECTS SHOULD NOT BE GIVEN LIVE VACCINES OR BLOOD PRODUCTS THAT ARE NOT IRRADIATED

ANJALI SUBBASWAMY, MD

WHAT TO DO – MAKE A DECISION

Live attenuated virus vaccines (measles, mumps, rubella, varicella, bacille Calmette-Guérin) could be lethal in individuals with T cell defects and should not be administered. The replication of vaccine viruses can be enhanced in persons with immune deficiencies, such as leukemia, lymphoma, generalized malignancy, or patients under therapy with alkylating agents, antimetabolites, radiation, large doses of corticosteroids. Case reports have linked measles vaccine and measles infection to subsequent death in severely immunocompromised children.

The immune system is classically divided into two responses, the innate and the adaptive responses. The innate immune system is comprised of neutrophils, macrophages, natural killer cells, and complement proteins, which respond rapidly to infections in a manner that is relatively nonspecific to any particular infection. The adaptive immune system is composed primarily of T and B cells, and typically responds to infections more slowly than the innate immune system. The adaptive immune system is much more specific to particular infections than the innate immune system due to a mechanism known as memory.

The adaptive immune system has been defined further into the humoral and cellular immune arms. The humoral immune system primarily involves B cells and their production of immunoglobulins, whereas the cellular immune system classically involves T cells and their ability to produce various cytokines. The humoral and cellular immune systems are functionally dependent on each other in mounting effective immune responses.

Blood administration also carries particular risks for the immunocompromised patient. Patients with pure B cell immunodeficiency have few transfusion-related problems. Those with T cell defects are susceptible to transfusion-associated graft-versus-host disease (TaGvHD). Three factors create this situation: (a) immunocompetent donor T cells, (b) histoincompatibility between donor and recipient, and (c) the inability of the recipient to reject donor T cells. There are risks with red blood cells,

© 2008 by Lippincott Williams & Wilkins, a Wolters Kluwer business

platelets, granulocytes and fresh liquid plasma. Previously, frozen products such as fresh frozen plasma did not carry the same risk. Lymphocyte viability declines with age, so older red blood cells carry reduced risk. TaGvHD can present from 4 days to 1 month posttransfusion. The symptoms include rash, diarrhea, hepatitis, fever, lymphadenopathy, and bone marrow suppression, leading to thrombocytopenia and anemia. Diagnosis requires demonstration of human leukocyte antigen chimerism and the treatment includes high-dose corticosteroids and supportive therapies. Irradiation of blood products can prevent TaGvGHD.

SUGGESTED READINGS

Badami KG. The immunocompromised patient and transfusion. *Postgrad Med J.* 2001;77:230–234.

Recommendations of the Advisory Committee on Immunization Practices (ACIP): use of vaccines and immune globulins in persons with altered immunocompetence. *MMWR Recomm Rep.* 1993;42(RR-4):1–18.

Verbsky JW, Grossman WJ. Cellular and genetic basis of primary immune deficiencies. *Pediatr Clin North Am.* 2006;53(4):649–684.

REMEMBER THAT ERYTHEMA MULTIFORME (EM) MAY BE A SIGN OF UNDERLYING HYPERSENSITIVITY AND MAY PROGRESS TO STEVENS-JOHNSON SYNDROME (SJS), WHICH CAN REQUIRE AGGRESSIVE FLUID AND SKIN CARE

MADAN DHARMAR, MD

WHAT TO DO — INTERPRET THE DATA

EM represents a syndrome of inflammatory skin eruptions that can manifest as a mild self-limiting form or as a life-threatening condition requiring aggressive lifesaving and critical care therapies.

EM-minor, or the mild form of EM, is characterized by the occurrence of characteristic skin lesions, which are described as target lesions, iris lesions, or iris erythema. The skin lesions follow a symmetric distribution and commonly seen on the extensor surfaces of the extremities, back of hands, feet, palms, and soles. The trunk and head are usually spared. Cutaneous symptoms consist of itching, stinging, and burning sensations; occasionally, general symptoms, such as mild fever and chill, are present.

The "erythema multiforme disease spectrum" comprises four distinct, severe, clinical subvariants: (a) bullous erythema multiforme (bullous-EM), (b) SJS, (c) SJS–toxic epidermal necrolysis (TEN)-overlap syndrome, and (d) TEN.

EM-major or bullous EM, in addition to the characteristic target lesions in symmetric distribution, consists of atypical, raised target lesions with some degree of moderate epidermal detachment involving <10% of the body surface.

In SJS, the cutaneous lesions are more extensive, with flat-atypical targets and macules that predominate over classic target lesions, and predominately in the trunk and face. When epidermal necrolysis becomes a dominant feature, with involvement of up to 10% of the body surface, EM-major merges into SJS. Blistering of individual skin lesions as well as erosions/detachment become delineating features. Moreover, these patients develop severe and extensive mucosal lesions of the oral, conjunctival, and genital mucous membranes, which then determine the course of the disease. These lesions are painful and consist of desquamation, erosions, and superficial ulcerations. This disease is often complicated by extensive percutaneous

© 2008 by Lippincott Williams & Wilkins, a Wolters Kluwer business

loss of electrolytes and fluids, and there is a high risk for scarring and milia and synechia formation, especially on the eyes, upper gastrointestinal tract, trachea, and genitalia. Patients are also at risk of serious bacterial infections from their erosions.

In SJS/TEN-overlap, patients have widespread macules or flat targets with 10% to 30% of the body surface area involved. TEN presents similarly to SJS, but involves at least 30% of body surface. EM, SJS, SJS/TEN overlap, and TEN not only have similar clinical features but also are caused by similar exposure to drugs or infection. The pathophysiological mechanisms in the diverse variants of the EM/SJS/TEN disease spectrum are only partially understood. The immunopathologic pattern of early lesions suggests a cell-mediated cytotoxic reaction against the epidermal cells with the epidermis infiltrated by activated lymphocytes, mainly CD8 cells, and macrophages. An immune reaction against drug-reactive metabolites produced in excess may be responsible. Because infiltrating cells are present in only moderate numbers, it is unlikely that these cells are the principal cause of epidermal necrosis. Cytokines, released by activated mononuclear cells and keratinocytes, may contribute to local cell death, fever, and malaise. The diagnosis of all of these disorders is primarily clinical, based on the characteristic lesion on the skin and mucous membranes. Skin biopsy is also helpful in making the diagnosis; it shows full thickness epidermal necrosis, which is characteristic of the diseases.

Early recognition of the disease, immediate withdrawal of any potential causative agent, and initiation of intravenous fluid replacement is essential in the management of this disease. All patients must be examined to access the extent of detachment of the epidermis and for an imbalance of fluid, protein, and electrolyte homeostasis on a daily basis. Considering the massive loss of fluid via denuded skin, fluid resuscitation should be initiated immediately after hospitalization, similar to burn victims. Any disturbance should be adequately treated with electrolyte solutions, blood products (e.g., erythrocytes, fresh frozen plasma), and albumin. Surgical débridement and whirlpool therapy are recommended to remove the necrotic epidermis. Regular ophthalmic examination and ophthalmic care using artificial tears or lubricating ointment is recommended.

The management of SJS involves aggressive fluid and electrolyte management, nutritional support, pain control, and necessary precautions to avoid super infections similar to the treatment for burn patients. Treatment with corticosteroids is controversial because it might aggravate the condition or increase risk of secondary infections. Some consider the use of early intravenous immunoglobulin to be of benefit, although to date, there has not been a randomized control trial demonstrating its efficacy.

SUGGESTED READINGS

Bastuji-Garin S, Rzany B, Stern RS, et al. Clinical classification of cases of toxic epidermal necrolysis, Stevens-Johnson syndrome, and erythema multiforme. *Arch Dermatol.* 1993;129(1):92–96.

Marvin JA, Heimbach DM, Engrav LH, et al. Improved treatment of the Stevens-Johnson syndrome. *Arch Surg.* 1984;119(5):601–605.

Roujeau JC, Stern RS. Severe adverse cutaneous reactions to drugs. *N Engl J Med.* 1994;(331):1272–1285.

PROVIDE SUPPORTIVE THERAPY FOR PATIENTS WITH HENOCH-SCHÖNLEIN PURPURA (HSP)

EMILY RIEHM MEIER, MD

WHAT TO DO – TAKE ACTION

Steroids should be considered only in the setting of severe gastrointestinal or renal involvement or painful cutaneous edema.

HSP is a vasculitis almost always affecting children younger than 20 years of age. It commonly presents as abdominal pain with nonthrombocytopenic palpable purpura on the lower extremities and buttocks following a viral upper respiratory infection. In most cases, it is a self-limited problem, resolving without intervention. Because of potential renal and serious gastrointestinal complications, careful monitoring is warranted. Renal complications can range from mild hematuria to glomerulonephritis. Gastrointestinal complications can range from self-limited abdominal pain to intussusception. Renal impairment is the most significant long-term complication in children with HSP. After careful study, children with a normal urinalysis at diagnosis are not at increased risk for chronic renal problems. On the other hand, children with nephrotic or nephritic syndrome at presentation have more than a 10-fold increase in long-term renal sequelae. These findings raise the question: Can anything be done to prevent long-term complications of HSP?

A recent prospective, placebo-controlled, double-blind study addressing this question was published by Ronkainen et al. in 2006. Because HSP is rare, a study of this nature is difficult. The investigators compared patients with HSP who were treated with prednisone (1 mg/kg/day) versus placebo for the first 2 weeks following diagnosis, followed by a taper for two more weeks. The primary outcome measure was renal involvement at different time points following diagnosis. Secondary outcomes included improvement of abdominal and joint pain and resolution of the purpuric rash.

The authors noted no significant differences between the treatment and placebo groups in either rash resolution or in rash recurrence after 1 month. Only a small percentage (8%) of children had debilitating abdominal pain during the acute phase of illness. In this small group, prednisone improved the pain. More significant than pain control, though, was an improvement in renal function in the prednisone-treated group. Forty-three

© 2008 by Lippincott Williams & Wilkins, a Wolters Kluwer business

percent of patients enrolled in the study had renal involvement, either at the time of diagnosis or within the first 6 months following diagnosis. Although prednisone did not prevent the development of renal complications, it was effective in altering the progression of renal disease. Patients treated with prednisone had a more rapid resolution of renal symptomatology than the placebo group.

Ronkainen's study demonstrated that early steroid therapy should not be used for each child diagnosed with HSP. Instead, early steroid treatment should be aimed at children who are at the highest risk for renal involvement, namely those who are older than 6 years of age at diagnosis or those with renal symptoms at diagnosis.

SUGGESTED READINGS

Ballinger S. Henoch-Schönlein purpura. *Curr Opin Rheumatol.* 2003;15:591–594.

Narchi H. Risk of long term renal impairment and duration of follow up recommended for Henoch-Schönlein purpura with normal or minimal urinary findings: a systematic review. *Arch Dis Child.* 2005;90:916–920.

Ronkainen J, Koskimies O, Ala-Houhala M, et al. Early prednisone therapy in Henoch-Schönlein Purpura: a randomized, double-blind, placebo-controlled trial. *J Pediatr.* 2006;149:241–247.

PATIENTS WHO NOTE A SEAFOOD OR IODINE ALLERGY CAN SAFELY RECEIVE INTRAVENOUS (IV) CONTRAST

CRAIG DEWOLFE, MD

WHAT TO DO – GATHER APPROPRIATE DATA

A previous reaction to seafood, povidone iodine, or other iodine-containing substance does not have any predictive value beyond a reaction to contrast material. The practitioner may also counsel the patients who have had a reaction to contrast material that they can continue to ingest iodine-containing foods or drugs. The false link between iodine-containing foods and contrast material can be traced to two studies in the early 1970s that reported a 6% rate of reaction in patients with a reported seafood allergy. Subsequent reports have not confirmed these findings. Instead, oversight committees, such as the one sponsored by the American College of Radiology, have regularly counseled that a seafood allergy should be considered in the same category as any other allergy when considering the individual risk of contrast material to the patient. Unfortunately, reports firmly establish that physicians resist performing needed studies in patients with a seafood allergy. In 2004, Confino-Cohen and Goldberg reported that 77% of physicians would have unnecessarily withheld radiocontrast material in patients with a history of a seafood allergy or rash after local application of iodine-containing antiseptics. Moreover, 69% of them would have taken various irrelevant precautions when using iodine-containing antiseptics in patients who have had a history of reaction to an iodinated contrast media (ICM).

ICM is regularly used for opacification in computed tomography, excretory urographic, and angiographic studies. ICM is classified into two groups: ionic high-osmolality contrast media and nonionic low-osmolality contrast material. The former is associated with a 5% to 12% incidence of adverse reactions, whereas the latter is associated with a 1% to 3% incidence, but because they both contain iodine, the discrepancy is related to another property of the media.

ICM reactions are related to either an anaphylactoid or a chemotoxic effect of the media. Anaphylactoid reactions occur spontaneously and independently of the dose or concentration of the material. Symptoms include

© 2008 by Lippincott Williams & Wilkins, a Wolters Kluwer business

urticaria, swelling of the mucus membranes, bronchospasm, hypotension, convulsions, and cardiac arrest. Reactions are generally thought to be caused by a combination of histamine release and activation of vasoactive cascade system.

Chemotoxic reactions are related to the concentration and dose of the ICM. Common symptoms include a hot, flushed, or tingly sensation; metallic taste; and nausea. Rarer but more serious reactions include acute renal failure, convulsions, cardiac arrhythmias, or cardiac failure. The reactions are caused by physiochemical effects of the injected agent on a specific organ.

There are several risk factors that increase the likelihood for a reaction to ICM. Sicker patients are more likely to have an adverse reaction associated with a chemotoxic effect, whereas patients with allergic tendencies are at increased risk for an anaphylactoid reaction. Studies suggest that patients with a history of an allergy to any substance are twice as likely to have an allergy to ICM, whereas patients with a history of asthma may have five times the risk. Patients with a past reaction to ICM may be at three to eight times the risk of the general population. A detailed screening of the patient for hemodynamic, neurologic, and general nutritive status in addition to history of allergies, asthma, and the use of beta-blockers should occur prior to ordering or administering the ICM. Higher-risk patients should receive low-osmolar, non-ICM. Corticosteroids and antihistamines should also be considered, although the need for the latter has been called into question by a recent meta-analysis. In addition, the practitioner should be prepared for the development of a reaction, usually within the first 20 minutes of the infusion. Fortunately, because of the greater awareness and preparation for reactions, the mortality rate associated with ICM has dropped to 0.9 per 100,000 administrations.

A reaction to seafood or iodine should not be treated differently than another allergic reaction when considering the risk of ICM. Iodine is an essential element for life, thus it is unlikely that a patient has a reaction to elemental iodine alone. Rather, in some rare cases, an iodine/protein complex triggers the reaction, but the reaction is not predictive beyond the fact that the patient is prone to allergic reactions. If a patient has a severe reaction that appears to be anaphylactoid to an iodine-containing product, then pretreatment with corticosteroids and antihistamines for subsequent exposure to ICM would be indicated. Less-significant reactions would likely not benefit from treatment.

In summary, patients who note a seafood or povidone iodine allergy can safely receive ICM. Similarly, those patients who have reacted to ICM can continue to ingest iodine-containing products.

SUGGESTED READINGS

American College of Radiology. Committee on Drugs and Contrast Media. Manual on contrast media version 5.0; 2004. Available at: http://www.acr.org/SecondaryMainMenu Categories/quality_safety/contrast_manual/FullVersionofManualonContrastMedia Doc12.aspx. Accessed February 1, 2007.

Bush WH, Swanson DP. Acute reactions to intravascular contrast media: types, risk factors, recognition, and specific treatment. *AJR Am J Roentgenol.* 1991;157:1153–1161.

Confino-Cohen R, Goldberg A. Safe administration of contrast media: what do physicians know? *Ann Allergy Asthma Immunol.* 2004;93:166–170.

95

MANY PATIENTS DO NOT RECEIVE CEPHALOSPORINS DUE TO THEIR PENICILLIN ALLERGY; MOST OF THESE PATIENTS WILL NOT HAVE AN ALLERGIC RESPONSE AND CAN RECEIVE THESE DRUGS SAFELY

DOROTHY CHEN, MD

WHAT TO DO – GATHER APPROPRIATE DATA

Many patients do not receive cephalosporins due to their penicillin allergy; most of these patients will not have an allergic response and can receive these drugs safely.

Penicillin is a commonly used antibiotic in pediatrics. The penicillins consist of a β-lactam ring and a side chain. The β-lactam ring provides the antimicrobial activity by inhibiting the bacterial penicillin-binding proteins. The side chains determine the spectrum of activity. Penicillin is often prescribed for common childhood infections, such as otitis media and sinusitis. Approximately 1% to 10% of patients who take β-lactam antibiotics report adverse reactions. These reactions are often assumed to be allergic reactions that limit their future use.

Adverse reactions can include a wide spectrum of symptoms: nausea, emesis, diarrhea, rash, or anaphylaxis. Many of these are nonimmunologic effects. It is important to elicit the details of the symptoms to differentiate between side effects and a true immunoglobulin (Ig)E-mediated reaction. Type I allergic reactions are IgE-mediated and present with signs ranging from urticaria to anaphylaxis. They typically occur from 1 to 72 hours after ingestion of the medication. Skin testing can be performed to confirm IgE-mediated reactions and is approximately 60% predictive of a reaction. Type II (IgG), III (IgG or IgM-mediated), and IV reactions to penicillin do occur, but these are not allergic (IgE-mediated) reactions.

Penicillins and cephalosporins both have a β-lactam ring. However, penicillins have a 5-membered thiazolidine ring and cephalosporins have a 6-membered dihydrothiazine ring. When these antibiotics degrade, their structures are quite different. Penicillins preserve the thiazolidine ring, whereas cephalosporins degrade both the β-lactam and dihydrothiazine rings, the cross-reactivity between the β-lactam rings is minimal. The American Academy of Pediatrics supports cephalosporin use in patients with non-IgE mediated reactions to penicillin.

© 2008 by Lippincott Williams & Wilkins, a Wolters Kluwer business

Skin rashes are the most common reaction to cephalosporins and occur in 1% to 3% of patients. Anaphylaxis is a rare reaction. In penicillin-allergic patients, a reaction to cephalosporins can be a primary cephalosporin reaction, and thus their concordant reactions can be a coincidence. Many studies have researched the effect of cephalosporin in penicillin-allergic patients. The use of the term *allergic* varies, so the studies do not focus solely on IgE-mediated reactions. The cross-reactivity between cephalosporins and penicillin reactions depends on the specific generation of cephalosporin.

Caution should be used when administering a cephalosporin, such as cefoxitin, which has a similar 7-position side chain on the β-lactam ring, to a patient with a severe IgE-mediated reaction to penicillin. However, evidence supports the American Academy of Pediatrics' recommendation to give ceftriaxone to patients with non-IgE mediated reactions to penicillin. A careful history of the prior "reaction" to penicillin remains the most important determinant in prescribing other classes of antibiotics.

SUGGESTED READINGS

Malik ZA, Litman N. The penicillins. *Pediatr Rev.* 2006;27(12):471–473.

Pichichero ME. A review of evidence supporting the American Academy of Pediatrics Recommendation for prescribing cephalosporin antibiotics for penicillin-allergic patients. *Pediatrics.* 2005;115(4):1048–1057.

Ponvert C, Le Clainche L, de Blic J, et al. Allergy to B-lactam antibiotics in children. *Pediatrics.* 1999;104(4):e45.

96

Proper Vaccine Administration is Crucial to Achieve the Anticipated Results. Know the Methods for Administering Vaccines

Dorothy Chen, MD

What to Do – Gather Appropriate Data

Childhood immunizations have reduced the incidence of many infectious diseases. The global eradication of smallpox in 1977 and the eradication of poliomyelitis from North and South America are both examples of the successful use of immunizations. Vaccine response is determined by the antigen's chemical and physical nature, mode of administration, and host factors.

In addition to the proper storage and handling of vaccines, it is important to use the proper technique for vaccine administration (*Table 96.1*). The current routes of immunization are oral, intranasal, and parenteral. The primary route for vaccines is parenteral, either intramuscular or subcutaneous, depending on the method that demonstrates maximum efficacy and safety. Live vaccines, such as polio, can be given orally. This enables replication at the mucosal surfaces and the induction of secretory immunoglobulin A. However, currently, inactivated poliovirus is recommended for use in the United States. The live-attenuated influenza vaccine is the only approved intranasal vaccine.

In addition to the route of administration, the appropriate site and needle size should be determined for age. The anterolateral thigh and deltoid are commonly used sites. Vaccines with adjuvants such as aluminum need to be injected deep into the muscle. The American Academy of Pediatrics' *Redbook 2006*, outlines the recommended site and needle size for intramuscular administration of commonly used vaccines. Subcutaneous vaccines can be administered in the pinched-fold of the anterolateral outer thigh or upper outer triceps at a 45-degree angle. Multiple vaccines can be given simultaneously, but at least 1 inch apart. In the event of a local reaction, this will facilitate the identification of the causative agent. When vaccines are given inappropriately, their efficacy can be decreased. For example, hepatitis B vaccine should be given intramuscularly in the deltoid muscle;

© 2008 by Lippincott Williams & Wilkins, a Wolters Kluwer business

TABLE 96.1 VACCINES LICENSED FOR IMMUNIZATION AND DISTRIBUTED IN THE UNITED STATES AND THEIR ROUTES OF ADMINISTRATION[a]

VACCINE	TYPE	ROUTE
BCG	Live	ID (preferred) or SC
Diphtheria-tetanus (DT, Td)	Toxoids	IM
DTaP	Toxoids and inactivated bacterial components	IM
DTaP, hepatitis B, and IPV	Toxoids and inactivated bacterial components, recombinant viral antigen, inactivated virus	IM
Hepatitis A	Inactivated viral antigen	IM
Hepatitis B	Recombinant viral antigen	IM
Hepatitis A-hepatitis B	Inactivated and recombinant viral antigens	IM
Hib conjugates	Polysaccharide-protein conjugate	IM
Hib conjugate-DTaP (PRP-T reconstituted with DTaP)	Polysaccharide-protein conjugate with toxoids and inactivated bacterial components	IM
Hib conjugate (PRP-OMP) -hepatitis B	Polysaccharide-protein conjugate with recombinant viral antigen	IM
Influenza	Inactivated viral components	IM
Influenza	Live attenuated virus	Intranasal
Japanese encephalitis	Inactivated virus	SC
Measles	Live attenuated virus	SC
Meningococcal	Polysaccharide	SC
Meningococcal	Polysaccharide	SC
Meningococcal	Polysaccharide protein conjugate	IM
MMR	Live attenuated viruses	SC
MMRV	Live attenuated virus	SC
Mumps	Live attenuated virus	SC
Pneumococcal	Polysaccharide	IM or SC
Pneumococcal	Polysaccharide protein conjugate	IM
Poliovirus (IPV)	Inactivated virus	SC or IM
Rabies	Inactivated virus	IM
Rotavirus	Live attenuated virus	Oral
Rubella	Live attenuated virus	SC
Tdap	Toxoids and inactivated bacterial components	IM
Tetanus	Toxoid	IM
Varicella	Live attenuated	SC
Yellow Fever	Live attenuated	SC

BCG, bacille Calmette-Guérin; DT, diphtheria and tetanus toxoids (for children younger than 7 years of age); DTaP, diphtheria and tetanus toxoids and acellular pertussis, adsorbed; ID, intradermal; IM, intramuscular; Hib, *Haemophilus influenzae* type b; IPV, inactivated poliovirus; MMR, live measles-mumps-rubella; MMRV, live measles-mumps-rubella-varicella; PRP-T, polyribosylribitol phosphate-tetanus toxoid; PRP-OMP, polyribosylribitol phosphate-meningococcal outer membrane protein; SC, subcutaneous; Td, diphtheria and tetanus toxoids (for children 7 years of age or older and adults); Tdap, tetanus toxoid, reduced diphtheria toxoid, and acellular pertussis.
[a]Other vaccines licensed in the United States but not distributed include anthrax, smallpox, rhesus tetravalent rotavirus, and oral poliovirus (OPV) vaccines. The U.S. Food and Drug Administration maintains a Web site listing currently licensed vaccines in the United States (www.fda.gov/cber/vaccine/licvacc.htm). The American Academy of Pediatricians maintains a Web site (www.aapredbook.org/news/vaccstatus.shtml) showing status of licensure and recommendations for new vaccines.

subcutaneous administration in the buttocks has been shown to lower sero-conversion rates.

SUGGESTED READING

American Academy of Pediatrics. Committee on Infectious Diseases (COID). *Red Book 2007 Report of the Committee on Infectious Diseases*. 27th ed. Elk Grove Village, IL: American Academy of Pediatrics: 2007. www.aapredbook.org/news/vaccstatus.shtml. Accessed December 20, 2007.

97

DO NOT ROUTINELY TEST CHILDREN FOR TUBERCULOSIS (TB) EXPOSURE

YOLANDA LEWIS-RAGLAND, MD

WHAT TO DO – GATHER APPROPRIATE DATA

Mycobacterium tuberculosis (MTB) is an infectious agent that usually attacks the lungs, but can attack almost any part of the body. It is spread from person to person through the air by droplets when a person with MTB in their lungs or throat coughs, laughs, sneezes, or even talks. However, significant and repeated contact is usually required for infection. The routine universal testing of all children is no longer recommended because the conditions under which most infections are spread, including poverty and overcrowding, are well described. After a known exposure, high-risk or symptomatic patients are encouraged to undergo screening.

TESTING

The tuberculin skin test is one method to determine if a person has TB. Although there are several skin tests available, the preferred method is known as the Mantoux test, which involves intradermal administration of 0.1 mL of 5 tuberculin units (TU) as a partial protein derivative (PPD), usually at the flexor surface (dorsal or volar) of the forearm. The test should be read 48 to 72 hours after administration, and the transverse diameter of induration should be measured in millimeters.

PPD INTERPRETATION

The interpretation of the PPD result is determined by the risk factor(s) of the tested individual. Three levels, based on the size of the induration, have been recommended for defining a positive tuberculin reaction. Patients at highest risk for developing TB (usually immunocompromised), have a recommended threshold level of ≥ 5 mm, whereas those individuals with low to no risk factors have a threshold level of > 15 mm. A reaction of ≥ 10 mm should be considered positive for those with an increased probability

© 2008 by Lippincott Williams & Wilkins, a Wolters Kluwer business

of recent infection or conditions that increase the risk for TB (i.e., recent immigrants from high-prevalence countries).

DIAGNOSIS

There is a difference between infection with MTB and having active disease. Infected patients have the bacterium in their body. The body's defenses are protecting them from being symptomatic with the bacteria and the individuals do not appear sick. This is referred to as latent TB infection (LTBI). Alternatively, patients with active disease experience symptoms such as cough, fever, chills, and weight loss. These patients can spread the disease to others and require treatment as soon as possible. Once a person experiences a positive PPD (depending on their risk factors), the next step is to determine whether they have TB disease. This is done by obtaining a chest x-ray and testing the patient's sputum for *Mycobacterium*.

TREATMENT

Isoniazid is the most-widely used of the antituberculosis agents—it is bactericidal, relatively nontoxic, easily administered, and inexpensive. It is often given in combination with other drugs like rifampin (which has some important side effects, including hepatitis and thrombocytopenia), and pyrazinamide (which also adversely affects the liver). Multidrug resistance can become a problem in treating TB, especially if a proper regimen is not implemented and adhered to. For these reasons, directly observed therapy and the simultaneous use of multiple agents has become common.

SUGGESTED READINGS

American Lung Association. Tuberculosis (TB). Available at: www.lungusa.org/site/pp.asp?c= dvLUK9O0E&b=35778. Accessed November 14, 2007.
Centers for Disease Control and Prevention. http://www.cdc.gov/tb/surv/default.htm.
World Health Organization. Tuberculosis. Available at: www.who.int/mediacentre/factsheets/ fs104/en/. Accessed November 14, 2007.

98

DO NOT AVOID ANTIBIOTIC USE IN PATIENTS WITH SERIOUS INFECTIONS BECAUSE OF THEORETICAL LIMITATIONS

YOLANDA LEWIS-RAGLAND, MD

WHAT TO DO – TAKE ACTION

The American Academy of Pediatrician's evidence-based guidelines endorse the use of cephalosporin antibiotics for patients with reported allergies to penicillin for the treatment of acute bacterial sinusitis and acute otitis media. Many physicians, however, remain reluctant to prescribe such agents because of a fear of cross-reactivity between the two drug classes. Although these concerns are understandable, a lack of consistent data regarding exactly what constitutes an initial penicillin-allergic reaction and subsequent cross-sensitivity to cephalosporins may possibly prevent patients from receiving optimal antibiotic therapy.

This topic is one of great importance because true allergic reactions to penicillin can be extremely varied. Allergic responses occurring with a penicillin allergy range from annoying rashes to life-threatening reactions, such as difficulty anaphylaxis.

SIGNS AND SYMPTOMS OF PENICILLIN ALLERGY

Common signs and symptoms of penicillin allergy include:

- Rash
- Hives
- Itchy eyes
- Swollen lips, tongue, or face (angioedema).

The most serious allergic reaction to penicillin, however, is anaphylaxis, which has a high mortality if untreated. Anaphylactic reactions develop immediately after penicillin exposure in highly sensitized people and cause bronchoconstriction, hypotension, and loss of consciousness. Other serious signs and symptoms include:

- Wheezing
- Lightheadedness
- Slurred speech
- Rapid or weak pulse

© 2008 by Lippincott Williams & Wilkins, a Wolters Kluwer business

- Cyanosis, including circumoral and nail beds
- Diarrhea
- Nausea and vomiting.

ARE CEPHALOSPORINS A REAL THREAT?

Cephalosporin antibiotics are important in infectious diseases and, like penicillins, are widely prescribed for common infections such as bronchitis, otitis media, pneumonia, and cellulitis. They are also administered as first-line prophylaxis for many types of surgical procedures. A *relative* contraindication to these agents has been a history of allergy to penicillin. In this situation, many clinicians would select a different class of antibiotic, such as a macrolide or vancomycin. However, the emergence of antimicrobial-resistant organisms demands that the selection of antibiotics be made only after careful evaluation.

In light of this, investigators have performed extensive studies with both experimental and clinical trials. The results indicate that if a cephalosporin with a side chain that is different from the penicillin is used. The risk of suffering an allergic reaction by administering cephalosporins to penicillin-allergic patients is very low.

SUGGESTED READINGS

Mayo Foundation for Medical Education and Research. Penicillin Allergy. December 22, 2005. Available at: www.cnn.com/HEALTH/library/DS/00620.html. Accessed November 14, 2007.

Novalbos A, Sastre J, Cuesta J, et al. Lack of allergic cross-reactivity to cephalosporins among patients allergic to penicillins. *Clin Exp Allergy*. 2001;31(3):438–443.

Romano A, Guéant-Rodriquez R-M, Viola M, et al. Summaries for patients. Cephalosporin allergy in patients with penicillin allergy. *Ann Intern Med*. 2004;141(1):I48.

99

KNOW THAT PINWORMS ARE A COMMON CAUSE OF HELMINTHIC INFECTION IN THE UNITED STATES AND MAY PRESENT WITH GENERIC ABDOMINAL SYMPTOMS IN CHILDREN

ESTHER FORRESTER, MD

WHAT TO DO – GATHER APPROPRIATE DATA

Parasites that infect the intestine cause morbidity in >25% of the world's population. Prevalent intestinal parasites within the United States include *Enterobius vermicularis*, *Giardia lamblia*, *Ancylostoma duodenale*, *Necator americanus, and Entamoeba histolytica*. In the United States, high-risk groups include international travelers, refugees, recent immigrants, and international adoptees.

The most prevalent of the previously listed helminthic organisms in the United States is *E. vermicularis*, or the pinworm. It has the largest geographic range of any helminth. As many as 30% of children and 10% of adults are infected worldwide. The ubiquitous infection occurs when eggs are ingested via fecal-oral route or via oral contact with contaminated hands or fomites. Infection can also occur when eggs are exposed to the air, aerosolized, and ingested. Slumber parties are an excellent source of cross infestation. The eggs hatch in the duodenum and the larvae mature as they migrate to the large intestine. The worms live primarily in the cecum, from which the pregnant female travels out of the anus at night and lays up to 15,000 eggs on the perineum. Male pinworms measure 2 to 5 mm; females measure 8 to 13 mm. Pinworms typically exit to lay eggs between 10 PM and 11 PM. It is easy to see why autoinoculation and reinfection are common. Most eggs dehydrate within 72 hours. If autoinoculation does not occur, the infestation usually resolves in 4 to 6 weeks.

Infection with *E. vermicularis* results in a spectrum of symptoms, and is often confused and misdiagnosed as another disease or condition (i.e., inflammatory bowel disease, sexual abuse). Infected patients typically present with irritation of the perineal, perianal, and vaginal areas. They experience pruritus as a result of egg deposition, and the constant itching severely disrupts sleep (egg deposition occurs at night). Therefore, suspicion of pinworm infection should arise for any child presenting with perianal pruritus and sleep disturbance. Due to the location of irritation seen with pinworm infections,

ⓒ 2008 by Lippincott Williams & Wilkins, a Wolters Kluwer business

it may present as vulvovaginitis, and possibly associated with sexual abuse. In addition, *E. vermicularis* infestation must be considered as a cause of non-specific colitis in patients presenting with symptoms of inflammatory bowel disease. Children with pinworms present with abdominal pain, chronic diarrhea, rectal bleeding, urinary tract infections, or weight loss. In some cases, pinworms are associated with appendicitis and intraperitoneal granulomas.

The diagnostic standard is direct visualization of the adult worm or microscopic detection of eggs. However, only 5% of individuals infested have eggs in their stool. The cellophane tape test may be used for a quick diagnosis, but its level of sensitivity is questionable. This test involves placing a piece of tape on a slide with the adhesive surface exposed, and then placing the tape on the perianal region several times. The slide and affixed tape are then removed and placed under the microscope for visualization of the eggs. Three days of consecutive testing increases the test's sensitivity.

The treatment of choice for pinworms is mebendazole, 100 mg orally once. Pyrantel pamoate 11 mg/kg orally once or albendazole 400 mg orally once, may be used as secondary choices. If the infection is persistent, repeating the treatment in 2 weeks is acceptable. Some clinicians repeat treatment in 2 weeks regardless of persistence. All family members should also receive treatment, and all linen should be cleaned.

SUGGESTED READINGS

Bernard D, Peters M, Makoroff K. The evaluation of suspected pediatric sexual abuse. *Clin Pediatr Emergency Med.* 2006;7:161–169.

Kucik CJ, Martin GL, Sortor BV. Common intestinal parasites. *Am Fam Physician.* 2004;69: 1161–1168.

Moon TD, Oberhelman RA. Antiparasitic therapy in children. *Pediatr Clin North Am.* 2005;52: 917–948.

Walshe T, Kavanagh DO, Bennani F, et al. The escaped worm. *J Am Coll Surg.* 2006;203(4):579.

100

ASSURE COVERAGE FOR RESISTANT *STREPTOCOCCUS PNEUMONIAE* WITH VANCOMYCIN IF THERE IS A CONCERN FOR MENINGITIS

YOLANDA LEWIS-RAGLAND, MD

WHAT TO DO – INTERPRET THE DATA

The first penicillin-resistant *Streptococcus pneumoniae* strain was isolated in 1967. Since then, however, there have been many reports of treatment failure in patients with pneumococcal infections caused by strains resistant to penicillin and other antimicrobial agents such as chloramphenicol, macrolides, trimethoprim-sulfamethoxazole, and cephalosporins. As a result, the selection of antimicrobial agents for the treatment of infections caused by these organisms has become increasingly difficult. In particular, the emergence of pneumococci-resistant to broad-spectrum cephalosporins has limited the antibiotic choices for the treatment of pneumococcal meningitis.

MENINGITIS SIGNS AND SYMPTOMS

Patients with central nervous system (CNS) infections, regardless of the etiology (bacterial, viral, or other), generally present with similar clinical features. The systemic signs of CNS infection include fever, malaise, and impairment of essential organs (heart, lung, liver, or kidney function). For older children and adults, the classic signs and symptoms suggesting CNS infection include headache; stiff neck; fever or hypothermia; changes in mental status, including hyperirritability evolving into lethargy and coma; seizures; and focal sensory and motor deficits.

Infants and young children, however, may lack obvious signs of meningitis, and present with simple temperature instability rather than fever. Otherwise, lethargy, irritability, vomiting, and poor feeding are often signs of CNS involvement in this group. Nuchal rigidity or a bulging fontanelle is present in <50% of infants and young children with meningitis.

RISK FACTORS FOR DEVELOPING MENINGITIS

Conditions that predispose the patient to infection of the CNS should be sought. One of the most common causes of meningitis is an infection of the sinuses or other structures in the head or neck region that results in direct extension of infection into the intracranial compartment. Open head injuries,

© 2008 by Lippincott Williams & Wilkins, a Wolters Kluwer business

recent neurosurgical procedures, immunodeficiency, and the presence of a mechanical shunt may likewise predispose individuals to intracranial infection.

MANAGEMENT OF BACTERIAL MENINGITIS

The broad-spectrum cephalosporins, cefotaxime and ceftriaxone, have traditionally been used as standard therapy for bacterial meningitis in infants and children. However, in the past decade, penicillin- and cephalosporin-resistant pneumococcal meningitis has been reported. In fact, cultures of cerebrospinal fluid (CSF) were positive for 3 to 14 days after the initiation of therapy. Therefore, in an attempt to identify an effective therapy, several antibiotic regimens including vancomycin, chloramphenicol, rifampin, erythromycin, and imipenem, alone and in combination were given to patients to identify an ideal anti–pneumococcal meningitis regimen.

Researchers concluded that on the basis of data from the pneumococcal meningitis models and limited clinical experience, it was impossible to make a single recommendation for initial empiric treatment that would be suitable for all patients with suspected or proven pneumococcal meningitis. However, the following guidelines could be considered in managing such patients:

- Physicians should be aware of the *S. pneumoniae* susceptibility patterns in their area and request their hospital laboratories to perform dilution susceptibility tests on any pneumococcal isolates recovered from usually sterile body sites.
- Because penicillin-resistant pneumococci have been identified in many areas of the United States, initial empiric therapy for bacterial meningitis should be based on the possibility that it is the etiology of the patient's illness. The recommended therapy is therefore ceftriaxone or cefotaxime *and* vancomycin (60 mg/kg/day divided in four doses), in addition to dexamethasone.
- A repeat lumbar puncture in patients with pneumococcal meningitis to document eradication of the pathogen should be performed 24 to 36 hours after the start of therapy, primarily in patients in whom the organism is cephalosporin resistant.
- Alteration of the initial antimicrobial regimen should be based on the clinical response of the patient and on the results of the CSF culture and susceptibility studies from the second lumbar puncture. In the event that the patients' clinical condition has worsened or that the follow-up Gram-stained smear or culture of CSF indicates failure to substantially reduce or eradicate the organism, substitution of rifampin for vancomycin in the therapeutic regimen is recommended.
- Patients without complications should be treated for a minimum of 10 days.

SUGGESTED READINGS

Heyderman RS, Klein NJ. Emergency management of meningitis. *J R Soc Med.* 2000;93:225–229.

Phillips EJ, Simor AE. Postgraduate medicine: symposium: bacterial meningitis in children and adults. Changes in community-acquired disease may affect patient care. *Postgrad Med.* 1998;103(3):102–117.

Wise KA, Bedford M, Wadhwa SS, et al. Meningitis caused by *Streptococcus pneumoniae* showing high level resistance to penicillin. *Pathology.* 1995;27(2):165–167.

101

Children Who Have Suffered an Infection for Meningococcus Should Receive a Workup for an Immunodeficiency (Specifically a Terminal Complement Disorder)

LINDSEY ALBRECHT, MD

What to Do – Gather Appropriate Data

The complement pathways make up an important part of the body's innate immune system. Complement proteins play a key role in defense against pyogenic organisms, and most congenital and acquired complement deficiencies are associated with an increased risk of infection. The complement system has three pathways: classical, alternative, and lectin. These are triggered separately but converge at complement protein C3. Activated C3 can itself activate more C3, generating amplification of this process. Clusters of C3b are ultimately deposited on the particular target, which allows the formation of a membrane attack complex comprised of components C5b through 9. The membrane attack complex then creates perforations in cellular membranes, thus exerting killing power over certain invading organisms.

Deficiencies in the terminal complement proteins (C5–C9) are associated with an increased risk of *Neisseria meningitides* infection. One pediatric study performed in New York showed that 18% of pediatric patients with a first episode of systemic meningococcal infection had an underlying complement deficiency; other estimates range between 1% and 15%. Patients with recurrent disease, a family history of disease, or disease caused by an uncommon meningococcal serotype are considered more likely to have a complement deficiency. Of patients who are known to be homozygous for terminal complement mutations (with resultant deficiencies in C5, C6, C7, C8 or C9), 50% to 60% will develop systemic meningococcal infection. This indicates that the membrane attack complex is critical for host defense against meningococcal infection. Interestingly, bacterial meningitis or septicemia caused by *N. meningitides* may be the first and only manifestation of an underlying congenital terminal complement deficiency. Late complement deficiencies are generally transmitted in an autosomal recessive manner.

In addition to terminal complement protein deficiencies, systemic *Neisseria* infection may more rarely be associated with properidin deficiency.

© 2008 by Lippincott Williams & Wilkins, a Wolters Kluwer business

Properidin is a serum protein that promotes activation of the alternate complement pathway. Unlike the complement deficiencies, properidin deficiency is frequently transmitted in an X-linked fashion. Given this, patients often have a family history of male members with a history of meningococcal infection.

Because of the significant association of terminal complement deficiency with systemic *N. meningitides* infection, screening is indicated in patients with systemic meningococcal infection. Screening for late complement deficiencies can be performed with a CH50 assay, a test that primarily evaluates the classical pathway of the complement cascade. Reduction of the CH50 occurs when individual complement components are deficient; a reduced CH50 is an indication for testing of individual complement components. Because properidin activates the alternative pathway, properidin deficiency will result in a normal CH50. The AP50 screening test of the alternative pathway may be abnormal, but often is in the low normal range. If this diagnosis is suspected, specialized testing of properidin is indicated.

Diagnosis of terminal complement deficiencies and properidin deficiency is important because it allows for counseling of the patient and the patient's physician with respect to management of future febrile illnesses. It also allows for the identification of other family members who might be affected and at risk for systemic meningococcal infection. Even if unaffected, family members may be carriers of a disease causing mutation and may pass this mutation on to their offspring. Genetic counseling is certainly appropriate in these families. The administration of the currently available quadrivalent meningococcal vaccine will likely reduce the morbidity and mortality associated with systemic meningococcal disease in these patients.

In conclusion, systemic meningococcal infection in children calls for an evaluation of the complement cascade. Diagnosis of complement or properidin deficiency allows for improved care of the affected patient and the potential identification of family members at risk for meningococcal disease.

SUGGESTED READINGS

Leggiadro RJ, Winkelstein JA. Prevalence of complement deficiencies in children with systemic meningococcal infections. *Pediatr Infect Dis J.* 1987;6(1):75–76.

Linton SM, Morgan BP. Properdin deficiency and meningococcal disease–identifying those most at risk. *Clin Exp Immunol.* 1999;118(2):189–191.

Mathew S, Overturf GD. Complement and properidin deficiencies in meningococcal disease. *Pediatr Infect Dis J.* 2006;25(3):255–256.

Overturf GD. Indications for the immunological evaluation of patients with meningitis. *Clin Infect Dis.* 2003;36(2):189–194.

CONSIDER THE DIAGNOSIS OF KAWASAKI DISEASE IN CHILDREN WITH DESQUAMATION, FEVER, AND RASH

LINDSEY ALBRECHT, MD

WHAT TO DO – INTERPRET THE DATA

Kawasaki disease is an acute systemic vasculitis manifested by fever and mucocutaneous inflammation that occurs primarily in early childhood. It is currently the most common cause of acquired heart disease in childhood in the United States and other developed countries. Although features of Kawasaki disease suggest an infectious cause and a genetic predisposition is likely, the etiology of the disorder is unclear. The incidence of Kawasaki disease varies according to ethnic group, with incidence highest in Asians and Pacific Islanders and lowest in whites. Because there is no specific diagnostic test available, diagnosis is based on well-established clinical criteria as well as supportive additional findings and laboratory data. Accurate diagnosis is important, as properly initiated treatment can significantly reduce the morbidity and mortality associated with the potential cardiac sequelae.

Classic diagnosis of Kawasaki disease requires fever for 5 or more days and four or more of the five major clinical features. These features include extremity changes, rash, oral mucosal changes, bilateral nonexudative conjunctivitis, and cervical lymphadenopathy. Extremity changes are particularly distinctive and include erythema or the palms and soles in the acute period. Edema of the hands and feet may also occur; induration when present is sometimes painful. Two to 3 weeks after disease onset, patients may have desquamation of the fingers and toes beginning in the periungual region. The rash of Kawasaki disease is typically a nonspecific maculopapular rash, though urticarial, scarlatiniform, and erythema multiforme-like varieties have been described. Conjunctival injection is usually painless and begins shortly after fever onset. The bulbar region of the conjunctivae is preferentially affected. Uveitis may coexist and is typically mild. Oral mucosal changes included generalized mucosal erythema; strawberry tongue; and peeling, redness, or cracking of the lips. Of the principal features, cervical lymphadenopathy is the least common; to meet diagnostic criteria the lymphadenopathy must be >1.5 cm in diameter and is most often unilateral.

© 2008 by Lippincott Williams & Wilkins, a Wolters Kluwer business

In addition to these classic features, other associated clinical findings include aseptic meningitis; sterile pyuria; abdominal symptoms, such as pain and diarrhea; arthritis; and Raynaud phenomenon. Coronary artery aneurysms are the most common cardiac sequelae, occurring in one of every four to five children who do not receive treatment. Aneurysms may lead to cardiac ischemia, infarction, and sudden death. Almost all deaths from Kawasaki disease are due to the cardiac manifestations, with the highest risk of myocardial infarction occurring in the first year following onset of disease.

In "incomplete" or "atypical" cases of Kawasaki disease, patients do not fulfill all classic criteria. Laboratory findings, if consistent with those typically seen in Kawasaki disease, may be helpful in supporting the diagnosis. These lab findings often include elevated erythrocyte sedimentation rate, C-reactive protein, leukocytosis, anemia, hypoalbuminemia, and elevated serum transaminases. Thrombocytosis is characteristic in the subacute period. Incomplete Kawasaki disease should be considered in all pediatric patients with fever for 5 or more days and two or three of the major clinical features. The level of suspicion should be highest for young infants, who may present only with fever. When incomplete Kawasaki disease is suspected, an echocardiogram should be obtained to evaluate for coronary artery anomalies.

Treatment of Kawasaki disease is with a single dose of intravenous immunoglobulin (IVIG) (2g/kg) in the acute phase to reduce the incidence of coronary artery aneurysms from 15% to 25% to approximately 5% of cases. It may be administered beyond day 7 to 10 of illness when there is persistent fever or the presence of coronary artery aneurysms in the face of ongoing inflammation. A repeat IVIG dose is recommended for the roughly 10% of patients who remain febrile following initial treatment. High-dose aspirin is additionally given in the acute phase for its anti-inflammatory and anti-platelet effects. Low-dose aspirin is given following high-dose therapy until there is no evidence of coronary artery anomalies by weeks 6 to 8 after disease onset. It may be continued much longer if there are coronary artery changes detected on echocardiogram. Management of coronary artery aneurysms, should they occur, depends on their size and whether or not a clot is present. Unsurprisingly, the degree of coronary artery involvement dictates the long-term follow-up plan in patients with Kawasaki disease.

SUGGESTED READINGS

Newburger JW, Fulton DR. Kawasaki disease. *Curr Opin Pediatr.* 2004;16:505–514.

Newburger JW, Takahashi M, Gerber MA, et al. Diagnosis, treatment, and long-term management of Kawasaki disease: a statement for health professionals from the Committee on Rheumatic Fever, Endocarditis, and Kawasaki Disease, Council on Cardiovascular Disease in the Young, American Heart Association. *Pediatrics.* 2004;114:1708–1731.

DO NOT FORGET TO USE BROAD ANTIMICROBIAL COVERAGE FOR PATIENTS WITH OSTEOMYELITIS

MADAN DHARMAR, MD

WHAT TO DO – MAKE A DECISION

Osteomyelitis is an infection of the bone. The three different modes of acquiring the infection are hematogenous, direct inoculation, and local invasion. In children, osteomyelitis is mostly hematogenous in origin and is usually caused by a bacterial infection. Risk factors for the hematogenous osteomyelitis in children are sepsis, hemoglobinopathies, and immunodeficiency disorders. The anatomic characteristic feature of the growing bone in children plays an important role in the pathogenesis and clinical feature of the disease. In children, the most common site of hematogenous osteomyelitis are in the long bones.

In children, osteomyelitis presents with nonspecific, systemic symptoms of low-grade fever and malaise, which is gradual in onset over several days to weeks. As the infection progresses, the patient presents with local symptoms of warmth, swelling, pain, and decreased mobility. The most common organisms causing hematogenous osteomyelitis in the normal host is *Staphylococcus aureus*. Other organisms causing hematogenous osteomyelitis are group A and B *Streptococcus*. Among children with sickle cell disease (SCD), *Salmonella* and other gram-negative organisms, such as *Escherichia coli*, can also cause osteomyelitis in addition to the typical organisms described above.

Osteomyelitis in SCD: Infections are a major cause of morbidity and mortality for patients with SCD. SCD patients are more susceptible to bacterial infections due to factors such as defective opsonins, and early loss of splenic function. These patients are more susceptible to osteoarticular infections, and osteomyelitis is one of the common infectious complications presenting in children with SCD.

Although *S. aureus* is the most common infectious agent causing osteomyelitis in the normal host, there still exists a controversy as to whether *S. aureus* or *Salmonella* is the most common infectious agent causing osteomyelitis in SCD patients. In their reviews, Burnett et al. and Chamber et al. have concluded that *Salmonella* is more common pathogen, followed

© 2008 by Lippincott Williams & Wilkins, a Wolters Kluwer business

by *S. aureus* in causing osteomyelitis infection in SCD. This has important implications for both the diagnosis and treatment of the disease.

Clinical Features and Diagnosis: The clinical diagnosis of osteomyelitis is often difficult because the presenting symptoms are similar to other common complications in these children (e.g., vaso-occlusive crisis). Both of these complication present with warmth, swelling, and local tenderness. Osteomyelitis should be considered in any patient who has fever, long-lasting pain, and decreased mobility associated with the above symptoms.

Blood tests, such as white blood cell count, erythrocyte sedimentation rate, and C-reactive protein, should be performed in suspected cases of osteomyelitis, even though they are not specific. Blood cultures should also be performed for suspected osteomyelitis, even though they are only positive in 50% of the cases. Bone biopsy, aspirations, and cultures are usually diagnostic and are the procedures of choice for suspected osteomyelitis.

Plain radiography is usually negative for the first 7 to 10 days except for soft tissue swelling, but can show destruction and new bone formation after 10 days. Magnetic resonance imaging is highly sensitive and specific for detecting bone involvement in suspected osteomyelitis. A bone scan with gallium or magnetic resonance imaging can help distinguish an infection from infarction.

The empirical antibiotic therapy for suspected osteomyelitis is based on the knowledge of the common pathogens causing the infection in SCD patients. Recommended regimens include treatment with a broad-spectrum cephalosporin, such as ceftriaxone or cefotaxime, in addition to an anti-*Staphylococcus* drug. If a specific pathogen is identified in culture, then antibiotic therapy needs to be specifically tailored. If the patient is responding to antibiotics, then the initial therapy is continued. The duration of intravenous antibiotic therapy is case-dependent based on the organisms identified and the clinical course of the disease. The key to diagnosis and treatment of osteomyelitis is to consider clinical symptoms, a positive culture, an abnormal imaging study, and the response to empirical antibiotic therapy.

SUGGESTED READINGS

Burnett MW, Bass JW, Cook BA. Etiology of osteomyelitis complicating sickle cell disease. *Pediatrics.* 1998;101(2):296–297.

Chambers JB, Forsythe DA, Bertrand SL, et al. Retrospective review of osteoarticular infections in a pediatric sickle cell age group. *J Pediatr Orthop.* 2000;20(5):682–685.

Gill FM, Sleeper LA, Weiner SJ, et al. Clinical events in the first decade in a cohort of infants with sickle cell disease. Cooperative Study of Sickle Cell Disease. *Blood.* 1995;86(2):776–783.

Goergens ED, McEvoy A, Watson M, et al. Acute osteomyelitis and septic arthritis in children. *J Paediatr Child Health.* 2005;41(1–2):59–62.

Karwowska A, Davies HD, Jadavji T. Epidemiology and outcome of osteomyelitis in the era of sequential intravenous-oral therapy. *Pediatr Infect Dis J*. 1998;17(11):1021–1026.

Lampe RM. Osteomyelitis and suppurative arthritis. In: Behrman RE, Kliegman R, Jenson HB. *Nelson Textbook of Pediatrics*. 17th ed. Philadelphia: Saunders; 2004, pages 2297–2302.

Lew DP, Waldvogel FA. Osteomyelitis. *Lancet*. 2004;364(9431):369–379.

KNOW WHAT TO DO FOR PUNCTURE WOUNDS AND THE APPROPRIATE ANTIBIOTIC THERAPY FOR PEDIATRIC PATIENTS

LAURA HUFFORD, MD

WHAT TO DO – MAKE A DECISION

Puncture wounds are a common form of minor trauma in the pediatric population. Although they are painful, these wounds usually heal easily and do not require medical attention. Complications of puncture wounds include retained foreign bodies and secondary infections. The most common organisms to cause secondary infections are *Staphylococcus* and *Streptococcus* species. Additionally, plantar puncture wounds are at risk for anaerobic infections, including those organisms likely seeded from the soil, a foreign body, or shoe. *Pseudomonas aeruginosa* infection can cause invasive, debilitating disease, such as osteochondritis and osteomyelitis.

Physical examination should be performed, looking for changes in sensation or motor function, erythema, swelling, and increased warmth, which suggests injury or infection. Initial management includes irrigation and close inspection for a retained foreign body. If there is high degree of suspicion for a foreign body and it cannot be easily visualized, radiographic studies and possible surgical exploration may be indicated.

Patients presenting within a day of the puncture rarely demonstrate signs of infection and thus management should be limited to rest and frequent foot soaks. However, patients presenting >24 hours often have pain, erythema, and swelling. Once the possibility of a retained foreign body has been eliminated, the clinician should consider whether the patient should receive oral antistaphylococcal antibiotics. Typically, if the puncture wound is shallow, no antibiotic prophylaxis is recommended; however, if the wound is "dirty" or deep, as are those more typically occurring in the foot, antibiotic prophylaxis is recommended. These patients should return for re-evaluation within 48 hours. If symptoms persist, hospital admission should occur for parenteral antibiotic therapy including coverage for *P. aeruginosa*.

Of note, oral fluoroquinolones are not indicated for prophylaxis of plantar puncture wounds. During the development of fluoroquinolones, the drugs were found to cause irreversible arthropathy in growing animals. Thus, there are few U.S. Food and Drug Administration-licensed pediatric indications

© 2008 by Lippincott Williams & Wilkins, a Wolters Kluwer business

for these medications. The American Academy of Pediatrics Committee on Infectious Diseases, 2004–2005 stated that parenteral treatment of osteomyelitis or osteochondritis caused by *P. aeruginosa* is an appropriate use of fluoroquinolone medications.

SUGGESTED READINGS

Baldwin G, Colbourne M. Puncture wounds. *Pediatr Rev.* 1999;20(1):21–23.
Chachad S, Kamat D. Management of plantar puncture wounds in children. *Clin Pediatr.* 2004; 43:213–216.
Committee on Infectious Disease. The use of systemic fluoroquinolones. *Pediatrics.* 2006;118: 1287–1292.

105

Children with Recurrent Infections, Unusually Severe Manifestations of Common Infections, or Atypical Infections Should Be Evaluated for Immunodeficiency

Emily Riehm Meier, MD

What to Do – Interpret the Data

The immune system is a complicated web of defenses needed to protect the human body. It can be broadly divided into four categories: cellular (affecting T cell function), humoral (affecting B cell function, most notably antibody production), phagocytic, and complement. Even though defects in humoral immunity are most common, deficiencies can occur in isolation or combination in any of the four categories. The type, severity, and number of infections that a child has all provide clues as to which part of the immune system is deficient. Multiple parts of the immune system may need to be evaluated, however, because overlap does exist.

Patients with an isolated humoral immunodeficiency usually present after 6 months of age, when placentally transferred maternal antibody levels start to decline. Recurrent bacterial respiratory tract infections (≥ 8 episodes of otitis media or ≥ 2 severe episodes of sinusitis or pneumonia in 1 year), enteroviral infections, or serious bacterial infections (including sepsis) are hallmarks of defects in humoral immunity. Isolated cellular immune defects most commonly present with *Salmonella* or nontuberculous *Mycobacterium* infections, although other intracellularly dividing organisms can also be involved. Recurrent fungal infections or *Pneumocystis carinii* also suggest a cellular immune defect. A combination of defects in cellular and humoral immunity represents the most serious type of immunodeficiency; it is commonly known as severe combined immunodeficiency (SCID). In most cases, SCID presents with failure to thrive, chronic diarrhea, opportunistic infections (*Pneumocystis jiroveci* [previously known as *Pneumocystis carinii*] pneumonia [PCP] and disseminated cytomegalovirus), and chronic respiratory infections.

Mouth ulcers, chronic skin abscesses, and recurrent *Staphylococcus aureus* or *Aspergillus* infections are the hallmarks of phagocytic defects of the immune system. Birth history may also reveal delayed separation of the umbilical cord (<1 month). Chronic granulomatous disease (CGD) is characterized

ⓒ 2008 by Lippincott Williams & Wilkins, a Wolters Kluwer business

by failure to produce a bactericidal oxidative burst and is the most classic phagocytic defect. Complement deficiencies are the least common immunodeficiencies and are usually characterized by recurrent *Neisseria* infections.

A complete history and physical examination should be performed on all patients with a suspected immunodeficiency. Special attention should be given to the number and type of infections the patient has had, birth and family history, consanguinity in the family (because most immunodeficiencies are autosomal recessive), signs of failure to thrive, dysmorphic features (possibly a sign of DiGeorge or Down syndrome), skin rashes (paying special mind to eczema, associated with Wiskott-Aldrich syndrome). Diagnostic workup for immunodeficiency is complex, but a few screening tests can guide clinicians. A chest x-ray can reveal an abnormally shaped heart or absent of thymus in infants. A complete blood count can reveal lymphopenia, neutropenia, thrombocytopenia, or anemia—all signs of immunodeficiencies. Blood cultures and other serologic studies help to determine which organism is involved in the infection. Immunoglobulin levels (age appropriate normal values should be used when interpreting these results), T cell subsets and CH50 are other tests that can be used to screen for immunodeficiency.

SUGGESTED READINGS

Bonilla FA, Geha RS. Primary immunodeficiency diseases. *J Allergy Clin Immunol.* 2003;111: S571–S581.

Tangsinmankong N, Bahna SL, Good RA. The immunologic workup of the child suspected of immunodeficiency. *Ann Allergy Asthma Immunol.* 2001;86:362–369.

106

CONSIDER METHICILLIN-RESISTANT *STAPHYLOCOCCUS AUREUS* (MRSA) IN PATIENTS WITH COMMUNITY-ACQUIRED *STAPHYLOCOCCUS AUREUS* INFECTIONS

SARIKA JOSHI, MD

WHAT TO DO – INTERPRET THE DATA

MRSA has increased in prevalence throughout the world. In addition to being resistant to methicillin, these organisms are also resistant to all β-lactam antibiotics, including cephalosporins. Although they are often thought of as a nosocomial pathogen, MRSA has been increasing in incidence in the community, as well. It is imperative for physicians to recognize MRSA as an important pathogen, and to understand the different characteristics of nosocomial versus community-acquired microbes.

In the United States, there is a high occurrence of MRSA among hospitalized patients. According to the Surveillance and Control of Pathogens of Epidemiologic Importance database, the frequency of MRSA responsible for nosocomial bacteremia increased more than 30% from 1995 to 2001. Significant risk factors for nosocomial MRSA include prolonged hospitalization, prior antibiotic therapy, and proximity to a patient with MRSA. In addition, the incidence of MRSA is pronounced in patients requiring intensive care, with burns, and with surgical wound infections. In children, other documented risk factors for acquisition of nosocomial MRSA are the presence of a central venous catheter or tracheostomy and the undergoing of frequent surgical procedures. The Hospital Infection Control Practices Advisory Committee, the Centers for Disease Control and Prevention, and the Society for Healthcare Epidemiology of America have established guidelines to help prevent the spread of nosocomial MRSA. As the most common route of transmission for nosocomial MRSA is on the hands of health care personnel, these recommendations include good hand hygiene and contact precautions.

The prevalence of community-acquired MRSA varies substantially by geographic region. Certain areas have incidences as high as 35% to 83%, with the highest occurrence in children younger than 2 years of age. Community-acquired MRSA is genetically distinct from nosocomial MRSA. Although nosocomial MRSA often causes respiratory and urinary tract infections, community-acquired MRSA is associated with skin and soft tissue infections.

© 2008 by Lippincott Williams & Wilkins, a Wolters Kluwer business

Risk factors for community-acquired MRSA include skin trauma, shaving, and physical contact with or sharing equipment with a person who has MRSA. Transmission often occurs within families or within a group of children in day care. Practical recommendations for reducing the spread of community-acquired MRSA are keeping nails short, using antimicrobial soaps, and changing sleep wear and towels daily.

The first step in the treatment of MRSA is identification and removal of potential foci of infection, such as indwelling catheters and abscesses. For nosocomial MRSA, intravenous vancomycin is the drug of choice. In children, the dose of vancomycin is 40 to 60 mg/kg/day divided in three to four doses. Other agents that have been used to treat nosocomial MRSA include clindamycin, although resistance may be readily induced; and linezolid. For community-acquired MRSA, trimethoprim-sulfamethoxazole (for skin and soft tissue infections) and clindamycin are recommended. In children, the dose of oral trimethoprim-sulfamethoxazole is 8 to 10 mg/kg/day divided in two doses for minor infections and 20 mg/kg/day divided in three to four doses for severe infections. The dose of oral clindamycin in children is 10 to 30 mg/kg/day divided in three to four doses. Other agents that have been used to treat community-acquired MRSA include linezolid and minocycline (for children younger than 8 years of age). Because antibiotic susceptibility of community-acquired MRSA can vary substantially by region, physicians need to be aware of local resistance patterns. Susceptibilities of wound cultures should be followed after initiation of empiric antibiotic therapy.

MRSA infections can be acquired in the hospital or in the community. Nosocomial and community-acquired organisms have differing antibiotic resistance patterns and are associated with distinct infections. Vancomycin is the treatment of choice for nosocomial MRSA, whereas trimethoprim-sulfamethoxazole and clindamycin are recommended for community-acquired MRSA.

SUGGESTED READINGS

Moran GJ, Krishnadasan A, Gorwitz RJ, et al. Methicillin-resistant *S. aureus* infections among patients in the emergency department. *N Engl J Med*. 2006;355:666–674.

Naimi TS, LeDell KH, Como-Sabetti K, et al. Comparison of community- and health care-associated methicillin-resistant *Staphylococcus aureus* infection. *JAMA*. 2003;290:2976–2984.

Sattler CA, Mason EO Jr, Kaplan SL. Prospective comparison of risk factors and demographic and clinical characteristics of community-acquired, methicillin-resistant versus methicillin-susceptible *Staphylococcus aureus* infection in children. *Pediatr Infect Dis J*. 2002;21:910–917.

107

KNOW THE DIFFERENCE BETWEEN EPSTEIN-BARR VIRUS (EBV) AND STREP PHARYNGITIS

SARIKA JOSHI, MD

WHAT TO DO – INTERPRET THE DATA

Sore throat is a common complaint from children and adolescents that often prompts physician visits. Many infectious agents are known to cause pharyngitis, and most require only supportive care. Two important causes of pharyngitis that should be recognized by clinicians are group A streptococcus (GAS, *Streptococcus pyogenes*) and EBV.

GAS pharyngitis occurs most commonly in school-aged children and accounts for 15% to 30% of all cases in children ages 5 to 15 years. The peak seasons for GAS pharyngitis are late fall, winter, and early spring. Classically, GAS pharyngitis has an abrupt onset and is associated with fever, headache, and abdominal pain. The common symptoms of viral upper respiratory infections, such as cough, rhinorrhea, and nasal congestion, are typically absent. Only 15% of patients will present with the classical constellation of signs and symptoms of acute pharyngitis with edema, erythema or exudates, and sometimes palatal petechiae and anterior cervical lymphadenopathy. Spontaneous resolution usually occurs in 3 to 5 days.

A throat culture is the gold standard method for the diagnosis of GAS pharyngitis. The throat culture, performed by sampling both tonsillar pillars and the posterior pharynx without touching the buccal mucosa or tongue, is incubated for at least 18 to 24 hours. Because of this delay, most physicians perform both a rapid antigen detection test and a throat culture. The specificity of the rapid test is very high, meaning that there are few false positives, but the sensitivity can be as low as 65%, which is why it is also imperative to send the throat culture to the laboratory. It is important to note that neither of these tests can distinguish between acute infection versus chronic carriage of GAS.

Appropriate antibiotic treatment of GAS pharyngitis helps to prevent the local suppurative complications, as well as the nonsuppurative complication of acute rheumatic fever (ARF). Local suppurative complications include otitis media, sinusitis, lymphadenitis, and retropharyngeal and peritonsillar abscesses. Antibiotic treatment has not been shown to prevent

© 2008 by Lippincott Williams & Wilkins, a Wolters Kluwer business

glomerulonephritis, another known nonsuppurative complication of GAS infection. Treatment with oral penicillin is the current first-line recommendation for GAS infections. Recommended treatment for penicillin-allergic patients is with erythromycin.

EBV is the usual etiologic agent for infectious mononucleosis, which occurs most commonly in adolescents. Despite high rates of exposure, children develop clinical infection <10% of the time, whereas adolescents develop symptoms >50% of the time. Classically, infectious mononucleosis presents with fever, pharyngitis, and posterior cervical lymphadenopathy, although lymph node involvement may be more generalized. Unlike GAS pharyngitis, the onset of infectious mononucleosis is often insidious with a prodrome of malaise and headache. The patient's exam reveals acute pharyngitis with edema, erythema or exudates, and sometimes palatal petechiae, similar to GAS pharyngitis; however, the edema with infectious mononucleosis may be so severe as to cause airway impingement. Other associated findings with infectious mononucleosis include splenomegaly and severe fatigue. The acute symptoms generally resolve in 1 to 2 weeks, but the fatigue may persist for months.

The diagnostic workup for infectious mononucleosis starts with blood work—a white blood cell count with differential and a heterophile antibodies test. Characteristically, there are 60% to 70% lymphocytes with >10% atypical lymphocytes, although these are not specific for EBV infection. Heterophile antibodies are the test of choice, since they are both sensitive and specific, about 85% and 100%, respectively. If heterophile antibodies are negative and the clinical suspicion for infectious mononucleosis is strong, EBV-specific antibodies may be drawn.

The mainstay for treatment of infectious mononucleosis is supportive care. If a patient is misdiagnosed (i.e., with GAS pharyngitis) and treated with amoxicillin or other antibiotics, a nonspecific rash may develop. Corticosteroids may be warranted in severe cases with impending airway obstruction. A rare but important complication of EBV infection is splenic rupture, which is spontaneous more than 50% of the time and usually occurs in the first 3 weeks of symptomatic illness. Due to this potential risk of splenic rupture, return to sports is a common clinical question. In general, noncontact sports can be resumed 3 weeks after symptom onset, whereas contact sports require a minimum of 4 weeks, if the patient does not have splenomegaly.

GAS and EBV are important pathogens of pharyngitis in children and adolescents. Diagnosis and appropriate antibiotic treatment for GAS helps to prevent the complication of ARF. Diagnosis of EBV infection alerts the physician to watch for the potentially life-threatening complications of airway obstruction and splenic rupture.

SUGGESTED READINGS

Bisno AL. Acute pharyngitis: etiology and diagnosis. *Pediatrics.* 1996;97(6 Pt 2):949–954.

Del Mar CB, Glasziou PP, Spinks AB. Antibiotics for sore throat. *Cochrane Database Syst Rev.* 2000;(4):CD000023.

Rea TD, Russo JE, Katon W, et al. Prospective study of the natural history of infectious mononucleosis caused by Epstein-Barr virus. *J Am Board Fam Pract.* 2001;14:234–242.

108

REMEMBER TO SCREEN FOR TORCH IN BABIES WHO PRESENT IN THE NEWBORN PERIOD WITH PATHOLOGY

ELLEN HAMBURGER, MD

WHAT TO DO – GATHER APPROPRIATE DATA

Perinatal infections are a significant cause of fetal and neonatal mortality and an important contributor to early and later childhood morbidity. The TORCH acronym originally grouped five pathogens with similar clinical findings. *TORCH* refers to *t*oxoplasmosis, *o*ther agents, (syphilis, etc.), *r*ubella, *C*ytomegalovirus (CMV), and *h*erpes simplex virus (HSV). Over time, many microbes, including human immunodeficiency virus (HIV), parvovirus B19, and enteroviruses, have been placed into the TORCH acronym. Although the term is useful in generating a differential diagnosis, the indiscriminate use of TORCH "titers" or battery as a diagnostic tool has limited utility due to low yield, difficulty in interpreting single serum samples. Furthermore, more sensitive and specific methods now exist to diagnose perinatal infections. In one study of almost 1,200 TORCH screens, only 1.4% were positive and only 0.7% were associated with confirmed disease.

The sole reliance on antibody response for diagnosis is difficult because maternal immunoglobulin (Ig)G can cross the placenta, leading to a falsely positive test, and neonatal IgM is technically difficult to perform, leading to a falsely negative test. In patients where perinatal infection is highly suspected, the clinician should consider cultures, polymerase chain reaction (PCR) methods, as well as specific serologic tests to confirm a diagnosis. Organ-specific tests, such as head computed tomography, funduscopic exam, and auditory tests, may provide important diagnostic information.

Neonatal infections with CMV, *Toxoplasma*, rubella, HSV, and syphilis present a diagnostic dilemma because their clinical features overlap and initially may be indistinguishable. Some infants may be infected without overt symptoms. Additionally, infection is subclinical in >95% of mothers with CMV, toxoplasmosis, hepatitis B, Parvovirus B19, and herpesvirus type 6. Symptoms suggestive of a perinatal infection from one of the TORCH organisms include intrauterine growth retardation, anemia, neutropenia, thrombocytopenia, petechiae, purpura, ocular signs (chorioretinitis, cataracts, keratoconjunctivitis, glaucoma, or microphthalmos), and central nervous system signs (microcephaly, hydrocephaly, intracranial calcifications). Other

ⓒ 2008 by Lippincott Williams & Wilkins, a Wolters Kluwer business

organ system involvement may include pneumonia, myocarditis, nephritis, hepatitis with hepatosplenomegaly, jaundice, and nonimmune hydrops. Once suspected, specific tests for each potential pathogen should be considered. For some infections, such as syphilis, a presumptive diagnosis with initiation of treatment prior to isolation of the organism is warranted. Specific therapies for many TORCH pathogens now exist, including ganciclovir for CMV, acyclovir for HSV, and penicillin for syphilis.

SUGGESTED READINGS

Cullen A, Brown S, Cafferkey M, et al. Current use of the TORCH screen in the diagnosis of congenital infection. *J Infect.* 1998;36(2):185–188.

Newton ER. Diagnosis of perinatal TORCH infections. *Clini Obstet Gynecol.* 1999;42(1):59–70.

109

FOLLOW PATIENTS WITH *STAPHYLOCOCCAL AUREUS* BACTEREMIA CLOSELY FOR DEVELOPMENT OF A NEW MURMUR

ELLEN HAMBURGER, MD

WHAT TO DO – GATHER APPROPRIATE DATA

In the past several decades, *S. aureus* has become the primary pathogen responsible for infective endocarditis (IE). Improved dental care, hygiene, and the growing incidence of nosocomial infections and intravascular devices are associated with this bacteriologic shift. Among children with staphylococcal bacteremia, as many as 20% develop endocarditis, including patients with no predisposing cardiac valvular disease. Given this high complication rate, any patient with staphylococcal bacteremia should be followed closely for the development of a new murmur or other signs of endocarditis. Those patients with a new or changed murmur should undergo echocardiography. Persistent fever despite appropriate antibiotic therapy should also prompt the search for cardiac involvement even when patients have other foci of infection (such as skin) or the absence of clear signs of IE.

Definitive diagnosis of IE is made by pathologic or clinical criteria. Pathologic diagnosis requires positive histology or microbiology of tissue obtained at autopsy or cardiac surgery (valve tissue, vegetations, embolic fragments, or intracardiac abscess content). Without pathologic material, definitive clinical diagnosis can be difficult. Several sets of diagnostic criteria to evaluate patients for endocarditis have been developed. Studies have verified that the most recent criteria, the Duke criteria, are superior to older criteria for diagnosing infective endocarditis in children. The criteria are based on the microbiology of endocarditis and evidence of endocardial involvement by exam or echocardiography.

Major criteria include:

1. Positive blood culture for IE
   a. Two positive blood cultures with organisms that typically cause infective endocarditis (*Viridans streptococci*, *Streptococcus bovis*, and HACEK organisms–*Haemophilus* species, *Actinobacillus actinomycetemcomitans*, *Cardiobacterium hominis*, *Eikenella*, *corrodens*, *Kingella kingae*)
   b. Persistent bacteremia from two blood cultures taken >12 hours apart or three or more positive blood cultures where the pathogen is less specific, such as *Staphylococcus aureus* and *Staphylococcus epidermidis*

© 2008 by Lippincott Williams & Wilkins, a Wolters Kluwer business

   c. Positive serology for *Coxiella burnetii, Bartonella* species, or *Chlamydia psittaci*

   d. Positive molecular assays for specific gene targets

2. Positive evidence of endocardial involvement

   a. Echocardiograph (transthoracic or transesophageal) showing oscillating mass, abscess formation, new valvular regurgitation, or dehiscence of prosthetic valves

   b. Clinical evidence of new valvular regurgitation

Minor criteria are:

3. Predisposing heart disease or intravenous drug use
4. Fever >38°C
5. Immunological phenomena such as glomerulonephritis, Osler nodes, Roth spots, or positive rheumatoid factor
6. Microbiological evidence not fitting major criteria
7. Elevated C reactive protein or erythrocyte sedimentation rate
8. Vascular phenomena such as major emboli, splenomegaly, clubbing, splinter hemorrhages, petechiae, or purpura

By these criteria, a definite case of endocarditis is made when a patient has positive pathologic criteria, two major criteria, one major and two minor criteria, or five minor criteria. Possible cases are those with one major and one minor criteria, or three minor criteria.

In summary, clinicians following patients with Staph A bacteremia must be vigilant for signs of infective endocarditis, knowledgeable in the Duke criteria for diagnosis, and aware that more than one fourth of these patients do not have underlying cardiac or valvular abnormalities.

SUGGESTED READINGS

Beynon RP, Bahl VK, Prendergast BD. Infective endocarditis. *BMJ*. 2006;333(7563):334–339.

Di Filippo S, Delahaye F, Semiond B, et al. Current patterns of infective endocarditis in congenital heart disease. *Heart*. 2006;92(10):1490–1495.

Friedland IR. du Plessis J, Cilliers A. Cardiac complications in children with *Staphylococcus aureus* bacteremia. *J Pediatr*. 1995;127(5):746–748.

Hoen B. Epidemiology and antibiotic treatment of infective endocarditis: an update. *Heart*. 2006;92(11):1694–1700.

Prendergast BD. The changing face of infective endocarditis. *Heart*. 2006;92(7):879–885.

CONSIDER PERICARDITIS IN THE TACHYCARDIC, TOXIC CHILD WITH RESPIRATORY DIFFICULTY EVEN IN THE ABSENCE OF A PERICARDIAL FRICTION RUB

CRAIG DEWOLFE, MD

WHAT TO DO – INTERPRET THE DATA

Bacterial pericarditis most often presents in a nonspecific pattern in the young child, and the practitioner should strongly consider the diagnosis when evaluating patients with unexplained tachycardia and tachypnea. Fever, agitation, and precordial chest pain are common presenting symptoms. The pericardial friction rub is the pathopneumonic physical finding in older patients, but diminished heart sounds rather than a friction rub may be found in patients with large effusions. Most pediatric cases of bacterial pericarditis present in children younger than 2 years of age and classic signs are not present, such as a friction rub or chest pain. Practitioners, therefore, should have a low index of suspicion in toxic patients. They should workup patients with tachycardia out of proportion to the fever and respiratory distress not fully explained by a septic or pulmonic process.

Pericardial effusions develop rapidly in patients with acute bacterial pericarditis. Cardiac filling is impaired as pericardial fluid accumulates, producing signs of congestion and diminished cardiac output. Patients with rapid accumulation of fluid will present with cardiogenic shock. Conversely, congestive symptoms, such as hepatomegaly, jugular venous distention, and pulmonary edema, will predominate in patients with a slower accumulation of pericardial fluid. Patients with constrictive pericarditis resulting from viral myopericarditis, cat-scratch disease, tuberculosis, or sequelae of purulent pericarditis may also present with congestive heart failure. In patients with tamponade, systemic perfusion is maintained by an increase in heart rate and systemic vascular resistance. The increased systemic vascular resistance produces a narrow pulse pressure, as opposed to a wide pulse pressure commonly seen in severe sepsis. Ultimately, in patients with purulent pericarditis, if the effusion remains undrained, systemic hypotension and cardiovascular collapse will result.

Bacterial pericarditis generally develops as a secondary infection; most often as a direct extension of an adjacent pulmonic process or as

ⓒ 2008 by Lippincott Williams & Wilkins, a Wolters Kluwer business

hematogenous seeding from a distant bacterial site. Additional etiologies of large pericardial effusions include viral, fungal, or tuberculosis pericarditis, as well as autoimmune disorders, drugs, trauma, malignancy, rheumatic fever, Kawasaki syndrome, and postoperative irritation. Pericarditis of all causes occurs in 1 out of every 850 hospitalized patients. Moreover, myocarditis or endocarditis may also accompany the infection, depending on the causative agent.

In patients who have an effusion, plain chest film radiographs may demonstrate an enlarged heart with a globular shadow, whereas in patients with constrictive pericarditis the cardiac silhouette is small. An electrocardiogram (ECG) may show sinus tachycardia, low voltage QRS complexes, and ST segment elevations with or without PR segment depression and T wave inversion, or electrical alternans. But, the image of choice is the ECG because of its sensitivity, specificity, and ability to quantify the amount of pericardial fluid for drainage. Equally as important, the ECG can guide the pericardiocentesis.

Draining the pericardial fluid is critical for the appropriate evaluation and treatment of the patient with pericarditis. Pericardial fluid should be sent for cell count, chemistries, culture, and cytology as indicated. Over 50% of patients with purulent pericarditis will have a positive culture. The most common causative organisms include *Staphylococcus aureus, Streptococcus pneumoniae, Streptococcus pyogenes, Haemophilus influenzae,* and *Neisseria meningitides.*

The treatment of choice for infectious pericarditis is drainage of the pericardial space and intravenous antimicrobial therapy. Temporary measures to stabilize patients prior to pericardiocentesis include volume expansion and inotropic drugs for hypotension. Therapies that cause vasodilation or reduced preload should be avoided. The practitioner should ideally obtain blood and pericardial fluid cultures prior to treatment. Rapid referral for pericardiocentesis is required for any patient with hemodynamic instability, as delay can quickly lead to tamponade and death. Empiric treatment of bacterial pericarditis should consist of vancomycin and a third- or fourth-generation cephalosporin. Treatment is generally offered for 3 to 4 weeks. Complicating conditions or unusual organisms, including fungus or tuberculosis, may extend the therapy or warrant the use of steroids. Serial ECG scans may be used postoperatively to screen for occult dysrhythmias or myocardial involvement. Mortality rates depend on early identification and treatment, but range from 2% to 20% in a recent case series. Constrictive pericarditis may present as a sequelae to bacterial infection, often weeks after treatment, but is generally rare and if develops warrants a pericardiectomy.

In summary, pericarditis is a rare but lethal condition that requires a high index of suspicion. The classic presenting findings of a pericardial friction rub and chest pain often do not apply to the most common pediatric population afflicted with the condition: the infant and toddler. Instead, the practitioner should consider pericarditis in the tachycardic child with respiratory distress not fully explained by a septic or pulmonic process.

SUGGESTED READINGS

Berger J. Pericarditis, Bacterial. In: Gessner I, Windle M, et al. (eds). eMedicine Journal (emedicine.com), 2001. Last updated March 30, 2006. Accessed January 7, 2008.
Demmler GJ. Infectious pericarditis in children. *Pediatr Infect Dis J.* 2006;25:165–166.
Towbin JA. Myocarditis and pericarditis in adolescents. *Adolesc Med.* 2001;12:47–67.

111

PROVIDE APPROPRIATE TRAVEL PROPHYLAXIS FOR FOREIGN TRAVEL BASED ON THE INDIGENOUS ORGANISMS AND GEOGRAPHIC LOCATION

MINDY DICKERMAN, MD

WHAT TO DO – TAKE ACTION

Immunizations and preventative medicines are an important part of travel preparation and reducing the risk of acquiring infections while traveling internationally. Travel prophylaxis for foreign travel should be based on the individual's risks for exposure to specific travel related diseases, the epidemiology of vaccine-preventable diseases, and the time available before trip departure. Travel prophylaxis includes updating and boosting routine immunizations, administering legally required vaccinations, and prescribing recommended vaccines and medicines to help prevent diseases. A physician also needs to be knowledgeable about the adverse events and contraindications associated with each vaccine and medication.

The first step in prescribing appropriate travel prophylaxis is a thorough assessment of a patient's risk of travel-related disease. The details of the planned travel are important, including the itinerary, all geographic destinations, type of lodging booked, planned activities, particular season of travel, duration of stay, and anticipated contact with local residents. This information needs to be integrated with an assessment of the patient's general health, medical problems, allergies, and current medications. It is important to identify travelers at high risk for acquiring travel-related illnesses. Patients considered at high risk are backpackers, those who are immunocompromised, or those currently living in the United States but born in another country who are traveling back to their country of origin. Consultation with a travel clinic may be advisable and early consultation when planned travel is to developing countries is encouraged. Consultations need to be based on current epidemiology and can be obtained from the Centers for Disease Control and Prevention in an annual publication or via their Web site at http://www.cdc.gov/travel. The World Health Organization (WHO) operates a similar Web site: http://www.who.int/ith/en.

© 2008 by Lippincott Williams & Wilkins, a Wolters Kluwer business

It is very important to review and update a patient's routine immunizations prior to international travel. If 5 or more years have elapsed since the last tetanus immunization and the patient is traveling to an area where postexposure tetanus immunization may be unavailable, a booster dose of tetanus should be considered. Measles is still endemic in many developing nations, and children 6 to 11 months of age should receive one dose of measles, mumps, rubella vaccine if traveling to highly endemic areas and must receive two doses after 12 months to be considered fully immunized. Polio is also still found in several countries around the world, including in India and Pakistan. Travelers to these countries may need a single booster of the polio vaccine. Varicella immunity and hepatitis B immunity should be reviewed and the vaccines given if necessary. Pneumovax should be considered for patients with chronic illnesses or who are immunocompromised. The influenza vaccine is recommended for all international travelers during influenza season, which peaks in different months in the Northern and Southern hemispheres.

There are some vaccines that are required for entry into endemic areas. Many yellow fever-endemic countries require proof of vaccination for entry. Yellow fever is a potentially fatal viral infection that is endemic in equatorial African and South America, and is transmitted by day-biting mosquito vectors. The yellow fever vaccine is recommended for any patient older than 8 months at least 10 days prior to traveling to areas where yellow fever is reported. The vaccination is not recommended in pregnancy. It is a live-attenuated virus given in a single subcutaneous injection. Immunity may be lifelong but revaccination is required at 10-year intervals. Country-specific epidemiology and requirements can be obtained from the CDC.

The inactivated hepatitis A virus vaccine is recommended for many international travelers, including travelers to areas in Mexico. Vaccination is preferred 4 weeks prior to departure, and a booster is needed 6 to 12 months later to provide protective antibody levels for >10 years. Japanese encephalitis virus is an arboviral infection transmitted by mosquitoes that is prevalent in the Indian subcontinent and other Asian countries. The vaccine should be offered to patients who plan to remain for 30 days or longer in an endemic area during the transmission season or to short-term travelers who are planning to engage in extensive outdoor activities. Primary immunization consists of three doses given on days 0, 7, and 30, and should ideally be completed at least 10 days prior to trip departure, due to the risk of reaction. Typhoid fever immunization is recommended for travelers to areas in Central and South America, the Indian subcontinent, and Africa. The two types of typhoid vaccines are only 50% to 80% effective and, therefore, cannot substitute for careful selection of food and drink. There is an intramuscular and an oral regimen, depending on the age of the patient. Meningococcal vaccine is recommended for travelers to areas in sub-Saharan Africa during certain times of the year. Pre-exposure rabies vaccination should be considered for travelers to certain areas that are planning to engage in certain activities. It is extremely important for a physician to provide appropriate prevention for malaria as well.

SUGGESTED READINGS

Center for Disease Control and Prevention. Traveler's Health. Available at: www.cdc.gov/travel/contentVaccinations.aspx. Accessed January 7, 2008.

Chen LH. Vaccines for travel: hepatitis A, meningococcal disease, and typhoid fever. *Clin Fam Pract.* 2005;7:675–696.

Lo Re V 3rd, Gluckman SJ. Travel immunizations. *Am Fam Physician.* 2004;70:89–99.

112

KNOW THAT PRIMARY PERITONITIS (SPONTANEOUS BACTERIAL PERITONITIS) OCCURS IN THE ABSENCE OF A VISCERAL PERFORATION, ABSCESS, OR OTHER LOCALIZED INTRA-ABDOMINAL INFECTION

SOPHIA SMITH, MD

WHAT TO DO – INTERPRET THE DATA

Peritonitis is defined as an inflammation of the peritoneum, the thin membrane that lines the abdominal wall and covers most of the organs of the body. It is often caused by the introduction of an infection into the otherwise sterile peritoneal environment as a result of perforated bowel, such as a ruptured appendix or colonic diverticulum. The disease may also be caused by introduction of a chemically irritating material, such as gastric acid from a perforated ulcer or bile from a perforated gall bladder or a lacerated liver.

Peritonitis is often clinically seen as a constellation of signs and symptoms, which includes abdominal pain, tenderness on palpation, abdominal wall muscle rigidity, and systemic signs of inflammation of an infection. It is often caused by the introduction of an infectious agent into the otherwise sterile peritoneal environment. The peritoneum reacts to a variety of pathologic stimuli, with a fairly uniform inflammatory response. Depending on the underlying pathology, the resultant peritonitis may be infectious or sterile (i.e., chemical or mechanical).

The most common etiology of primary peritonitis is spontaneous bacterial peritonitis (SBP) due to chronic liver disease. The common etiologic entities of secondary peritonitis (SP) include perforated appendicitis; perforated gastric and duodenal ulcer disease; perforated (sigmoid) colon caused by diverticulitis, volvulus, or cancer; and strangulation of the small bowel. Tertiary peritonitis represents the persistence or recurrence of peritoneal infection following apparently adequate therapy of SBP or SP, often without the original visceral organ pathology. Patients with tertiary peritonitis usually present with an abscess, or phlegmon, with or without fistulization. In secondary and tertiary peritonitis, systemic antibiotic therapy is the second mainstay of therapy. In SBP, the initial empiric therapy with a third-generation cephalosporin and then tailored therapy according to the culture results is of critical importance. Patients with chronic liver disease

© 2008 by Lippincott Williams & Wilkins, a Wolters Kluwer business

are at an increased risk for nephrotoxicity with aminoglycoside use, but these agents may be indicated for the appropriate antimicrobial spectrum.

Rapid diagnosis is also important. X-rays are taken with the patient supine and standing. Free gas in the abdominal cavity can be seen on x-rays and may indicate a bowel wall rupture. Occasionally, a needle may be used to withdraw fluid from the abdominal cavity so that laboratory personnel can detect and identify any infectious organisms and test its sensitivity to various antibiotics.

SUGGESTED READING

Hyams JS. Peritonitis, Chapter 352. In: Behrman RE, Kliegman RM, Jensen HB, eds. *Nelson Textbook of Pediatrics* 17th ed. Philadelphia: Saunders; 2004.

113

CONSIDER THE DIAGNOSIS OF LYME DISEASE (LD) IN ANY PATIENT WITH ARTHRITIS

SONYA BURROUGHS, MD

WHAT TO DO – INTERPRET THE DATA

LD has become the most common vector-borne disease in North America. The highest prevalence occurs in patients aged 2 to 15 years and 30 to 59 years. In the United States, most LD is localized to three highly endemic areas: (a) the Northeast (Maine to Maryland), (b) the Midwest (Minnesota and Wisconsin), and (c) the West (Northern California and Oregon).

LD or lyme borreliosis is caused by members of the genus *Borrelia*. *B. burgdorferi* is the only species causing disease in the United States. *B. afzelii* and *B. garinii* are the predominant species infecting humans in Europe and Asia. *B. burgdorferi* is the most arthritogenic of the three *Borrelia* species that result in human disease. Pathogenic *Borrelia* are carried and transmitted by the *Ixodes ricinus* complex of ticks. The clinical manifestations of LD vary based on the stage of infection. Infection is divided into three stages: early localized, early disseminated, and late chronic. *Table 113.1* provides the clinical features at different stages.

Symptoms typically develop between 7 to 10 days after a tick bite, but ranges of 1 to 36 days have been reported. The most common manifestation in children is erythema migrans rash followed by arthritis, facial nerve palsy, carditis, and aseptic meningitis.

Lyme meningitis in children may be subtle and usually occurs without meningismus. The presentation typically involves less fever, when compared with viral meningitis. As mentioned previously, arthritis is a common symptom found in LD. This diagnosis should be considered in any patient with arthritis, especially if they live or have recently traveled to an endemic area. Early diagnosis is essential because untreated infection may lead to more advanced disease involving the heart, central nervous system, and joints.

ⓒ 2008 by Lippincott Williams & Wilkins, a Wolters Kluwer business

TABLE 113.1	CLINICAL FEATURES OF LYME DISEASE		
SYSTEM	STAGE 1 (EARLY) LOCALIZED	STAGE 2 (EARLY) DISSEMINATED	STAGE 3 (LATE) CHRONIC
Skin	Erythema migrans	Secondary annular lesions	
Musculoskeletal	Myalgia, arthralgia	Migratory pain in joints; brief arthritis attacks	Prolonged arthritis attacks, chronic arthritis
Neurologic	Headache	Meningitis, Bell palsy, cranial neuritis, radiculoneuritis	Encephalopathy, polyneuropathy, leukoencephalitis
Cardiac		Atrioventricular block, myopericarditis, pancarditis	
Constitutional	Flulike symptoms	Malaise, fatigue	Fatigue
Lymphatic	Regional lymphadenopathy	Regional or generalized lymphadenopathy	

Lyme arthritis may impersonate juvenile idiopathic arthritis. The arthritis associated with LD is a monoarthritis or oligoarthritis, usually affecting the knee. Sudden pain and swelling with massive effusions are common, and attacks are usually intermittent. Even without antibiotic therapy, arthritic flares due to LD gradually become less severe, occur less often, and eventually resolve completely. It is distinctly rare to have flares beyond 5 years of the diagnosis. Juvenile idiopathic arthritis is a clinical diagnosis made in a child younger than 16 years of age with arthritis for >6 weeks' duration, with other identifiable causes of arthritis excluded. Serology testing is necessary to rule out a diagnosis of LD or other arthritic-causing infections in the clinical scenario of arthritis.

The diagnosis of Lyme arthritis is based primarily on clinical findings. An estimate of the likelihood of LD is based on geographic location and the signs and symptoms of the patient, referred to as the pretest probability of disease; it is a key factor in the diagnosis of this disease. It also assists with the decision making on when to order tests and how to interpret laboratory findings (*Table 113.2*).

When laboratory testing is utilized, enzyme-linked immunoabsorbent assay (ELISA) is used primarily for screening, and the Western blot is used as confirmation. Synovial fluid should be obtained from all patients with suspected Lyme arthritis. White blood cell counts of the synovial fluid usually ranges from 1,000 to 50,000 cells/mm.

TABLE 113.2	ESTIMATING PRETEST PROBABILITY AND USING IT TO GUIDE INTERPRETATION OF SEROLOGIC TESTING		
ENDEMICITY OF LYME DISEASE	OBJECTIVE CLINICAL SIGNS AND SYMPTOMS	PRETEST PROBABILITY	LABORATORY TESTING
High, moderate, or low	Absent	Very low	NOT recommended (high false-positive rate)
Low	Absent, but has prolonged, unexplained nonspecific symptoms	Very low	NOT recommended
Moderate/high	Absent, but has prolonged, unexplained nonspecific symptoms	Moderately low	Should be considered
Moderate	Present without erythema migrans	Moderate	Recommended
Moderate/low	Erythema migrans present	Moderate-high	NOT recommended (high false-negative rate); diagnosis of Lyme disease based on clinical grounds alone
High	Erythema migrans present	High	NOT recommended (high false-negative rate); diagnosis of Lyme disease based on clinical grounds alone

SUGGESTED READINGS

DePietropaolo DL, Powers JH, Gill JM, et al. Diagnosis of Lyme disease. *Am Fam Physician* 2005;72:297–304.
Hu L. Lyme arthritis. *Infect Dis Clin North Am.* 2005;19:947–961.
Foy AJ, Studdiford J. Lyme disease. Clinics in family practice. 2005;7:191–208.

114

ALTHOUGH MANY PROVIDERS WILL OBTAIN AN ANTINUCLEAR ANTIBODY (ANA) TO RULE OUT SYSTEMIC LUPUS ERYTHEMATOSUS (SLE), THE ANA IS AN EXTREMELY SENSITIVE TEST, BUT NOT VERY SPECIFIC, AND SHOULD BE FOLLOWED UP BY MORE DEFINITIVE TESTS SUCH AS THE ANTI-DS-DNA OR ANTI-SMITH ANTIBODY

SONYA BURROUGHS, MD

WHAT TO DO – GATHER APPROPRIATE DATA

SLE is an autoimmune disorder that affects multiple organ systems. The cause is unknown, but the hallmark of the disease is the production of autoantibodies to the cell nucleus. The incidence of SLE varies significantly among various ethnic groups. Incidence also varies based on sex. Data suggests that the incidence rates of SLE with onset <19 years is 6 to 18.9/100,000 in white females, with higher rates in African American (20–30/100,000) and Puerto Rican females (16–36.7/100,000). The male:female ratio is 1:4.4.

Although the cause is unknown, there is a strong genetic component to SLE, with a 25% to 50% concordance rate in monozygotic twins. Approximately 10% to 16% of patients have a first- or second-degree relative with the disorder. An association with human leukocyte antigen has been found. The high female-to-male ratio, coupled with the fact that pregnancy frequently causes flares and worsens nephritis, strongly suggests that female hormones may play a role in development of the disease. Several drugs are known to induce lupuslike disease including, but not limited to, hydralazine, procainamide, isoniazid, minocycline, and D-penicillamine.

The clinical findings of SLE are a result of inflammation and blood vessel abnormalities. Bland vasculopathy, vasculitis, and immune-complex deposition have all been described. Patients frequently present with complaints of fever, diffuse hair loss, weight loss, fatigue, and arthralgias or arthritis (especially of small joints and wrists). Lymphadenopathy and hepatosplenomegaly may also be present. The differential diagnosis should include malignancy, infection, or other autoimmune disorders (i.e., rheumatoid arthritis, and Sjögren syndrome).

© 2008 by Lippincott Williams & Wilkins, a Wolters Kluwer business

ANAs are seen in up to 95% of patients with SLE. ANA testing is sensitive, but not very specific for SLE. ANA also occurs in up to 5% of the normal population. Antibodies to double-stranded DNA (anti-ds DNA) and to the Sm nuclear antigen (anti-Sm) are found only in patients in SLE.

The diagnosis is based on history, physical exam, and laboratory findings. Diagnostic criteria have been established by the American Academy of Rheumatology. These criteria are sensitive (78% to 96%) and specific (89% to 96%) for SLE. See *Table 114.1.*

TABLE 114.1   1997 REVISED/REVISED CLASSIFICATION CRITERIA FOR SYSTEMIC LUPUS ERYTHEMATOSUS (SLE)

Before a patient can be classified as having definite SLE, at least four of the following 11 disorders must be present at some time in the disease course:

- **Malar rash:** Fixed erythema, flat or raised, over the malar eminences, tending to spare the nasolabial folds
- **Discoid rash:** Erythematous raised patches with adherent keratotic scaling and follicular plugging
- **Photosensitivity:** Unusual skin rash due to reaction to sunlight, by patient history or physician observation
- **Oral ulcers:** Oral or nasopharyngeal ulceration, usually painless, observed by physician
- **Arthritis:** Nonerosive arthritis involving two or more peripheral joints, characterized by swelling, tenderness, or effusion
- **Serositis:** Pleuritis by convincing history or pleuritic pain or rub heard by a physician or evidence of pleural effusion

OR pericarditis documented by ECG, rub, or evidence of pericardial effusion

- **Renal disorder:** Persistent proteinuria >0.5 g/day or >3+ or cellular casts, which may be red cell, hemoglobin, granular, tubular, or mixed
- **Neurologic disorder:** Seizures or psychosis in the absence of offending drugs or known metabolic derangements (uremia, ketoacidosis, or electrolyte imbalance)
- **Hematologic disorder:** Hemolytic anemia with reticulocytosis, OR leukopenia <4000/mm^3 on two or more occasions, OR lymphopenia <1500/mm^3 on two or more occasions OR thrombocytopenia <100,000/mm^3 in the absence of offending drugs
- **Immunologic disorder:** Positive antiphospholipid antibody or anti-dsDNA antibody or anti-Sm antibody or false-positive serologic syphilis test known to be positive for at least 6 months and confirmed by negative *Treponema pallidum* immobilization or fluorescent treponemal antibody absorption test
- **Antinuclear antibodies:** An elevated titer of antinuclear antibody by immunofluorescence or an equivalent assay at any point in time and in the absence of drugs known to be associated with "drug-induced lupus" syndrome

ECG, electrocardiogram
Adapted with permission from Tan EM, Cohen AD, Fries JF, et al. The 1982 revised criteria for the classification of systemic lupus erythematosus. *Arthritis Rheum.* 1982;25:1274, and Hochberg MC. Updating the American College of Rheumatology revised criteria for the classification of systemic lupus erythematosus. *Arthritis Rheum.* 1997;40:1725, with permission.

The management of SLE is based on symptoms and organ involvement. The treatment can be extremely challenging due to treatment side effects. Corticosteroids are a mainstay of SLE therapy. Symptoms treated with
this modality include constitutional symptoms, arthritis, serositis, nephritis,
cerebritis, vasculitis, and hematologic abnormalities. Despite the fact that
corticosteroids are useful anti-inflammatory agents, their adverse effects and
withdrawal must not be forgotten. SLE is one of many conditions in which
high dose (1–2 mg/kg/day) corticosteroid treatment is necessary. Toxicity
often accompanies this therapy. Cushingoid appearance, obesity, and hypertension are commonly seen as a result of moderate-to-high-dose steroid
therapy. Growth suppression may also occur in children, as does steroid
myopathy. The risk of developing avascular necrosis associated with SLE
is increased further by long-term steroid therapy (4–6 months of continuous use). Other side effects include osteopenia, increased risk of infection,
peptic ulceration, posterior subcapsular cataracts, mood swings, depression, and emotional lability. Remember, sudden withdrawal of prolonged
and high-dose corticosteroid therapy may result in life-threatening adrenal
insufficiency. Patients may exhibit high fever in the absence of infection, hypotension, nausea, vomiting, confusion, hyponatremia, hyperkalemia, and
hypoglycemia. Steroid supplementation may also be needed in these patients
to prevent addisonian crisis.

SUGGESTED READINGS

Gedalia A, Shetty AK. Chronic steroid and immunosuppressant therapy in children. *Pediatr Rev.* 2004;25:425–434.

Gottlieb BS, Ilowite NT. Systemic lupus erythematosus in children and adolescents. *Pediatr Rev.* 2006;27:323–330.

Taylor ML, Gill JM. Lupus and related connective tissue diseases. *Clin Fam Prac.* 2005;7:209–224.

115

Do not prescribe ibuprofen in patients with systemic Lupus erythematosus (SLE) because it can cause ibuprofen-induced aseptic meningitis

Johann Peterson, MD

What to Do – Make a Decision

Nonsteroidal anti-inflammatory drugs (NSAIDs) are commonly used in many rheumatologic diseases, including SLE. Despite their common use and over-the-counter status, they are a potential cause of adverse reactions and should be prescribed with caution.

Aseptic meningitis refers to the clinical picture of meningeal inflammation (stiff neck, headache, fever, photophobia, Kernig and Brudzinski signs) and pleocytosis of the cerebrospinal fluid (CSF), but without an infectious agent identified in the CSF. It is, therefore, a diagnosis of exclusion, and most cases will require empiric antibiotic coverage while cultures and viral studies are pending. With the development of sensitive viral assays, many cases that previously would have been classified as aseptic meningitis are probably now being diagnosed as viral meningitis. Enteroviral infections (coxsackievirus, echovirus, polio) are a common cause of viral meningitis in children. Mumps and California virus are also possible. Localized infections, such as an epidural abscess, cranial osteomyelitis, and sinusitis, can cause meningeal inflammation, mimicking aseptic meningitis. And other infectious agents, such as mycobacteria, malaria and other parasites, fungi, spirochetes, and *Rickettsiae*, can cause meningitis and may not be identified with the usual CSF testing.

There are a number of recognized causes of aseptic meningitis, including drug reactions, autoimmune diseases, meningeal involvement with tumors, *Borrelia burgdorferi* infection (Lyme disease), and the acute retroviral syndrome. Ibuprofen is the most common medication responsible for drug-induced aseptic meningitis, and the risk appears to be greater among patients with SLE or other autoimmune diseases. Other NSAIDs have been implicated, as well as trimethoprim with or without sulfamethoxazole, cephalosporins and other antibiotics, intravenous immunoglobulin (IVIG), and other agents. Not surprisingly, a number of intrathecal medications and contrast agents have also been responsible. NSAID-induced aseptic meningitis can occur after only one dose, and typically occurs shortly after ingestion

© 2008 by Lippincott Williams & Wilkins, a Wolters Kluwer business

of ibuprofen, but it can be delayed until after 2 years of regular use. Some patients have suffered multiple episodes until the relationship was recognized. In most cases, patients can be successfully treated with another NSAID, but there are some reports of patients who developed aseptic meningitis with multiple different NSAIDs.

There is insufficient published data to estimate a quantitative risk of aseptic meningitis in healthy patients or in patients with rheumatologic disease. In one recent literature review, 39% of published cases were in patients with SLE. In patients with lupus, avoiding ibuprofen as a first-line agent may be useful. Screening for autoimmune disease in otherwise-healthy patients who develop NSAID meningitis may also be important.

Clinically, most patients have a typical meningitis syndrome, although some have encephalitic features including focal neurologic deficits, Babinski sign, syndrome of inappropriate secretion of antidiuretic hormone (SIADH), sensorineural hearing loss, and even coma. There are no reports of permanent neurologic sequelae. The CSF findings usually include pleocytosis (9–5,000 white blood cells [WBCs]/μL), which is often mostly neutrophils, but occasionally monocytes or eosinophils predominate. Protein is often elevated, but CSF glucose is usually normal. No CSF findings have been shown to reliably exclude bacterial meningitis. Symptoms may resolve rapidly (1–2 days) after stopping ibuprofen, but CSF abnormalities may last longer. Factors that may help distinguish Lyme meningitis from aseptic meningitis of another cause are a more subacute course, and longer duration of headache, history of facial weakness or cranial neuropathy, and, of course, the erythema migrans rash.

SUGGESTED READINGS

Eppes SC, Nelson DK, Lewis LL, Klein JD. Characterization of Lyme meningitis and comparison with viral meningitis in children. *Pediatrics*. 1999;103(5 Pt 1):957–960.

Jolles S, Sewell WA, Leighton C. Drug-induced aseptic meningitis: diagnosis and management. *Drug Saf*. 2000;22(3):215–226.

Rodriguez SC, Olguín AM, Miralles CP, et al. Characteristics of meningitis caused by Ibuprofen: report of 2 cases with recurrent episodes and review of the literature. *Medicine (Baltimore)*. 2006;85(4):214–220.

116

KNOW THE IMPORTANT DIFFERENCES BETWEEN RHEUMATIC DISEASES AND HOW TO RECOGNIZE AND MAKE AN APPROPRIATE DIAGNOSIS

NAILAH COLEMAN, MD

WHAT TO DO – GATHER APPROPRIATE DATA

Rheumatic diseases include both primary vascular disorders, as well as disorders of connective tissues. Almost any organ can be affected, from the heart and lungs to the bones, joints or skin, and the clinical presentation can vary greatly, depending on the site involved. Three of the most common rheumatic disorders that can present in childhood are juvenile idiopathic arthritis (JIA, also known as juvenile rheumatoid arthritis), systemic lupus erythematosus (SLE), and juvenile dermatomyositis (JDMS).

Although there can be some overlap between these three diseases, they each have distinct criteria that should be met for accurate diagnosis. In JIA, children younger than 16 years of age must exhibit the presence of arthritis in at least one joint for more than 6 weeks, and other types of childhood arthritis should have been excluded. Common classifications include pauciarticular JIA (involvement of four or fewer joints during the first 6 months of illness), polyarticular JIA (involvement of five or more joints during the first 6 months of illness; may be associated with mild systemic symptoms, such as fever or malaise), and systemic-onset JIA (extra-articular manifestations, such as fever or rash, tend to precede the onset of articular symptoms, and complications, like pericarditis and pleuropericarditis, are more common).

The diagnosis of SLE is made if the clinician can detect the presence of four or more of the 11 criteria as proposed by the American College of Rheumatology. These criteria are as follows: malar rash, discoid rash, photosensitivity, oral ulcers, arthritis, serositis, renal, neurologic, hematologic, or immunologic disorders, and/or the presence of antinuclear antibodies (ANAs).

JDMS can have diagnostic similarities to other rheumatic diseases. Many patients with JDMS can have a characteristic rash that may be confused with the malar rash of SLE. Unlike in SLE, patients with JDMS also present with symmetric proximal muscle pain and/or weakness, involving the shoulder and pelvic girdles, and fatigue.

© 2008 by Lippincott Williams & Wilkins, a Wolters Kluwer business

Blood tests are often used in conjunction with the history and physical to support a particular diagnosis. ANAs, one of the diagnostic criteria of SLE, may be present in any number of rheumatic diseases, as well as non-rheumatic diseases, such as neoplasms or infections. It can also be seen in up to 15% to 30% of the normal population, making it a nonspecific finding. ANA is also used to stratify the risk of certain disease complications; for example, patients with JIA that are ANA-positive are at a greater risk of development uveitis. Anti-double-stranded DNA or anti-Smith antibodies may be present in SLE. Both are less sensitive, but much more specific than ANA for SLE. Rheumatoid factor may be seen in both rheumatic and nonrheumatic diseases, but its presence in JIA can be associated with more severe erosive joint disease and poorer functional outcomes. Children with JDMS often have elevated muscle enzymes (i.e., creatine kinase, aspartate aminotransferase, lactate dehydrogenase, and aldolase), nonspecific markers of muscle inflammation that may be elevated in a number of diseases.

As mentioned previously, rheumatic disorders can affect any organ, resulting in a variety of complications. Nonetheless, the physician should be familiar with some of the more common complications:

- **Uveitis:** An inflammatory condition of the anterior eye, often seen in JIA, that may lead to impaired vision or blindness. It is often asymptomatic and requires regular screening.
- **Lupus cerebritis:** A condition that may present with headache, psychosis, depression, or altered mental status; however, children on immunosuppressive therapy for their lupus may have similar symptoms due to an acute infection (i.e., meningitis) and must be evaluated accordingly.
- **Serositis:** An inflammation of the pericardium or pleural spaces that may lead to cardiac tamponade or pulmonary effusions and compromised cardiopulmonary function that can be life-threatening in severe cases.
- **Libman-Sacks endocarditis:** An inflammation of the endocardium that may result in the formation of sterile vegetations, increasing the risk of infectious endocarditis. These patients require infective endocarditis prophylaxis prior to invasive procedures.
- **Lupus nephritis:** Renal disease, graded based on pathology seen on renal biopsy, and a major cause of morbidity and mortality that can lead to hypertension and/or renal failure.
- **Raynaud phenomenon:** A vasculopathy of the digits that is often exacerbated by cold, emotional stress, caffeine or tobacco smoke; severe disease may require treatment with a vasodilator or even lead to infarction of the digit.

- **Esophageal dysmotility**: Disordered esophageal motion, often seen with JDMS. In severe cases, associated reflux may lead to severe or recurrent aspiration pneumonitis.

The treatment of rheumatic disorders is tailored to the organ or system involved, but the goals of therapy are common to all diseases. In each case, the clinician should work to maximize mobility. Both arthritis and myositis can lead to impaired musculoskeletal function and decreased mobility. Physical therapy, occupational therapy, and splint applications are used in preserving function and limiting the development of contractures. Any patients with arthritis should have their pain addressed and adequately treated. First-line options for pain relief are nonsteroidal anti-inflammatory drugs (NSAIDs), although these medications do not necessarily alter disease progression. Patients with chronic NSAID use must also be given gastrointestinal prophylaxis, with the use of antacids, histamine blockers, or proton-pump inhibitors. With a multitude of evidence that a number of rheumatic disorders are related to altered immune function, immunomodulators are often used. As such, the use of steroids, methotrexate, antitumor necrosis factor receptors or anti-interleukin agents can be used in some or all of these diseases. Patients on immunomodulators are considered immunocompromised, with an increased susceptibility to a number of infections, particularly tuberculosis, listeriosis, and histoplasmosis, as well as the more common pathogens, and should be treated accordingly:

- Whenever possible, ensure live vaccines (i.e., varicella as well as measles, mumps, and rubella) are given prior to the initiation of treatment.
- Patients should be screened for latent tuberculosis, as the initiation of these medications may lead to reactivation of the disease.
- Immunomodulators should not be initiated until malignancies or neoplasms have been ruled out.

All patients should be monitored for disease progression as well as for adverse effects of treatment. Patients on chronic steroids should be monitored for growth delays and osteopenia; patients on methotrexate should be given folic acid supplements to prevent oral ulcers and vitamin deficiencies. Whenever an exacerbating factor can be identified, instruct patients to take appropriate precautions. For example, exposure to sunlight may lead to a disease flare in patients with JDMS or SLE. These patients must be instructed to wear sunscreen at all times, including with exposure to indoor light. In all cases, early and aggressive interventions lead to better outcomes.

SUGGESTED READINGS

Goldmuntz EA, White PH. Juvenile idiopathic arthritis: a review for the pediatrician. *Pediatr Rev.* 2006;27(4):e24–e32.

Gottlieb BS, Ilowite NT. Systemic lupus erythematosus in children and adolescents. *Pediatr Rev.* 2006;27(9):323–330.

Pachman LM. Juvenile dermatomyositis: a clinical overview. *Pediatr Rev.* 1990;12(4):117–125.

Wikipedia. Rheumatism. Available at: http://en.wikipedia.org/wiki/Rheumatic_diseases. Accessed November 16, 2007.

117

KNOW THAT THE FIRST URINARY ABNORMALITY IN CHILDREN WITH COLLAGEN VASCULAR DISORDERS IS HEMATURIA, ALTHOUGH IT MAY PRESENT WITH PROTEINURIA AND NEPHROTIC SYNDROME

SOPHIA SMITH, MD

WHAT TO DO – INTERPRET THE DATA

Collagen Vascular Disorders and Hematuria. Hematuria is one of the most common urinary findings that bring children to the attention of the pediatric nephrologist. It is defined as the presence of >5 red blood cells (RBCs) per high-power field in three of three consecutive centrifuged specimens obtained <1 week apart. The hematuria may be overtly bloody or microscopic. It may be symptomatic or asymptomatic, transient or persistent, and either isolated or associated with proteinuria and other urinary abnormalities.

The etiology of this hematuria may be the result of a structural disruption in the integrity of the glomerular basement membrane caused by inflammatory or immunologic processes. But other causes, such as chemicals, may cause disruptions of the renal tubules and calculi that may cause mechanical erosion of mucosal surfaces in the genitourinary tract, resulting in hematuria. Collagen vascular disease is a somewhat antiquated term used to describe diseases of the connective tissues that typically include diseases associated with blood vessel abnormalities. Collagen represents 30% of body protein and shapes the structure of tendons, bones, and connective tissues. These collagen vascular disorders are a diverse group of diseases that affect the supporting tissues of the body. Some collagen vascular diseases include: rheumatoid arthritis, systemic lupus erythematosus, scleroderma, dermatomyositis, and polyarteritis nodosa.

The clinical manifestations of nephritis associated with collagen vascular diseases are not different from other forms of glomerulonephritis and include a nephritic sediment (dysmorphic erythrocytes and erythrocyte casts), proteinuria or nephrotic syndrome, and hematuria. Immune complex glomerulonephritides are a diverse group of conditions that develop in patients with pre-existing glomerular disease and histopathologic studies consistent with collagen vascular disease.

© 2008 by Lippincott Williams & Wilkins, a Wolters Kluwer business

Systemic lupus erythematosus is one of a number of collagen vascular disorders with renal involvement. Lupus itself is an autoimmune vasculitis characterized by antinuclear antibodies and widespread immunocomplex-mediated inflammation. The renal lesions are the most important clinically and affect prognosis. Glomerular changes vary from minimal involvement to diffuse proliferative disease. This results in a focal or diffuse proliferative glomerulonephritis. Patients may develop chronic renal failure, but the prognosis has been improved with immunosuppressive treatment (steroids, azathioprine or cyclophosphamide). In gathering a patient physical exam, a history of joint pains, skin rashes, and prolonged fever, in addition to a diagnosis of hematuria in an adolescent strongly suggests a collagen vascular disorder. The presence of anemia cannot be accounted for by hematuria alone. Other disease processes should be considered, such as a bleeding diathesis. But with finding anemia in a patient with hematuria and pallor, systemic lupus erythematosus should be considered.

SUGGESTED READING

Barratt TM and Niaudet P. Clinical Evaluation, Chapter 20. In: Avner ED, Harmon WE and Niaudet P. *Pediatric Nephrology* 5th Edition. Philadelphia: Lippincott Williams & Wilkins, 2004.

118

REMEMBER TO THINK BROADLY ABOUT THE DIFFERENTIAL DIAGNOSIS OF SYNCOPE IN CHILDREN

ANJALI SUBBASWAMY, MD

WHAT TO DO – GATHER APPROPRIATE DATA

Syncope/Long QT. Syncope is a loss of consciousness related to decreased cerebral perfusion to the areas of the brain necessary for consciousness, which include the brainstem, reticular activating system, and the bilateral cerebral cortices. International incidence was reported in 126 of the 100,000 children monitored, with peak incidence between the ages 15 to 19. Neurocardiogenic syncope and neurologic disorders were the most common etiologies, representing 80% and 9%, respectively. Other causes included psychological, cardiac, respiratory, toxicologic, and metabolic problems (*Table 118.1*). Neurocardiogenic and disease-related syncope were easily identified or suspected by history and physical examination.

Vasovagal syncope may be characterized by the sudden loss of vasomotor tone with resultant systemic hypotension (the vasodepressor response), accompanied by significant bradycardia or asystole, known as the cardioinhibitory response. Most episodes occur when the patient is in the upright position, either during a prolonged period of standing (such as in church, gym/military drill), or during the rapid change from supine or sitting position to standing. There may be an emotional component and symptoms often occur in the setting of fatigue, hunger, concurrent illness, and dehydration. The loss of consciousness typically lasts <1 to 2 minutes.

Syncope during exercise or physical activity should always raise the question of a cardiac abnormality in which the patient is unable to maintain cardiac output to meet increased demands. A family history of syncope, seizures, or unexplained sudden death may also identify those at risk for long QT syndrome (LQTS), hypertrophic obstructive cardiomyopathy,

© 2008 by Lippincott Williams & Wilkins, a Wolters Kluwer business

TABLE 118.1   CAUSES OF SYNCOPE IN CHILDREN

Autonomic
Vasovagal (fainting): Most common cause in children
Excessive vagal tone: Athletes, adolescents
Reflex:
   Situational: Cough, micturition, hair grooming
   Pallid breath holding
Orthostatic: Dehydration, blood loss
Cardiac:
   Obstructive lesions: Aortic stenosis, hypertrophic obstructive cardiomyopathy, primary
     pulmonary hypertension
   Arrhythmia: Supraventricular tachycardia, ventricular tachycardia, heart block
   Hypercyanosis: Tetralogy of Fallot spells
   Miscellaneous: Pump dysfunction, myocardial infarction, anomalous coronary anatomy
Noncardiac:
   Neurologic: Seizures, migraine
   Metabolic: Hypoglycemia
   Hyperventilation
   Hysterical: Audience, complete absence of trauma
   Vascular: Cervical anomalies, vertebrobasilar insufficiency

Wolf-Parkinson-White syndrome, or arrhythmogenic right ventricular dysplasia. Those with LQTS may demonstrate prolongation of the QT interval during physical exercise, intense emotion (e.g., fright, anger, or pain), or by a startling noise. The classic example is of a child who jumps into a pool, and the sudden cold triggers the arrhythmia. This can lead to syncope and in some instances drowning. This may be the initial presentation of the arrhythmia. Clues for the suspicion of LQTS include a corrected QT interval (QTc) >0.44 seconds, unexplained syncope, seizures, or cardiac arrest preceded by emotion or exercise or family history of LQTS. It is important to calculate the QTc (beginning of QRS complex to end of the T wave) by hand and not rely on the autocalculation by the electrocardiographic machine. The average age of first syncopal episode in LQTS is 14 years. The 1-year mortality after first syncopal episode is 20%, emphasizing the need for a high index of suspicion. There is a rare, autosomal recessive disorder of congenital sensory deafness associated with a prolonged QT interval called the Jervell and Lange-Nielsen syndrome.

SUGGESTED READINGS

Garson A Jr, Dick M 2nd, Fournier A, et al. The long QT syndrome in children. An international study of 287 patients. *Circulation.* 1993;87:1866–1872.
Massin MM, Bourguignont A, Coremans C, et al. Syncope in pediatric patients presenting to an emergency department. *J Pediatr.* 2004;145(2):223–228.
Prodinger RJ, Reisdorff EJ. Syncope in children. *Emerg Med Clin North Am.* 1998;16(3):617–626.

119

DO NOT FORGET TO PRESCRIBE PROPHYLAXIS AGAINST ENDOCARDITIS FOR PATIENTS WITH HEART DISEASE

SARIKA JOSHI, MD

WHAT TO DO – TAKE ACTION

Antibiotic prophylaxis for patients with certain types of heart disease (e.g., rheumatic heart disease, infective endocarditis, and congenital heart disease [CHD]) is part of standard medical therapy in most developed nations. Infective endocarditis (IE) is less common in children than in adults. Although the incidence of rheumatic heart disease in developed countries has decreased, it appears that the incidence of IE in children has been increasing, due to, in part, improved survival of potentially at-risk children, such as those with CHD and those with indwelling venous catheters. In the developed world, CHD is the most common risk factor for IE.

Cardiac endothelial damage is the initiating factor for IE. In children with CHD, shear forces from high-velocity aberrant blood flow can damage the cardiac endothelium. Alternatively, damage may be caused by catheter-induced trauma. A thrombus can form at the site of damage. If a child subsequently has transient bacteremia with an organism capable of causing endocarditis, the thrombus may become infected. The most common etiologic organisms for IE in children are streptococci and staphylococci, especially viridans group streptococci and *Staphylococcus aureus*. Bacterial proliferation results in the formation of vegetations. The goal of antibiotic prophylaxis is to prevent or quickly treat bacteremia and prevent IE in susceptible patients. Despite its widespread practice, no study has ever demonstrated that antimicrobial prophylaxis in at-risk individuals prior to invasive procedures definitively prevents IE.

Because the presentation of IE is generally insidious with fever and other nonspecific systemic complaints (e.g., weakness, fatigue and weight loss) physicians must have a high degree of suspicion in the appropriate clinical circumstance. Once suspected, the Duke criteria, comprised of major and minor criteria, can be used to assist in diagnosing IE in children. The major Duke criteria are as follows:

- Two separate positive blood cultures with a typical etiologic agent for IE
- Evidence of cardiac involvement (e.g., a positive finding on echocardiography or new valvular regurgitation).

ⓒ 2008 by Lippincott Williams & Wilkins, a Wolters Kluwer business

The minor Duke criteria include:

- A predisposing condition (i.e., CHD, indwelling catheter)
- Fever
- Vascular complications (i.e., Janeway lesions)
- Immunologic complications (i.e., Osler nodes, Roth spots)
- Microbiologic evidence that does not meet major criteria
- Echocardiographic evidence that does not meet major criteria.

Using these clinical criteria, definite IE is diagnosed with two major criteria, one major criterion and three minor criteria, or five minor criteria. Echocardiography is the primary imaging modality used in the diagnosis of IE.

The American College of Cardiology and the American Heart Association have established guidelines to assist physicians with deciding when to prescribe antibiotic prophylaxis for IE. Patients are stratified into high-risk, moderate-risk, and low-risk groups. Antimicrobial prophylaxis is recommended for high- and moderate-risk groups prior to an invasive procedure. Common invasive procedures requiring antibiotic prophylaxis include oral and dental procedures, including routine dental cleanings, and genitourinary and gastrointestinal procedures. As the risk of bacteremia is highest for oral and dental procedures, maintaining good dental hygiene is especially important in children at risk for IE.

Children's risk for IE can be determined using the American College of Cardiology and the American Heart Association guidelines. Those at high risk for IE are those with prosthetic heart valves, a previous history of IE, complex cyanotic CHD (i.e., tetralogy of Fallot) and surgically constructed systemic or pulmonary conduits. Children at moderate risk for IE include those with other types of CHD, excluding children older than 6 months after surgical repair of atrial septal defect, ventricular septal defect and patent ductus arteriosus, and isolated secundum atrial septal defect; acquired valvular dysfunction or prior valvular repair; hypertrophic cardiomyopathy with obstruction; mitral valve prolapse with regurgitation or thickened leaflets; and intracardiac defects repaired within the last 6 months.

Recommended antibiotic prophylaxis regimens vary with the type of invasive procedure. For oral, dental, and upper respiratory tract procedures, one dose of amoxicillin (50 mg/kg/dose, maximum 2 g/dose) 1 hour prior to the procedure is suggested. For genitourinary and gastrointestinal procedures, ampicillin (50 mg/kg/dose, maximum 2 g/dose) and gentamicin (1.5 mg/kg/dose) 30 minutes prior to the procedure, followed by a second dose of ampicillin or amoxicillin 6 hours later is suggested for high-risk patients. For moderate-risk individuals, ampicillin or amoxicillin within 30 minutes of starting the procedure is suggested. Physicians should be alert to the need for antimicrobial prophylaxis against IE in the appropriate clinical scenario, such as children with CHD prior to dental procedures.

SUGGESTED READINGS

Bonow RO, Carabello BA, Chattergee K, et al. ACC/AHA 2006 guidelines for the management of patients with valvular heart disease: a report from the American College of Cardiology/ American Heart Association Task Force on Practice Guidelines (writing committee to revise the 1998 guidelines for the management of patients with valvular heart disease) developed in collaboration with the Society of Cardiovascular Anesthesiologists endorsed by the Society for Cardiovascular Angiography and Interventions and the Society of Thoracic Surgeons. *J Am Coll Cardiol.* 2006;48:e1–e148.

Ferrieri P, Gewitz MH, Gerber MA, et al. Unique features of infective endocarditis in childhood. *Pediatrics.* 2002;109:931–943.

120

DO NOT IGNORE REGURGITANT MURMURS, THEY ARE PATHOLOGIC

RUSSELL CROSS, MD

WHAT TO DO – TAKE ACTION

There are many ways to classify murmurs that can aid in determining whether any given one is pathologic. Systolic murmurs should be classified according to their timing within systole as being either ejection or regurgitant. Systolic murmurs that begin immediately after the first heart sound (S_1) are called regurgitant, whereas those that have a delay in onset timing after S_1 are called ejection. The S_1 sound is created by closure of the mitral and tricuspid valves that occurs at the beginning of ventricular contraction. Systolic regurgitant murmurs begin immediately after S_1. Blood in a higher pressure ventricle can immediately begin to flow into a lower pressure area as soon as the ventricle contracts. The delay between an S_1 and a systolic ejection murmur occurs because the ventricular pressure must first rise higher than the pressure in another area before flow can begin. It is important to determine the onset timing of systolic murmurs, as this can help to differentiate the cause of the murmur.

During systole, blood leaving a ventricle can flow either into the corresponding atrium or great vessel or into the other ventricle. When one thinks of normal cardiac physiology, the left ventricle is typically at higher pressure than the right, and both ventricles are at higher pressure than their corresponding atria. Thus, systolic regurgitant murmurs are created by atrioventricular valve regurgitation (tricuspid or mitral valve regurgitation) or by a ventricular septal defect. Regurgitant murmurs are also typically described as "harsh" in quality or "pansystolic" in timing. Although it is important to make use of other murmur characteristics such as location, quality, intensity, and radiation to determine the cause of a murmur, any murmur that can be defined as regurgitant is by its nature pathologic and should not be ignored.

Ejection murmurs, on the other hand, are created by obstruction to flow into the great vessels because pressure in the ventricle must rise above the pressure in its corresponding great vessel before ejection can begin. Ejection murmurs are those that are typically described as "crescendo-decrescendo" or "diamond shaped." Careful attention to other abnormal cardiac sounds such as an ejection click, fixed split S_2, or gallop will distinguish benign ejection murmurs from pathologic ones.

© 2008 by Lippincott Williams & Wilkins, a Wolters Kluwer business

There are many types of innocent or nonpathologic murmurs that can be heard in the pediatric population. These include the peripheral pulmonary artery stenosis murmur of the newborn, aortic and pulmonary flow murmurs, venous hums, and a Still murmur. All of these murmurs are typically graded as having intensity 1 to 2 on a scale of 6, and tend to be less harsh in nature. The murmur of peripheral pulmonary artery stenosis is a 1 to 2 out of 6 systolic ejection type murmur that is typically heard in the corresponding axilla. The key to identifying this murmur is that it is typically heard in infants younger than 6 months of age and is only heard in the axilla and not in the chest or back. This is compared to the more pathologic pulmonary stenosis murmur, which is heard in the chest and typically radiates to the back.

The benign pulmonary flow murmur is frequently heard in the child, adolescent, and young adult age groups. It is a 1 to 2 out of 6 systolic ejection murmur that is heard at the upper left sternal border, but is not associated with any other abnormal findings such as splitting of the second heart sound, an ejection click, the presence of a thrill, or radiation to the back, as would be present in pathologic pulmonary valve stenosis. The presence of a fixed split S_2 raises the index of suspicion for an atrial septal defect. The benign aortic flow murmur is similar but is heard at the right upper sternal border and is heard at times of increased cardiac output, such as fever, anemia, nervousness, and may also occur during the adolescent growth surge. The benign aortic flow murmur again has no other pathologic characteristics associated with it. The venous hum is a continuous murmur heard in the upper chest due to turbulent flow in systemic veins draining the head and upper extremities. It is louder when the patient is upright, and may disappear when the patient lies down. The intensity of the venous hum can be diminished by turning the patient's head or by light compression on the corresponding jugular vein.

The Still murmur is the most common innocent murmur of childhood, occurring most frequently between the ages of 2 and 6, although it can be heard at any age. It was first described by George Still in 1909. The Still murmur is heard along the left lower sternal border during early systole and is 1 to 2 out of 6 in intensity. It is low-pitched and frequently described as vibratory, "twanging," or musical in nature. The classic characteristic of the Still murmur is that it diminishes in intensity when the patient moves from supine to sitting or standing, a characteristic that is not present with any of the pathologic murmurs.

SUGGESTED READINGS

Mahnke CB, Nowalk A, Hofkosh D, et al. Comparison of two educational interventions on pediatric resident auscultation skills. *Pediatrics*. 2004;113(5):1331–1335.

McConnell ME, Adkins SB 3rd, Hannon DW. Heart murmurs in pediatric patients: when do you refer? *AmFamPhys*. 1999;60(2):558–565.

Poddar B, Basu S. Approach to a child with a heart murmur. *Indian J Pediatr*. 2004;71:63–66.

121

IDENTIFY ATRIAL FLUTTER IN CHILDREN, IT IS ONE OF THE MOST COMMONLY MISSED TACHYCARDIAS

RUSSELL CROSS, MD

WHAT TO DO – GATHER APPROPRIATE DATA

Atrial flutter is an uncommon arrhythmia in the pediatric population, particularly in those without congenital heart disease. Atrial flutter is easily missed in this age group because of its rarity and the fact that it can masquerade as other rhythms depending on the extent of atrioventricular (AV) conduction. Atrial flutter is characterized on electrocardiogram by the appearance of flutter waves, which classically have a "saw tooth" pattern (*Fig. 121.1*). Flutter waves typically have an atrial rate of 240 to 360 beats per minute (bpm), but the rate can be slower. The ventricular response to atrial flutter can be highly variable depending on the conduction through the AV node. The ventricular response is typically described as the ratio of flutter waves to conducted QRS complexes (2:1, 3:1, 4:1, etc.). The most common AV conduction ratio is 2:1. In atrial flutter, the QRS complexes have a normal morphology but occur at a fraction of the atrial flutter rate depending on the degree of AV block.

When significant AV nodal block is present, the diagnosis of atrial flutter can be readily made because the flutter waves on electrocardiogram are more evident between the conducted QRS complexes. When there is less AV nodal block, such as 2:1 or 3:1 conduction, the flutter waves can be harder to differentiate (*Fig. 121.2*). In these cases, the rhythm may appear to be sinus in origin, with the flutter waves appearing to be the P and T waves of sinus tachycardia. In patients with 2:1 AV conduction, the second flutter wave is often concealed by the QRS complex. Alternatively, atrial flutter may also be confused with supraventricular or AV reentrant tachycardia because of the similarity in the electrocardiogram tracings. Infants who often have rapid AV conduction are frequently misdiagnosed as having either sinus tachycardia or supraventricular tachycardia. A key differentiating feature between sinus tachycardia and either sinus tachycardia or reentrant tachycardia is that the rate of sinus tachycardia is variable, whereas the rate of atrial flutter and reentrant tachycardia is fixed. Thus, close observation of the patient's heart rate over time, along with treatment of patient specific causes of sinus tachycardia

© 2008 by Lippincott Williams & Wilkins, a Wolters Kluwer business

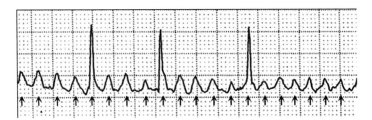

FIGURE 121.1. Atrial flutter with variable high-grade atrioventricular (AV) block (flutter rate approximately 300 beats per minute). Atrial flutter waves are readily seen, as indicated by arrows.

(e.g., fluid bolus, analgesics, or antipyretics if indicated), may help to clarify that sinus tachycardia is present.

It can be more difficult to differentiate cases of atrial flutter with rapid ventricular response compared to supraventricular or reentrant tachycardia. Both of these arrhythmias can lead to hemodynamic compromise or congestive heart failure if left untreated. Additionally, there is a risk of development of atrial thrombi in the case of prolonged atrial flutter. The differentiation of atrial flutter versus re-entrant tachycardia can be aided by the administration of adenosine. Adenosine is an endogenous nucleoside that affects cellular potassium conductance and also has an indirect antiadrenergic effect. Adenosine results in slowing of the sinus node as well as depression of AV nodal conduction. It is this slowing of AV nodal conduction that can be used to differentiate atrial flutter from reentrant tachycardia. In the case of supraventricular or re-entrant tachycardia, adenosine will slow conduction through the AV node, a component of the re-entrant circuit creating the tachycardia, and will terminate the arrhythmia. On the other hand, adenosine has relatively little effect on conductance of atrial tissue itself, and thus will not terminate atrial flutter. However, adenosine can be a diagnostic aid in

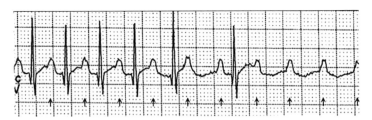

FIGURE 121.2. Atrial flutter at approximately 150 bpm, initially with 1:1 ventricular conduction. Note that initial tracing could be mistaken for sinus tachycardia, but flutter waves become apparent at end of tracing when AV conduction is blocked. Atrial flutter waves are indicated by arrows.

the case of atrial flutter as it will produce higher degrees of AV nodal block, thus slowing the ventricular response and unmasking the saw tooth flutter pattern on the electrocardiogram (*Fig. 121.2*).

Adenosine has a half-life of <10 seconds as it is rapidly metabolized by erythrocytes as well as vascular endothelium. Thus, it must be administered as a rapid bolus into a reasonably central vein. Side effects of adenosine bolus include flushing, lightheadedness, chest pain, and dyspnea, but these are self-limited due to the drug's short half-life. Adenosine should be administered in a setting with readily available access to emergency equipment, as it can induce other arrhythmias such as atrial fibrillation.

SUGGESTED READINGS

Bink-Boelkens MT. Pharmacologic management of arrhythmias. *Pediatr Cardiol.* 2000;21:508–515.

Engelstein ED, Lippman N, Stein KM, et al. Mechanism-specific effects of adenosine on atrial tachycardia. *Circulation.* 1994;89:2645–2654.

Texter KM, Kertesz NJ, Friedman RA, et al. Atrial flutter in infants. *J Am Coll Cardiol.* 2006;48:1040–1046.

122

KNOW THE THERAPEUTIC USES FOR NITRIC OXIDE (NO)

WHAT TO DO — GATHER APPROPRIATE DATA

NO was first identified as an endogenous endothelial-derived vasodilator in 1987, and is now widely used for the treatment of pulmonary hypertension. NO is a colorless, odorless gas that can easily be blended into various types of respiratory gas therapies. After inhalation, NO is rapidly absorbed from the alveolar space into the adjacent capillary where it activates guanylate cyclase in the pulmonary vascular smooth muscles. Activated guanylate cyclase in turn promotes the conversion of guanosine triphosphate (GTP) to cyclic guanosine monophosphate (c-GMP), which promotes the relaxation of vascular smooth muscle. A key feature of inhaled NO therapy is its selectivity for the pulmonary vascular bed due to the rapid binding of NO by hemoglobin. In the blood, NO reacts with oxyhemoglobin to form methemoglobin, and with deoxyhemoglobin to form iron-nitrosyl-hemoglobin. Ultimately, approximately 70% of inhaled NO is excreted in the urine as nitrate. Certain phosphodiesterase inhibiting drugs, such as sildenafil and others, allow for a higher level of activated c-GMP, which in turn promotes pulmonary vasodilatation.

In clinical use, inhaled NO can be administered through a mechanical ventilator, nasal cannula, or mask. In the past, doses of 5 to 80 ppm were used, but subsequent evaluation has shown that doses >20 ppm do not produce greater hemodynamic effects. One of the common uses of NO is for the treatment of pulmonary hypertension of the newborn (PPHN). PPHN can be seen in association with meconium aspiration, neonatal pneumonia, pulmonary hypoplasia of various etiologies, prematurity, and premature ductal closure, as well as other idiopathic causes. Profound hypoxemia can result from PPHN when patients have a persistent patent ductus arteriosus or patent foramen ovale, which allows for right-to-left shunting of deoxygenated venous blood into the systemic circulation. In cases where the ductus arteriosus and foramen ovale have closed, the right ventricle will be unable to pump blood through the high pressure pulmonary bed and, heart failure and shock will ensue. Although PPHN was treated with aggressive hyperventilation in the past, current initial treatment includes vasoactive agents and volume expansion to support cardiac function, treatment of metabolic acidosis, and treatment of underlying disorders. In patients with refractory

© 2008 by Lippincott Williams & Wilkins, a Wolters Kluwer business

PPHN, inhaled NO has been shown to improve oxygenation and to reduce the need for initiation of extracorporeal membrane oxygenation (ECMO), a costly and invasive but lifesaving mechanical support therapy for refractory PPHN. On the basis of multicenter randomized trials, the U.S. Food and Drug Administration have approved inhaled NO as treatment for respiratory failure in neonates with clinical or echocardiographic evidence of pulmonary hypertension.

Other clinical applications of inhaled NO include acute respiratory distress syndrome, postoperative cardiac surgery, and postlung transplantation. Acute pulmonary hypertensive episodes following corrective surgery for congenital heart disease are a significant cause of mortality and morbidity. Cardiopulmonary bypass causes endothelial dysfunction and diminished endogenous NO production, that leads to potentially lethal pulmonary hypertensive crises. Data from several small studies demonstrates that inhaled NO improves cardiac function and potentially reduces incidence of pulmonary hypertension crises. The role of inhaled NO in patients with severe respiratory disease is less clear. The predominant mechanism for hypoxemia is intrapulmonary shunting and parenchymal lung disease. Several clinical studies have demonstrated improvements in oxygenation, but not differences in mortality or duration of mechanical ventilation. Because mortality in severe lung disease is related to multisystem organ dysfunction, whether transient improvements in oxygenation is important remains an open question. Inhaled NO is also used in the cardiac catheterization laboratory as a means to selectively evaluate the pulmonary vascular reactivity potential in patients with pulmonary hypertension, as a means to predict the patient's ability to respond to other vasodilating agents. The side effects of inhaled NO are minimal and inhalation of low doses has been shown to be safe. However, close monitoring of its major byproducts, nitrogen dioxide (NO_2) and methemoglobin, is required to minimize their undesired toxic side effects. NO_2 formation is dependent on the concentration of inspired O_2 and the amount of time the two gases commingle. NO_2 has been demonstrated to increase airway reactivity in concentrations >1.5 ppm, and higher concentrations can result in pulmonary edema and death. Inhaled NO also combines with hemoglobin in the blood and is ultimately metabolized to methemoglobin. NO binds to hemoglobin with a much greater affinity than oxygen, and as a result tissue hypoxemia can ensue when there are significant levels of circulating methemoglobin. In clinical practice, blood levels of methemoglobin and the concentration of inspired NO_2 are closely monitored, but significant toxicity is uncommon at inhaled NO doses of <80 ppm.

Another important clinical aspect of the use of inhaled NO is the phenomena of rebound pulmonary hypertension. Rapid discontinuation of inhaled NO can cause profound elevations in pulmonary vascular resistance and reduced oxygenation. The exact mechanism of this rebound pulmonary hypertension is unclear, but studies suggest decreased endogenous NO production and up-regulation of vasoconstrictors, such as endothelin play a significant role. In clinical practice, inhaled NO should be weaned in a stepwise process over the course of 1 to 2 days in patients who exhibit symptoms of rebound response. If rebound hypertension persists despite increased inspired levels of oxygen, the NO wean is typically slowed to an even greater extent.

SUGGESTED READINGS

Clark RH, Kueser TJ, Walker MW, et al. Low-dose nitric oxide therapy for persistent pulmonary hypertension of the newborn. Clinical Inhaled Nitric Oxide Research Group. *N Engl J Med*. 2000;342(7):469–474.

Ichinose F, Roberts JD Jr, Zapol WM. Inhaled nitric oxide: a selective pulmonary vasodilator: current uses and therapeutic potential. *Circulation*. 2004;109:3106–3111.

Steudel W, Hurford WE, Zapol WM. Inhaled nitric oxide: basic biology and clinical applications. *Anesthesiology*. 1999;91:1090–1121.

123

KNOW HOW TO CHARACTERIZE THE SECOND HEART SOUND (S₂) BECAUSE IT MAY BE PATHOLOGIC

RUSSELL CROSS, MD

WHAT TO DO – INTERPRET THE DATA

The S_2 should be considered as an essential component of every pediatric cardiac exam, and should not be overlooked. The timing and characterization of S_2 can in some cases be the only exam finding suggesting a cardiac problem, particularly in the newborn that still has a patent ductus arteriosus. It is important that the examiner perform a deliberate, stepwise evaluation each time auscultation is performed. The S_2 is created by closure of the aortic and pulmonic valves at the end of systole, and is typically described as having an aortic (A_2) and pulmonic (P_2) component. The important characterizing aspects of S_2 are the intensity of its components, their timing and relationship to each other. Characterization of the S_2 sound can be diagnostic of congenital heart abnormalities such as atrial septal defects, more serious congenital heart disease such as pulmonary atresia, and hypoplastic left heart syndrome, and can also reveal evidence for pulmonary hypertension.

In the normal heart, the S_2 timing varies with respiration. At end expiration, the A_2 valve closes at the same time as or slightly before the pulmonary valve closes. The negative intrathoracic pressure that is created during inspiration draws slightly more blood into the right ventricle from the systemic veins; this small increase in right ventricular volume takes slightly longer to exit the right ventricle during the systolic contraction. This longer emptying time creates a relative delay of the P_2 closure component compared to A_2. As a result, the listener will hear an increased splitting of S_2 during inspiration, compared to a more narrowly split or single S_2 during expiration. The variation in S_2 splitting will be obvious in many cases, whereas it is described as a muffling of the crisp S_2 heard during expiration in others.

Another important feature of the S_2 that should be evaluated is its intensity or loudness. Normally the P_2 intensity will be significantly diminished when compared to the A_2 component. This relates to the fact that in the normal individual the pulmonary pressure is significantly lower than aortic pressure–typically about 25% of the systemic pressure. The P_2 component of the S_2 is, therefore, softer compared to the A_2 component because the pressure closing the pulmonary valve is lower than the pressure closing the

ⓒ 2008 by Lippincott Williams & Wilkins, a Wolters Kluwer business

aortic valve. The intensity of the S_2 can, therefore, give great insight into the status of the pulmonary pressure.

The most common congenital heart lesion for which evaluation of the S_2 can be diagnostic is the atrial septal defect. When there is significant left-to-right shunting at the atrial level, the S_2 will be more prominently split than usual and will also have less variation with respirations. This alteration relates to the fact that it takes a longer period of time for the increased volume of the right ventricle to be ejected during systole compared to that of the left ventricle. A wide split S_2 is pathognomonic of an atrial septal defect and should be readily recognized by any individual performing pediatric cardiac auscultation.

A more subtle, but equally important, abnormal ausculatory finding is that of the single S_2. Several different forms of congenital heart disease can result in a single S_2, but they all can be similarly classified as a result of the single S_2 being created by the absence or severe diminishment of one of its components—that is, either the aortic component or pulmonary component of the S_2 may be missing. One example is that of pulmonary atresia. In this disease, there is no pulmonary valve to create a P_2 component of the S_2, so the S_2 is single and no respiratory variation can be appreciated. Any form of congenital heart disease that results is absence or extreme hypoplasia of the pulmonary valve will result in a single S_2. Likewise, aortic atresia or hypoplastic left heart syndrome will result in a single S_2 as a result of the loss of the aortic component. These severe forms of congenital heart disease will ultimately result in other findings, such as hypoxemia and poor perfusion, but these changes will not occur until the ductus arteriosus closes at several hours to days of life. This, again, makes it imperative that those performing pediatric cardiac examinations be capable of detecting a single S_2, as it can be an early sign of serious heart disease that ideally would be detected prior to the physiologic changes that ensue following ductal closure.

Another form of congenital heart disease that can result in a single S_2 is transposition of the great arteries. In transposition, the aortic and pulmonary arteries are switched and arise from the wrong ventricle. The lesion usually results in profound hypoxemia. On physical examination, one can frequently appreciate a single S_2, which in this case does not result from the absence of a semilunar valve, but rather is caused by the fact that the pulmonary valve lies much deeper in the chest than normal, and cannot be heard due to its lower intensity. As mentioned earlier, close attention to the characteristics of the second heart sound can also be important for diagnosing pulmonary hypertension. Regardless of the etiology, pulmonary hypertension will result in a loud P_2 component. In the older child or teenager, pulmonary hypertension sometimes presents with vague complaints such as lethargy, malaise, and shortness of breath. In such cases, detection of the loud P_2 can be an important finding, separating pulmonary hypertension from the more commonplace and less serious presentation of these symptoms.

Evaluation of the S_2 and the ability to detect abnormalities in its components takes significant practice and close attention to detail. It is important that the ausculatory exam be performed in a methodical stepwise fashion, paying deliberate attention to the timing and intensity of its components as they can give important insight into pathology.

SUGGESTED READINGS

Gaskin PR, Owens SE, Talner NS, et al. Clinical auscultation skills in pediatric residents. *Pediatrics*. 2000;105:1184–1187.

O'Toole JD, Reddy PS, Curtiss EI, et al. The mechanism of splitting of the second heart sound in atrial septal defect. *Circulation*. 1977;56:1047–1053.

124

WHEEZING INFANTS MAY HAVE ASTHMA, BUT BE ALERT FOR HEART FAILURE AS WELL

RUSSELL CROSS, MD

WHAT TO DO – INTERPRET THE DATA

Wheezes are coarse whistling sounds generated by vibration of a narrowed airway from turbulent airflow. Wheezing often is equated with asthma, reactive airways disease, bronchiolitis, or other respiratory disease. Wheezing, however, is also a common finding in infants and children with congestive heart failure. Cardiac asthma may be defined as the clinical syndrome induced by acute passive congestion and edema of the lungs. The classic explanation for wheezing during pulmonary edema is that bronchial wall edema and intraluminal edema fluid cause narrowing of the small airways, but bronchial hyperresponsiveness also plays a part. This bronchoconstriction is mediated by unmyelinated C-fiber nerve endings in bronchi, pulmonary vasculature, and lung parenchyma (J or juxtacapillary receptors). In animal studies, these receptors, which are carried in the vagus nerve, have increased their activity fivefold as a result of pulmonary edema.

In infants, heart failure may be difficult to identify. Infants whose bronchioles are proportionately narrow as compared to adults will not typically have crackles with pulmonary edema but rather wheezes. Consequently, the signs of cardiac-induced pulmonary congestion may be indistinguishable from bronchiolitis or asthma. A history of feeding disturbance, slow weight gain, diaphoresis should raise the suspicion of cardiac disease. Further confounding the diagnosis, pneumonitis with or without atelectasis, especially in the right middle and lower lobes is common in children with heart disease due to bronchial compression by the enlarged heart. Physical exam findings can help distinguish heart failure from respiratory disease. Hepatomegaly is a common finding in infants and children with heart failure. The cardiac exam will show increased precordial activity. Auscultation may reveal a gallop or murmur. The presence of these features should prompt further workup with an electrocardiogram and chest x-ray. Cardiomegaly is very frequent in children with significant heart disease.

When presented with the older child with a first episode of acute wheezing, assessment for heart disease is equally important. Myocarditis or dilated

© 2008 by Lippincott Williams & Wilkins, a Wolters Kluwer business

cardiomyopathy can present similarly as RAD. Consideration of heart disease is especially important in children who do not seem to respond to bronchodilator therapy. A history of exercise intolerance, weight loss or gain, or a negative family history of asthma or allergies raises the suspicion of heart disease. Again, the clinician should make note of the presence or absence of hepatomegaly or jugular venous distention.

The chest radiograph is an important tool for the pediatrician in distinguishing cardiac versus respiratory disease. Cardiomegaly is frequent in children with heart disease, and this finding, whether unexpected or not, requires further workup for myocardial or pericardial disease. Additional findings on chest radiograph include increased pulmonary vascularity. Infants and children with large left-to-right shunts have exaggeration of the pulmonary arterial vessels to the periphery of the lung fields, whereas patients with cardiomyopathy may have a relatively normal pulmonary vascular bed early in the course of disease. Fluffy perihilar pulmonary markings suggestive of venous congestion and acute pulmonary edema are seen only with most severe degrees of heart failure.

TABLE 124.1   ETIOLOGY OF HEART FAILURE BY AGE GROUP

Fetal
  Severe anemia (hemolysis, fetomaternal transfusion, parvovirus B 19-induced anemia,
    hypoplastic anemia
  Supraventricular tachycardia
  Ventricular tachycardia
  Complete heart block

Premature Neonate
  Fluid overload
  Congenital heart defects (patent ductus arteriosus, ventricular septal defect)
  Cor pulmonale associated with bronchopulmonary dysplasia
  Hypertension

Full-term Neonate
  Myocardial dysfunction (asphyxia, arrhythmia, sepsis)
  Arteriovenous malformation (vein of Galen)
  Left-sided obstructive lesions (coarctation of the aorta, hypoplastic left heart syndrome)
  Large mixing cardiac defects (single ventricle, truncus arteriosus)
  Viral myocarditis
  Dilated cardiomyopathy

Infant–Toddler
  Left to right cardiac shunts (ventricular septal defect, patent ductus arteriosus)
  Hemangioma (arteriovenous malformation)
  Anomalous left coronary artery from the pulmonary artery
  Metabolic cardiomyopathy
  Acute hypertension (hemolytic uremic syndrome)
  Supraventricular tachycardia
  Kawasaki disease
  Viral myocarditis

The differential diagnosis for children with congestive heart disease is long and age-dependent (*Table 124.1*). The age of the patient is a very important feature. For instance, immediately after birth, congestive heart failure or cardiogenic shock is most frequently related to myocardial dysfunction from sepsis, asphyxia, arrhythmia, or a primary cardiomyopathy. Children with large left-to-right shunts from a ventricular septal defect or patent ductus arteriosus do not present until the pulmonary vascular resistance falls, typically around 4 to 6 weeks of life. Older children develop congestive heart failure from primary or secondary cardiomyopathies. Secondary cardiomyopathy can develop from prolong runs of supraventricular tachycardia. Approximately half of patients with incessant supraventricular tachycardia lasting >48 hours will have heart failure. Cardiology consultation should be considered in any child with heart failure or cardiomegaly.

SUGGESTED READINGS

Krieger BP. When wheezing may not mean asthma. Other common and uncommon causes to consider. *Postgrad Med.* 2002;112(2):101–102, 105–108, 111.

McColley SA. Extrapulmonary Disease with Pulmonary Manifestations. In: Behrman RE, Kliegman RM, Jenson HB, eds. *Nelson Textbook of Medicine.* 17th ed. Philadelphia: Saunders; 2004: pages 1471–1472.

125

DEFIBRILLATE FIRST IN VENTRICULAR TACHYCARDIA (VT) OR VENTRICULAR FIBRILLATION (VF)

RUSSELL CROSS, MD

WHAT TO DO – TAKE ACTION

There are distinct differences in the causes of cardiopulmonary arrest between pediatric and adult patients. In both patient populations, cardiopulmonary arrest can be preceded by multiple causes such as respiratory insufficiency of various etiologies–including airway obstruction, metabolic abnormalities, noncardiogenic shock, and arrhythmias. However, adults are more likely than a child to have a cardiopulmonary arrest secondary to a primary cardiac cause, most commonly myocardial infarction. Adults are approximately twice as likely to present in cardiopulmonary arrest with VF compared to the pediatric population. In out-of-hospital cardiac arrests, approximately 40% of adults will have VF as the first-monitored rhythm. Studies of in-hospital arrest demonstrate that approximately 25% of adults will have VT or fibrillation as their first documented rhythm in a pulseless arrest, compared to about half as many in children. Pulseless VT and VF are lethal arrhythmias, unless treated quickly. In both situations, the initial treatment is rapid defibrillation, followed by further treatment of the primary cause of the cardiac arrest. Although the approach to a patient in cardiopulmonary arrest differs when comparing pediatric to adult patients, a paramount tenet is that a patient who is in pulseless VT or VF should receive lifesaving cardiac defibrillation as soon as possible; studies in adults show the probability of survival declines for each minute without defibrillation and cardiopulmonary resuscitation (CPR). In the pediatric age group, primary cardiac arrest is rare, and more typically, cardiac arrest in children is a terminal event resulting from respiratory failure or shock. To that extent, Pediatric Advanced Life Support (PALS) recommendations focus heavily on the primary establishment of an airway with good ventilation techniques, along with chest compressions and fluid resuscitation, whereas Adult Advanced Cardiovascular Life Support (ACLS) focuses more on rapid along with ensuring adequate airway, ventilation, and circulation (CPR). It must be remembered, however, that in the event of a *pulseless* arrest in a child, the PALS algorithm calls for rapid determination of whether the patient has a "shockable rhythm," pulseless VT or VF, at the same time that other basic

© 2008 by Lippincott Williams & Wilkins, a Wolters Kluwer business

life-support measures are being performed. In the event that a pediatric patient is identified to have a shockable rhythm, then defibrillation at a dose of 2 Joule/kg should be immediately delivered. Health care providers must have efficient coordination of CPR and defibrillation with minimal interruptions for rhythm analysis and shock delivery.

One multicenter study looking at cardiac arrest outcomes showed that slightly less than one third of both adult and pediatric patients whose first monitored rhythm was VF or pulseless VT survived to hospital discharge. This same study showed that pediatric patients are more likely than adult patients to survive to hospital discharge following a cardiac arrest with asystole or pulseless electrical activity (24% vs. 11%). Regardless of whether dealing with a pediatric patient or an adult patient in an arrest situation, rapid determination of the heart rhythm must be performed so that defibrillation is achieved in <5 minutes for those patient who are in VF or pulseless VT.

SUGGESTED READINGS

American Heart Association. 2005 American Heart Association Guidelines for Cardiopulmonary Resuscitation and Emergency Cardiovascular Care: part 12: Pediatric Advanced Life Support. *Circulation.* 2005;112:IV-167–IV-187.

American Heart Association. 2005 American Heart Association Guidelines for Cardiopulmonary Resuscitation and Emergency Cardiovascular Care: part 4: Adult Basic Life Support. *Circulation.* 2005;112: IV-19–IV-34.

American Heart Association. 2005 American Heart Association Guidelines for Cardiopulmonary Resuscitation and Emergency Cardiovascular Care: part 4: Advanced Life Support. *Circulation.* 2005;112:III-25–III-54.

Nadkarni VM, Larkin GL, Peberdy MA, et al. for the National Registry of Cardiopulmonary Resuscitation Investigators. First documented rhythm and clinical outcome from in-hospital cardiac arrest among children and adults. *JAMA.* 2006;295:50–57.

126

MEASURE GROWTH PATTERNS AT EACH WELL-CHILD VISIT AND EACH HEALTH CARE ENCOUNTER

ANJALI SUBBASWAMY, MD

WHAT TO DO – GATHER APPROPRIATE DATA

Normal patterns and variations of growth will assist clinicians in understanding subtle changes in body chemistry that may not manifest themselves for considerable periods of time (e.g., hypothyroidism, other endocrine problems). Discuss normal variations in growth.

Assessing a child's growth pattern gives a picture of the child's overall health. In fact, some suggest that growth be viewed as a vital sign. It is a sensitive indicator of general health. Abnormal growth may be the first manifestation of pathology. Despite this fact, a survey of primary care practices in the United States showed that 10% of pediatric practices and 40% of family practices did not measure children at well-child visits. It is often difficult to distinguish between normal and abnormal growth. Short stature may represent a normal variant or signify underlying disease.

In utero growth is influenced by nutrition, uterine size, and the metabolic environment. Insulin, insulinlike growth factor (IGF), and their binding proteins are important for fetal growth. Growth hormone (GH) and thyroid hormone do not have a role in growth in utero; however, they are major influences for normal postnatal growth. GH circulates free and bound and induces growth of chondrocytes at the growth plate. It also stimulates secretion of IGF-1, which mediates many of GH's growth-promoting actions. During the postnatal period, there is rapid linear growth velocity that declines after birth. A child's linear growth velocity averages 25, 12, and 8 cm/year during the first 3 postnatal years. From this time until the onset of puberty, linear growth occurs steadily at a rate of 4 to 7 cm annually; weight gain averages 2.5 kg annually. At puberty, sex hormones (testosterone and estrogen), coupled with GH, thyroid hormone, and nutrition, result in an accelerated rate of growth—the pubertal growth spurt. In girls, this

---

© 2008 by Lippincott Williams & Wilkins, a Wolters Kluwer business

usually occurs during sexual maturity rating (SMR) 3 for breast; the growth spurt in boys typically occurs during SMR 4 in boys. Following puberty, growth ultimately ceases secondary to closure of the epiphyseal plates due to the effects of estrogen. Growth represents an intricate connection between genetics, hormones, nutrition, and environment. Physicians must accurately assess growth during every well-child visit and know when further evaluation is needed.

When evaluating a child with a possible growth problem, the accurate analysis of the growth curve is crucial. Four aspects of the growth curve should be evaluated:

1. Reliability of measurements.
2. Absolute height relates to the likelihood of an existing pathologic condition (i.e., a child with an absolute height 3 standard deviations (SDs) below the mean is more likely to have underlying disease than one with an absolute height 1 SD below the norm).
3. Height velocity refers to the observation of a child's height over time. It is the most important of the four aspects, and requires at least 4 to 6 months of observation. A deceleration in height velocity (crossing percentiles) between 3 and 12 to 13 years is pathologic until proven otherwise. A normal height velocity regardless of absolute height is usually not pathologic.
4. A weight to height relationship assists in evaluating the cause of growth delay in the short child. Systemic disorders are associated with lower weight to height ratios (impairment of weight gain greater than that of linear growth). Endocrine disorders are usually associated with preservation of weight gain (higher weight to height ratios).

Target height is also useful in determining a patients genetic potential for growth. It is calculated by the following equations:

Target height in boys =

$$(\text{father's height [cm]} + \text{mother's height [cm]} + 13)/2$$

Target height in girls =

$$(\text{father's height [cm]} + \text{mother's height [cm]} - 13)/2$$

Most children reach heights within 10 cm of the target. Bone age is a method of evaluating bone and skeletal maturity by comparing the patients epiphyseal centers obtained via radiograph with age-appropriate standards. The commonly used method assesses the bones of the hand and wrist. If there is short stature, and a delayed bone age, the short stature is somewhat "reversible." However, a normal bone age and short stature is a greater concern.

Assessing the upper-to-lower body segment (U/L) ratio demonstrates if the short stature is proportional. Skeletal dysplasias involving the spine typically have decreased U/L ratio for age; those involving the long bones (i.e., achondroplasia) typically have increased U/L ratio. Precocious puberty may present with an increased U/L ratio for age. A decreased ratio may be seen in Klinefelter or Kallmann syndrome.

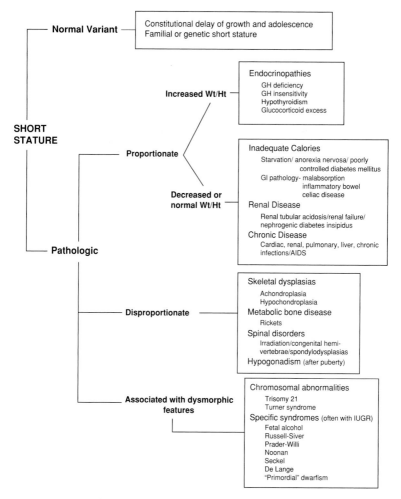

FIGURE 126.1. Causes of growth delay/retardation. AIDS, acquired immunodeficiency syndrome; GH, growth hormone; GI, gastrointestinal; IUGR, intrauterine growth restriction.

Constitutional delay of growth (CDGA) and familial short stature (FSS) are considered normal variations of growth. In CDGA, growth is characterized by: (a) normal birth length; (b) slowing linear growth during the first 3 years of life (weight and height decline across percentiles); (c) normal or near-normal rate of linear growth below but parallel to fifth percentile during prepubertal years; (d) delayed bone age and pubertal maturation coincides with bone age, not chronologic age; and (e) final adult height is usually normal. This is the "late bloomer." Typically, the father of the child was a short child and experienced puberty late. Bone age is always delayed. The growth pattern of FSS is quite similar to CDGA until puberty. They have normal height and weight at birth, and tend to cross linear growth percentiles during the first 2 years of life (fulfilling genetic appropriate growth). At this point, a child with FSS has steady growth below, but parallel to, normal growth curve. Puberty coincides with chronologic age, and final adult height is short, but appropriate based on parental height. Bone age is typically normal. See *Figure 126.1* below for causes of growth delay/retardation.

SUGGESTED READINGS

Grimberg A. "Growth Curves: Are we missing the picture?" American Academy of Pediatrics Section on Endocrinology. 2003 vol 11 p. 15. http://www.aap.org/sections/endocrinology/Endonewsspring03.pdf. Accessed January 7, 2008.

Rose SR, Vogiatzi MG, Copeland KC. A general pediatric approach to evaluating a short child. *Pediatr Rev.* 2005:26:410–420.

Vogiatzi MG, Copeland KC. The short child. *Pediatr Rev.* 1998;19:92–99.

127

BEFORE INITIATING TREATMENT FOR RICKETS, IT IS IMPORTANT TO OBTAIN BASELINE TESTS FOR RENAL FUNCTION, HYDROXYVITAMIN D, AND DIHYDROXYVITAMIN D LEVELS TO RULE OUT RICKETS SECONDARY TO RENAL DISEASES AND OTHER CAUSES

ANJALI SUBBASWAMY, MD

WHAT TO DO – GATHER APPROPRIATE DATA, MAKE A DECISION

Rickets is a disease entity that was first described more than 2,000 years ago, and it is often mistakenly considered a diagnosis of the past or of developing countries. There has been a recent resurgence of this disease in the United States and Europe. The United States did witness the eradication of nutritional rickets when it was discovered in the 1930s that vitamin D was antirachitic. It is difficult to ascertain the current prevalence of this condition due to the lack of ongoing national surveillance. Current estimates of the prevalence of nutritional rickets range from 5 to 9 per 1,000,000 children aged 6 months to 5 years.

In general terms, rickets results from the failure of bone to mineralize. Calcification of the cartilaginous growth plate is delayed in children whose epiphyses have yet to fuse. It is usually delayed due to an inadequate supply of calcium or phosphate to the growth plate. The causes of rickets can be grouped into three categories: (a) inability to maintain serum calcium-calcipenic, (b) inability to maintain serum phosphorus-phosphonpenic, and (c) causes that inhibit mineralization of the growth plate and osteoid. Vitamin D-deficiency rickets is a calcipenic form of rickets, as well as any abnormalities of vitamin D metabolism. The many forms of impaired renal phosphate reabsorption are included as phosphopenic types of rickets. Vitamin D is a prohormone and has two sources: cholecalciferol and ergocalciferol. When the skin is exposed to ultraviolet light, 7-dehydrocholesterol is converted into cholecalciferol (vitamin D_3). Ergocalciferol or vitamin D_2 is obtained from the diet. Vitamin D is hydroxylated in the liver to 25-hydroxyvitamin D, and then in the kidney, 25-hydroxyvitamin D is hydroxylated to 1,25 dihydroxyvitamin D. 1,25-dihydroxyvitamin D, or calcitriol, ensures

© 2008 by Lippincott Williams & Wilkins, a Wolters Kluwer business

TABLE 127.1   THE DIFFERENT TYPES OF RICKETS, THEIR CAUSES, FEATURES, AND TREATMENTS

TYPE	CAUSES	CLINICAL FEATURES	TREATMENT
Vitamin D deficiency	Vitamin D deficiency, phosphorus or calcium deficiency (rare), inadequate sunlight exposure, secondary to malabsorption syndromes (IBD, celiac disease, cystic fibrosis [rarely])	Skeletal findings, abnormal gait, hypocalcemic tetany/seizures, developmental delay, failure to thrive	Replace the deficient nutrient orally; may need to administer vitamin D intramuscularly if rickets secondary to malabsorption
Vitamin D–dependent rickets			
Type I or pseudovitamin D-deficiency rickets	Deficiency of renal 25(OH) D₃–1–α–hydroxylase	Younger than 2 years, hypocalcemic tetany, severe bony changes, seizures	Calcitriol (Rocaltrol)
Type II or hereditary 1-α, 25-dihydroxyvitamin D-resistant rickets	Defective interaction between calcitriol and receptor	Younger than 1 year, severe bony changes, alopecia	Massive doses of calcitriol and calcium
Vitamin D–resistant rickets			
Familial hypophosphatemic rickets or X-linked hypophosphatemic rickets	Impaired proximal renal tubular reabsorption of phosphorus and inappropriately normal calcitriol levels	Short stature, leg bowing, dental abnormalities	Oral phosphate and calcitriol
Hereditary hypophosphatemic rickets with hypercalciuria	Impaired proximal renal tubular reabsorption of phosphorus and increased calcitriol	Bone pain, muscular weakness	Oral phosphate
Miscellaneous			
Renal rickets or renal osteodystrophy	Loss of functional renal parenchyma caused by chronic renal failure leads to mineral derangements and decreased calcitriol production	Bone pain, arthralgias, fractures, muscle weakness, failure to thrive	Vitamin D and phosphate–binding compound
Rickets of prematurity	Multifactorial	Osteopenia, fractures	Replace dietary deficiencies and minimize iatrogenic causes

IBD, irritable bowel disease.

adequate absorption of calcium from the intestines and meets the requirements of a growing child.

Because of the pathogenesis of rickets, it is easy to understand that vitamin D-deficiency rickets is more common in children of color (decreased production of vitamin D in the skin), infants exclusively breastfed (vitamin D supplementation only recently advised in breastfed infants; vitamin D content in breast milk directly proportional to maternal 25-hydroxyvitamin D levels), and those with decreased vitamin D and calcium intake (i.e., strict vegan diets). Rickets typically follows a particular course. As 25-hydroxyvitamin D levels fall, parathyroid hormone (PTH) levels increase. This, in turn, leads to increased mobilization of calcium from bone. With low vitamin D levels, intestinal calcium absorption is decreased and serum calcium levels fall. This precedes the decrease in serum phosphate levels. Again, PTH increases due to the low serum calcium and phosphaturia increases (serum phosphate levels fall). It is at this time that clinical features of rickets are seen.

Clinical manifestations of this disease include decreased linear growth, bowing of legs, developmental delay, seizures, and tetany. Often, it is diagnosed as an incidental finding on radiography or physical exam. Skeletal and radiographic findings associated with rickets include craniotabes, costochondral beading (rachitic rosary), dental abnormalities, and flaring of the ribs at the level of the diaphragm (Harrison groove).

Rickets can also be vitamin D-dependent or vitamin D-resistant. Type I vitamin D-dependent rickets is caused by a defect in 25(OH) D_3-1-α-hydroxylase. Type II vitamin D-dependent rickets is caused by a defect in the vitamin D receptor. Vitamin D-resistant rickets, or familial hypophosphatemic rickets, is the most common heritable form. In this disorder, there is renal wasting of phosphorus at the proximal tubule level and resultant hypophosphatemia. Rickets that results from renal disease is secondary to disturbances in calcium and phosphorus regulation, as well as, calcitriol production. As one can see, there are many causes of rickets, and the use of a diagnostic algorithm is extremely helpful. See *Table 127.1* for various types of rickets and treatment.

SUGGESTED READINGS

Joiner TA, Foster C, Shope T. The many faces of vitamin D deficiency rickets. *Pediatr Rev.* 2000;21:296–302.

Nield LS, Mahajan P, Joshi A, et al. Rickets: not a disease of the past. *Am Fam Physician.* 2006;74:619–626.

Pettifor JM. Rickets and vitamin D deficiency in children and adolescents. *Endocrinol Metab Clin North Am.* 2005;34:537–553.

128

DO NOT DISMISS GENERIC COMPLAINTS WITHOUT CONSIDERING POSSIBLE THYROID CONDITIONS

LINDSEY ALBRECHT, MD

WHAT TO DO – GATHER APPROPRIATE DATA

Deficiency of thyroid hormone leads to a generalized slowing of metabolic processes in the body. Signs and symptoms of hypothyroidism depend upon the underlying etiology, degree of deficiency, and the patient's age. Although the diagnosis may be apparent in a child with the classic symptoms and physical exam findings, occasionally children and adolescents will present with a vague complaint of feeling unwell. In these cases, it is important to have a high index of suspicion for the disease.

Children may be affected by congenital or acquired hypothyroidism. Congenital forms are present at birth and are typically due to dysgenesis of the thyroid gland, though many other causes exist. Because thyroid hormone plays a critical role in early growth and central nervous system (CNS) development, unrecognized congenital hypothyroidism leads to irreversible mental retardation. Additional findings may include prolonged neonatal jaundice, enlarged fontanelles, macroglossia, hoarse cry, constipation, and poor weight gain. Newborn screening allows early diagnosis of congenital hypothyroidism; properly instituted treatment with thyroid hormone replacement allows for normal cognitive outcomes.

Acquired forms of hypothyroidism typically occur in older children, though there are rare reports of onset in infancy. Acquired hypothyroidism may be due to a primary disorder of the thyroid gland, or may be due to central deficiencies in either thyroid-stimulating hormone (TSH) or thyrotropin-releasing hormone (TRH). Primary hypothyroidism is associated with decreased levels of free thyroxine (T_4) and elevated TSH, the major factor controlling thyroid hormone synthesis and secretion. Normal or low TSH in a hypothyroid patient usually indicates a central cause.

Chronic autoimmune thyroiditis is the most common cause of acquired hypothyroidism in childhood and may occur with or without goiter. In this case, laboratory testing will reveal elevated titers of thyroid antibodies (thyroid peroxidase antibody and thyroglobulin antibody). Acquired hypothyroidism is less commonly due to irradiation of the thyroid gland, postsurgical effects, excessive iodide intake, subacute thyroiditis, and drug effects. In these

© 2008 by Lippincott Williams & Wilkins, a Wolters Kluwer business

cases, the history often suggests the particular etiology. In developing parts of the world, iodide deficiency may result in acquired hypothyroidism.

Findings associated with acquired hypothyroidism in childhood include goiter, deceleration of growth or short stature, constipation, muscle weakness, delayed tooth eruption or delayed primary tooth shedding, and precocious sexual development, given that elevated serum TSH can act on follicle-stimulating hormone (FSH) receptors, causing gonadotropic effects. Slipped capital femoral epiphysis is also associated with hypothyroidism and is suggested by hip or knee pain. Older children are more likely to report generalized malaise and some may present only with difficulties concentrating or worsening school performance. Attention deficit hyperactivity disorder (ADHD) may be suspected in some children, given their difficulties focusing on a particular task. Other CNS symptoms may include chronic fatigue, headaches, and slowed speech.

Treatment of acquired hypothyroidism is with thyroid hormone replacement. Dosages are based on age and body weight, with adjustments made to account for differences in hormone metabolism. Monitoring of TSH in patients with primary hypothyroidism and free thyroxine (FT_4) in patients with central hypothyroidism allows for detection of under- or overtreatment, as well as for monitoring of medication compliance. In the older child with hypothyroidism, treatment with thyroid hormone will lead to a return to baseline neurologic function and a resolution of most other symptoms. Failure to achieve expected adult height is common in patients with a delayed diagnosis.

Thus, the diagnosis of acquired hypothyroidism in childhood should be suspected when a patient presents with decreased growth velocity, decreased energy, goiter, or other symptoms of thyroid deficiency. These symptoms may be vague, and may include generalized malaise and decreased ability to concentrate. Early diagnosis and treatment will ensure maximal linear growth and lead to resolution of other symptoms.

SUGGESTED READINGS

Rose SR, Brown RS, Foley TP, et al. Update of newborn screening and therapy for congenital hypothyroidism. *Pediatrics.* 2006;117(6):2290–2303.
Foley TP Jr. Hypothyroidism. *Pediatr Rev.* 2004;25(3):94–100.
Greenspan FS. The thyroid gland. In: Greenspan FS, Gardner DG, eds. *Basic and Clinical Endocrinology.* 7th ed. New York: McGraw-Hill; 2004:251–259.

129

KNOW THE NORMAL PATTERNS OF PUBERTY AND ENSURE THAT PUBERTAL DEVELOPMENT IS PROCEEDING APPROPRIATELY

MICHAEL CLEMMENS, MD

WHAT TO DO – GATHER APPROPRIATE DATA, INTERPRET THE DATA

Precocious, delayed, or atypical patterns of pubertal development may be a sign of underlying pathology or disease.

Puberty is a normal developmental process that results in reproductive capability and sexual maturity. Initiation of puberty and normal progression through its stages requires an intact hypothalamic-pituitary-gonadal (HPG) axis. The onset of puberty follows the return of pulsatile secretion of gonadotropin-releasing hormone (GnRH) from the hypothalamus. GnRH stimulates the release of leuteinizing hormone (LH) and follicle-stimulating hormone (FSH) from the pituitary gland, which in turn stimulate the gonads to mature. This process is termed gonadarche, and results in the production of sex steroids, predominantly testosterone and estradiol. Concurrently, the zona reticularis of the adrenal gland matures, resulting in the production of adrenal androgens. These hormones produce the secondary sex characteristics, such as pubic hair, axillary hair, body odor, and acne. The exact triggers for adrenarche are not known.

Traditionally, the expert consensus regarding the normal timing of puberty and the stages of pubertal development have been based on studies done by Marshall and Tanner more than 40 years ago in Britain. These studies documented that most girls experienced breast development and menarche between the ages of 8.5 to 13 years, and most boys showed signs of genital development between the ages of 9.5 to 13.5 years. In girls, thelarche, or breast development, is usually the first sign of puberty and occurs at an average age of approximately 11 years. Menarche typically occurs 2.5 years after thelarche, at an average age 13.5 years. In boys, increased testicular volume is typically the first sign of puberty and occurs at an average age of nearly 12 years. Enlargement of the penis occurs 6 to 18 months later. Of note, the timing of the growth spurt associated with puberty occurs later for boys than for girls. In general, the variable timing of the onset and progression of puberty is primarily related to genetic factors, but several environmental factors also play a role. The five stages of puberty are reviewed in *Table 129.1.*

© 2008 by Lippincott Williams & Wilkins, a Wolters Kluwer business

STAGE	FEMALE BREAST DEVELOPMENT	MALE GENITAL DEVELOPMENT	PUBIC HAIR DEVELOPMENT
I	Elevation of papilla only	Immature male genitalia	Vellus hair only
II	Elevation of breasts and papilla (breast budding), increased diameter of areolae	Increase in testicular volume, scrotal sac enlarges and changes texture	Sparse, long, pigmented hair on labia in females, at base of penis in males
III	Continued enlargement of breasts and areolae, no separation of contour	Growth in length and then circumference of penis, continued growth of testes and scrotum	Hair darker, coarser, curlier, meets in the midline
IV	Areolae and papillae elevate above level of breasts (secondary mound), continued enlargement of breasts	Growth in length and circumference of penis, development of glans penis, continued growth of testes and scrotum	Inverted triangle in distribution, but not on medial surface of thighs
V	Mature female breasts	Mature male genitalia	Adult distribution, including medial surface of thighs

TABLE 129.1   STAGES OF PUBERTAL DEVELOPMENT

Data from several large studies in the United States have described a recent trend towards earlier pubertal development, particularly among girls. These studies documented a mean age for both breast development and pubic hair of approximately 10 years for white girls and approximately 9 years for black girls. Among experts, there is a great deal of controversy regarding the validity of these results, related in part to the methodology of the investigations. A full discussion of the issues is beyond the scope of this brief review, but an abundance of information exists in the references provided. One absolute is that the newest data was collected as the prevalence of overweight and obesity among children was increasing, and there is a relationship between increased adiposity and earlier sexual maturation in girls.

Aberrations from the normal pattern of pubertal development should alert the clinician to the possibility of underlying pathology. Most experts define precocious puberty as the onset of puberty before age 8 years in girls and 9 years in boys. Taking the newest information about the timing of puberty into account, some would relax the definition for girls to include the occurrence of breast development before age 7 years in white girls and 6 years in black girls. However, one must also consider the rate of pubertal progression

TABLE 129.2   CAUSES OF PRECOCIOUS PUBERTY

CENTRAL (GnRH-DEPENDENT)	PERIPHERAL (GnRH-INDEPENDENT)
Idiopathic	Congenital adrenal hyperplasia
CNS tumors	Tumors producing testosterone or estrogen
CNS infection	Tumors producing gonadotropin or hCG
Head trauma	Exogenous exposure to androgen or estrogen
Iatrogenic (chemotherapy, radiation, etc.)	McCune-Albright syndrome
CNS malformations	Ovarian cysts
CNS Ischemia	Hypothyroidism
	Other

CNS, central nervous system; GnRH, gonadotropin-releasing hormone; hCG, human chorionic gonadotropin.

and the overall rate of growth. Girls younger than 8 years with rapid progression of breast development or documented growth acceleration over 6 to 12 months are more likely to have an abnormal pattern of pubertal development. *Table 129.2* lists general causes of precocious puberty. Central

TABLE 129.3   CAUSES OF DELAYED PUBERTY

CATEGORY	EXAMPLE
Constitutional delay of growth and maturation	n/a
Functional hypogonadotropic hypogonadism	Systemic illness
	Endocrinopathy
	Excessive exercise
	Undernutrition
Permanent hypogonadotropic hypogonadism	CNS tumor or infiltrative disease
	Genetic defects or syndrome (e.g., Kallmann, Prader-Willi)
	CNS infections
	Iatrogenic (chemotherapy, radiation, etc.)
	Midline defects
	Trauma
Permanent hypergonadotropic hypogonadism	Genetic syndromes (e.g., Turner Syndrome)
	Cryptorchidism
	Gonadal dysgenesis
	Iatrogenic (chemotherapy, radiation, etc.)
	Metabolic disorder
	Gonadal infection, trauma, torsion
	Androgen insensitivity

CNS, central nervous system.

precocious puberty results from early reactivation of the HPG axis and resultant gonadarche. In girls, central precocious puberty is likely idiopathic. However, approximately 60% of boys with central precocious puberty have an underlying problem. Peripheral precocious puberty occurs less frequently than central precocious puberty. Premature thelarche or premature adrenarche can occur, but typically these processes do not lead to progressive pubertal development. Delayed puberty is defined as the absence of pubertal development by age 13 years in girls and 14 years in boys. The most common cause is constitutional delay of growth and maturation (CDGM), especially in boys. Children with CDGM have no underlying pathology and eventually undergo spontaneous pubertal development. There is a strong genetic predisposition for CDGM. Other causes of delayed puberty are listed in *Table 129.3*. Functional hypogonadotropic hypogonadism can result from systemic illness, such as inflammatory bowel disease or cystic fibrosis, endocrinopathies such as diabetes or hypothyroidism, excessive exercise, and malnutrition. In some cases, delayed puberty may be the only presenting sign of an underlying problem.

SUGGESTED READINGS

Fenichel P. Delayed puberty. *Endocr Dev.* 2004;7:106–128.

Kaplowitz P. Precocious puberty: update on secular trends, definitions, diagnosis, and treatment. *Adv Pediatr.* 2004;51:37–62.

Muir A. Precocious puberty. *Pediatr Rev.* 2006;27:373–381.

Nathan BM, Palmert MR. Regulation and disorders of pubertal timing. *Endocrinol Metab Clin North Am.* 2005;34:617–641.

130

WORKUP HYPOTHYROIDISM IN PATIENTS WITH SHORT STATURE AND DEVELOPMENTAL DELAY

ELIZABETH WELLS, MD

WHAT TO DO – GATHER APPROPRIATE DATA

Growth is one of the most important measures of health in pediatrics. The American Academy of Pediatrics recommends that a child's height and weight be measured at each well-child visit. Short stature is defined as being more than two standard deviations below the mean sex-matched height for age. The two most common causes of short stature are genetic short stature, in which the child is growing within the parental target range, and constitutional growth delay, in which the bone age is delayed. Children with endocrine disorders are usually overweight-for-height, in contrast to children with nutritional deficiencies who are underweight-for height. Hypothyroidism is a cause of growth failure in children. Hypothyroidism in infancy and early childhood is also one of the most common preventable causes of mental retardation. Pediatricians must include hypothyroidism in their differential diagnosis of patients with short stature and developmental delay.

Hypothyroidism in children with developmental delay may be either congenital or acquired. Congenital hypothyroidism (CH), an irreversible disorder that affects 1 in 4,000 live births, usually results from an abnormality in thyroid gland development (dysgenesis or agenesis) or an inborn error in thyroid hormonogenesis. Less commonly, CH may result from a pituitary or hypothalamic abnormality. Most neonates with CH have a normal appearance and no detectable physical signs. Timely newborn screening, and thyroid therapy started within 2 weeks of delivery, can ensure normal cognitive development. Persistent hypothyroidism, as defined by delayed return of serum thyroxine (T_4) levels to normal after initiation of treatment, may lead to adverse cognitive outcomes; therefore, a history of treated CH may not exclude hypothyroidism as a cause of short stature and developmental delay.

Worldwide, the most common cause of hypothyroidism is iodine deficiency. Acquired hypothyroidism in children in the United States usually results from chronic autoimmune thyroiditis (AKA Hashimoto thyroiditis), with goiter being a more common presentation of this disease than thyroid

© 2008 by Lippincott Williams & Wilkins, a Wolters Kluwer business

atrophy. Children with some chromosomal abnormalities, such as trisomy 21, Turner syndrome, and Klinefelter syndrome, as well as children with Type 1 diabetes mellitus have an increased risk for chronic autoimmune thyroiditis. Another cause of hypothyroidism is thyroid injury, which may result from tumors of the head and neck region, craniospinal radiation, and radioiodine treatment for Graves' hyperthyroidism. Hypothalamic or pituitary disease causes central hypothyroidism, and should be suspected when the thyroid-stimulating hormone (TSH) is low.

Developmental delay from congenital hypothyroidism may occur even in infants who have normal T_4 and TSH newborn screening results. CH may manifest or be acquired after newborn screening. There are some proponents of retesting after 4 weeks in all neonates with low and very low birth weight; therefore, clinicians should not hesitate to repeat thyroid screening.

The workup for hypothyroidism should include measurements of serum TSH and free T_4. Children with primary hypothyroidism will have high serum TSH and low serum free T_4 levels, whereas children with central hypothyroidism will have normal, or low, serum TSH and low serum free T_4 values. Most children with chronic autoimmune thyroiditis will have high serum anti-thyroid peroxidase (TPO) antibody concentrations. The measurement of TSH alone may miss central hypothyroidism. Brain magnetic resonance imaging and tests of other pituitary hormones should be performed in patients who are suspected of having central hypothyroidism.

Thyroid hormone (T_4) is the treatment of choice in children with hypothyroidism. The goal of treatment is to normalize thyroid function rapidly, to restore normal growth and development, and to minimize central nervous system exposure to low thyroid levels in infants with CH.

The longer the diagnosis of CH is delayed (i.e., the longer CH is left untreated), the higher the risk of mental retardation and other neurologic sequelae. The association between acquired hypothyroidism and brain development in older children has not been systematically studied. Thyroid hormone is clearly important for brain development in infancy and early childhood, but it may play a role in adolescent brain activity and maturation, as well. For instance, one study showed improvement in intelligence quotient scores associated with improved compliance with T_4 in adolescent patients with CH.

In terms of physical growth, many children with hypothyroidism may achieve normal growth potential with treatment, as their skeletal age is usually as delayed as their height age. Studies suggest that catch-up growth is optimal, when hypothyroidism is diagnosed early and before puberty. Additionally, pediatricians should be aware of gender biases in levels of clinical suspicion. Studies have suggested that that sex differences in short stature referrals may delay the diagnosis of the disease in girls, while promoting overzealous evaluations of healthy boys who do not appear to be tall enough.

SUGGESTED READINGS

Rose SR, Brown RS, et al. Update of newborn screening and therapy of congenital hypothyroidism. *Pediatrics.* 2006;117:2290–2303.

American Academy of Pediatrics Policy Statement. Committee on practice and ambulatory medicine. Recommendations for preventive pediatric health care. *Pediatrics.* 2000;105:645.

Büyükgebiz A. Newborn screening for congenital hypothyroidism. *J Pediatr Endocrinol Metab.* 2006;19(11):1291–1298.

Chiesa A, Gruñeiro de Papendieck L, et al. Final height in long-term primary hypothyroid children. *J Pediatr Endocrinol Metab.* 1998;11(1):51–58.

Committee on Practice and Ambulatory Medicine. Recommendations for preventive pediatric health care. *Pediatrics.* 1995;96(2 Pt 1):373–374.

Grimberg A, Kutikov JK, Cucchiara AJ. Sex differences in patients referred for evaluation of poor growth. *J Pediatr.* 2005;146(2):212–216.

Holtzman C, Slazyk WE, Cordero JF, et al. Descriptive epidemiology of missed cases of phenylketonuria and congenital hypothyroidism. *Pediatrics.* 1986;78:553–558.

New England Congenital Hypothyroidism Collaborative. Correlation of cognitive test scores and adequacy of treatment in adolescents with congenital hypothyroidism. *J Pediatr.* 1994;124:383–387.

Rivkees AS, Bode HH, Crawford JD. Long-term growth in juvenile acquired hypothyroidism: the failure to achieve normal adult stature. *N Eng J Med.* 1988;318(10):599–602.

Rose SE, Brown RS. Update of newborn screening and therapy of congenital hypothyroidism. *Pediatrics.* 2006;117:2290–2303.

Tylek-Lemańska D, Kumorowicz-Kopiec M, Starzyk J. Screening for congenital hypothyroidism: the value of retesting after four weeks in neonates with low and very low birth weight. *J Med Screen.* 2005;12(4):166–169.

Yordam N, Ozon A. Neonatal thyroid screening: methods-efficiency-failures. *Pediatr Endocrinol Rev.* 2003;1(Suppl 2):177–184; discussion 184.

Zois C, Stavrou I, Svarna E, et al. Natural course of autoimmune thyroiditis after elimination of iodine deficiency in Northwestern Greece. *Thyroid.* 2006;16:289–293.

131

CONSIDER KETOTIC HYPOGLYCEMIA WHEN EVALUATING INFANTS AND TODDLERS FOR HYPOGLYCEMIA

WILLIAM GIASI, JR., MD

WHAT TO DO – INTERPRET THE DATA

In infants and toddlers, signs and symptoms of hypoglycemia can often be vague and subtle. Given the subtle and nonspecific findings of the signs and symptoms, the detection of hypoglycemia is dependent on a high index of suspicion.

Symptoms of hypoglycemia can be characterized into two physiologic categories: activation of the autonomic nervous system characterized by an adrenergic symptoms and neuroglycopenic (cerebral glycopenia) symptoms. When serum glucose levels are <40 mg/dL, it may produce hunger and trigger an adrenergic response. Common adrenergic symptoms include jitteriness, anxiety, sweating, tachycardia, pallor, weakness, nausea, and emesis. Neuroglycopenic symptoms include headache, dizziness, mental dullness, fatigue, difficulty concentrating, confusion, personality changes, visual changes, seizures, and coma. Neonatal symptoms include those seen in children, such as tremors, jitteriness, and tachycardia, but may also present with nonspecific signs, such as tachypnea, apnea, cyanosis, hypotonia, feeding difficulty, abnormal cry, seizures, and coma.

The differential diagnosis and management of hypoglycemia is extensive and requires an understanding of the pathogenesis. Hypoglycemia may result from disorders of gluconeogenesis, glycogen metabolism, lipid oxidation, or amino acid metabolism.

The serum glucose should be measured to confirm hypoglycemia. Determining whether a patient is ketotic is an important decision for generating a differential diagnosis. There are two major categories: nonketotic hypoglycemia and ketotic hypoglycemia.

Those disorders that result in nonketotic hypoglycemia involve the inability to produce glucose and appropriate forms of energy despite appropriate glycogen storage. A prominent effect of insulin and counterregulatory hormones is to suppress lipolysis and ketogenesis. Therefore, those etiologies that involve high levels of insulin or lack of counterregulatory hormones do not generate high levels of ketones. These etiologies include hyperinsulinism for islet cell adenomas or overproduction, infants of diabetic mothers,

© 2008 by Lippincott Williams & Wilkins, a Wolters Kluwer business

congenital panhypopituitarism, congenital adrenal hyperplasia, fatty oxidation defects, and Beckwith-Wiedemann syndrome.

Hypoglycemia with resulting ketosis is often secondary to insufficient glycogen stores. Etiologies include ketotic hypoglycemia, metabolic diseases (galactosemia, hereditary fructose hypoglycemia, glycogen storage disease type 1), ingestions (ethanol, insulin, salicylates, propanolol), liver failure, and sepsis. Ketotic hypoglycemia is the most common etiology for hypoglycemia in children from 18 months to 5 years of age. The hypoglycemic episodes occur most often when food intake is limited and the child experiences a prolonged fast; for example during periods of illness. Children with ketotic hypoglycemia are frequently smaller than their peers and have a history of transient neonatal hypoglycemia. The classic history is a child who misses an evening meal and then is difficult to arouse the following morning. In children with ketotic hypoglycemia, fasting for 12 to 18 hours will result in hypoglycemia, ketonemia, and ketonuria. Normal children may withstand fasting up to 24 to 48 hours, at which time they develop similar symptoms.

The etiology and pathogenesis of ketotic hypoglycemia is unknown. It is believed that there is a defect in complex process of protein catabolism. The smaller muscle mass and defects in processing compromise the supply substrates to gluconeogenic pathways, thus predisposing the patient to develop hypoglycemia more rapidly. The child with ketotic hypoglycemia will classically have ketonuria, ketonemia, appropriately low levels of insulin, and low levels of serum alanine at the time of hypoglycemia. The presence of ketones is reflective of the child's inability to use protein and the bodies' attempt to use alternative energy sources for gluconeogenesis. Treatment of ketotic hypoglycemia requires frequent high-protein, high-carbohydrate meals. In addition, during periods of illness or a decrease in caloric intake, the child's urine should be monitored for ketones.

It is important to emphasize that hypoglycemia is a symptom rather than a diagnosis. Furthermore, because many of the signs and symptoms of hypoglycemia are nonspecific and subtle, the clinician must maintain a high suspicion for hypoglycemia. Laboratory evaluation may assist the clinician in the establishing the etiology of the hypoglycemia. It is essential to confirm the presence of hypoglycemia by measuring the serum glucose. Furthermore, it is critical at the time of hypoglycemia include a urinalysis, insulin, cortisol, growth hormone levels, serum ketones, and electrolytes. Additional labs to consider if metabolic etiologies are on the differential include ammonia, lactate, free fatty acids, acylcarnitine profile, and organic acid. The history and laboratory data can inform the differential diagnosis, evaluation, and management.

SUGGESTED READINGS

Claudius I, Fluharty C, Boles R. The emergency department approach to newborn and child-hood metabolic crisis. *Emerg Med Clin North Am.* 2005;23:843–883.

Gruppuso PA, Schwartz R. Hypoglycemia in children. *Pediatr Rev.* 1989;11(4):117–124.

Sperling M. Hypoglycemia. In: Behrman EM, Kliegman RE, Jenson HB, eds. *Nelson Textbook of Pediatrics,* 17th ed. Philadelphia: Saunders; 2004:505–518.

Sperling MA, Menon RK. Differential diagnosis and management of neonatal hypoglycemia. *Pediatr Clin North Am.* 2004;51:703–723.

Sunehag A, Haymond MW. Etiology of hypoglycemia in infants and children. UpToDate. 2007.

132

REMEMBER TO PROVIDE BOTH ALPHA AND BETA BLOCKADE FOR CHILDREN WITH PHEOCHROMOCYTOMA

CYNTHIA GIBSON, MD

WHAT TO DO – TAKE ACTION

Pheochromocytomas are rare disorders in children. It is a tumor that arises from the adrenal medulla and secretes excessive catecholamines. Intermittent hypertension is the classic presentation but sustained hypertension with or without paroxysms is also seen clinically. A common description of paroxysms refers to the "5 Ps" –pressure (sudden increase in blood pressure), pain (headache, chest, abdomen), perspiration, palpitations, and pallor. Children are more at risk than adults for malignant disease, and about 10% of diagnoses occur in the pediatric population. Children are also more likely to have recurrent disease especially in those with familial pheochromocytoma.

Appropriate screening should be performed when there is a high index of suspicion. Initial diagnosis is made by 24-hour urine collection and measurement of free catecholamines (norepinephrine and epinephrine) or their metabolites (vanillylmandelic acid [VMA] and total metanephrine). Plasma metanephrine measurements may also be useful in children who may provide an inaccurate 24-hour urine sample. Several imaging techniques, such as computed tomography, magnetic resonance imaging, or nuclear scan, can localize the lesion.

Preoperative management should be done in a critical care setting. Treatment includes starts with the use of α-adrenergic blockade with phenoxybenzamine. The dosing is started low and increased until symptoms and blood pressure are controlled and mild orthostasis is induced. A beta-blocking agent is then added to compensate for the tachycardia. Beta blockers should never be used first, as their use may lead to a hypertensive crisis due to unopposed alpha receptor stimulation. Preparation for surgery usually takes about 10 to 14 days. With removal of tumor tissue, catecholamine secretion returns to normal, with normalization of blood pressure within 1 week. Metastatic disease should be treated with surgical debulking and continued medical therapy with alpha blockade. Pheochromocytoma, although rare, can be a life-threatening situation requiring proper blood pressure management with alpha and beta blockade. Surgery is curative, with a low recurrence rate of about 10%.

© 2008 by Lippincott Williams & Wilkins, a Wolters Kluwer business

SUGGESTED READINGS

Benn D, Gimenez-Roqueplo AP, Reilly JR, et al. Clinical presentation and penetrance of pheochromocytoma/paraganglioma syndromes. *J Clin Endocrinol Metab.* 2006;91(3):827–836.

Brouwers F, Eisenhofer G, Lenders JW, et al. Emergencies caused by pheochromocytoma, neuroblastoma, or ganglioneuroma. *Endocrinol Metab Clin North Am.* 2006;35:699–724.

Young W. Pheochromocytoma in Children. Up to Date, Jan 2007, version 15.1.

133

REMEMBER THAT CONGENITAL ADRENAL HYPERPLASIA (CAH) IS IN THE DIFFERENTIAL DIAGNOSIS FOR CHILDREN PRESENTING WITH FAILURE TO THRIVE, SHOCK, LETHARGY, VOMITING, OR CIRCULATORY COLLAPSE

CYNTHIA GIBSON, MD

WHAT TO DO – INTERPRET THE DATA

Infants may present with CAH at birth with ambiguous genitalia or at 1 to 2 weeks of life, with acute adrenal salt wasting crisis. They often have nonspecific symptoms of failure to thrive with poor feeding, lethargy, irritability, and vomiting. Or symptoms may be severe, with dehydration, hypotension, seizures, or even profound shock and may progress to death if not treated. Any neonate presenting with these symptoms should be considered to be in acute adrenal crisis and treated appropriately.

The initial workup should include evaluation of electrolytes and glucose. Classic findings include hyperkalemia, hyponatremia with hypoglycemia, and acidosis. If suspicion for CAH exists, a steroid profile should be sent prior to treatment unless the patient is too unstable.

Emergency management should include attention to the ABCs and correction of shock, with fluid resuscitation. Intravenous hydrocortisone is the mainstay of emergency treatment, providing glucocorticoid and some mineralocorticoid effect. Patients will require fludrocortisone for long-term therapy. Electrolyte correction often occurs with volume and glucocorticoid replacement.

SUGGESTED READINGS

Perry R, Kecha O, Paquette J, et al. Primary adrenal insufficiency in children: twenty years experience at the Sainte-Justine Hospital, Montreal. *J Clin Endocrinol Metab.* 2005;90:3243–3250.

van der Kamp HJ, Wit JM. Neonatal screening for congenital adrenal hyperplasia. *Eur J Endocrinol.* 2004;151(Suppl 3):U71–U75.

© 2008 by Lippincott Williams & Wilkins, a Wolters Kluwer business

134

MONITOR MENTAL STATUS IN PATIENTS WITH DIABETIC KETOACIDOSIS (DKA) DURING FLUID AND ELECTROLYTE REPLACEMENT

MINDY DICKERMAN, MD

WHAT TO DO – GATHER APPROPRIATE DATA

Cerebral edema is the most feared complication of DKA in children. Clinically apparent cerebral edema occurs in 1% of childhood DKA. One third to one half of children who develop cerebral edema as a consequence of DKA die and another one-third suffer severe permanent neurologic disability. It is unclear if asymptomatic or subclinical cerebral edema occurs commonly in pediatric DKA or if it is present prior to the initiation of treatment. Cerebral edema is more commonly seen in children presenting with severe DKA, a new onset type 1 diabetic, younger age, and a child with longer duration of symptoms prior to treatment.

A number of possible mechanisms may contribute to cerebral edema in DKA. There is uncertainty about whether the pathophysiology is a result of vasogenic edema or cytotoxic edema. Some studies have suggested that cerebral hypoperfusion and subsequent reperfusion may play a role in the pathogenesis of cerebral edema. It is thought the reperfusion, in addition to the breakdown of the blood–brain barrier endothelium, causes vasodilatation and vasogenic edema. Other studies have proposed the edema formation is due to cytotoxic edema from increased brain osmolality where, in a chronic hyperosmolar state due to hyperglycemia, cerebral cells compete with the osmotic force of serum by storing intracellular osmoles.

Clinically, significant cerebral edema may develop at any time during the first 24 hours of treatment. The diagnosis of this complication must be based on clinical bedside criteria. Children may present with abnormal motor or verbal response to pain, decorticate or decerebrate posturing, cranial nerve palsies, an abnormal neurogenic respiratory pattern, altered mentation, sustained bradycardia, vomiting, headache, and/or lethargy. Because the symptoms can be vague, it is critical to have a high index of suspicion for cerebral edema.

A child with DKA should be cared for in a hospital environment with an experienced nursing staff and where frequent neurologic evaluations can be performed. The treatment of cerebral edema should be treated as soon as it is suspected and should not be delayed in order to obtain a computed

© 2008 by Lippincott Williams & Wilkins, a Wolters Kluwer business

tomography scan. The rate of intravenous fluid should be reduced. Intra-venous mannitol should be administered at a dose of 0.5 to 1 g/kg over 20 minutes. Intubation may be necessary for a patient with impending respiratory failure or neurologic compromise.

SUGGESTED READINGS

Agus MS, Wolfsdorf JI. Diabetic ketoacidosis in children. *Pediatr Clin North Am.* 2005;52:1147–1163.

Glaser NS, Wootton-Gorges SL, Marcin JP, et al. Mechanism of cerebral edema in children with diabetic ketoacidosis. *J Pediatr.* 2004;145:164–171.

135

BE AWARE OF HYPOGLYCEMIA IN DIABETIC PATIENTS TAKING INSULIN

SOPHIA SMITH, MD

WHAT TO DO – GATHER APPROPRIATE DATA

Type 1 diabetes mellitus is a condition resulting from destruction of the beta cells in the islets of Langerhans of the pancreas. This results in medically significant symptoms of hyperglycemia, dehydration, and acidosis, producing derangements in intermediary metabolism. This can lead to diabetic ketoacidosis, diabetic coma, or even death from absolute or relative insulin deficiency. Exogenous insulin replacement is the only therapy for this.

Hypoglycemia occurs when the body's blood glucose level drops too low to provide enough energy for the body's activities. This is a common side effect of patient's with Type 1 diabetes and relates to excess insulin administration. Hyperinsulinemic hypoglycemia describes the effects of low blood glucose caused by excessive insulin. It is the most common type of severe but transient hyperinsulinemic hypoglycemia occuring accidentally in persons who take insulin.

Although hypoglycemia can occur suddenly, it can also usually be treated quickly, bringing the blood glucose level back to normal. If the hypoglycemia is mild, it is easily treated by eating or drinking foods containing carbohydrate. If left untreated, the hypoglycemia can become severe and lead to a loss of consciousness. In these extreme circumstances, food cannot be eaten, but glucagon can be injected to quickly raise the blood glucose level.

There are uncommon cases of more persistent harm, and rarely even death due to severe hypoglycemia. One reason hypoglycemia caused by excessive insulin can be dangerous is that insulin reduces the glucose available for the brain's energy requirement and brain damage can occur. The conditions range from focal effects to impaired memory and thinking. Children with prolonged or recurrent hyperinsulinemic hypoglycemia in infancy can experience harm to their brains and developmental delay. Therefore, the immediate recognition and intervention of hypoglycemia are important for a successful outcome.

Hypoglycemia can also occur while asleep. If there are noted periods of crying out or nightmares; damp pajamas or sheets from perspiration; or complaints of feeling tired, irritable, or confused upon waking, there should be a high suspicion for hypoglycemia. The Somogyi phenomenon is a

© 2008 by Lippincott Williams & Wilkins, a Wolters Kluwer business

paradoxical situation of insulin-induced, posthypoglycemic hyperglycemia. It occurs often in children and adolescents. It is the result of the body's defense mechanisms against hypoglycemia. It is a hypoglycemia-induced hyperglycemia, such that if too much insulin is received, the body will try to protect itself and respond by releasing glucagon from the liver and secreting diabetogenic hormones, which induce hyperglycemia.

Nocturnal hypoglycemia is dealt with by a readjustment in the timing and dose of insulin. The failure of the Somogyi phenomenon to occur puts insulin-dependent diabetic patients at increased risk to potential lethal consequences of nocturnal hypoglycemia.

SUGGESTED READING

Saleh M, Grunberger G. Hypoglycemia: An excuse for poor glycemic control? *Clinical Diabetes* 2001;19:161–167.

136

REMEMBER, IN HYPERGLYCEMIC STATES, A "FACTITIOUS HYPONATREMIA" OCCURS

ESTHER FORRESTER, MD

WHAT TO DO – MAKE A DECISION

To have a thorough understanding of fluid and electrolyte issues, one must truly understand the body's composition of solutes and water and how equilibrium is maintained in normal circumstances. Water is the most plentiful compound within the human body. Its percentage changes with age and body composition. It accounts for 80% of body weight in severely preterm infants, 70% in term infants, 65% in young children, and approximately 60% in older children and adolescents. There are two compartments for body water: intracellular and extracellular compartments.

Intracellular water (ICW) accounts for approximately 40% of body weight, or two thirds of total body water. Extracellular water (ECW) refers to interstitial and intravascular fluid volumes, collectively. Interstitial fluid is the water bathing the cells; serum is the water part of blood. ECW accounts for approximately 20% to 25% of body weight, or one third of total body water. Water movement between the interstitial and intravascular areas (i.e., water movement within ECW) is governed by starling forces. The equation is as follows:

$$\text{Fluid movement} = K^*[(P_c - P_i) - (II_c - II_i)]$$

where K = capillary filtration coefficient, P_c = capillary hydrostatic pressure, P_i = interstitial hydrostatic pressure, II_c = capillary oncotic pressure, and II_i = interstitial oncotic pressure.

The movement of fluid across a capillary membrane is governed by the permeability of that membrane and the difference in hydrostatic and oncotic pressures on each side of the membrane. When normal homeostasis is disrupted (i.e., dehydration), the net movement of fluid is from the interstitial compartment into the intravascular compartment in the hopes of regaining homeostasis and maintaining blood pressure. On the other hand, the net

© 2008 by Lippincott Williams & Wilkins, a Wolters Kluwer business

movement of water is from the intravascular space into the interstitium when there is intravascular volume overload or hypoalbuminemia.

Movement of water between fluid compartments (i.e., between the intracellular and extracellular space) occurs based on osmotic gradients. The osmolality of each compartment is reflective of the amounts and types of solutes in each space. Osmolality is defined as the number of milliosmoles of solute per kilogram of water. Extracellular homeostasis is regulated by the kidney. Intracellular homeostasis is regulated by a variety of transport mechanisms. Water flows freely (across semipermeable cell membrane) between the intracellular and extracellular compartments to equalize osmolality. Sodium and chloride are the major extracellular solutes. Glucose and urea nitrogen also play a significant role in extracellular osmolality, and the following equation estimates serum osmolality:

$$2 \times Na^+(mEq/L) + \frac{[BUN\,(mg/dL)]}{2.8} + \frac{[Glucose\,(mg/dL)]}{18}$$

where BUN = blood urea nitrogen.

Based on the above equation, one can see how hypernatremia creates hyperosmolality; however, hyponatremia is not synonymous with hypo-osmolality (urea, glucose, or other osmoles contribute to serum osmolality).

Glucose does not cross cell membranes easily. Therefore, a high serum glucose (remember, serum reflects the extracellular compartment) results in an osmotic gradient with the movement of fluid from the intracellular into the extracellular compartment. This leads to a lower serum sodium concentration and is sometimes referred to as "factitious hyponatremia." In hyperglycemic states, the movement of fluid results in a 1.6 mEq/L decrease in levels of serum sodium for every 100 mg/dL elevation in glucose above normal. The calculation to estimate the "true" serum sodium is:

$$[Na^+] + \frac{[Glucose\,(mg/dL) - 100]}{100} \times 1.6$$

Similarly, severe hyperlipidemia and hypernatremia can result in a pseudohyponatremia. Correction of the hyperglycemia, hyperlipidemia, and/or hyperproteinemia results in a diffusion of water back into the intracellular compartment and normalization of serum sodium levels. Although the intracellular and extracellular compartments are separate, they play off of one another; if the extracellular osmolality increases, water will "exit" from the intracellular space for example. Cell function is also affected and may be compromised. Intracellular edema or contraction can result in deadly effects. For example, brain cells have an extremely low tolerance for swelling or contraction. In diabetic ketoacidosis, there is movement of fluid from the intracellular into the extracellular space (due to hyperglycemia), which can

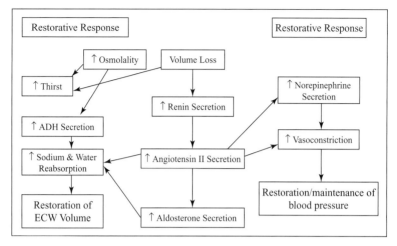

FIGURE 136.1. The protective and restorative responses to volume loss. When the kidney senses a decrease in the ECW, it secretes renin, which initiates a cascade of responses that ultimately leads to increased systemic vasoconstriction and the maintenance or restoration of blood pressure. At the same time, volume loss (particularly if associated with increased osmolality) leads to increased thirst and ADH secretion. Increasing ADH levels are associated with increased water reabsorption, while ADH, along with angiotensin II and aldosterone, increases sodium and water reabsorption. In the absence of continuing losses, these responses lead to the restoration of the ECW volume. ADH, antidiuretic hormone; ECW, extracellular water.

lead to cerebral dysfunction. Thankfully, the body has protective mechanisms to protect and restore homeostasis. For example, see *Figure 136.1*, which depicts how the body responds to volume loss.

SUGGESTED READINGS

Mortiz ML, Ayus JC. Disorders of water metabolism in children: hyponatremia and hypernatremia. *Pediatr Rev.* 2002;23:371–380.

Ruth JL. Wassner SJ. Body composition: salt and water. *Pediatr Rev.* 2006;27:181–187; quiz 188.

137

IT IS LIKELY WORSE TO TREAT YOUNG INFANTS AND TODDLERS WITH HYPOTONIC INTRAVENOUS (IV) FLUID (D5 1/2 OR D5 1/3), BECAUSE HYPO-OSMOTIC FLUIDS CAN LEAD TO IATROGENIC HYPONATREMIA

MADAN DHARMAR, MD

WHAT TO DO – MAKE A DECISION

Acute gastroenteritis is one of the common illnesses affecting infants and children throughout the world. Correction of dehydration is the mainstay of treatment, which is given as oral rehydration therapy (preferably) or intravenous fluids, depending on the severity of dehydration and various other factors. It is imperative to correctly choose the type of fluid to avoid electrolyte disturbances that might lead to dangerous complications.

Among children in the United States, acute gastroenteritis remains a major cause of morbidity and hospitalization, accounting for >1.5 million outpatient visits, 200,000 hospitalizations, and approximately 300 deaths per year.

The volume of fluid lost through stools can vary from 5 mL/kg body weight per day, which is approximately normal, to ≥200 mL/kg body weight per day, which is severe diarrhea. Dehydration and electrolyte losses associated with untreated diarrhea are the main reason for morbidity in acute gastroenteritis. History, physical examination, and dehydration assessment are the main features in the assessment of diarrhea. Treatment usually includes two phases: rehydration and maintenance. The rehydration phase involves quick replacement of fluids usually within 3 to 4 hours. The maintenance phase is the phase in which maintenance calories and fluids are administered. IV fluids are the mainstay of management in cases of severe dehydration.

IV fluid administration to maintain water and electrolyte balance in an individual was first described by Holliday and Segar in 1957. They had based the free water requirement on evidence that it equated the energy expenditure in healthy children. However, sodium and potassium requirements (3.0 and 2.0 mEq/100 kcal/24 hour, respectively) were rationalized based on intake of electrolytes by infants receiving breast and cow milk. Use of hypotonic IV fluids was based on the above recommendations. Although these recommendations may be appropriate for the healthy child, they do not necessarily apply in acute illness, where energy expenditure and electrolyte

ⓒ 2008 by Lippincott Williams & Wilkins, a Wolters Kluwer business

requirements deviate significantly from that of a normal healthy individual. The calculation based on this recommendation could overestimate the hypotonic solution needs in patients.

Hyponatremia occurs when the water to sodium ratio is increased, which means that the plasma sodium concentration is <136 mM. This can be either due to decrease in sodium or an increase in the water. This could occur when there is a positive balance of electrolyte free water in the body due to increased input of water than excretion of water. A decrease in the water output usually occurs secondary to antidiuretic hormone (ADH) secretion. In normal individuals, ADH is controlled by osmotic stimuli and hence water diuresis occurs only when the plasma sodium level falls below 136 mM (due to ADH suppression). However, hospitalized pediatric patients have multiple causes for nonosmotic stimuli for ADH secretion, and hence when the plasma sodium level falls below 136 mM, water diuresis does not take place due to the presence of ADH (nonosmotic stimuli) and this increases the available electrolyte free water in the body. Administration of hypotonic solution would further contribute to the electrolyte free water, leading to hyponatremia in these patients. It has been shown that patients admitted with gastroenteritis have obligate urinary sodium losses irrespective of initial serum sodium. The urinary tonicity at presentation of these patients is approximately equal to normal saline. Therefore, infusion of a hypotonic solution, which is lower in tonicity than that of urine passed, is predictive of a decrease in subsequent serum sodium.

Hyponatremia can cause water to move into the intercellular compartment, thereby causing the cells to swell. The expansion of intracellular fluid volume is of major importance in the central nervous system, as the brain is confined in a rigid bony cage and has only limited ability to expand. Thus, brain cell swelling is very likely to increase intracranial pressure and predispose to brain herniation. Children are at greater risk of this sequela because their brains have a larger intracellular fluid volume per total skull volume. The incidence of permanent brain damage is higher in children with symptomatic hyponatremia when compared to adults. Symptoms of cerebral edema include nausea, vomiting, agitation, headache, seizures, and coma. Choong et al. state that "based on published case reports of deaths and neurological injury from acute hyponatremia that the administration of hypotonic solutions to children with a P_{Na}, 138 mmol/L is potentially hazardous, given that ADH is likely to be acting."

The administration of isotonic maintenance solution in certain cases has resulted in a more rapid return of ADH to normal concentrations, when compared to hypotonic fluids. Isotonic crystalloid solutions, such as lactated Ringer and normal saline, expand the fluid space and improve circulating volume without exacerbating hyponatremia, thereby decreasing the risk of cerebral edema. Isotonic fluids could cause hyponatremia during the perioperative period in a person who had been given Ringer lactate solution to prevent a fall in blood pressure by the process of desalination. However, administration of isotonic fluids in individuals who produced hypotonic urine could cause positive sodium, leading to hypernatremia.

In conclusion, the current recommendation for IV fluid management is not based on clinical experiment on hospitalized patients but rather was derived based on the normal homeostatic mechanisms in healthy individuals. There is evidence that, at least in some pediatric patients, hypotonic solutions exacerbate the risks of hyponatremia, whereas isotonic solutions may be protective. Taking these into account a judicious choice of fluid type should be made in the management of dehydration based on individual needs.

SUGGESTED READINGS

Choong K, Kho ME, Menon K, et al. Hypotonic versus isotonic saline in hospitalised children: a systematic review. *Arch Dis Child.* 2006;91(10):828–835.

Holliday MA, Segar WE. The maintenance need for water in parenteral fluid therapy. *Pediatrics.* 1957;19(5):823–832.

King CK, Glass R, Bresee JS, et al. Managing acute gastroenteritis among children oral rehydration, maintenance, and nutritional therapy. *MMWR Recomm Rep.* 2003;52(RR-16):1–16.

Moritz ML, Ayus JC. Prevention of hospital-acquired hyponatremia: a case for using isotonic saline. *Pediatrics.* 2003;111(2):227–230.

Shafiee MA, Bohn D, Hoorn EJ, et al. How to select optimal maintenance intravenous fluid therapy. *QJM.* 2003;96(8):601–610.

World Health Organization. *The Treatment of Diarrhoea: A Manual for Physicians and Other Senior Health Workers.* Geneva, Switzerland: World Health Organization; 2005.

138

ACCURATELY MEASURE THE BLOOD PRESSURE (BP) IN ALL PEDIATRIC PATIENTS OLDER THAN AGE 3 AND IN YOUNGER HIGH-RISK PATIENTS

JENNIFER MANISCALCO, MD

WHAT TO DO – GATHER APPROPRIATE DATA

Hypertension during childhood is not rare, with an estimated prevalence ranging from 1% to 5.8%. Children with hypertension may develop early abnormalities in target organs systems, even in the absence of signs and symptoms. Furthermore, childhood hypertension is a strong risk factor for adult hypertension. An aggressive surveillance system to detect hypertension in children can lead to prompt diagnosis and management, prevention of target organ damage, and a reduced risk of adult hypertension. Recent guidelines suggest that all children older than 3 years should have their BP checked. Younger children should have their BP checked if risk factors for hypertension are present (*Table 138.1*).

Hypertension in the pediatric population is defined as an average systolic blood pressure (SBP) or diastolic blood pressure (DBP) $\geq 95\%$ for age, gender, and height, measured on at least three separate occasions. Appropriate technique in BP measurement is required to diagnose hypertension accurately. Auscultation using mercury sphygmomanometry is the gold standard, but many oscillometric devices have been validated for use in children. Regardless of the device employed, the correct cuff size is essential for the accurate measurement of BP. The width of the cuff bladder should be approximately 40% of the arm circumference measured at the midpoint of the upper arm. The length of the cuff bladder should be 80% to 100% of the arm circumference.

Hypertension in children can be classified as primary or secondary. Primary hypertension, also called essential hypertension, does not have an identifiable cause, but rather results from a combination of genetic and environmental factors. It occurs more commonly in adolescents than younger children, and it is associated with overweight, obesity, and other cardiovascular risk factors. Individuals with primary hypertension are often asymptomatic and without evidence of target organ damage at presentation.

Secondary hypertension is more common in younger children and results from an underlying disease process. At presentation, these children are

© 2008 by Lippincott Williams & Wilkins, a Wolters Kluwer business

TABLE 138.1	CONDITIONS UNDER WHICH THE CHILD YOUNGER THAN AGE 3 SHOULD HAVE THEIR BLOOD PRESSURE CHECKED

History of prematurity, very low birth weight, umbilical artery catheter placement, or other neonatal condition requiring intensive care
Congenital heart disease
Recurrent urinary tract infections, hematuria, or proteinuria
Known renal disease or urologic malformation
Family history of congenital renal disease
Solid-organ transplant
Malignancy or bone marrow transplant
Treatment with drugs known to raise blood pressure
Other systemic illnesses associated with hypertension
Evidence of elevated intracranial pressure

Adapted from National High Blood Pressure Education Program Working Group on High Blood Pressure in Children and Adolescents. The fourth report on the diagnosis, evaluation, and treatment of high blood pressure in children and adolescents. *Pediatrics.* 2004;114(2 Suppl):555–576.

more likely to have dramatic elevations of BP, symptoms of hypertension, and evidence of target organ damage. The most common cause of secondary hypertension is renal disease. Renal parenchymal disease is more common than renovascular disease. Other causes of secondary hypertension include cardiac diseases such as coarctation of the aorta, medications, and poorly controlled pain. Primary endocrine disorders are rare and include hyperthyroidism, Cushing disease, and endocrine tumors such as pheochromocytoma and neuroblastoma. *Table 138.2* provides the common causes of hypertension by age group.

The evaluation of a child with hypertension begins with a thorough history and physical exam. The focus should be on the signs and symptoms of diseases that cause hypertension as well as comorbid conditions and evidence of target organ damage. For older children and adolescents, family history should focus on hypertension and its comorbid conditions. The social history should address diet, physical activity, smoking, and recreational drug use. Laboratory evaluation of children with hypertension should include complete blood count, chemistries, blood urea nitrogen, creatinine, complete urinalysis, and urine culture. A renal ultrasound should be obtained. Specialized tests such as renin, steroid and catecholamine levels, and renovascular imaging may be obtained as the clinical situation dictates. Evidence of target organ damage should be documented. Ophthalmologic consultation may reveal retinal changes, and echocardiography may reveal left ventricular hypertrophy. Comorbid conditions, such as dyslipidemia, glucose

TABLE 138.2	COMMON CAUSES OF HYPERTENSION IN CHILDREN, GROUPED BY AGE, IN DESCENDING ORDER	
AGE	**CAUSES OF HYPERTENSION**
Newborn	Renal artery thrombosis Renal artery stenosis Renal venous thrombosis Congenital renal abnormalities Coarctation of the aorta Bronchopulmonary dysplasia Patent ductus arteriosus Intraventricular hemorrhage
1–12 months	Coarctation of the aorta Renovascular disease Renal parenchymal disease
1–6 years	Renal parenchymal disease Renovascular disease Coarctation of the aorta Endocrine causes Essential hypertension
6–12 years	Renal parenchymal disease Renovascular disease Essential hypertension Coarctation of the aorta Endocrine causes Iatrogenic (medications, etc.)
12–18 years	Essential hypertension Iatrogenic Renal parenchymal disease Renovascular disease Endocrine causes Coarctation of the aorta

Adapted from Bartosh SM, Aronson AJ. Childhood hypertension. An update on etiology, diagnosis, and treatment. *Pediatr Clin North Am.* 1999;46:235–252; Varda NM, Gregoric A. A diagnostic approach for the child with hypertension. *Pediatr Nephrol.* 2005;20:499–506.

intolerance, and hyperuricemia, should be sought in children who are overweight or who have essential hypertension.

SUGGESTED READINGS

Bartosh SM, Aronson AJ. Childhood hypertension. An update on etiology, diagnosis, and treatment. *Pediatr Clin North Am.* 1999;46:235–252.

National High Blood Pressure Education Program Working Group on High Blood Pressure in Children and Adolescents. The fourth report on the diagnosis, evaluation, and treatment of high blood pressure in children and adolescents. *Pediatrics.* 2004;114(2 Suppl):555–576.

Varda NM, Gregoric A. A diagnostic approach for the child with hypertension. *Pediatr Nephrol.* 2005;20:499–506.

139

ASSESS THE VOLUME STATUS AND ELECTROLYTES IN CHILDREN WITH POSTSTREPTOCOCCAL GLOMERULONEPHRITIS

BRIAN KIT, MD

WHAT TO DO – GATHER APPROPRIATE DATA

Acute poststreptococcal glomerulonephritis (APSGN) is a sequela of group A β-hemolytic streptococci (GAS) infection of the skin or pharynx with strains of GAS that are nephrogenic. The onset of disease depends on the location of initial infection, with an average presentation of 10 days following pharyngitis and 3 weeks following a cellulitis. The etiology of the kidney damage is from deposition of antigen-antibody complexes in the glomeruli.

In the majority of cases of APSGN, the typical clinical presentation is a nephritic syndrome, including hematuria, mild proteinuria, edema, and hypertension with or without oliguria. Classically, the presentation of hematuria is heralded as "cola-colored" urine. The edema is typically noted first in the periorbital areas. Orthopnea, dyspnea, and cough may be other associated complaints related to volume overload. There may also be associated non-specific findings including lethargy, anorexia, vomiting, fever, or headache.

Most clinicians start their evaluation of APSGN with analysis of the urine, which almost always reveals hematuria. Proteinuria is often present, correlating with the amount of blood in the urine. Additional laboratory evaluation may reveal signs of acute renal failure, including an elevation in the creatinine. Hyperkalemia and acidosis may also result.

Confirming the diagnosis of APSGN requires documentation of a previous GAS infection. Bacterial cultures of the skin or pharynx will likely not be helpful because they are rarely positive at the time of presentation. Antistreptolysin O (ASO) titer is elevated when the disease is preceded by pharyngitis but is rarely elevated in preceding skin infections. Antideoxyribonuclease B (anti-DNAse B) titers provide advantages over ASO for documenting previous GAS skin infections. ASO and anti-DNAse B titers are often elevated sufficiently at the time of presentation to confirm a previous GAS infection. In almost all cases, there is a suppressed C3 level at the time of presentation, which returns to baseline in 6 weeks.

Treatment is directed at the patient's symptoms. All patients should have salt and water restriction. Attention to the potassium is important for

© 2008 by Lippincott Williams & Wilkins, a Wolters Kluwer business

preventing cardiac complications, as a result of hyperkalemia. For treatment of hypertension, loop diuretics are often used, which may also be helpful in reducing the hyperkalemia, if present. In the presence of severe hypertension or oliguria, other antihypertensives, including a calcium channel blocker or a beta blocker may be useful. Angiotensin-converting enzyme inhibitors should be used cautiously because hyperkalemia is a known adverse event associated with this class of antihypertensives. In severe cases with profound renal failure, hemodialysis or peritoneal dialysis may be necessary. Although antibiotic therapy does not affect the clinical course of APSGN, appropriate GAS treatment is recommended to eradicate GAS on the individual level and to reduce the risk of transmission of nephrogenic GAS to other members of the community.

The prognosis of APSGN in children is favorable. Hypertension and gross hematuria usually resolve over several weeks, although microscopic hematuria may persist for several years. Proteinuria resolves over several months. There is a return to their baseline creatinine in 3 to 4 weeks. A C3 level should be repeated at 6 to 8 weeks. If the C3 level does not return to normal, referral to a pediatric nephrologist should be initiated to consider other etiologies of glomerulonephritis, including lupus nephritis and membranoproliferative glomerulonephritis.

SUGGESTED READINGS

Berrios X, Lagomarsino E, Solar E, et al. Post-streptococcal acute glomerulonephritis in Chile– 20 years of experience. *Pediatric Nephrol.* 2004;19(3):306–312.

Johnston F, Carapetis J, Patel MS, et al. Evaluating the use of penicillin to control outbreaks of acute poststreptococcal glomerulonephritis. *Pediatr Infect Dis J.* 1999;18(4):327–332.

Rodriguez-Iturbe B. Postinfectious glomerulonephritis. *Am J Kidney Dis.* 2000;35(1):XLVI– XLVIII.

140

CALCULATE AN OSMOLAL GAP IN THE SETTING OF ANION GAP METABOLIC ACIDOSIS

JENNIFER MANISCALCO, MD

WHAT TO DO – INTERPRET THE DATA

Metabolic acidosis develops when there is an accumulation of hydrogen ions in or an excessive loss of bicarbonate from the bloodstream. There are numerous causes of metabolic acidosis, and determination of the anion gap can narrow the differential diagnosis considerably. The anion gap refers to the unmeasured anions in the bloodstream which, in conjunction with chloride and bicarbonate, counteract the main cation sodium (*Table 140.1*). An increase in the anion gap occurs with increased production of endogenous acids, as in diabetic or starvation ketoacidosis; decreased excretion of fixed acids, as in uremia or chronic renal insufficiency; or ingestion of exogenous acids, such as salicylates. Toxic alcohol ingestion with methanol and ethylene glycol can also result in increased exogenous acids as the parent alcohol gets broken down into its metabolites.

Toxic alcohol ingestion from methanol or ethylene glycol results in predictable clinical toxidromes. Both toxidromes are characterized by extensive central nervous system, cardiopulmonary, and gastrointestinal involvement (*Table 140.2*). Ethylene glycol intoxication also involves the kidneys, while methanol intoxication has extensive ophthalmologic involvement. However, clinical manifestations of intoxication by either substance are often delayed until significant metabolism of the parent alcohol has occurred. This makes the initial diagnosis more difficult, especially in the absence of an ingestion history. The presence of an anion gap metabolic acidosis without alternative explanation can provide a clue to the diagnosis of toxic alcohol ingestion.

Furthermore, both methanol and ethylene glycol intoxication can result in an elevation of the osmolal gap. Other causes of anion gap metabolic acidosis do not. Serum osmolality refers to the total amount of osmotically active particles in the blood stream. It is influenced primarily by small molecules that are present in high concentrations such as sodium, potassium, chloride, bicarbonate, urea, and glucose. Several formulas exist for the calculation of the serum osmolality, and a common formula is listed in Table 140.1. The osmolal gap represents the difference between the measured and the calculated serum osmolality. Both methanol and ethylene glycol are osmotically

© 2008 by Lippincott Williams & Wilkins, a Wolters Kluwer business

TABLE 140.1	COMMON FORMULAS RELATED TO THE ANION GAP AND THE OSMOLAL GAP

Anion Gap $= (Na^+ + K^+) - (Cl^- + HCO_3^-)$
Normal value $= 8 - 16 \text{ mEq/L}$
Calculated Osmolality $= 2(Na^+) + (\text{glucose} \div 18) + (BUN \div 2.8)$
Osmolal Gap $=$ Measured Osmolality $-$ Calculated Osmolality
Normal value $\leq 10 \text{ mmol/L}$

BUN, blood urea nitrogen.

TABLE 140.2	CLINICAL MANIFESTATIONS OF ETHYLENE GLYCOL AND METHANOL INGESTIONS	
	ETHYLENE GLYCOL	METHANOL
Onset of toxicity	4–12 hours	≤ 30 hours
Central nervous system	Intoxication, stupor, coma, seizures, cerebral edema, herniation syndromes, cranial nerve palsies (ophthalmoplegia, pupillary deficits, facial weakness, hearing loss, dysarthria, dysphagia)	Alert, intoxication, headaches, dizziness, agitation, stupor, coma, seizures, cerebral edema, herniation syndromes, basal ganglia infarcts or hemorrhages
Cardiopulmonary (usually preterminal findings)	Hypertension, tachycardia, ECG changes (related to hypocalcemia), hyperpnea, Kussmaul respirations, pulmonary edema	Hypertension, tachycardia, hyperpnea, Kussmaul respirations, pulmonary edema
Gastrointestinal	Nausea, vomiting	Nausea, vomiting, abdominal pain, pancreatitis, elevated liver transaminases
Renal	Acute tubular necrosis, acute renal failure, calcium oxalate crystalluria	–
Ophthalmologic	Pupillary deficits	Normal vision, blurred vision, hazy vision described as a "snowstorm," photophobia, visual hallucinations, blindness, papillary deficits, papilledema, hyperemic optic discs, retinal edema or hemorrhages
Other	Hypocalcemia, myoclonic jerks, tetany, myositis	

ECG, electrocardiogram.

active substances that increase the serum osmolality and subsequently the osmolal gap.

However, the results of the osmolal gap must be interpreted with caution. Because it is the methanol and ethylene glycol, and not their metabolites, that are osmotically active and increase the osmolal gap, the measured osmolality and hence the osmolal gap decrease as the parent compound is metabolized. A patient with toxic alcohol ingestion may have a normal osmolal gap if a significant amount of metabolism has already occurred. In addition, the accuracy of the measured serum osmolality is dependent on the technique used to perform the test, the preferred technique being the freezing point depression method. The calculated serum osmolality is also variable, depending on the formula used to obtain the measurement. Finally, coingestion with ethanol or another osmotically active substance will alter the measured serum osmolality and the osmolal gap.

Initial management of methanol or ethylene glycol ingestion centers on supportive care. Because the toxicity of both parent alcohols is related to their metabolites, treatment is aimed at inhibiting the rate-limiting enzyme in the metabolic process, alcohol dehydrogenase. Ethanol and fomepizole (4-methylpyrazole) are both competitive inhibitors of alcohol dehydrogenase and are frequently used for this purpose. Hemodialysis is indicated in cases of markedly elevated serum methanol or ethylene glycol levels, significant metabolic acidosis, metabolic acidosis unresponsive to bicarbonate infusion, and impaired renal function.

SUGGESTED READINGS

Ford MD, McMartin K. Ethylene glycol and methanol. In: Ford MD, Delaney KA, Ling LJ, et al. (eds). *Clinical Toxicology*. 1st ed. Philadelphia: WB Saunders; 2001:757–768.

Glaser DS. Utility of the serum osmol gap in the diagnosis of methanol and ethylene glycol ingestion. *Ann Emerg Med.* 1996;27:343–346.

Michael JB, Sztajnkrycer MD. Deadly pediatric poisons: nine common agents that kill at low doses. *Emerg Med Clin North Am.* 2004;22:1019–1050.

141

CALCULATE THE CREATININE CLEARANCE FOR CHILDREN WITH RENAL INSUFFICIENCY SO DRUGS THAT ARE EXCRETED BY A RENAL MECHANISM ARE APPROPRIATELY DOSED

MICHAEL S. POTTER AND ANTHONY SLONIM, MD

WHAT TO DO – INTERPRET THE DATA

The glomerular filtration rate (GFR) has become the standard means of evaluating renal function and has traditionally been estimated from creatinine clearance or the serum creatinine concentration. Unfortunately, both of these estimations are frequently inaccurate, particularly in children. For creatinine clearance measurements, a carefully timed urine sample is required, the results of which are often inaccurate. Serum creatinine concentration is affected by factors other than GFR, such as the production of creatinine, which is primarily related to muscle mass. Because of the variability among children in size and body habitus, this measure can also result in erroneous GFR readings.

Over the years, several calculations have been developed for estimating GFR, all of which have their shortcomings when used on various populations and under various circumstances (*Table 141.1*). For example, the Cockcroft and Gault formula, which has been the most commonly used formula, systematically overestimates GFR values in obese and edematous people. A better formula was developed by Levey et al. that reduces variability in measurement among different population types. Special studies have been conducted to analyze the effectiveness of using traditional GFR estimation strategies on pediatric patients. In a 2003 study, Hogg et al. identified several metrics for more accurately measuring creatinine clearance in children and adolescents given conditions such as diabetes. Two formulae in particular were found to be much more practical for pediatric use (*Table 141.2*). If renal insufficiency exists in a pediatric patient, it is essential to remember that renal impairment may require drug dosage alterations or therapeutic drug monitoring. Detailed alterations specific to each drug can be found in various pharmacological textbooks or databases. Therapeutic drug monitoring can also be used to measure the changes in drug levels administered to patients suffering from renal insufficiency or failure. For example, Livernese et al. studied the use of antibacterial agents in renal failure and provided good information about drug management in patients with renal failure.

© 2008 by Lippincott Williams & Wilkins, a Wolters Kluwer business

TABLE 141.1 — FORMULAS FOR ESTIMATING GLOMERULAR FILTRATION RATE USING SERUM CREATININE AND OTHER CLINICAL PARAMETERS

FORMULA (MALE)	FORMULA (FEMALE)	UNITS	REFERENCES
$\dfrac{100}{Cr} - 12$	$\dfrac{100}{Cr} - 7$	$mL/min/1.73\,m^3$	Jelliffe & Jelliffe
$\dfrac{Wt \times (29.3 - 0.203 \times Age)}{Cr \times 14.4}$	$\dfrac{Wt \times (25.3 - 0.175 \times Age)}{Cr \times 14.4}$	mL/min	Mawer et al., Kampmann et al.
$\dfrac{98 - 16 \times (Age - 20)}{(20/Cr)}$	$\left[\dfrac{98 - 16 \times (Age - 20)}{(20/Cr)}\right] \times 0.90$	$mL/min/1.73\,m^3$	Jelliffe
$\dfrac{(140 - Age) \times Wt}{72 \times Cr}$	$\left[\dfrac{(140 - Age) \times Wt}{72 \times Cr}\right] \times 0.85$	mL/min	Cockroft & Gault
$\dfrac{(140 - Age)}{Cr} - 3$	$\left[\dfrac{(140 - Age)}{Cr} - 3\right] \times 0.85$	$mL/min/70\,kg$	Hull et al.
$\dfrac{27 - (0.173 \times Age)}{Cr}$	$\dfrac{25 - (0.175 \times Age)}{Cr}$	mL/min	Bjornsson et al.
$\dfrac{7.58}{Cr \times 0.0884} - (0.103 \times Age) + (0.096 \times Wt) - 6.66$	$\dfrac{6.05}{Cr \times 0.0884} - (0.080 \times Age) + (0.080 \times Wt) - 4.81$	$mL/min/1.73\,m^3$ (height^2)	Walser et al.
$170 \times Cr^{-0.999} \times Age^{0.278} (\times 0.762$ for female and/or $\times 1.180$ for black$) \times SUN^{-0.278} \times Alb^{0.225}$		$mL/min/1.73\,m^3$	Levey et al.

Age, in years; *Alb*, serum albumin (g/dL); *Cr*, serum creatinine (mg/dL); *SUN*, serum urea nitrogen (mg/dL); *wt*, body weight (kg)
Cr, creatinine; Wt, weight.
(Used with permission from Brenner BM, Rector FC, eds. *Brenner & Rector's The Kidney.* 6th ed. Philadelphia: WB Saunders Company; 2000.)

TABLE 141.2   ESTIMATION OF GLOMERULAR FILTRATION RATE IN CHILDREN USING SERUM CREATININE AND HEIGHT

AUTHOR (NO. OF SUBJECTS)	FORMULA
Schwarts et al ($N = 186$)	$C_{Cr}\,(mL/min/1.73\,m^2) = \dfrac{0.55 \times Height\,(cm)}{S_{Cr}\,(mg/dL)}$
Counahan et al ($N = 108$)	$GFR\,(mL/min/1.73\,m^2) = \dfrac{0.43 \times Height\,(cm)}{S_{Cr}\,(mg/dL)}$

C_{Cr}, creatinine clearance; S_{Cr}, serum creatinine.
In the Schwarts equation, the constant to be used in young children (<1 year of age) is 0.45, in adolescent boys the value of the constant changes to 0.7. To convert serum creatinine in $\mu mol/L$ to mg/dL, the value in $\mu mol/L$ is multiplied by 0.0113.
(Used with permission Hogg RJ, Furth S, Lemley KV, et al. National Kidney Foundation's Kidney Disease Outcomes Quality Initiative clinical practice guidelines for chronic kidney disease in children and adolescents: evaluation, classification, and stratification. *Pediatrics.* 2003;111(6 Pt 1):1416–1421.)

Formulas for measuring renal health are imperfect, but being aware of some of the differences in formulaic constructs that have been developed can help in applying the correct formula to each situation. For example, Cockroft and Gault's formula may be appropriate for adult patients, whereas Levey and colleagues' formula is more suited for patients of African American descent. For pediatric patients, the Schwarts et al. and Counahan et al. formulae have been shown to be more appropriate. Finally, an awareness of the effects that renal insufficiency can have on patient drug regimens is important. Utilizing appropriate dose adjustment and therapeutic drug monitoring when necessary can assure that renal complications do not influence the outcome of the child.

SUGGESTED READINGS

DynaMed Editorial Team. Acute renal failure–renal disease. Last updated June 14, 2007. Available at: www.ebscohost.com/dynamed. Accessed July 4, 2007.
Guignard JP and Santos F. Chapter 21. In: Avner ED, Harmon WE and Niaudet P. *Pediatric Nephrology.* 5th ed. Philadelphia: Lippincott Williams & Wilkins; 2004.
Hogg RJ, Furth S, Lemley KV, et al. National Kidney Foundation's Kidney Disease Outcomes Quality Initiative clinical practice guidelines for chronic kidney disease in children and adolescents: evaluation, classification, and stratification. *Pediatrics.* 2003;111(6 Pt 1):1416–1421.
Livernese LL Jr, Slavin D, Gilbert B, et al. Use of antibacterial agents in renal failure. *Infect Dis Clin North Am.* 2004;18:551–579.
Silkensen JR, Kasiske BL. Laboratory assessment of kidney disease: clearance, urinalysis, and kidney biopsy. In: Brenner BM. *Brenner & Rector's The Kidney.* 7th ed. Philadelphia: Saunders; 2004;1107–1150.
Wuyts B, Bernard D, Van Den Noortgate N, et al. Reevaluation of formulas for predicting creatinine clearance in adults and children, using compensated creatinine methods. *Clin Chem.* 2003;49(6 Pt 1):1011–1014.

142

Do not treat factitious hyperkalemia, treat the underlying disorder

Craig DeWolfe, MD

What to Do – Make a Decision

Although hyperkalemia can be a serious disorder associated with serious consequences, the inattention to, or inappropriate treatment of, factitious hyperkalemia can result in its own set of unnecessary and potentially dangerous interventions. One should suspect factitious hyperkalemia when the patient lacks kidney disease and does not show the typical signs and symptoms of muscle weakness or electrocardiographic abnormalities associated with true hyperkalemia. If suspicious, the clinician should obtain a more accurate specimen or account for leukocytosis, thrombocytosis, or genetic factors when weighing the importance of the measured value. Secondary, nonrenal causes of hyperkalemia should also be considered since the disruption may be iatrogenic or a result of an equally serious underlying disorder.

Factitious hyperkalemia, or pseudohyperkalemia, reflects an artificially high measured potassium level resulting from its release just before or after phlebotomy. Venous stasis from a tourniquet, fist clenching, straining, or hyperventilating can cause a potassium efflux from cells. Specimens obtained using a small-gauge needle, stored on ice, or processed after a considerable delay may also cause falsely elevated potassium results. In vitro potassium will be released from clots of white blood cells and platelets once the blood has been drawn and will be exacerbated by significant cases of leukocytosis ($>100 \times 10^9$/L) or thrombocytosis ($>1,000 \times 10^9$/L) commonly found in myeloproliferative disorders or Kawasaki syndrome. Finally, familial pseudohyperkalemia, a genetic condition passed as an autosomal dominant trait on chromosome 16 may predispose affected patients to factitious hyperkalemia as a result of an abnormal leakage of ions across the red blood cell membranes. Any combination of these factors may raise the measured potassium level by 2 mEq/L; the practitioner should consider how the specimen was processed while examining the patient for symptoms. Important diagnostic studies include measures of renal function tests, an electrocardiogram, and a repeat specimen. If the repeat level is normal, the practitioner should be reassured; however, if the potassium remains persistently elevated, further investigation and treatment may be warranted.

© 2008 by Lippincott Williams & Wilkins, a Wolters Kluwer business

Secondary, nonrenal causes of hyperkalemia are extensive. Often these disruptions are mild, but in patients with renal insufficiency or when known causes of hyperkalemia are left unmonitored and unmanaged, the elevations in potassium can result in significant morbidity or mortality. Iatrogenic causes of hyperkalemia include medications and the induction of metabolic acidosis. Acute metabolic acidosis may result in hyperkalemia due to an efflux of potassium ions out of the cells, as excess protons are buffered inside the cells. The use of ammonium chloride to manage alkalosis can cause up to a 1.5 mEq/L rise in the potassium concentration for every 0.1 unit reduction in arterial blood pH. Other drugs may temper the body's normal catecholamine and mineralocorticoid response to hyperkalemia. For example, beta-blockers, angiotensin-converting enzyme inhibitors, or angiotensin-receptor antagonists may precipitate hyperkalemia in patients during periods of exercise. Cytotoxic drugs may cause a tumor lysis syndrome in patients with a significant tumor burden found in certain cases of lymphoma or neuroblastoma. Succinylcholine works as a muscle relaxant by depolarizing muscle cells and can lead to significant increases in potassium in susceptible patients including those with neuromuscular disease or extensive burns cannot handle a significant potassium load. In fact, elevations of 6 mEq/L have been documented. Finally, digoxin toxicity inhibits the cellular Na^+-K^+-ATPase and can cause a potassium leak from cells.

Exogenous and endogenous potassium loads are also of concern. Clearly, overdoses of oral or intravenous potassium are concerning, but intravenous penicillin preparations and red blood cell products over 5 days old may result in markedly elevated potassium levels. Also, endogenous potassium loads after intravascular coagulation, sickle cell hemolysis crisis, rhabdomyolysis, trauma, burns, and massive gastrointestinal bleeds may result in hyperkalemia. In these cases, the practitioner should treat the underlying cause of the disruption while surveying the risk of the potassium level.

Generally, potassium levels >8 mEq/L with electrocardiographic changes and muscle weakness should be considered an emergency and treated with a combination of potassium antagonists (calcium gluconate), redistribution compounds (glucose and insulin, sodium bicarbonate), and agents directed at eliminating the potassium (sodium polystyrene sulfonate resin, furosemide, albuterol). A combination of treatments is recommended due to the variable onsets of action and the ultimate need to eliminate the excess potassium.

In cases where cardiac complications are not of immediate concern, the practitioner should quickly investigate the etiology of hyperkalemia by recognizing the various factitious and reversible secondary causes and treat them accordingly.

SUGGESTED READINGS

Schwartz GJ. Potassium. In: Avner ED, et al. eds. *Pediatric Nephrology*. 5th ed. Philadelphia: Lippincott Williams & Wilkins; 2004;147–188.

Wiederkehr MR, Moe OW. Factitious hyperkalemia. *Am J Kidney Dis.* 2000;36:1049–1053.

143

CONSIDER THE COEXISTENCE OF HYPOMAGNESEMIA WHEN TREATING REFRACTORY HYPOCALCEMIA OR HYPOKALEMIA

CRAIG DeWOLFE, MD

WHAT TO DO – INTERPRET THE DATA

Magnesium, calcium, and potassium are three of the four most abundant cations in the human body. A disturbance in any one may affect the other. In the case of refractory hypokalemia or hypocalcemia, the clinician should investigate for hypomagnesemia and treat if present, because repleting magnesium stores will likely facilitate corrections of the other electrolyte disturbances.

Concurrently low serum levels of potassium and magnesium are frequently seen in patients and are well documented in the literature. Studies have suggested that 42% of cases of hypomagnesemia are associated with hypokalemia and that hypokalemia itself may lead to excessive renal losses of magnesium. Although pediatric studies are limited, adult patients with low magnesium and potassium levels have a higher mortality rate than severity matched patients with normal magnesium levels. Possible etiologies of the excess mortality include cardiac dysrhythmias, coronary vasospasms, and cardiac arrests. The administration of magnesium can reduce arrhythmias and the mortality rate after adult myocardial infarctions by 25% to 74%. Additional medical studies suggest that efforts to maintain high-normal concentrations of magnesium will lead to a positive potassium homeostasis and less need for potassium infusions. This is important because magnesium infusions are considerably safer than infusions of potassium. Although rapid infusions of magnesium can lead to hypotension arrhythmia and flushing, potassium infusions have a significantly higher risk of cardiac dysrhythmia, phlebitis, pain, and tissue necrosis in the event of extravasation.

Magnesium and calcium are also highly interdependent. Low levels of both result in neuromuscular weakness, fasciculations, tetany, and seizures. Their combined deficiency makes the manifestations more prominent and more refractory to treatment. Combined deficiencies can occur from genetic defects as well as acquired causes such as sepsis. In familial hypomagnesemia, the hypomagnesemia resulting from a defect in its gut absorption produces hypocalcemia by diminishing the production, release, or responsiveness to

© 2008 by Lippincott Williams & Wilkins, a Wolters Kluwer business

parathyroid hormone and an impaired formation of 25-dihydroxyvitamin D3. The same hormonal responses have been identified in other clinical scenarios with hypomagnesemia and hypocalcemia such as sepsis. In sepsis, intracellular calcium levels rise as tissue magnesium falls and that this relationship leads to cell death. One third of adult intensive care patients with hypomagnesemia also have hypocalcemia. When this is the case, the clinician will not be able to correct a calcium deficiency until magnesium has first been given.

Hypomagnesemia can occur in cases of chronic diarrhea or vomiting, celiac disease, hyperaldosteronism, increased urinary losses from nephrotoxic drugs, or incomplete supplementation during prolonged parenteral nutrition. Additional cases can occur in infants of diabetic mothers, polycythemia of infancy, the short bowel syndrome, and in other various specific genetic conditions affecting magnesium homeostasis. Studies suggest that 13% of critically ill children and 32% of critically ill neonates may have hypomagnesemia. As described above, the ramifications of its delayed identification and treatment are profound especially when it is manifested as hypokalemia and hypocalcemia. The practitioner should be aware, however, that serum concentrations of magnesium may not accurately reflect intracellular stores and that current lab techniques do not allow for the accurate measure of physiologically active free magnesium. The practitioner, therefore, should consider magnesium supplementation when treating hypocalcemia and hypokalemia when replacement alone has failed.

SUGGESTED READINGS

Hamill-Ruth RJ, McGory R. Magnesium repletion and its effect on potassium homeostasis in critically ill adults: results of a double-blind, randomized, controlled trial. *Crit Care Med.* 1996;24:38–45.

Khilnani P. Electrolyte abnormalities in critically ill children. *Crit Care Med.* 1992;20:241–250.

Noronha JL, Matuschak GM. Magnesium in critical illness: metabolism, assessment, and treatment. *Intensive Care Med.* 2002;28:667–679.

Visudhiphan P, Visudtibhan A, Chiemchanya S, et al. Neonatal seizures and familial hypomagnesemia with secondary hypocalcemia. *Pediatr Neurol.* 2005;33:202–205.

144.

AVOID OVERAGGRESSIVE CORRECTION OF HYPONATREMIA AS THIS CAN PUT YOUR PATIENT AT RISK FOR CEREBRAL DEMYELINATION

CRAIG DEWOLFE, MD

WHAT TO DO – MAKE A DECISION

Hyponatremia may present in many medical conditions and requires careful assessment, treatment, and monitoring in order to prevent consequences of rapid fluid shifts in the brain. Sodium (Na) concentrations are maintained physiologically between 135 to 145 mEq/L by a balance of salt and water intake and excretion. Cells throughout the body respond to different serum concentrations of sodium by shifting water through an osmotic process, but nowhere in the body are the shifts as delicate as in the cells of the brain. If a patient has had an acute manifestations of hyponatremia, often seen during a course of intravenous hydration and demonstrates symptoms of hyponatremic encephalopathy, he or she would most benefit from a rapid correction of the serum sodium level. However, if a patient has developed hyponatremia slowly, he or she could be relatively asymptomatic but be at risk for cerebral demyelination (i.e., central pontine myelinolysis) related to sudden corrections in serum sodium levels. Taking a good history and having an understanding of the acuity of hyponatremia will help protect the patient from any devastating consequences of overly rapid correction.

Patients who are dehydrated, have had a recent operation, or have a contributing pulmonary or central nervous system disorder and have been treated with hypotonic fluids are at risk of developing hyponatremic encephalopathy from rapid fluid shifts resulting in cerebral edema. They often present acutely with lethargy, restlessness, seizure, respiratory arrest, or coma. In these circumstances, rapid treatment with 3% saline under the guidance of a specialist is beneficial. The treatment should be directed at increasing the serum sodium by 1 mEq/L/hr until the patient is alert and free of seizures, the serum sodium has increased by 20 mEq/L or a serum sodium level of 125 mEq/L has been achieved. One mL/kg of 3% sodium chloride will raise the serum sodium by approximately 1 mEq/L. Hypertonic (3% saline) should not be used in asymptomatic hyponatremia due to the risk of rapid fluid shifts.

© 2008 by Lippincott Williams & Wilkins, a Wolters Kluwer business

Patients who develop hyponatremia over a period of 24 to 48 hours or more should have their sodium levels corrected slowly. Animal and retrospective clinical data suggest a slow correction of sodium levels by no more than 0.5 mEq of Na per hour, with a goal correction of 15 to 20 mEq in 48 hours will limit the risk of cerebral demyelination. Cerebral demyelination, when isolated to the pontine region is called central pontine myelinolysis and is characterized by a 2- to 7-day delay in symptoms. Patients may exhibit dysarthria, dysphagia, spastic paraparesis, and a pseudocoma with a "locked-in stare." Lesions outside of the pontine region tend to present in a more variable manner, with movement disorders such as ataxia and altered mental status, including coma. In either region, serious disruptions can lead to death. Careful calculation of sodium and water needs and ongoing losses in addition to regular electrolyte checks, as often as every hour at the start of treatment, will help protect the patient from these neurologic syndromes. In addition, fluid restriction may help in certain cases of chronic hyponatremia associated with hyper or euvolemia.

The hydration status of the patient and urine spot sodium concentrations are helpful components in the diagnostic and treatment process. If a patient is dehydrated and has a dilute urine (Na <30 mEq/L), the differential diagnosis includes dermal losses through sweating or burns or gastrointestinal losses such as vomiting and diarrhea. If the hypovolemic patient has high urine sodium levels (urine Na >30 mEq/L), the practitioner should consider diuretics, cerebral or nephrogenic salt wasting, or mineralocorticoid deficiency as the etiology. In patients with hypovolemia, restore the intravascular volume with 1 to 3 normal saline boluses prior to adjusting the concentration of sodium in the fluids. In the hypervolemic patient with a low urine sodium, consider congestive heart failure or nephrotic syndrome in the differential, whereas a high urine sodium should lead the practitioner to consider chronic renal failure. In each of these cases, the practitioner should treat the underlying cause and use fluid restriction. Finally, in the euvolemic patient, the practitioner should consider syndrome of inappropriate secretion of antidiuretic hormone, hypopituitarism, hypothyroidism, or water intoxication through primary polydipsia or iatrogenic administration of hypotonic fluid as the cause. In these patients, fluid restriction is the mainstay of treatment.

The cause and acuity of the hyponatremia can effectively and safely dictate the rate of sodium correction. If the patient is acutely symptomatic, one should treat rapidly until the symptoms have resolved or until a 20 mEq/L increase in serum sodium concentration or concentrations of 120 to 125 mEq/dL have been achieved, whichever comes first. Thereafter, proceed cautiously with the sodium correction, ensuring that sodium levels are not altered >0.5 mEq/L/hr. This will help protect the patient from any devastating consequences of the initial insult and the correction.

SUGGESTED READINGS

Moritz ML, Ayus JC. Preventing neurological complications from dysnatremias in children. *Pediatr Nephrol.* 2005;20:1687–1700.

Reynolds RM, Padfield PL, Seckl JR. Disorders of sodium balance. *BMJ.* 2006;332:702–705.

145

AVOID OVERAGGRESSIVELY CORRECTING HYPERNATREMIA AS THIS CAN PUT YOUR PATIENT AT RISK FOR CEREBRAL EDEMA, CONVULSIONS, COMA, AND DEATH

CRAIG DEWOLFE, MD

WHAT TO DO – MAKE A DECISION

The principles of correcting hypernatremia are similar to those for correcting hyponatremia. Sodium is a functionally impermeable solute, and thus, it is the main contributor to cellular osmolarity and causes shifts of water across cell membranes. These fluid shifts may cause cells to expand or shrink more rapidly than the body can withstand. Rapid decreases in brain cell size caused by hypernatremia can lead to brain injury due to brain tissue separation from the meninges, rupture of the bridging veins, and venous sinus thromboses. Rapid correction of severe hypernatremia can also lead to significant brain injury from increased intracranial pressure and herniation, caused by rapid cellular expansion within the fixed capacity of the intracranial vault. Often, rapid iatrogenic corrections of hypernatremia cause more serious complications than the original disorder. Studies suggest that a patient with chronic hypernatremia is at a high risk for cerebral edema when the sodium drops >0.5 mEq/L/hr. To manage the rate of sodium decline, the practitioner needs to be aware of the general fluid status of the patient, select the appropriate initial fluid concentration, and be prepared to frequently alter its rate and concentration based on frequent checks of the serum sodium concentration and ongoing fluid losses.

Hypernatremia is defined as a serum sodium concentration >145 mEq/L. It represents a deficit of water in relation to the body's sodium stores and occurs as a result of a net water loss, or less commonly, a net sodium gain. It should be considered in patients who present with anorexia, restlessness, weakness, a high-pitched cry, hyperpnea, nausea, and vomiting. The greater and more rapid the water and salt disruption, the more significant the patient's clinical manifestations. Patients with sodium concentrations >170 mEq/L may have severe neurologic symptoms, including stupor or coma. Practitioners should have a high index of suspicion for hypernatremia when evaluating infants and other patients who have an impaired ability to control their free water intake.

© 2008 by Lippincott Williams & Wilkins, a Wolters Kluwer business

Hypernatremia invariably denotes hypertonic hyperosmolality and results in cellular dehydration, at least transiently. Cell shrinkage in the brain can result in vascular rupture, with cerebral bleeding or subarachnoid hemorrhages. Brain shrinkage is countered within hours as water moves from the cerebrospinal fluid into brain cells and electrolytes enter the brain cells. Normalization of the brain volume is complete within days as organic osmolytes (e.g., myoinositol) complete the osmotic restoration. Although brain water may be restored, the hyperosmolality of the brain persists. During rehydration, the brain can rapidly release the accumulated electrolytes but the loss of osmolytes occurs much more slowly, a phenomenon that acts to hold water within the cells. Therefore, slow correction of hypernatremia allows the brain to release accumulated osmolytes and prevent cerebral edema. In the case of overly aggressive treatment with hypotonic fluids, cerebral edema may lead to coma, seizures, and death.

To treat hypernatremia, the practitioner should consider the underlying cause and hydration status of the patient before determining the appropriate fluid resuscitation. Hypernatremic patients may be dehydrated from vomiting, diarrhea, or excessive sweating in addition to diuresis from medications, relief of a urinary tract obstruction, chronic renal disease, or hyperglycemia-induced diuresis. In each of the cases, attention to ongoing losses is paramount to treating the hypernatremia. Conversely, a hypernatremic patient may be hypervolemic from the use of hypertonic saline, tube feedings, or high sodium-containing antibiotics in addition to hyperaldosteronism. Finally, in the euvolemic patient one should consider fever, hyperventilation, and mechanical ventilation as well as diabetes insipidus if the patient has had unrestrained access to free water.

The goal of treatment is to safely but expeditiously correct fluid losses and re-establish sodium concentrations to 145 mEq/L. Practitioners can treat hypernatremia that develops over hours, for example, after emergent sodium bicarbonate loads during resuscitation procedures, by dropping the plasma sodium content by 1 mEq/L as it improves the patient's prognosis without putting him or her at risk for cerebral edema and convulsions. If the hypernatremia developed more chronically or if the time course of developing hypernatremia is unknown, then the hypernatremia should be corrected more judiciously at a rate of <0.5 mEq/L/hr or 10 mEq/day. Administering salt and water orally or by feeding tube is the preferred route of rehydration and as a result, the practitioner should be aware of the common salt and sugar contents of commercially available rehydration products (e.g., Pedialyte has the salt content of 25% normal saline [NS]). Emergent management of vascular compromise should be treated with boluses of NS (generally limited to 2–3), but once hemodynamics are restored, it is best to treat with D5¼% to D5½% NS to replace fluid losses, provide maintenance fluid needs, and manage the sodium disruption. Useful formulas for treating hypernatremia in the pediatric population are listed below. The formulas estimate the effect of 1 L of infusate (where NS consists of 154 mEq of Na per liter of fluid) on the calculated serum sodium.

$$\text{Change in serum Na} = (\text{infusate Na} - \text{serum Na})/(0.6 \times \text{wt in kg}) + 1$$

$$\text{Change in serum Na} = (\text{infusate Na} + \text{infusate K})$$
$$- \text{serum Na}/(0.6 \times \text{wt in kg}) + 1$$

where K = potassium, NA = sodium, and wt = weight.

Frequent early checks of the electrolyte concentrations cannot be overemphasized as the corrections do not take into account continued water and salt losses.

In summary, the practitioner should judiciously treat hypernatremia, maintenance fluid needs, and ongoing losses to ensure that sodium concentrations do not fall >0.5 mEq/L/hr and to prevent cerebral edema, seizures, coma, or death.

SUGGESTED READINGS

Adrogué HJ, Madias NE. Hypernatremia. *N Engl J Med.* 2000;342:1493–1499.
Moritz ML, Ayus JC. Preventing neurological complications from dysnatremias in children. *Pediatr Nephrol.* 2005;20:1687–1700.
Reynolds RM, Padfield PL, Seckl JR. Disorders of sodium balance. *BMJ.* 2006;332:702–705.

146

USE REPLACEMENT FLUIDS WITH APPROPRIATE ELECTROLYTE CONCENTRATIONS TO REPLACE THE FLUIDS BEING LOST

MICHAEL S. POTTER AND ANTHONY SLONIM, MD

WHAT TO DO – MAKE A DECISION

Pediatric patients may experience fluid loss and dehydration in a number of ways. The gastrointestinal tract represents one of the most significant sources of water and electrolyte losses that can result in dehydration and electrolyte imbalance. Accompanying these fluid and electrolyte losses are resulting acid–base disturbances that occur through bicarbonate loss in the stool or acid losses through vomiting.

There are several sources of electrolyte imbalance that occur through the loss of body fluids. *Table 146.1* provides the electrolyte concentrations for common gastrointestinal secretions. Being mindful of these electrolyte concentrations can assist providers in appropriately selecting replacement fluids and replenishing deficits.

To correct electrolyte imbalances caused by sodium, potassium, and chloride losses in stool and urine, maintenance fluids are frequently selected to augment the body's homeostatic mechanisms and compensate for the electrolyte imbalance. The general maintenance requirements for sodium are 2 to 3 mEq/kg/24 hour and the requirement for potassium is 1 to 2 mEq/kg/24 hour. As long as at least half of these elements are bound as a chloride salt, the chloride requirements will automatically be satisfied due when disassociation of the ions occurs. Most commercially available intravenous solutions are adequate for replacement and are much less expensive and error-prone than customized solutions. *Table 146.2* provides the electrolyte profiles for commonly available intravenous solutions.

© 2008 by Lippincott Williams & Wilkins, a Wolters Kluwer business

TABLE 146.1	ELECTROLYTE CONCENTRATIONS IN GASTROINTESTINAL SECRETIONS (mEq/L)					
SECRETION	[NA$^+$]	[K$^+$]	[CL$^-$]	[HCO$_3^-$]	[H$^+$]	RATE (mL/D)
Salivary	50	20	40	30	–	100–1,000
Gastric						
Basal	100	10	140	–	30	1,000
Stimulated	30	10	140	–	100	4,200
Bile	140	5	100	–	–	500–1,000
Pancreatic	140	5	75	–	–	1,000
Duodenum	140	5	80	–	–	100–2,000
Ileum	140	5	70	–	–	100–2,000
Colon	60	70	15	–	–	–

Cl$^-$, chloride ion; H$^+$, hydrogen ion; HCO$_3^-$, bicarbonate; K$^+$, potassium ion; Na$^+$, sodium ion.
(Used with permission from Wait RB, Seymour NE. Fluids, electrolytes, and acid-base balance. In: Mulholland MW, Maier RV, Lillemoe KD, et al. *Greenfield's Surgery: Scientific Principles and Practice.* 4th ed. Philadelphia: Lippincott Williams & Williams; 2006:224.)

TABLE 146.2	COMPOSITION OF INTRAVENOUS SOLUTIONS				
FLUID	[NA$^+$]	[CL$^-$]	[K$^+$]	[CA^{2+}]	[LACTATE$^-$]
Normal saline (0.9% NaCl)	154	154	–	–	–
$^1/_2$ Normal saline (0.45% NaCl)	77	77	–	–	–
$^1/_4$ Normal saline (0.225% NaCl)	38.5	38.5	–	–	–
Ringer lactate	130	109	4	3	28

Ca^{2+}, calcium ion; Cl$^-$, chloride ion; K$^+$, potassium ion; Na$^+$, sodium ion.
(Used with permission from Greenbaum LA. Pathophysiology of body fluids and fluid therapy. In: Behrman RE, Kliegman RM, Jenson HB. *Nelson Textbook of Pediatrics.* 17th ed. Philadelphia: Saunders; 2004.)

SUGGESTED READINGS

Greenbaum LA. Pathophysiology of body fluids and fluid therapy. In: Behrman RE, Kliegman RM, Jenson HB, eds. *Nelson Textbook of Pediatrics.* 17th ed. Philadelphia: Saunders; 2004.

Schiller LR, Sellin JH. Diarrhea. In: Feldman M, Friedman LS, Brandt L. *Sleisenger & Fordtran's Gastrointestinal and Liver Disease: Pathophysiology/Diagnosis/Management.* 8th ed. Philadelphia: Saunders; 2006.

Wait RB, Seymour NE. Fluids, electrolytes, and acid-base balance, Chapter 45. In: Mulholland MW, Maier RV, Lillemoe KD, et al. *Greenfield's Surgery: Scientific Principles and Practice.* 4th ed. Philadelphia: Lippincott Williams & Williams; 2006:224;191–242.

147

ADVISE THE INTAKE OF WATER TO INFANTS, THEY DO NOT HAVE THE RENAL CONCENTRATING ABILITY TO APPROPRIATELY MANAGE HYPOTONIC FLUIDS

CAROLINE RASSBACH, MD

WHAT TO DO – TAKE ACTION

Parents should be advised to feed their babies breast milk or infant formula exclusively for the first 4 months of life. They should be specifically advised not to give free water to their babies. Newborns do not have the renal concentrating ability that they will have later in life, and can suffer from hyponatremia if free water is given.

The newborn kidney has a lower glomerular filtration rate (GFR) and, therefore, a lesser ability to concentrate urine than the mature kidney does. At birth, the serum creatinine level is reflective of the mother's serum creatinine. This level then falls over a period of 7 to 10 days by about 50%, to a new level of approximately 0.5 mg/dL. The serum creatinine then continues to drop at a slower rate until 4 to 6 weeks of age, when the level is about 0.3 mg/dL. Although muscle mass increases with growth, the creatinine level remains stable during the first 2 years of a child's life. This is because of an increased GFR, which causes the creatinine level to stay the same despite an increased muscle mass. Beyond 2 or 3 years of age, any further increase in muscle mass is reflected by a rise in serum creatinine concentration.

The GFR at birth is approximately 40 mL/min/1.73 m². By 2 to 3 years of age, the GFR is at the adult rate of 100 to 120 mL/min/1.73 m². The serum creatinine level approximately doubles for every 50% reduction in GFR. Serum osmolality is maintained in a narrow range of 280 to 290 mOsm/kg. With increased osmolality, antidiuretic hormone (ADH) is released by the hypothalamus, resulting in tubular water reabsorption. With decreased osmolality, ADH release is inhibited and distal tubular water reabsorption is decreased. The hypothalamic response to changes in osmolality is fully mature in newborns. In fact, the kidney's ability to dilute urine is established early in gestation. However, the ability of the kidney to produce dilute urine depends not only on suppression of ADH, but also on adequate GFR. Therefore, in young babies, the ability of the kidney to dilute urine after a free water load may be delayed by the low GFR. Newborns

© 2008 by Lippincott Williams & Wilkins, a Wolters Kluwer business

are, thus, susceptible to water retention and hyponatremia after a free water load.

In healthy newborns, hyponatremia most commonly results from overdilution of infant formula or from feeding free water. Hyponatremia is characterized clinically by vomiting, weakness, seizures, and altered mental status. With progressive encephalopathy, respiratory arrest and cerebral herniation may occur.

Because of their relatively high GFR, newborns are not able to promptly and adequately dilute their urine to compensate for a free water load. They should, therefore, not consume free water during the first few months of life, but should instead consume breast milk or properly mixed infant formula exclusively.

SUGGESTED READINGS

Atiyeh BA, Dabbagh SS, Gruskin AB. Evaluation of renal function during childhood. *Pediatr Rev.* 1996:17(5):175–180.

Ruth JL, Wassner SJ. Body composition: salt and water. *Pediatr Rev.* 2006:27(5):181–187, quiz 188.

148

KNOW WHEN TO WORK UP PROTEINURIA IN CHILDREN

WILLIAM GIASI, JR., MD

WHAT TO DO – GATHER APPROPRIATE DATA

Detection of protein on routine urinalysis is a common finding. Its presence may be a benign condition or may be an ominous sign of renal parenchymal disease and renal failure. Therefore, the practitioner should be aware of the differential and follow a logical sequence to differentiate among the different etiologies.

In the normal kidney, the glomerular basement membrane allows for the passage of small molecules into the renal tubule while restricting the passage of macromolecules. Normal protein excretion is affected by the permeability of the glomerular basement membrane and tubular reabsorption mechanisms. Injury to the kidney that increases the permeability or decreases tubular reabsorption will result in increased loss of protein. Glomerular injury results in the loss of intermediate-weight proteins (i.e., albumin) and larger macromolecules. Tubular injury results in increased excretion of low molecular weight proteins secondary to decreased reabsorption.

The upper limit of daily protein excretion is 100 mg/m^2/day. In adults the limit of normal protein excretion is defined as 150 mg/day. Approximately half of the protein that is excreted originates from the plasma, with albumin representing the largest fraction. The upper limit of albumin excretion is 30 mg/day.

Proteinuria is detected by several methods. The most common test is the urine dipstick. The urine dipstick can only measure the concentration of albumin and can not quantify the amount of protein excreted. The dipstick commonly is reported as negative, trace, 1+ (approximately 30 mg/dL), 2+ (approximately 100 mg/dL), 3+ (approximately 300 mg/dL), and 4+ (approximately 2,000 mg/dL). In contrast, the sulfosalicylic acid test can detect the concentration of all proteins in the urine.

A quantitative measurement of urine protein excretion can be obtained via a 24-hour urine collection. A semiquantitative measurement can be obtained by a urine protein/creatinine ratio. Urinary protein excretion >100 mg/m^2/day or a urine protein/creatinine of 0.5 protein/mg in children younger than 2 years of age, or 0.2 mg protein/mg in children older than 2 years of age is abnormal. A urine protein/creatinine ration >3 is suggestive

© 2008 by Lippincott Williams & Wilkins, a Wolters Kluwer business

of nephrotic range proteinuria. Nephrotic range proteinuria is defined as $>1,000 \text{ mg/m}^2/\text{day}$.

Asymptomatic proteinuria is defined as a level of protein excretion above the upper limits for the child's age and generally <1 g/day without clinical manifestations such as edema, hematuria, oliguria, and hypertension. The prevalence of asymptomatic proteinuria on random samples ranges widely from 5 % to 10%. Asymptomatic proteinuria can be classified into several categories: transient, orthostatic or postural, and persistent.

Transient asymptomatic proteinuria occurs can be found in 30% to 50% of children. It commonly occurs in association with exercise, stress, fevers, congestive heart failure, extreme cold, and following abdominal surgery or a seizure.

Orthostatic or postural proteinuria is defined as increased excretion of protein while erect compared with while recumbent. This situation occurs under normal circumstances; however, the level of protein excretion is normally below the threshold for detection. The proteinuria usually does not exceed 1 to 1.5 g daily. It may be present in 60% to 70% of children with proteinuria.

Persistent asymptomatic proteinuria is characterized by excretion of protein for long periods without symptoms or clinical evidence of renal disease and by the absence of orthostatic proteinuria. The absence of other renal signs does not exclude renal disease. The differential diagnosis includes benign proteinuria, acute glomerulonephritis, minimal change disease, focal segmental glomerulosclerosis, membranous glomerulonephropathy, membranoproliferative glomerulonephritis, lupus, Henoch-Schönlein, chronic interstitial nephritis, hydronephrosis, polycystic kidney disease, renal hypoplasia/dysplasia, and reflux nephropathy.

Evaluation of proteinuria should begin with a complete medical history and physical looking for signs and symptoms of renal disease. At least two additional urinalyses should be performed on a patient with proteinuria; a urine protein/creatinine ratio on the first morning specimen and a urinalysis from the office visit. If the urine protein/creatinine ratio is within normal limits and the urinalysis is normal, then it is likely the patient has transient proteinuria. A normal urine protein/creatinine on the first morning void and the presence of dipstick positive proteinuria in the office is indicative of orthostatic proteinuria. Lastly, if both the first morning void protein/creatinine ratio and urinalysis are abnormal, it is indicative possible persistent proteinuria and requires further evaluation.

SUGGESTED READINGS

Bergstein JM. A practical approach to proteinuria. *Pediatr Nephrol.* 1999;13(8):697–700.

Feld L, Morris S, Frederick K. Evaluation of the child with proteinuria. *Pediatr Rev*. 1984;5(8): 248–253.

Gagnadoux Marie. Evaluation of proteinuria in children. UpToDate.

Hogg RJ, Portman RJ, Milliner D, et al. Evaluation and management of proteinuria and nephrotic syndrome in children: recommendations from a pediatric nephrology panel established at the National Kidney Foundation conference on proteinuria, albuminuria, risk, assessment, detection and elimination (PARADE). *Pediatrics*. 2000;105(6):1242–1249.

149

KNOW THE ETIOLOGY FOR METABOLIC ACIDOSIS BECAUSE IT CAN INFORM THE TREATMENT

MEGHA SHAH FITZPATRICK, MD

WHAT TO DO – GATHER APPROPRIATE DATA

Acid–base disorders are common in hospitalized and critically ill children. More specifically, metabolic acidosis is perhaps the most common acid–base disorder seen in children with illness. Patients with a metabolic acidosis have a low serum bicarbonate level with or without a correlating change in serum carbon dioxide levels. Normal serum pH is between 7.35 and 7.45; therefore, an acidosis is a pH of 7.35. The metabolic acidosis itself is only a sign of an underlying illness or problem that needs to be corrected for the acidosis to be treated. The three basic mechanisms causing metabolic acidosis are loss of bicarbonate from the body, impaired ability to excrete acid by the kidney, and addition of exogenous or endogenous acid to the body. Types of metabolic acidosis are divided into two main categories: with an anion gap and without an anion gap. The anion gap is calculated by subtracting the serum chloride plus the serum bicarbonate from the serum sodium value. A normal anion gap is ≤ 16. Serum albumin and phosphorus levels also can affect the anion gap but are generally not accounted for unless extremely abnormal.

Metabolic acidosis without an anion gap has two major causes in pediatrics. Diarrhea is the most common, causing a loss of bicarbonate from the body. If diarrhea persists, it can also lead to a lactic acidosis secondary to volume loss and hypoperfusion. The second cause of nonanion gap metabolic acidosis is renal tubular acidosis, which occurs in three forms: distal (type I), proximal (type II), and hyperkalemic (type IV).

Metabolic acidosis with an anion gap has several causes including methanol poisoning, renal failure/uremia, diabetic ketoacidosis, inborn errors of metabolism, lactic acidosis, ethanol or ethylene glycol poisoning, and salicylate poisoning. The basic dogma in treating an anion gap metabolic acidosis is to treat the underlying cause. Acidosis is thought to have a deleterious effect on cellular function and hemodynamics, such as depressed responsiveness of adrenergic receptors to circulating catecholamines, leading to decreased cardiac output. Other detrimental effects of severe academia (pH <7.2) include but are not limited to insulin resistance, increased free radical formation, increased protein degradation, gut barrier dysfunction,

© 2008 by Lippincott Williams & Wilkins, a Wolters Kluwer business

and potentially hemodynamically significant serum electrolyte disturbances, such as serum calcium and potassium. Some types of metabolic acidosis have specific treatments, such as insulin and fluids for patients with diabetic ketoacidosis. Insulin helps convert ketone bodies (acetoacetic acid and β-hydroxybutyrate) formed via increased beta oxidation of fatty acids during insulin-deficient states into bicarbonate, correcting the acidosis. Fluid helps correct intravascular volume depletion caused by glucosuria-mediated diuresis. Similarly, treatment of distal renal tubular acidosis with sodium bicarbonate helps buffer the academia secondary to the kidney's impaired ability to secrete acid into the urine. Treatment of lactic acidosis is not quite as straightforward.

Although it is very tempting to use sodium bicarbonate to treat a lactic acidosis in the setting of a severe academia, there are many side effects of sodium bicarbonate used in this setting to be considered. When sodium bicarbonate is administered, it is converted to carbonic acid then to carbon dioxide. If a patient's alveolar ventilation is limited, build up of carbon dioxide after sodium bicarbonate administration can cause a paradoxical academia. Another important consideration is that although arterial pH can be normalized with sodium bicarbonate administration, the body is composed of multiple compartments separated by membranes with differing permeabilities. Specifically, the carbonic acid formed after sodium bicarbonate administration diffuses easily across the blood–brain barrier, whereas bicarbonate diffuses more slowly. This can result in a drop in the pH of the cerebrospinal fluid and have a vasodilatory effect (specifically secondary to increased carbon dioxide on cerebral vasculature). If the patient is at risk for increase intracranial pressure or other intracerebral derangements, administration of sodium bicarbonate may contribute to further central nervous system deterioration. Finally, carbonic acid also diffuses more readily across cell membranes, so intracellular pH may fall instead of rise as the desired response would be to bicarbonate administration.

In conclusion, because of the potential deleterious effects of sodium bicarbonate use as outlined above, the use of sodium bicarbonate to treat a lactic acidosis is not recommended. Instead, it is prudent to determine the underlying etiology of the lactic acidosis and attempt to reverse this. In cases where the patient is severely academic (pH <7.2), the potential side effects of correcting the acidosis with sodium bicarbonate must be weighed carefully against any potential benefit of the treatment.

SUGGESTED READINGS

Behrman RE, Kliegman RM, Jenson HB, eds. *Nelson Textbook of Pediatrics*. 17th ed. Philadelphia: Saunders; 2004.

Furhman BP, Zimmerman J, eds. *Pediatric Critical Care*. 3rd ed. Philadelphia: Mosby Elsevier; 2006.

150

KNOW HOW TO DIAGNOSE AND TREAT METABOLIC ALKALOSIS

MEGHA SHAH FITZPATRICK, MD

WHAT TO DO – MAKE A DECISION

Alkalosis is a pathologic process that results in a decrease in the overall hydrogen ion concentration in the body. A metabolic alkalosis is the result of an elevated serum bicarbonate concentration. The normal serum bicarbonate level is 23 to 28 mEq/L. Therefore, a metabolic alkalosis is a serum bicarbonate level >28 mEq/L. The most common causes of metabolic alkalosis in children are emesis and diuretic use. The etiologies of metabolic alkalosis are divided into two categories based on the urine chloride level. A metabolic alkalosis can be thought of as a failure of the kidney to eliminate bicarbonate at a normal capacity.

If the urine chloride is <15 mEq/L, the metabolic alkalosis is considered to be chloride-responsive. This type of metabolic alkalosis usually exists with a concurrent potassium deficiency to decrease the glomerular filtration rate or enhance proximal fractional bicarbonate reabsorption or both. This combination of disorders evokes secondary hyperreninemic hyperaldosteronism. The alkalosis may be improved by correcting the chloride deficit through the administration of a chloride salt, either sodium chloride or potassium chloride. Common causes of chloride responsive metabolic alkalosis include gastric losses due to emesis or nasogastric suction, loop or thiazide diuretics, chloride-losing diarrhea, chloride-deficient formula, cystic fibrosis, and posthypercapnic states.

If the urine chloride is >20 mEq/L, the metabolic alkalosis is considered to be chloride-resistant and is generally secondary to hypermineralocorticoidism and hypokalemia. In this case, the alkalosis can be corrected by removing the excess mineralocorticoid. This type of metabolic alkalosis in children is then further divided into two groups based on normal and abnormal blood pressure. The etiology of chloride-resistant metabolic alkalosis with normal blood pressure in children includes adrenal adenoma or hyperplasia, renovascular disease, rennin-secreting tumors, Cushing syndrome, 17 α-hydroxylase deficiency, 11 β-hydroxylase deficiency, and Liddle syndrome, and an autosomal dominant disorder mimicking hyperaldosteronism. In children with normal blood pressures and chloride resistant metabolic alkalosis, common causes include Gitelman syndrome, Bartter syndrome

© 2008 by Lippincott Williams & Wilkins, a Wolters Kluwer business

(both renal tubular salt wasting disorders), and exogenous base administration.

The most useful diagnostic test to help determine the etiology of a metabolic acidosis in children is a spot urine chloride test. After the etiology of the alkalosis is determined, the treatment can be instituted by replacing chloride or removing the excess mineralocorticoid.

SUGGESTED READINGS

Behrman RE, Kleigman RM, Jenson HB, eds. *Nelson Textbook of Pediatrics.* 17th ed. Philadelphia: Saunders; 2004.

Brenner BM, Levine SA, eds. *Brenner and Rector's The Kidney.* 7th ed. Philadelphia: WB Saunders; 2004.

GASTROENTEROLOGY

151

PATIENTS WITH GASTROENTERITIS NEED A SLOW REINTRODUCTION OF FEEDS WHILE THE BRUSH BORDER OF THEIR GASTROINTESTINAL TRACT HEALS

ESTHER FORRESTER, MD

WHAT TO DO – MAKE A DECISION

Acute gastroenteritis (AGE) is an extremely common cause of morbidity and mortality in infants and children living in the United States and accounts for >1.5 million outpatient visits, 200,000 hospitalizations, and approximately 300 deaths/year. It is usually of viral etiology, most commonly rotavirus. Worldwide, diarrheal diseases result in 1.5 to 2.5 million deaths per year in children younger than 5 years. Rates of morbidity and mortality remain extremely high, but mortality has been dramatically decreased with the use of worldwide campaigns that promote the treatment of acute diarrhea with oral rehydration therapy (ORT). Although originally used in developing countries, the success of oral rehydration solutions (ORS) resulted in the first World Health Organization (WHO) guidelines for ORT. ORT is now the standard of care for acute gastroenteritis (clinically efficacious and cost-effective).

In AGE, vomiting usually precedes diarrhea by 12 to 24 hours. The patient may or may not have fever. Dehydration may exist, but its clinical symptoms may not be easy to detect depending on the degree of dehydration. Those at increased risk for dehydration include those who are younger than 12 months, have frequent stools (>8/day), have frequent episodes of emesis (>2/day), and who that are undernourished. Acute diarrhea is defined as ≥3 loose or watery stools per day. The volume can range from 5 mL per kilogram of body weight/day to ≥200 mL per kilogram of body weight/day. Viral diarrhea affects the small bowel and results in large amounts of watery diarrhea and midabdominal cramping. On the other hand, bacterial diarrhea results in smaller volumes of bloody, mucoid diarrhea, and lower abdominal pain. A bacterial etiology should especially be considered in children with

© 2008 by Lippincott Williams & Wilkins, a Wolters Kluwer business

TABLE 151.1	SEVEN PRINCIPLES OF APPROPRIATE TREATMENT FOR CHILDREN WITH DIARRHEA AND DEHYDRATION

1. Oral rehydration solutions (ORS) should be used for rehydration.
2. Oral rehydration should be performed rapidly (i.e., within 3–4 hours).
3. For rapid realimentation, an age-appropriate, unrestricted diet is recommended as soon as dehydration is corrected.
4. For breastfed infants, nursing should be continued.
5. If formula-fed, diluted formula is not recommended, and special formula usually is not necessary.
6. Additional ORS should be administered for ongoing losses through diarrhea.
7. No unnecessary laboratory tests or medications should be administered.

Adapted from Sandhu BK, European Society of Pediatric Gastroenterology, Hepatology and Nutrition Working Group on Acute Diarrhoea. Practical guidelines for the management of gastroenteritis in children. *J Pediatr Gastroenterol Nutr.* 2001;33(Suppl 2):S36–S39.

a history of travel, who have epidemic day care exposure, and who have high fevers, bloody stools, or severe cramping. Emesis may be the initial presentation of a variety of illnesses including appendicitis, urinary tract infection, volvulus, inborn errors of metabolism, diabetic ketoacidosis, and hemolytic uremic syndrome. Obtaining a thorough and accurate history is for the workup and diagnosis of AGE and should not be made prematurely.

Treatment of AGE with ORT often begins at home and begins with seven specific principles of therapy (*Table 151.1*). It is important to stress to parents that they have a supply of ORS in the home at all times for this reason. Early administration of ORS leads to fewer office and emergency department visits, and fewer hospitalizations. Parents should be encouraged to start this therapy as soon as diarrhea begins, and they should be trained to recognize signs of illness or treatment failure. Indications for medical intervention or evaluation include:

- Age younger than 6 months or weight <8 kg
- History of premature birth, chronic medical conditions, or concurrent illness
- Fever ≥38°C for infants younger than 3 months or ≥39°C for children aged 3 to 36 months
- Visible blood in stool
- High output, including frequent and substantial volumes of diarrhea
- Persistent vomiting
- Caregiver's report of signs consistent with dehydration (i.e., sunken eyes or decreased tears, dry mucous membranes, decreased urine output)

- Change in mental status (i.e., irritability, apathy, or lethargy)
- Suboptimal response to ORT already administered or inability of caregiver to administer

On initial presentation, the general condition of the patient must be assessed and an accurate weight and vital signs obtained (*Table 151.2*). A pre-illness weight may be approximated. The condition of the eyes, mouth, lips, and tongue will give an indication of hydration status. If deep respirations are present, it may indicate a metabolic acidosis; absent bowel sounds are consistent with hypokalemia. Recent studies show that the first signs of

TABLE 151.2	SYMPTOMS ASSOCIATED WITH DEHYDRATION		
SYMPTOM	MINIMAL OR NO DEHYDRATION (<3% LOSS OF BODY WEIGHT)	MILD TO MODERATE DEHYDRATION (3%–9% LOSS OF BODY WEIGHT)	SEVERE DEHYDRATION (>9% LOSS OF BODY WEIGHT)
Mental status	Well; alert	Normal, fatigued or restless, irritable	Apathetic, lethargic, unconscious
Thirst	Drinks normally; might refuse liquids	Thirsty; eager to drink	Drinks poorly; unable to drink
Heart rate	Normal	Normal to increased	Tachycardia, with bradycardia in most severe cases
Quality of pulses	Normal	Normal to decreased	Weak, thready, or impalpable
Breathing	Normal	Normal; fast	Deep
Eyes	Normal	Slightly sunken	Deeply sunken
Tears	Present	Decreased	Absent
Mouth and tongue	Moist	Dry	Parched
Skin fold	Instant recoil	Recoil in <2 seconds	Recoil in >2 seconds
Capillary refill	Normal	Prolonged	Prolonged; minimal
Extremities	Warm	Cool	Cold; mottled; cyanotic
Urine output	Normal to decreased	Decreased	Minimal

(Adapted from Duggan C, Santosham M, Glass RI. The management of acute diarrhea in children: oral rehydration, maintenance, and nutritional therapy. Centers for Disease Control and Prevention. *MMWR Recomm Rep.* 1992;41(No. RR-16):1–20; and World Health Organization. The treatment of diarrhoea: a manual for physicians and other senior health workers. Geneva, Switzerland: World Health Organization, 1995. Available at: www.who.int/child-adolescent-health/New_Publications/CHILD_HEALTH/WHO.CDR.95.)

dehydration might not be evident until 3% to 4% dehydration, increasing signs are present at 5% dehydration, and signs of severe dehydration are not evident until fluid losses reach 9% to 10%. Due to an overlapping threshold effect, updated recommendations group together cases of mild–moderate dehydration and show that signs of dehydration may be present over a wide range of fluid loss.

Laboratory evaluation should include a blood glucose level in those with prolonged vomiting or abdominal pain (to rule out diabetic ketoacidosis), and a urinalysis to rule out infection (especially in young females presenting with abdominal pain and vomiting). Electrolytes are generally *not* needed in a well-appearing patient. Stool cultures are also *not* necessary in most children presenting with vomiting and diarrhea.

Treatment includes two phases: rehydration and maintenance. During rehydration, the fluid deficit is replaced over 3 to 4 hours. At the end of this phase, clinical hydration is assessed. During the maintenance phase, maintenance calories plus fluids are given. The goal should be the quick return to a normal, age-appropriate, unrestricted diet. Gut rest is not indicated. Foods high in simple sugars should be avoided because they may worsen diarrhea (due to osmotic load); these foods include juice, carbonated soft drinks, and gelatin desserts. The BRAT (bread, rice, applesauce, toast) diet is *not* necessary or recommended in the treatment of AGE. In fact, it can result in suboptimal nutrition. Furthermore, the practice of "no food," for 24 hours is not indicated. Early refeeding is actually recommended in managing AGE. Luminal contents are a growth factor for enterocytes and help facilitate mucosal repair. Breastfeeding should be continued (even during the rehydration phase), and the diet should be increased as tolerated.

SUGGESTED READINGS

Dennehy PH. Acute diarrheal disease in children: epidemiology, prevention, and treatment. *Infect Dis Clin North Am.* 2005;19:585–602.

King CK, Glass R, Breese JS, et al. Centers for Disease Control and Prevention. Managing acute gastroenteritis among children: oral rehydration, maintenance, and nutritional therapy. *MMWR Recomm Rep.* 2003;52(RR-16):1–16.

McCollough M, Sharieff GQ. Abdominal pain in children. *Pediatr Clin North Am.* 2006;53:107–137.

152

CHRONIC LIVER DISEASE AND CIRRHOSIS HAVE A NUMBER OF ETIOLOGIES THAT ARE TREATABLE

MADAN DHARMAR, MD

WHAT TO DO – GATHER APPROPRIATE DATA, INTERPRET THE DATA, MAKE A DECISION

They present with a similar complex of symptoms including hepatosplenomegaly, nevi, varices, or hemorrhoids. The treatment principles need to be known and followed.

Injury to the liver results in alterations in hepatic structure and function due to cell (hepatocytes) injury. This results in inflammation or cell death, which leads to scar formation (fibrosis), and potentially nodule formation (regeneration). Chronic hepatitis is defined as a persistent inflammatory condition of the liver in which the biochemical and histopathological abnormalities are present for >6 months. Cirrhosis is the end result of virtually any progressive liver disease.

Chronic liver disease can be caused by a wide spectrum of etiologies including infectious, metabolic, genetic, drug-induced, idiopathic, structural, and autoimmune diseases. Many of these diseases have similar presentations and initial laboratory findings that definitive diagnosis can be made only by specialized laboratory tests and the histological examination of the liver tissue. Most acute hepatitis, if lasting >3 months, needs to be aggressively investigated to determine the etiology of the disease, because most of these diseases lead to chronic hepatitis, which may respond to specific medical therapy. Patients with chronic liver disease present with clubbing, spider telangiectasia, and hepatosplenomegaly (stigmata of chronic liver disease); and/or with evidence of severe liver disease (hepatic failure).

Based on the location of the inflammatory lesion on histopathology, chronic hepatitis can be chronic persistent hepatitis (CPH) or chronic active hepatitis (CAH). In CPH the inflammatory cells are limited to the portal triad preserving the lobular architecture, whereas in CAH, they are not restricted to the portal triad and enter the lobule thereby disturbing the lobular architecture. CPH is typically due to a slow resolving viral hepatitis, α_1-antitrypsin deficiency or Wilson disease. CPH is insidious in its presentation, with the patients being asymptomatic or with mild symptoms, whereas CAH presents with prominent clinical manifestations of liver disease.

ⓒ 2008 by Lippincott Williams & Wilkins, a Wolters Kluwer business

Cirrhosis is considered to be a clinical-pathologic state that represents the end stage of any chronic liver disease. Histologically, the liver shows scarring and regeneration nodules devoid of central veins, surrounded by bands of fibrous tissues which distorts the lobular architecture. The progressive scarring of the tissue in the liver leads to altered hepatic flow and increased resistance to portal blood flow, causing portal hypertension and loss of hepatic function. Patients with cirrhosis may be either in a compensated or decompensated state. In the compensated state, the patient is asymptomatic with physical findings of enlarged liver, spleen, or both; whereas in a decompensated state, patients present with symptoms of hepatic dysfunction, portal hypertension, or both.

Presentation and Diagnostic Workup. Chronic liver disease causes profound cholestasis, which can lead to nonspecific symptoms of liver disease such as fatigue, anorexia, abdominal pain, malnutrition and growth failure, and bleeding. These symptoms precede signs of jaundice, dark urine, and light-colored stools. The presence of physical signs of liver disease such as palmar erythema, spider angiomas, xanthomas, ascites, muscle wasting, and an enlarged firm liver and spleen indicates the chronic nature of the disease. Patients with cirrhosis present with splenomegaly, ascites, and gastroesophageal varices, which are indicative of portal hypertension. Hepatorenal syndrome is a functional renal failure in patients with end-stage liver disease. Hepatopulmonary syndrome is characterized by the triad of hypoxemia, intrapulmonary vascular dilations, and liver disease. Variceal bleeding and ascites are lethal complications of chronic liver disease and cirrhosis.

Evaluation for chronic liver disease involves a careful history and physical examination, and skillful interpretation of signs and symptoms. Previous history of acute hepatitis, jaundice during infancy, maternal and patient risk factors for hepatitis (transfusion, intravenous drug abuse, and ethnic background), family history of chronic liver disease and exposure to hepatotoxins. Initial laboratory evaluation includes a complete blood count; erythrocyte sedimentation rate; and liver function test, such as serum aminotransferases, total and fractionated bilirubin levels; alkaline phosphatase, and 5′ nucleotidase or gamma-glutamyltransferase. The hepatocellular function (synthetics ability) is specifically determined by measuring the serum albumin, and prothrombin time. These tests reveal the extent of liver disease and also help in determining the prognosis and response to therapy in a patient. These must be followed up with specific diagnostic test to determine the etiology of the liver disease.

Specialized diagnostic test to evaluate chronic liver disease includes measuring levels of serological markers for chronic hepatitis B virus (HBV) namely HBV DNA, hepatitis B surface antigen (HBsAg) and hepatitis E antigen (HBeAg). When these tests are negative, appropriate serological tests to diagnose other viral infections such as hepatitis C virus infection, cytomegalovirus infection, and Epstein-Barr virus infection need to be performed. Specific testing includes α_1-antitrypsin level in the blood to diagnose α_1-antitrypsin deficiency; serum ceruloplasmin level, a 24-hour urinary copper excretion to, and an examination of the eyes for Kayser-Fleischer rings or sunflower cataracts to diagnose Wilson disease. In addition, a normal sweat sodium level would rule out cystic fibrosis and autoantibodies for antinuclear, smooth muscle, mitochondrial and liver kidney microsome to help to make the diagnosis of autoimmune hepatitis.

Plain x-rays and abdominal ultrasonography help in determining the size and shape of the liver. Ultrasound may also help to define the architecture of the liver, the hepatobiliary tract and the blood flow in the liver. Ultrasound identifies anatomical abnormalities such as biliary atresia, and choledochal cysts and stones. Although computed tomography and magnetic resonance imaging may not play an important role in the initial diagnosis of liver disease, they do detect subtle differences in the parenchyma (storage disorders) and characterize liver masses clearly. Radionuclide scanning helps to detect abnormalities in liver uptake and parenchymal concentration and excretory abilities. Endoscopy is the most reliable method for detecting esophageal varices and bleeding. Liver biopsy (typically obtained percutaneously) is considered the definitive method by which to diagnose underlying liver disease. Histopathological examination of the liver tissue can identify the structural, genetic and metabolic disorders causing chronic liver disease.

Management of Chronic Liver Disease. The management of chronic liver disease involves mainly supportive or palliative care to relieve symptoms of the diseases. In patients with chronic viral hepatitis, interferon-α can induce long-term remission in 25% of treated children. In patients with Wilson disease, chelating agents such as penicillamine can increase the urinary copper excretion and slowly improve the clinical condition. The administration of ursodeoxycholic acid decreases xanthomas and relieves pruritus. In addition, it helps to decrease symptoms due to cholestasis by increasing bile flow. Patients must be treated for malabsorption that arises directly or indirectly from cholestasis and due to loss of hepatic function. Malnutrition due to malabsorption, and vitamin and micronutrient deficiencies are treated with dietary formula or supplements with medium-chain triglycerides, fat-soluble vitamins, calories, water-soluble vitamins, and micronutrients.

In patients with portal hypertension, a variety of surgical procedures allow diversion of portal blood flow and a reduction in portal pressure. Portocaval shunts and transjugular intrahepatic portosystemic shunt (TIPS) divert the portal blow flow and reduce pressure in the portal system. These procedures are prone to thrombosis and the diversion of the blood flow from the liver could also result in encephalopathy. Variceal bleeding is a life-threatening complication of portal hypertension which needs emergency treatment directed at prevention of initial and subsequent bleeding. Fluid resuscitation with crystalloid infusions, followed by the replacement of red blood cells must be performed with care because overresuscitation could increase bleeding. The correction of coagulopathy by the administration of vitamin K or the infusion of platelets or fresh frozen plasma may be required. In patients with prolonged bleeding, pharmacologic therapy to decrease portal pressure and endoscopic sclerosis of the esophageal varices need to be considered to stop bleeding. Ascites, another complication due to progressive liver disease is treated with salt restriction and spironolactone, the diuretic of choice in these patients. A paracentesis may be performed if the abdomen is tense, the child uncomfortable, or if abdominal distension causes respiratory distress. Central venous pressure should be monitored, and albumin provided in cases of low pressure.

Finally, liver transplantation with immunosuppression is the standard therapy for children with end-stage liver disease, life-threatening hepatic metabolic disorders, and cancers of the liver. The use of reduced-size transplants and living donors increases the ability to treat small children successfully. The prognosis for survivals is very encouraging. Most children have improvement in growth and development and the stigmata of chronic liver disease resolve.

SUGGESTED READINGS

Behrman RE, Kliegman R, Jenson HB, eds. *Nelson Textbook of Pediatrics*. 17th ed. Philadelphia: Saunders; 2004.

D'Agata ID, Balistreri WF. Evaluation of liver disease in the pediatric patient. *Pediatr Rev.* 1999;20(11):376–390.

Mews C, Sinatra F. Chronic liver disease in children. *Pediatr Rev.* 1993;14(11):436–444.

Rosenthal P, Lightdale JR. Laboratory evaluation of hepatitis. *Pediatr Rev.* 2000;21(5):178.

153

WATCH FOR GASTROESOPHAGEAL REFLUX (GER), WHICH CAN CAUSE SERIOUS PROBLEMS IF UNTREATED

ELLEN HAMBURGER, MD

WHAT TO DO – INTERPRET THE DATA

The presentation of GER can be varied, subtle, and differ considerably depending upon the child's age. GER is caused by transient lower esophageal sphincter relaxation, which allows passive flow of acidic and nonacidic gastric contents into the esophagus.

In infancy, reflux is likely to develop at approximately 1 month of age. Preterm infants may develop the condition even earlier. The incompetence of the lower esophageal sphincter allows the increasing volumes of breast milk or formula to wash up the esophagus, resulting in spitting up or frank vomiting. In addition to a motility disorder, there is now good evidence that food hypersensitivity is a cause of some cases of infant reflux. More severe symptoms occur in babies who reflux and swallow stomach contents, rather than spit up or vomit. These infants develop esophagitis from acidic stomach contents washing up and down the esophagus. Their clinical presentation is one primarily of arching and crying. In addition, they often have nasal congestion, frequent hiccups, and, less frequently, a cough. Parents often interpret the discomfort as "gas." In primary care settings, clinicians should ask about reflux symptoms at the 1 month well-child visit, because parents rarely recognize the fussiness associated with esophagitis as a symptom of reflux.

If the reflux progresses, untreated, feedings can be disrupted. After beginning to feed, babies pop off the nipple (breast or bottle) to arch and cry. Ultimately, feeding aversion and failure to thrive can result. Parents often report that the only time the babies will feed is when they are almost asleep. The more relaxed state seems to have a protective effect on the amount of refluxing. There is no clear association between apnea or apparent life-threatening events (ALTE) and reflux.

In older children, reflux can present with more classic symptoms of "heartburn" with chest pain and discomfort. Pulmonary symptoms, including recurrent pneumonia, exacerbation of asthma, or chronic cough can also develop. The interplay between asthma and reflux can be confusing. Cases of refractory asthma may warrant diagnostic evaluation for reflux or a diagnostic trial of acid-suppressant therapy.

© 2008 by Lippincott Williams & Wilkins, a Wolters Kluwer business

In infants, the diagnosis is made primarily by history. If weight gain is appropriate, further workup is often not necessary. For infants with accompanying symptoms of feeding difficulties or failure to thrive, diagnosis can often be achieved with a good history and a therapeutic trial as described below. When response to treatment is not adequate, further studies may be necessary to ensure correct diagnosis.

There is variability in the use of various diagnostic studies and are chosen in part based on symptoms. A barium swallow is advisable for infants refractory to treatment who have pulmonary symptoms such as cough, wheeze, or stridor. A barium swallow may demonstrate anatomic malformations such as a tracheoesophageal fistula, intestinal malrotation, or a vascular ring whose symptoms mimic reflux. In older children, it can demonstrate hiatal hernia and esophageal stricture. Children with dysphagia or odynophagia (painful swallowing) should also have a barium esophagram.

Esophageal pH monitoring is another valid and reliable measure of acid reflux. It can help in establishing the temporal association of symptoms and acid reflux as well as the adequacy of acid-suppressant therapy. For infants and children whose reflux is in large part nonacidic, it is not helpful. This may be particularly true for many asthma patients whose course is complicated by reflux. Finally, endoscopy and biopsy are useful to assess the presence and severity of esophagitis, strictures, and Barrett esophagus and to exclude other disorders such as eosinophilic or infectious esophagitis. It may be warranted in refractory asthmatics as well.

The initial treatment for infants includes conservative measures designed to keep the milk in the stomach; thickening feeds and the use of gravity. Feeding should be thickened with baby cereal (rice or oatmeal) starting with 1 teaspoon per ounce and increasing to as high as 3 teaspoons per ounce. Alternatively, there are commercial formula options that thicken on contact with stomach acid. Given the association of GER with food hypersensitivity, a trial of elimination of milk and soy from a breastfeeding mother's diet or feeding amino acid-based formula is worthwhile. Positioning should be either vertical in the caretaker's arms or lying supine on a surface placed at almost a 45-degree incline.

For older children and adolescents, conservative measures and lifestyle changes can provide relief. Positioning during sleep with the head elevated and lying on the left side can be beneficial. Further, these patients should avoid foods that exacerbate symptoms including caffeine, chocolate, alcohol, and spicy foods. Obesity and exposure to tobacco also have adverse effects on reflux.

In infants, if there are clearly signs of esophagitis (arching, crying, with or without excessive hiccups, nasal congestion), acid-suppressant therapy should be started before a feeding aversion develops. Older children with heartburn should also receive acid-suppressants. For infants and older children, proton pump inhibitors appear to be more effective in acid suppression and healing esophagitis than H2 blockers. Prokinetic agents have not proven useful. Surgical therapy for reflux is fundoplication. There are no good clinical trials comparing surgery to aggressive medical management comparing potential risks, benefits, and costs.

SUGGESTED READINGS

Heine RG. Gastroesophageal reflux disease, colic and constipation in infants with food allergy. *Curr Opin Allergy Clin Immunol.* 2006;6(3):220–225.

Nelson SP, Chen EH, Syniar GM, et al. Prevalence of symptoms of gastroesophageal reflux during infancy. A pediatric practice-based survey. Pediatric Practice Research Group. *Arch Pediatr Adolesc Med.* 1997;151:569–572.

Rudolph CD, Mazur LJ, Liptak GS, et al. North American Society for Pediatric Gastroenterology and Nutrition. Guidelines for evaluation and treatment of gastroesophageal reflux in infants and children: recommendations of the North American Society for Pediatric Gastroenterology and Nutrition. *J Pediatr Gastroenterol Nutr.* 2001;32(Suppl 2):S1–S31.

154

OBTAIN LIVER FUNCTION TESTS (LFTS) FOR A SPECIFIC INDICATION TO MORE SPECIFICALLY IDENTIFY LIVER FUNCTION ABNORMALITIES

DOROTHY CHEN, MD

WHAT TO DO – GATHER APPROPRIATE DATA

After a careful history and physical exam, concern for liver disease prompts many health care providers to order laboratory tests. LFTs are a commonly ordered panel when evaluating for liver disease. LFTs usually consist of aspartate aminotransferase (AST, serum glutamic-oxaloacetic transaminase-SGOT), alanine aminotransferase (ALT, serum glutamic-pyruvic transaminase-SGPT), alkaline phosphatase (AP), albumin, total and conjugated bilirubin, and total protein. However, all of these lab values are not always the best measure of liver function.

LFTs and other enzyme levels can help differentiate between two types of liver injury: (a) cholestasis or obstructive bile duct injury, and (b) hepatocellular injury. Therefore, if bile duct injury is suspected, it is valuable to measure the serum levels of substances that are normally excreted in bile such as alkaline phosphatase, bilirubin and gamma glutamyl transpeptidase. When there is toxic injury to the liver, enzymes that are normally within hepatocytes (i.e., aminotransferases) will be the most telling. However, to evaluate the liver's synthetic function, it is best to measure serum albumin and prothrombin time (PT), rather than LFTs.

The aminotransaminases include alanine and aspartate. ALT and AST facilitate the conversion of ketogluatarate to pyruvate and oxaloacetate, respectively. However, ALT is found primarily in the liver, whereas AST is found in the liver, erythrocytes, cardiac and skeletal muscle, the kidney, and pancreas. Serum levels of ALT and AST rise when there is either damage to the hepatocytes and other tissues containing transaminases, resulting in the enzymes being released or when there is an increased permeability of tissue, permitting leakage of the enzymes into the circulation. Given the concentration of ALT in the liver, it is more specific to liver damage than AST. The coenzyme for both aminotransaminases is vitamin B_6, so low levels of both enzymes may suggest vitamin B deficiency.

AP is primarily located in the canalicular membrane of the liver cell, so elevated AP levels often indicate obstructive liver disease. The highest

© 2008 by Lippincott Williams & Wilkins, a Wolters Kluwer business

concentrations of AP are in liver and bone (osteoblasts), and lower levels are present in the kidney, gastrointestinal tract, leukocytes, and the placenta. Sepsis and drugs can also affect the levels of AP. Other laboratory values should be considered in conjunction with AP when evaluating for liver function. For example, 5-nucleotidase and gamma-glutamyl transferase increase in liver disease, so coexistent elevations with AP assist in identifying the liver as the source of AP elevation.

Gamma-glutamyl transferase (GGT) is a mitochondrial enzyme found not only in the liver, but also the pancreas, spleen, brain, breast, small intestine, and kidney. In the liver, it is found within the centrilobular hepatocytes and the small bile ductule epithelium. In particular, it does not increase in bone disease, so it aids in differentiating the cause for elevated AP levels. Albumin is produced in the rough endoplasmic reticulum of hepatocytes. Therefore, synthetic liver function can be reflected in the serum level of albumin. However, it is also important to evaluate for other causes of hyper- or hypoalbuminemia and recognize that albumin levels decrease over time and often indicate chronic disease. The half-life of albumin, in contrast to many other proteins, is quite long (18 to 20 days).

Direct bilirubin is analogous to "conjugated" and "fractionated" bilirubin. The total bilirubin refers to unconjugated levels. A normal liver will remove unconjugated bilirubin from the blood and conjugate the bilirubin with glucuronic acid. The conjugated bilirubin can then be excreted in the bile. When hyperbilirubinemia is found, it is necessary to measure the conjugated and unconjugated levels of bilirubin. Elevated unconjugated bilirubin levels can result from either hemolysis or delayed conjugation in the hepatocytes, so it is not specific to liver function. In contrast, elevated levels of conjugated bilirubin raise concern for liver disease.

PT is one of the best short-term indicators of synthetic liver function. PT measures the time that is required for prothrombin (factor II) to be converted to thrombin. The half-life of serum prothrombin is short (3.5 days), in comparison to proteins such as albumin. Factors II, VII, IX, and X are vitamin K-dependent coagulation factors and require adequate liver function. Within the liver, vitamin K catalyzes the gamma-carboxylation of coagulation factors. Therefore, a damaged liver will not support these processes. PT that is not improved after vitamin K administration indicates that the liver is the primary source of the dysfunction, rather than vitamin K deficiency. When evaluating liver function when hepatic injury has occurred, factor VII has a half-life of 3 to 4 hours and, therefore, an improving PT represents improving liver function.

Ammonia is not produced in the liver but made from the action of bacteria on dietary proteins. However, the liver is active in the elimination of ammonia, so liver dysfunction can result in hyperammonemia. Ammonia requires proper collection and proper evaluation in the context of other laboratory values.

SUGGESTED READINGS

Bates MD, Balistreri WF. Development and function of the liver and biliary system. In: Behrman RE, Kliegman RM, Jenson HB, eds. *Nelson Textbook of Pediatrics.* 17th edition. Philadelphia: Saunders; 2004:1304–1308.

Corathers D. Focus on diagnosis: the alkaline phosphatase level: nuances of a familiar test. *Pediatr Rev.* 2006;27(10):382–384.

D'Agata ID, Balistreri WF. Evaluation of liver disease in the pediatric patient. *Pediatr Rev.* 1999;20(11):376–390.

Kaplan MM. Liver function tests that detect injury to hepatocytes. Available at: www.UpToDateonline.com Accessed on February 24, 2007.

Montgomery RR, Scott JP. Hemorrhagic and thrombotic diseases. In: Behrman RE, Kliegman RM, Jenson HB, eds. *Nelson Textbook of Pediatrics.* 17th ed. Philadelphia: Saunders; 2004:1654–1674.

Ng VL, Balistreri W. Manifestations of liver disease. In: Behrman RE, Kliegman RM, Jenson HB, eds. *Nelson Textbook of Pediatrics.* 17th ed. Philadelphia: Saunders; 2004:1308–1314.

155

DERANGED LIVER FUNCTION TESTS (LFTs) MAY REFLECT MUSCLE BREAKDOWN RATHER THAN A FAILING LIVER; THEREFORE, CHECKING A CREATINE KINASE IS IMPORTANT

CAROLINE RASSBACH, MD

WHAT TO DO – INTERPRET THE DATA

When checking LFTs, it is important to know that abnormalities may reflect a problem in a different organ system. "Liver function" is actually a misnomer, as only prothrombin time (PT) and albumin are actual measures of the liver's synthetic function. The other parameters are indirect measures of liver function. Deranged LFTs may represent muscle injury rather than liver damage, and checking a CK level is essential to determining the correct etiology.

The aminotransferases include aspartate transaminase (AST) and alanine transaminase (ALT). These enzymes are found within hepatocytes, are released during cell necrosis, and are the most sensitive tests of hepatocyte injury. Common insults include viral hepatitis, toxic injury (i.e., acetaminophen toxicity), and ischemic injury. The degree of elevation of the aminotransferases does not necessarily correlate with the severity of liver disease. The aminotransferases may rise slightly as a result of cholestatic jaundice because bile is hepatotoxic.

In addition to being present in the liver, AST is also found in cardiac and skeletal muscle, erythrocytes, and kidney and pancreatic tissue. Elevations of AST and ALT may represent muscle injury, with AST rising to a greater degree than ALT. Even strenuous exercise can result in mild elevations in the transaminases.

A CK level may be useful to help distinguish muscle disease from liver disease when aminotransferase levels are elevated. CK is a sensitive marker of muscle injury, as it is found predominately in skeletal and cardiac muscle. CK is composed of three types of dimers: MM is found mostly in skeletal muscle, MB in cardiac muscle, and BB is predominately in the brain and intestine. An elevated CK level is highly sensitive for muscle injury.

Other enzymes may also be helpful when interpreting LFTs. Lactate dehydrogenase (LDH) is present in blood cells and is elevated in hemolytic conditions. It is also released from the liver early in the course of viral

© 2008 by Lippincott Williams & Wilkins, a Wolters Kluwer business

hepatitis, and with space-occupying lesions of the liver. In addition, LDH is found in the lungs, kidney, brain, and skeletal and cardiac muscle.

Alkaline phosphatase (AP) is present in the canalicular membrane of hepatocytes and is elevated in obstructive jaundice. It rises to a lesser degree as a result of hepatocyte injury. It is also present in bone, kidney, and small intestine. During periods of rapid growth, AP will be elevated; therefore, age-specific reference ranges are important.

Unconjugated bilirubin is produced as a result of red blood cell breakdown and is conjugated by the liver. The serum unconjugated bilirubin may be elevated as a result of excess production, such as from hemolysis, or delayed conjugation, as in physiologic jaundice, breastfeeding jaundice, Crigler-Najjar syndrome, and hypothyroidism. Normally, bilirubin is conjugated by glucuronyl transferase in the liver and is excreted by the biliary tree. Conjugated bilirubin levels are elevated with biliary tract obstruction or infection.

Gamma-glutamyl transferase (GGT) is an enzyme present in the liver and biliary tree that rises in response to cholestasis. The level may also rise slightly in response to hepatocyte injury and to anticonvulsant drugs. It is present in lower concentrations in the pancreas, spleen, brain, breast, small intestine, and kidney. Because the GGT enzyme is very active in young children, age-dependent normals should be used for reference.

The two most direct measures of hepatic synthetic function are albumin and PT. Albumin is synthesized by hepatocytes, and levels fall as a result of decreased liver function. Decreased albumin levels usually occur late in the course of liver disease.

PT measures the time required for prothrombin (factor II) to be converted to thrombin. Because this conversion occurs in the liver, hepatocellular disease will result in a prolonged PT. The conversion of prothrombin to thrombin is vitamin K-dependent; therefore, any process that impairs vitamin K absorption, such as biliary obstruction where bile salts do not reach the intestine, will also result in a prolonged PT.

Finally, ammonia levels may be used to assess liver function. Ammonia is created in the colon as a result of the breakdown of dietary proteins. It is then eliminated by the liver under normal circumstances. An elevated ammonia level signifies a poorly functioning liver. Assessing liver function requires interpreting enzymes which are present in a number of tissues. It is important to know which tissues release each enzyme so as to accurately interpret the result. Specifically, when aminotransferase levels are elevated, a CK level will distinguish muscle disease from liver disease.

SUGGESTED READINGS

Digestive system disorders. In: Behrman RE, Kliegman RM, Jenson HB, eds. *Nelson Textbook of Pediatrics*. 17th ed. Philadelphia: Saunders; 2004:

Ng VL, Balistreri W. Manifestations of liver disease. In: Behrman RE, Kliegman RM, Jenson HB, eds. *Nelson Textbook of Pediatrics*. 17th ed. Philadelphia: Saunders; 2004:1308–1314.

Neuromuscular disorders: evaluation and investigation. In: Behrman RE, Kliegman RM, Jenson HB, eds. *Nelson Textbook of Pediatrics*. 17th ed. Philadelphia: Saunders; 2004:

D'Agata ID, Balistreri WF. Evaluation of liver disease in the pediatric patient. *Pediatr Rev* 1999;20(11):376–390.

Giboney PT. Mildly elevated liver transaminase levels in the asymptomatic patient. *Am Fam Physician*. 2005;71(6):1105–1110.

156

In Abdominal Pain, Performing a Complete Examination, Including Examination of the Genitals, is Important

Caroline Rassbach, MD

What to Do – Gather Appropriate Data

Testicular torsion and ectopic pregnancy present similarly to appendicitis, and both have serious morbidity if not quickly diagnosed.

The differential diagnosis for a child with abdominal pain is extensive. It includes problems from organs within the abdomen as well as from organs outside of the abdomen. Both testicular torsion and ectopic pregnancy can present with abdominal pain that mimicks appendicitis, and both can lead to significant morbidity if not quickly diagnosed. As a result, it is important to always perform a complete physical examination, including examining the genitals, when a child presents with abdominal pain.

Testicular torsion requires prompt diagnosis and intervention if the testicle is to be saved. Spermatogenesis may be lost within 4 to 6 hours of absent blood flow. It is the most common cause of testicular pain in boys older than 12 years, and is uncommon in boys younger than 10 years. Testicular torsion occurs in a testis that is inadequately fixated in the scrotum because of a redundant tunica vaginalis. This anatomical abnormality is called the bell-clapper deformity and is often bilateral. Testicular torsion usually presents with testicular pain and swelling, although in some cases may present with abdominal pain. The pain usually begins abruptly and without precipitating event. Occasionally there is a report of genital trauma prior to the onset of pain. The pain may be accompanied by nausea and vomiting. Physical examination will reveal swelling and erythema of the scrotal sac. The testis will be in a horizontal rather than vertical position and the cremasteric reflex will almost always be absent. Torsion of an undescended testis will present as abdominal pain; examination of the genitals will reveal an empty scrotal sac.

Suspicion of testicular torsion should lead to prompt intervention. In equivocal cases, a Doppler ultrasound may be useful and may reveal decreased blood flow to the affected testis. A ^{99m}Tc-pertechnetate testicular flow scan is a good alternative to Doppler ultrasound. False-negative studies can occur; therefore, highly suspicious cases should be treated immediately without

© 2008 by Lippincott Williams & Wilkins, a Wolters Kluwer business

waiting for radiologic imaging. When diagnosis occurs within 6 hours of the onset of torsion, as many as 90% of testes can be saved through either manual or surgical detorsion. Survival of the gonad depends on the amount of time elapsed since the onset of torsion, and on the degree of torsion. If the degree of torsion is <360 degrees, the testis may still be viable after 24 to 48 hours. Manual detorsion may be successful in approximately 25% of cases. Attempts at manual detorsion should not delay surgical consultation. Surgical intervention is indicated for failed manual detorsion, for removal of a nonviable testis, or as a first-line intervention for detorsion. Following detorsion, bilateral orchiopexy is necessary to prevent future episodes of torsion.

Ectopic pregnancy is another serious problem on the differential diagnosis for abdominal pain. If a delay in diagnosis occurs, the ectopic pregnancy may rupture leading to blood loss, hypotension, and possibly death. The mortality of patients with ectopic pregnancy is 5 in 10,000. Ectopic pregnancy occurs most often in sexually active patients with a history of pelvic inflammatory disease. As a result of pelvic inflammatory disease, these patients have inflammation, scarring, and adhesions in their fallopian tubes, leading to inability of the fertilized egg to pass to the uterus. Patients with a history of tubal surgery are also at risk for ectopic pregnancy.

Ectopic pregnancy can mimic appendicitis in presentation. Patients most often present with abdominal pain approximately 7 weeks after their last menstrual period, often with vaginal bleeding or spotting. Physical examination will reveal a normal or slightly enlarged uterus. Vaginal bleeding, an adnexal mass, and pelvic pain with manipulation of the cervix significantly increase the likelihood of ectopic pregnancy. A ruptured ectopic pregnancy may present with hypotension, significant abdominal pain, rebound, and guarding.

Ectopic pregnancy cannot be reliably excluded by physical examination alone. In order to diagnose ectopic pregnancy, a test for the β subunit of human chorionic gonadotropin (hCG) should be performed initially. This test turns positive within 1 week of conception, before an expected menstrual period is missed. Following a positive β-hCG, the patient should undergo ultrasound examination to determine whether the pregnancy is intrauterine or ectopic. Ectopic pregnancy should be suspected if the β-hCG level is >1,500 IU/L and the transvaginal ultrasound does not show an intrauterine gestational sac. Serial quantitative β-hCG levels can be used as an adjunct to diagnose ectopic pregnancy. With an intrauterine pregnancy, β-hCG levels will increase by at least 50% every 48 hours during the first 6 weeks of gestation. With an ectopic pregnancy, however, β-hCG levels do not rise to the same degree. Serial β-hCG levels may be helpful; however, diagnosis of ectopic pregnancy by this information alone is neither sensitive nor specific.

Once an ectopic pregnancy is diagnosed, it may be managed in several ways. An ectopic pregnancy with a low and declining hCG level, no fetal heartbeat, good follow-up care, and an ectopic mass <3 cm may be managed expectantly. When intervention is indicated, a nonruptured ectopic pregnancy may be treated medically with methotrexate or with surgery. Surgery is indicated in the case of ruptured ectopic pregnancy.

Both testicular torsion and ectopic pregnancy can cause significant morbidity if they are not quickly diagnosed. Both can present with abdominal pain and should be on the differential diagnosis for acute appendicitis. Therefore, a complete physical examination, including examination of the genitals, is necessary in the evaluation of abdominal pain in children.

SUGGESTED READINGS

Elder JS. Disorders and anomalies of the scrotal contents. In: Behrman RE, Kliegman RM, Jenson HB, eds. *Nelson Textbook of Pediatrics*. 17th ed. Philadelphia: Saunders; 2004:1817–1820.

Hartmann GE. Acute appendicitis. In: Behrman RE, Kliegman RM, Jenson HB, eds. *Nelson Textbook of Pediatrics*. 17th ed. Philadelphia: Saunders; 2004:1283–1285.

Lozeau AM, Potter B. Diagnosis and management of ectopic pregnancy. *Am Fam Physician*. 2005;72(9):1707–1714.

Paradise JE, Grant L. Pelvic inflammatory disease in adolescents. *Pediatr Rev*. 1992;13(6):216–223.

Ringdahl E, Teague L. Testicular torsion. *Am Fam Physician*. 2006;74(10):1739–1743.

157

PERFORM A DIGITAL RECTAL EXAMINATION ON EVERY YOUNG CHILD WITH CHRONIC CONSTIPATION TO EXCLUDE UNDERLYING ANATOMIC ABNORMALITIES THAT MIGHT ACCOUNT FOR THE CONSTIPATION

WILLIAM GIASI, JR., MD

WHAT TO DO – GATHER APPROPRIATE DATA

Perform a digital rectal examination on every young child with chronic constipation to exclude underlying anatomic abnormalities that might account for the constipation such as an imperforate anus with perineal fistula, intestinal obstruction (mass effect), or Hirschsprung disease.

Constipation accounts for 5% of pediatric office visits and up to 25% of referrals to pediatric gastroenterologists. In addition, this disorder may cause more anxiety and distress in the caregiver than the patient. Many caregivers worry that a child's constipation is a sign of a more serious medical problem. Constipation can be defined as the failure to completely evacuate the rectal vault of stool.

Functional constipation that results from fecal retention is the most common etiology of constipation in childhood, accounting for approximately 97% of cases. The differential diagnosis of constipation is lengthy. The common organic causes of constipation include anal stenosis, imperforate anus, anteriorly displaced anus, presacral teratoma, pelvic tumor or mass, spinal cord abnormalities, cerebral palsy, hypotonia, aganglionosis (Hirschsprung), hypothyroidism, celiac disease, and cystic fibrosis.

Although the likelihood of undertaking and extensive evaluation is small, an accurate history and complete physical exam is instrumental in establishing the etiology of constipation. The physician must be aware of red-flags in both the history and physical exam that would indicate an uncommon organic etiology.

The patient's history should begin from birth and include the birth history, timing of meconium passage, feeding history, changes in feeding type, and initiation of solid foods. In addition, it is important to gather accurate data on developmental milestones, such as the transition from diapers to toilet training, and a social history. The family history should be reviewed for evidence of genetic disorders such as cystic fibrosis, hypothyroidism, neurofibromatosis, or myopathies. The medical history should address

© 2008 by Lippincott Williams & Wilkins, a Wolters Kluwer business

previous surgeries and neonatal complications, such as necrotizing enterocolitis. The character of the stools should be reviewed and include the consistency, caliber, volume, and frequency.

In addition to plotting growth parameters and an abdominal and back examination, a complete rectal examination is instrumental in differentiating functional constipation from an organic etiology. As with other systems, the examination should begin with inspection of the perineum, looking for signs of infection, fissures, abscesses, fistulas, ulcerations, and anal wink. The positioning of the anal opening should be observed and documented if an anterior ectopic anus is suspected. The rectal exam should be performed with the child as comfortable as possible. The tone of the anal canal should be observed. The anal canal, although initially tight, should relax in the absence of a stenosis, stricture, or aganglionic segment. The normal rectal ampulla should be slightly dilated and may contain stool. The rectal ampulla should be palpated for the presence of internal fissures, pelvic mass, or tumor.

SUGGESTED READINGS

Abi-Hanna A, Lake AM. Constipation and encopresis in childhood. *Pediatr Rev.* 1998;19(1):23–30.

Biggs WS, Dery WH. Evaluation and treatment of constipation in infants and children. *Am Fam Physician.* 2006;73(3):469–477.

Di Lorenzo C. Pediatric anorectal disorders. *Gastroenterol Clin North Am.* 2001;30(1):269–287.

Fitzgerald JF. Constipation in children. *Pediatr Rev.* 1987;8(10):299–302.

158

USE OF ORAL MINERAL OIL AS A LAXATIVE IS CONTRAINDICATED IN INFANTS, BECAUSE ASPIRATION OF THIS MEDICATION CAN HAVE DEVASTATING CONSEQUENCES

DOROTHY CHEN, MD

WHAT TO DO – INTERPRET THE DATA

Constipation is a common phenomenon in children and can be very concerning to parents. It is the reason for over 3% of general pediatric visits and 30% of pediatric gastroenterologist visits. The consistency of stools, not the frequency, determines the diagnosis of constipation. Infants routinely have more than one stool daily. For older children, soft stools every 2 to 3 days can be normal; however, a hard stool with difficulty every 3 days is considered constipation.

The etiology of constipation can be either functional (nonorganic) or organic. When an anatomical abnormality or underlying disease process is not suspected, behavior and diet modifications are often used. Over-the-counter medications are also often tried by families. Oral mineral oil is one laxative that has been used to relieve constipation. However, mineral oil should be avoided due to the rare, but reported, complication of lipoid pneumonia.

Mineral oil, or liquid paraffin, is a hydrocarbon. It is tasteless and indigestible. Mineral oil acts as a laxative by decreasing the absorption of water from the intestine. However, the high viscosity of mineral oil depresses the normal cough reflex, even in patients with normal swallowing function. Patients with abnormal swallowing function are at even more increased risk of aspiration. Case reports of aspiration and subsequent lipoid pneumonia have been reported from mineral oil ingestion, rectal administration, and excessive lip balm application.

Once in the alveoli, mineral oil can result in chronic alveolar and interstitial inflammation, which then leads to exogenous lipoid pneumonia (ELP). The clinical presentation of ELP can be nonspecific and varies due to the amount of aspiration, frequency of aspiration, and age of patient. Diagnostic measures include computed tomographic scans, bronchoscopy, and open lung biopsy. Bronchoalveolar lavage that shows fat globules and lipid-laden macrophages is consistent with ELP.

Case reports of lipoid pneumonia have been reported in children and adults. There is no consistent clinical course; reported outcomes range from

ⓒ 2008 by Lippincott Williams & Wilkins, a Wolters Kluwer business

complete resolution, fibrosis, infection, and chronic lung disease to fatality. Treatment is primarily supportive, but there have been reports of administering prednisone and whole-lung lavage for diffuse pulmonary damage.

SUGGESTED READINGS

Bandla HP, Davis SH, Hopkins NE. Lipoid pneumonia: a silent complication of mineral oil aspiration. *Pediatrics.* 1999;103(2):E19.

Hoffman LR, Yen EH, Kanne JP, et al. Lipoid pneumonia due to Mexican folk remedies: cultural barriers to diagnosis. *Arch Pediatr Adolesc Med.* 2005;159(11):1043–1048.

159

IDENTIFY THE SOURCE OF
GASTROINTESTINAL (GI) BLEEDING

MINDY DICKERMAN, MD

WHAT TO DO – GATHER APPROPRIATE DATA

GI bleeding can be divided into upper GI hemorrhage (bleeding proximal to the ligament of Treitz) and lower GI hemorrhage (bleeding distal to that point). It is helpful to try and identify the site in the GI tract where the bleeding may originate from based on the color and nature of the bleeding, in context with the other presenting signs and symptoms.

The evaluation of a potential GI bleed should first establish the hemodynamic stability of the patient. Second, it is necessary to ensure that blood is present because many foods and drinks can discolor stool and vomit. The next step is to identify the bleeding source. A detailed history and physical examination with attention to the patient's age can clarify the source.

Upper gastrointestinal bleeding (UGIB) is an uncommon but potentially serious problem in children. Acute UGIB can present with hematemesis, which is defined as the vomiting of gross blood or coffee ground material, or with the passage of melena, maroon colored stools, or tarry stools. Occasionally, UGIB may present with hematochezia, blood per rectum, because the bleeding is very rapid and, therefore, not altered by the transit time through the digestive system. A nasogastric tube lavage that yields blood or coffee ground material confirms the diagnosis of an UGIB.

An initial priority when evaluating a child with suspected GI bleed is to assess both the hemodynamic stability and the severity of the bleeding, followed by resuscitation if necessary. A nasogastric tube may be helpful to assess extent of bleeding. Significant losses may be caused by hemorrhagic gastritis, esophageal varices, peptic ulcers, and vascular malformations. Both a gastroenterologist and a surgeon should be notified early on if a patient is suspected to have severe acute bleeding.

Many substances, such as red food coloring, fruit juices, beets, iron, and spinach, may color the stool or emesis red or black, and when ingested by children may be mistaken for blood. If unsure and if the color indicates blood, one should test the stool or the gastric contents by a guaiac test. Swallowed blood from the nasopharynx or respiratory tract may also be mistaken for UGIB and a physical exam may help clarify the source.

© 2008 by Lippincott Williams & Wilkins, a Wolters Kluwer business

In the United States, the most common causes of UGIB are gastric and duodenal ulcers, esophagitis, gastritis, and varices. It is helpful during the diagnostic evaluation to keep in mind the specific etiologies of GI bleeding at different ages. Common causes of UGIB in infants and toddlers include esophagitis, gastritis, ingestion of a foreign body, or swallowed maternal blood. Variceal bleeding is a possibility in a patient with portal hypertension. More rare causes are hemangiomas, aortoesophageal fistulas, hereditary hemorrhagic telangiectasia, Kasabach-Merritt syndrome, duplications cysts, parasites, vasculitis, gastric polyps, and systemic mastocytosis. Etiologies in older children and adolescents are similar to adults and include peptic ulcers, gastritis, Mallory-Weiss tears, varices, Dieulafoy lesions, and pill esophagitis.

Lower gastrointestinal bleeding (LGIB) is more commonly encountered than UGIB. Hematochezia, bright red blood or fresh clots per rectum, is usually a sign of a LGIB, typically from the colon.

As with UGIB, the etiology of LGIB varies depending on age. The most common diagnosis to consider in newborns are swallowed maternal blood, anorectal fissures, necrotizing enterocolitis, malrotation with midgut volvulus, Hirschsprung disease, and coagulopathy. Among older children, rectal polyps are the most common cause of rectal bleeding. Etiologies to consider among infants include anorectal fissures, milk/soy-induced enterocolitis, intussusception, Meckel diverticulum, hemolytic uremic syndrome, Henoch-Schönlein purpura, lymphonodular hyperplasia, and GI duplication. The most common causes of LGIB in the school-age child are infections, polyps, and inflammatory bowel disease. The age of the patients and the history and physical exam will narrow the diagnostic possibilities and guide the evaluation. A rectal exam is important to exclude anal fissures or polyps and obtain stool for guaiac testing. An abdominal examination for signs of portal hypertension, masses, or tenderness will aid in the differential diagnosis. Identifying malrotation is critical because it is life–threatening and requires emergent evaluation and treatment. The classic presentation is abdominal distention, bilious emesis, and melena, but this presentation only occurs in 10% to 20% of cases.

SUGGESTED READINGS

Arvola T, Ruuska T, Keränen J, et al. Rectal bleeding in infancy: clinical, allergological, and microbiological examination. *Pediatrics.* 2006;117(4):e760–e768.

Chawla S, Seth D, Mahajan P, et al. Upper gastrointestinal bleeding in children. *Clin Pediatr.* 2007;46:16–21.

Silber G. Lower gastrointestinal bleeding. *Pediatr Rev.* 1990;12(3):85–93.

Squires RH Jr. Gastrointestinal bleeding. *Pediatr Rev.* 1999;20(3):95–101.

160

OBTAIN A CONTRAST-ENHANCED COMPUTED TOMOGRAPHY (CT) SCAN AS THE GOLD STANDARD FOR DIAGNOSING PANCREATIC NECROSIS AND PERIPANCREATIC FLUID COLLECTIONS

MINDY DICKERMAN, MD

WHAT TO DO – GATHER APPROPRIATE DATA

Acute pancreatitis can be classified as edematous, interstitial pancreatitis (mild) or necrotizing pancreatitis (severe). Although most attacks of acute pancreatitis are mild and patients recover relatively quickly, severe necrotizing pancreatitis is associated with a high rate of morbidity and a significant mortality. Rarely, there are patients who present with early severe acute pancreatitis, consisting of extensive pancreatic necrosis and organ failure at admission.

Knowing the severity of pancreatitis helps determine the management and predicted outcome. Contrast-enhanced CT is the imaging modality of choice to assess the severity of acute pancreatitis and for detecting complications related to acute pancreatitis. Contrast-enhanced CT distinguishes between edematous and necrotizing pancreatitis because areas of necrosis and exudate do not enhance. CT is more accurate than ultrasonography for the diagnosis of severe pancreatic necrosis. It takes time for pancreatic necrosis to develop and is unlikely to be seen by contrast CT on the first day of illness. It is, therefore, more helpful to obtain a contrast CT if the initial diagnosis is unclear, if a child with acute pancreatitis is deteriorating, or is determined clinically or by outcome severity score to have severe pancreatitis. A radiologist is able to assign a CT severity index score based on the percentage of necrosis seen on contrast enhanced CT, which is used to predict outcome and dictate subsequent management in adults.

If necrosis is present, many adult centers will transfer a patient to the intensive care unit and initiate antimicrobial therapy with a broad-spectrum antibiotic such as imipenem. Infected pancreatic necrosis is associated with a high mortality (up to 80%). Surgical débridement of the pancreas is recommended if a patient is unstable or if there is evidence of infected pancreatic necrosis that is unresponsive to more conservative management.

Pancreatic injury from blunt trauma, although rare, is an important cause of pancreatitis and pancreas-related complications. Pancreatic injuries

ⓒ 2008 by Lippincott Williams & Wilkins, a Wolters Kluwer business

occur in <3% of children with blunt abdominal trauma. The typical mechanism of injury includes hitting bicycle handlebars, motor vehicle crashes, and direct blows to the abdomen (as may occur in child abuse). The pancreatic injury is thought to be from compression of the pancreas against the rigid spinal column or secondary to discrete intrusion forces. Young children, are more likely to sustain pancreatic abdominal injuries from blows to the abdomen than adults, because they have flatter diaphragms, thinner abdominal walls, and higher costal margins.

Children with pancreatic injuries due to blunt trauma may present with symptoms of vomiting or abdominal pain that radiates to the back. On examination, they may have epigastric tenderness that is persistent. Severe injury can lead to peritonitis and hypovolemia from leakage of pancreatic enzymes. If presentation is delayed, patients may have epigastric pain, palpable abdominal mass, and elevated amylase levels. It is important to know that children may or may not have bruising on their abdomen or back in the setting of significant abdominal organ injury.

Elevated serum amylase may indicate intra-abdominal injury but is not specific for pancreatic injury and, therefore, it is controversial in the management of children with blunt abdominal injury. The specific level has not been shown to correlate with severity of pancreatic injury on initial evaluation but is helpful when following serial levels if imaging is inconclusive. In the setting of abdominal trauma, pancreatic injury should be visualized by CT with an attempt to diagnose pancreatic ductal injury. Admission CT may not show pancreatic injuries and will likely not show a complicating pseudocyst. It is helpful to obtain repeat CT imaging if pancreatic injury is suspected. Although most patients do well with conservative management after pancreatic injury, those with ductal disruption may benefit from early operative management. The formation of pseudocyst does occur in a percentage of children after traumatic pancreatic injury.

SUGGESTED READINGS

Jobst MA, Canty TG Sr, Lynch FP. Management of pancreatic injury in pediatric blunt abdominal trauma. *J Pediatr Surg.* 1999;34:818–824.

Mattix KD, Tataria M, Holmes J, et al. Pediatric pancreatic trauma: predictors of nonoperative management failure and associated outcomes. *J Pediatr Surg.* 2007;42:340–344.

Mayerle J, Simon P, Lerch MM. Medical treatment of acute pancreatitis. *Gastroenterol Clin North Am.* 2004;33:855–869.

161

CONSIDER VON WILLEBRAND DISEASE (vWD) IN TEENAGE PATIENTS WITH MENORRHAGIA DURING MENARCHE

LINDSEY ALBRECHT, MD

WHAT TO DO — INTERPRET THE DATA

Menarche is often when the disease first presents in women.

vWD is the most common inherited bleeding disorder, with a prevalence of about 1.3% in the pediatric population. It can be caused by either a qualitative or quantitative defect in von Willebrand factor, a protein that plays an important role in both platelet adhesion and the transportation of clotting factor VIII. vWD is inherited in an autosomal manner; there is marked heterogeneity in the extent of bleeding symptoms, given the variance in possible underlying protein defects. Even in families with identical mutations, the extent of bleeding may vary. Symptoms of vWD may include easy bruising, heavy postoperative or postpartum bleeding, gingival bleeding, bleeding following dental procedures or extractions, and menorrhagia (heavy cyclic menstrual bleeding).

Menorrhagia is reported in the majority of women with vWD and may in fact be the only manifestation of the disorder. Menorrhagia beginning at the time of menarche is typical, with one large study showing that 65% of women with vWD report menorrhagia beginning at menarche (vs. 9% of women with menorrhagia without vWD). Menorrhagia often affects quality of life around the time of menstruation, and can be severe enough to result in red blood cell transfusion or even hysterectomy or other measures to prevent severe bleeding. In addition to menorrhagia, women with vWD have a longer duration of menstrual bleeding per menstrual cycle. Adolescent girls may be particularly prone to menorrhagia; the concentration of von Willebrand factor increases with age, potentially decreasing menstrual bleeding over time.

Among all women with menorrhagia, studies demonstrate that roughly 15% will have vWD. Smaller percentages may have other inherited forms of bleeding disorders, such as clotting factor deficiencies or platelet dysfunction.

© 2008 by Lippincott Williams & Wilkins, a Wolters Kluwer business

Given the significant proportion of vWD among women with menorrhagia, consideration of the disorder is appropriate, especially in the adolescent female presenting with heavy bleeding at or since the time of menarche.

History taking in a patient suspected of having vWD should include a detailed menstrual history, including how often the patient changes her tampon or pad on the heaviest day, how many tampons or pads are used for a typical menstrual cycle, and the length of a typical menstrual cycle. Because patients with vWD usually have heavy bleeding in regular cycles, irregular patterns of bleeding may imply another etiology involving hormonal imbalance. Quality-of-life issues, such as missed days of school, should also be assessed. A history of bleeding following procedures or interventions needed for bleeding (e.g., blood cell transfusion) should be elicited. A family history of bleeding may not be present but should be considered.

Basic coagulation studies are not sufficient as a laboratory investigation, as most women with vWD will have a normal activated partial prothrombin time (given adequate concentration and activity of factor VIII to produce a normal test result). International normalized ratio is typically normal and is not helpful in making the diagnosis. A von Willebrand profile, including von Willebrand factor antigen, ristocetin cofactor, and factor VIII level, is usually sufficient to make the diagnosis. A complete blood count should be performed to evaluate platelet numbers in patients with heavy bleeding but will also reveal anemia secondary to blood loss in many menstruating women with vWD. Additional laboratory testing, of course, should be performed as appropriate for the clinical situation, because many other scenarios can lead to heavy menstrual bleeding (i.e., hypothyroidism).

Adolescent patients with menorrhagia beginning at the time of menarche have an increased risk of having vWD. The diagnosis of this disorder is important because it allows the opportunity for minimization of a patient's bleeding risk prior to surgical procedures or childbirth. Additionally, because therapeutic options (such as intranasal desmopressin) exist, interventions can lead to the attenuation of monthly symptoms.

SUGGESTED READINGS

Kadir RA, Economides DL, Sabin CA, et al. Assessment of menstrual blood loss and gynecological problems in patients with inherited bleeding disorders. *Haemophilia.* 1999;5:40–48.

Kadir RA, Economides DL, Sabin CA, et al. Frequency of inherited bleeding disorders in women with menorrhagia. *Lancet.* 1998;351:485–489.

Kouides PA. Menorrhagia from a haemotologist's point of view. Part I: initial evaluation. *Haemophilia.* 2002;8:330–338.

Werner EJ, Broxson EH, Tucker EL, et al. Prevalence of von Willebrand disease in children: a multiethnic study. *J Pediatr.* 1993;123:893–898.

162

IN AN INFANT OR A CHILD WITH DEEP VEIN THROMBOSIS, BE SURE TO EVALUATE FOR A GENETIC PREDISPOSITION TO THROMBUS, SUCH AS METHYLENETETRAHYDROFOLATE REDUCTASE AND FACTOR V LEIDEN

EMILY RIEHM MEIER, MD

WHAT TO DO – GATHER APPROPRIATE DATA

Advances in the treatment of common childhood illnesses have led to an increase in the number of thromboembolisms (TEs) in children. Premature infants as well as children with congenital heart disease and cancer are at highest risk of having a TE, related to the use of central venous lines (CVLs) and other commonly used interventional therapies. CVLs account for most of TEs in children and are the reason childhood TEs are more common in the upper extremity vasculature than the lower extremity. *Table 162.1* lists common causes of TE in children. The incidence of TE is highest in two age groups: neonates, who have the highest rate, and adolescents, who have the highest incidence of spontaneous TE.

Physical exam findings are related to the location of a TE. Extremity clots are usually evidenced by localized painful edema and discoloration. Inferior vena cava or renal vein thromboses present with renal dysfunction or an abdominal mass associated with hematuria and thrombocytopenia. Pulmonary embolism classically presents with acute chest pain and respiratory distress. Common symptoms of stroke are hemiparesis in adolescents and seizures in neonates. CVL clots usually present with loss of patency or superior vena cava syndrome.

Imaging remains the gold standard in making the diagnosis of TE. The best imaging modality depends on the location of the TE. For example, an extremity TE is best detected by Doppler ultrasound, although a venogram may be required if a CVL-associated TE in the upper extremity is suspected. Suspected PE would warrant a spiral chest computed tomography scan or ventilation/perfusion scan. No laboratory test can confirm the presence of TE. However, in the last decade, numerous prothrombotic factors have been discovered. Unfortunately, little is known about the need for TE prophylaxis in the pediatric population based on these test results. Inherited prothrombotic factors can be divided into three groups: factors in the coagulation cascade, their natural inhibitors, or metabolic factors (*Table 162.2*).

ⓒ 2008 by Lippincott Williams & Wilkins, a Wolters Kluwer business

TABLE 162.1 CAUSES OF THROMBOEMBOLISM BY AGE

Infants
Catheter placement
Perinatal asphyxia
Infection/sepsis/disseminated intravascular coagulation
Congenital heart disease
Hypovolemia

Children and Adolescents
Trauma
Major surgery requiring immobilization
Nephrotic syndrome
Chronic steroid use
Medications (contraceptive use in adolescent girls)
Spontaneous

The most significant genetic risk factor for TE is the factor V Leiden mutation. It occurs in 5% to 15% of whites. Heterozygosity of this mutation, which causes factor V to be resistant to inactivation by activated protein C, increases the risk of thrombosis by six- to eightfold. Homozygotes for the mutation have 80 times the risk of clot formation compared to those without the mutation. Factor V Leiden mutations have been shown to be a risk factor in pediatric strokes. Prothrombin gene mutation also plays a role in pediatric stroke, but to a lesser degree. It is less prevalent than factor V Leiden mutation, occurring in 3% to 7% of whites. Prothrombin (factor II) levels can be increased by up to 30%, which leads to a prothrombotic state. Both factor V Leiden and prothrombin gene mutation cause venous thromboses in the majority of cases. Dysfibrinogemias are very rare and are inherited in an autosomal recessive pattern. They are usually associated with hemorrhage, but can cause thrombosis in 20% of cases due to faulty fibrinolysis.

TABLE 162.2 PROTHROMBOTIC FACTORS

Coagulation factors
Prothrombin gene mutation
Factor V Leiden
Fibrinogen (rare)

Inhibitors of Coagulation cascade
Protein C deficiency
Protein S deficiency
Antithrombin III deficiency

Metabolic factors
MTHFR/Hyperhomocysteinemia

MRHFR, methylenetetrahydrofolate.

Activated protein C is a vitamin K-dependent factor that inactivates factors V and VIII, effectively inhibiting thrombin formation. Deficiency of Protein C (PC) is inherited as autosomal dominant. Activated PC levels of <50% (normal 70%–100%) place children at increased of thrombosis. Heterozygotes are at increased risk of TE, especially during adolescence or their early 20s, Homozygotes for PC deficiency usually present in the neonatal period with purpura fulminans, disseminated intravascular coagulation, venous thrombosis of renal or mesenteric vasculature, or in utero strokes. Protein S (PS) is another vitamin K-dependent factor that enhances PC activity against activated factors V and VIII. Deficiency of PS is virtually indistinguishable from PC deficiency, with heterozygotes at increased risk for thrombosis and homozygotes having serious sequelae in the neonatal period.

Antithrombin (AT) inactivates factors IX, X, and XI, and thrombin. Children who are heterozygous for AT deficiency are at 10 times the risk of developing clots. These thromboses usually occur during adolescence. AT is the target of both heparin and low molecular weight heparin (LMWH). AT's effect on thrombin is increased 1,000-fold by heparin, whereas LMWH preferentially increases its effect on factor Xa.

Hyperhomocysteinemia causes TE mainly, although its actions on vascular endothelium, where it induces smooth muscle proliferation and decreases the effectiveness of heparin sulfate. Homocysteine metabolism is affected by MTHFR, which is important in remethylating homocysteine to methionine. Folic acid, cobalamin (vitamin B_{12}), and vitamin B_6 are important cofactors in this reaction. Homozygotes for MTHFR C677T mutation, and heterozygotes for the C677T and A1298C mutations, have mild hyperhomocysteinemia, but the true thrombotic risk of this is not well understood. Daily doses of the vitamin cofactors listed above have been shown to lower plasma homocysteine levels and potentially lower the risk of TE formation.

TE should be treated with anticoagulation to stop clot propagation and allow vessel recannulation. LMWH is the therapy of choice in children due to its decreased risk of bleeding complications, ease of administration, and minimal requirements for monitoring. Therapy should continue for 3 to 6 months following the event. In most cases, routine prophylaxis for TE is not recommended in children. The low risk of TE does not outweigh the risks of spontaneous bleeding associated with the prophylactic medications. However, neonates with homozygous PC or PS deficiency should receive fresh frozen plasma for PC replacement initially. They can then be transitioned to warfarin therapy. Oral contraceptives should be avoided in all patients with inherited prothrombotic conditions.

SUGGESTED READINGS

Cattaneo M. Hyperhomocysteinemia and venous thromboembolism. *Semin Thromb Hemost.* 2006;32:716–723.

Schneppenheim R, Greiner J. Thrombosis in infants and children. *Hematology Am Soc Hematol Educ Program.* 2006;:86–96.

Tormene D, Gavasso S, Rossetto V, et al. Thrombosis and thrombophilia in children: a systematic review. *Semin Thromb Hemost.* 2006;32:724–728.

163

PROVIDE FACTOR REPLACEMENT TO CHILDREN WITH HEMOPHILIA WHO ARE AT RISK FOR BLEEDING AFTER TRAUMA REGARDLESS OF THEIR CLINICAL SIGNS AND SYMPTOMS

EMILY RIEHM MEIER, MD

WHAT TO DO – MAKE A DECISION

Hemophilia A and B are bleeding disorders resulting from decreased levels of factor VIII and IX, respectively, and follow an X-linked inheritance pattern. Hemarthroses and intramuscular bleeds are the hallmarks of hemophilia. Even so, petechiae and mucosal bleeding can occur. Intracranial hemorrhage is the leading cause of death due to bleeding in hemophiliac patients, so special care must be taken with patients presenting with a history of head trauma or headache.

Normal levels of factor VIII and IX activity are 50% to 200%. Patients with <1% factor activity are considered severe hemophiliacs, those with 1% to 5% activity are considered moderate, and those with >5% activity are considered mild. Several types of factor replacement are available and used to treat patients with both hemophilia A and B. The vast majority of patients have a home supply of factor; it is of utmost importance to use of the brand of factor used at home whenever possible in an emergency situation. Hemophiliacs should be instructed to bring a home supply of factor with them if they have experienced trauma and need to seek care in an emergency department. If such a patient presents with a history of trauma and/or pain, factor should be infused immediately; even preceding diagnostic evaluation. This caveat is especially important if the pain and/or site of trauma is intracranial or intra-abdominal. These two sites are of special concern because of the risk of increased intracranial pressure with a head bleed and the risk of large amount of blood loss in the abdominal cavity before symptoms arise. Bleeding is the cause of pain in most hemophiliac patients and needs to be treated in a timely fashion to prevent long-term sequelae.

The dose of factor replacement is different for hemophilia A and B. The general rule for hemophilia A is 1 unit of factor replacement per kilogram of body weight to increase the factor VIII level by 2%, whereas for hemophilia B, 1 unit of factor replacement per kilogram increases the factor IX level by 1%. Joint, muscle, and other minor bleeding require 40% to 50%

© 2008 by Lippincott Williams & Wilkins, a Wolters Kluwer business

correction (meaning that type A hemophiliacs receive 25 U/kg of factor, whereas hemophilia B patients receive 50 U/kg); while head, ophthalmologic, or intra-abdominal trauma demand 100% correction (50 U/kg for hemophilia A and 100 U/kg for hemophilia B patients). Because the half-life of factor is fairly short (8–12 hours for factor VIII and 12–24 hours for factor IX), repeat infusion of replacement factor may be warranted, depending on the clinical situation.

SUGGESTED READINGS

Furie B, Limentani SA, Rosenfield CG. A practical guide to the evaluation and treatment of hemophilia. *Blood.* 1994;84:3–9.

Roberts HR, Eberst ME. Current management of hemophilia B. *Hematol Oncol Clin North Am.* 1993;7:1269–1280.

164

KNOW WHAT TO DO WHEN A SICKLE CELL PREP IS POSITIVE IN THE NEWBORN

HEIDI HERRERA, MD

WHAT TO DO – TAKE ACTION

Sickle cell disease (SCD) is the most common single gene disorder in African Americans. Other high-risk infant populations include the Mediterranean countries, Turkey, the Arabian and Indian subcontinent, Hispanic persons in the United States, and people from the Caribbean and South and Central America. SCD can now be diagnosed in the neonatal period and pediatricians should familiarize themselves with their particular state's screening program. A screening sample should always be obtained before blood transfusion regardless of gestational age.

A high-risk infant not screened at birth or who is missing documentation should be screened by hemoglobin electrophoresis as soon as possible. For infants with positive results, confirmatory testing should be performed at least before 2 months of age so that parents can be educated and penicillin prophylaxis started.

Confirmatory testing requires hemoglobin separation by electrophoresis (cellulose acetate and citrate agar), isoelectric focusing, or high-performance liquid chromatography. Solubility testing methods (Sickledex, Sicklequik) and sickle cell preparations are inappropriate diagnostic techniques for the newborn. These tests do not differentiate SCD from sickle cell trait. In addition, due to the predominance of fetal hemoglobin in newborns, it can cause false-negative results in infants with SCD. Solubility testing methods can always detect sickle hemoglobin in persons with severe anemia.

Most infants with SCD are healthy at birth and only become symptomatic later in infancy when fetal hemoglobin levels drop. Affected patients can present with painful swelling of the hands and feet (dactylitis), pneumonococcal sepsis or meningitis, severe anemia splenic enlargement, acute chest syndrome, pallor, or jaundice. Therefore, an early diagnosis can alert the parents before the disease becomes clinically apparent. Prophylactic penicillin should be started by 2 months of age and the heptavalent conjugated pneumococcal vaccine (Prevan). After 6 months of age, children can begin receiving influenza virus vaccines.

ⓒ 2008 by Lippincott Williams & Wilkins, a Wolters Kluwer business

SUGGESTED READINGS

American Academy of Pediatrics. Health supervision for children with sickle cell disease. *Pediatrics.* 2002;109(3):526–535.

Wethers DL. Sickle cell disease in childhood: part I. Laboratory diagnosis, pathophysiology and health maintenance. *Am Fam Physician.* 2000;62:1013–1020, 1027–1028.

165

KNOW THE DIFFERENCES IN TREATMENT FOR APLASTIC CRISIS AND APLASTIC ANEMIA

HEIDI HERRERA, MD

WHAT TO DO – MAKE A DECISION

Anemia can present in children who are otherwise healthy, or who have systemic disease or a known hematologic disorder. Anemia is defined as a reduction in red blood cell (RBC) mass or blood hemoglobin concentration, resulting in reduced oxygen-carrying capacity. Anemia can present as a single (infectious such as parvovirus B19) or multiple cell line defect, including bone marrow involvement (aplastic anemia). Therefore, children who present with anemia with associated symptoms should be carefully evaluated to promptly formulate a differential diagnosis, anticipate a life-threatening condition, confirm the diagnosis, and start appropriate therapies.

An aplastic crisis is an infection caused by human parvovirus B19 transmitted through exposure to infected respiratory droplets or other viruses that including cytomegalovirus, Epstein-Barr virus, and human immunodeficiency virus. The virus targets rapidly proliferating erythroid progenitor cells in the bone marrow and attaches to the P antigen receptor, resulting in reticulocytopenia and erythropoietic arrest. The RBC production is "turned off" for approximately 10 days. In patients with sickle cell disease, the RBCs only live for 10 to 15 days. Therefore, these patients are severely affected and will experience significant reductions in blood counts, with resulting congestive heart failure, cerebrovascular accident, and acute splenic sequestration. Confirmation of parvovirus B19 is performed with DNA testing. Patients with transient aplastic anemia or immunodeficiency will not test positive for immunoglobulin (Ig)M or IgG with the B19-specific antibody and remain contagious. Treatment includes simple blood transfusion to correct the severe anemia and prevent other organ complication or failure. After viral infection, patients will gain lifelong immunity with parvovirus B19, a one-time event for the patient.

Aplastic anemia is a condition of bone marrow failure characterized by peripheral pancytopenia and marrow hypoplasia. Aplastic anemia can be congenital (Fanconi anemia, Shwachman-Diamond, paroxysmal nocturnal hemoglobinuria, amegakaryocytic thrombocytopenia) or acquired (idiopathic, transfusional graft-versus-host disease, pregnancy, infectious: hepatitis, Epstein-Barr virus, human immunodeficiency virus, *Parvovirus,*

© 2008 by Lippincott Williams & Wilkins, a Wolters Kluwer business

mycobacteria). Aplastic anemia is also associated with exposure to substances such as benzene, and radiation, drugs (chloramphenicol, carbamazepine, phenytoin, quinine, phenylbutazone). Diagnosis can be confirmed with a bone marrow biopsy. The treatment includes suppression of the immune system or bone marrow transplantation for more severe cases. A short course of antithymocyte globulin and several months of cyclosporine to help modulate the immune system. Mild chemotherapy (cyclophosphamide and vincristine) may be effective. Steroids, although often used, are ineffective. Untreated aplastic anemia leads to rapid deterioration and death within 6 months. If promptly diagnosed and immediate therapy started, the survival rate increases dramatically over the next 5 to 10 years. A relapse of aplastic anemia is common.

Pediatricians should have a high index of suspicion with patients presenting with anemia as the primary event. A prompt and thorough evaluation of the acutely ill-appearing patient is imperative, with the aid of the physical and laboratory exams. Patients with aplastic crisis require simple blood transfusion until the marrow recovers. Children with aplastic anemia will require a bone marrow biopsy and aspirate to confirm diagnosis followed by prompt appropriate medical therapy.

SUGGESTED READINGS

Blackman SC, Gonzalez del Rey JA. Hematologic emergencies: acute anemia. *Clin Ped Emerg Med.* 2005;6:124–137.

Guinan EC. Clinical aspects of aplastic anemia. Aplastic anemia and stem cell biology. *Hematol Oncol Clin North Am.* 1997;1:1025–1044.

Wanki SO, Telen MJ. Transfusion management in sickle cell disease. *Hematol Oncol Clin North Am.* 2005;19:803–826.

166

CONSIDER METHEMOGLOBINEMIA IN INFANTS WITH DIARRHEA AS A CAUSE OF REDUCED OXYGEN SATURATIONS

CRAIG DEWOLFE, MD

WHAT TO DO – INTERPRET THE DATA

The differential diagnosis for the cyanotic infant should focus on pulmonary or cyanotic heart disease, but when the cyanosis does not respond to oxygen and the PaO_2 in the arterial blood gas is normal, methemoglobinemia should be considered as a potential diagnosis. Blood with significant amounts of methemoglobin (MHb) appears chocolate brown as opposed to dark red/violet, and the color does not lighten when exposed to oxygen (i.e., when placed on filter paper). The paradoxical elevation of PaO_2 despite a low saturation is a reflection of the normal oxygen diffusion into the blood with abnormal hemoglobin.

Pulse oximetry by measuring the absorbance at two light wavelengths only determines the saturation of functional hemoglobin: hemoglobin that is capable of carrying oxygen. Consequently, the pulse oximeter provides misleading results when significant amounts of carboxyhemoglobin or MHb are present in the blood. Co-oximeters, by using 4 to 6 wavelengths of light, are able to determine the ratio of oxygenated hemoglobin to all other hemoglobin types, including methemoglobin. MHb significantly absorbs light at both light wavelengths used in pulse oximeters, which is then interpreted by the photodetector as an increase in both oxyhemoglobin and reduced hemoglobin. Subsequent calculations lead to a reading in the mid-80s even as MHb rises to very high levels. Therefore, although levels of oxyhemoglobin are low, the reported saturation is falsely elevated. Co-oximetry, by contrast, is an accurate measure of MHb levels, because it measures this level directly.

Methemoglobinemia is a condition in which oxidized hemoglobin molecules cannot effectively bind oxygen and release it to the tissues. When ingested oxidants in food, drugs, or chemicals cause oxidation of ferrous iron (Fe^{2+}) in hemoglobin to the ferric state (Fe^{3+}), MHb is formed. Any increase in the percent of MHb will be manifest as a reduced oxygen-carrying capacity of red blood cells and can cause impaired aerobic respiration, metabolic acidosis, and death. Several physiologic reduction reactions, such as the cytochrome-b5-MHb reductase system, exist in the body to limit MHb to

© 2008 by Lippincott Williams & Wilkins, a Wolters Kluwer business

TABLE 166.1	SYMPTOMS OF METHEMOGLOBINEMIA BASED ON CONCENTRATION AND PERCENTAGE	
METHEMOGLOBIN CONCENTRATION IN G/DL	% TOTAL HEMOGLOBIN (ASSUMING HGB = 15 G/DL)	SYMPTOMS
<1.5	<10	None
1.5–3	10–20	Cyanotic skin discoloration
3–4.5	20–30	Anxiety, tachycardia
4.5–7.5	30–50	Lethargy, tachypnea, and increased tachycardia
7.5–10.5	50–70	Coma, seizures, arrhythmia, acidosis
>10.5	>70	Death

Hbg, hemoglobin.

<2% of normal circulating hemoglobin. In anemic patients with a given MHb level, the pathologic effects will be more severe, as the true effect of the condition relates to the remaining concentration of functioning hemoglobin rather than the percent of MHb (*Table 166.1*).

Methemoglobinemia can be a congenital or acquired disorder. In neonates, genetic deficiencies in the enzymes associated with the cytochrome-b5-MHb reductase system may cause congenital cyanosis. Agents such as nitrates (found in some well water, and in vegetables such as spinach, beets, and cabbages), as well as aniline dye, benzocaine, dapsone, and phenazopyridine (Pyridium) can lead to high levels of MHb and are the most common cause for methemoglobinemia in infants older than 6 months. But, in healthy infants younger than 6 months of age, there are several factors that put them at risk for methemoglobinemia even in absence of ingestion of large quantities of oxidants. First, infants do not achieve adult levels of the cytochrome-b5-MHb reductase enzymes until 4 months of life. Second, fetal hemoglobin is more easily oxidized than hemoglobin A. Finally, the higher gastric pH in infants allows gram-negative bacterial proliferation that convert dietary nitrates to nitrites which are potent oxidizing agents.

The most common cause of methemoglobinemia in infants younger than 6 months is multifactorial, but the common endpoint seems to be acidosis or diarrhea. Studies suggest that subclinical and clinically significant methemoglobinemia occurs more frequently in this population than previously known. Associated factors include dehydration, low chloride, and growth curves <10% for weight. The practitioner should have a high index of suspicion for methemoglobinemia when evaluating infants with diarrhea who appear dehydrated, cyanotic, tachypneic, or acidotic.

The first step in treating methemoglobinemia is removal of the oxidizing stress; whether that is hydration and providing bicarbonate in a patient with diarrhea and acidosis or eliminating the oxidizing source in a patient with ingestion. In addition, adequate glucose levels should be ensured in order to supply endogenous reducing enzymes with sufficient substrate. When the patient's MHb level reaches symptomatic states, between 15% and 30% depending on the baseline hemoglobin level, a trial of methylene blue (1% solution) is warranted. The dose is 1 to 2 mg/kg over 3 to 5 minutes. It can be repeated in 30 minutes if the MHb is still considered dangerously high. Patients with significant glucose-6-phosphate dehydrogenase (G6PD) deficiency may be at risk of hemolysis or paradoxical elevation in the MHb level when dosed methylene blue, but because patients most often only have a partial G6PD deficiency, it is still the first-line treatment in these patients for life-threatening disease. In patients with known G6PD deficiency, the dose of methylene blue is reduced to 0.3 to 0.5 mg/kg and titrated upward for positive effect. If the patient's condition worsens, then exchange transfusion is the second-line treatment.

In summary, methemoglobinemia should be considered in cyanotic patients who have diarrhea and are acidotic, especially for those with normal PaO_2 levels. Confirmation of the diagnosis should be obtained by measuring the methemoglobin and saturation level directly with a co-oximeter. The treatment is aimed at resolving the underlying etiology—normalization of pH and rehydration most often in infants younger than 6 months of age and detoxification in older children—and methylene blue for more significant disease.

SUGGESTED READINGS

Lebby T, Roco JJ, Arcinue EL. Infantile methemoglobinemia associated with acute diarrheal illness. *Am J Emerg Med.* 1993;11:471–472.

Pollack ES, Pollack CV Jr. Incidence of subclinical methemoglobinemia in infants with diarrhea. *Ann Emerg Med.* 1994;24:652–656.

Wright RO, Lewander WJ, Woolf AD. Methemoglobinemia: etiology, pharmacology, and clinical management. *Ann Emerg Med.* 1999;34:646–656.

Yano SS, Danish EH, Hsia YE. Transient methemoglobinemia with acidosis in infants. *J Pediatr.* 1982;100:415–418.

167

CONSIDER THE EXCESSIVE INGESTION OF COW'S MILK AS A CAUSE OF DRAMATIC ANEMIA IN TODDLERS

CAROLINE RASSBACH, MD

WHAT TO DO – INTERPRET THE DATA

Iron deficiency is the most common nutritional deficiency in children in the United States. Its prevalence in infants younger than 1 year of age has decreased owing to improved nutrition; however, iron deficiency in toddlers remains a significant problem. Excessive consumption of cow's milk and other iron-poor foods can lead to iron deficiency. Iron deficiency, in turn, can lead to remarkable anemia and to long-term cognitive deficits. Therefore, in toddlers with dramatic anemia, the excessive ingestion of cow's milk is a consideration.

Iron is necessary for hemoglobin production, which is required for oxygen transport. Healthy term infants are born with enough iron stores to last about 6 to 9 months. Dietary iron is required for growth and to replace daily iron losses. Inadequate dietary intake and poor absorption of iron contribute to iron deficiency.

The American Academy of Pediatrics (AAP) recommends that infants younger than 1 year of age consume breast milk or iron-fortified cow's milk formula. Breast milk contains less iron than does iron-fortified formula, yet it is better absorbed. Between 4 and 6 months of age, infants require an additional source of iron, such as an iron-fortified cereal. After 1 year of age, children should consume 16 oz/day of vitamin D-fortified whole milk and a variety of healthy table foods.

Risk factors for iron deficiency include early introduction of cow's milk at younger than 1 year of age and consumption of >24 oz/day of cow's milk. Cow's milk contains very little iron and often replaces foods that are rich in iron. In addition, cow's milk inhibits iron absorption from other food sources and can cause occult intestinal bleeding.

Most of the body's iron is in the form of hemoglobin. Iron is stored in the liver, spleen, and bone marrow as ferritin. Children who do not consume enough dietary iron will initially use their iron stores to continue hemoglobin production. The red cell distribution width detects anisocytosis and is usually the first detectable laboratory sign of anemia. A red cell distribution width >14.5% is consistent with iron-deficiency anemia. The red

© 2008 by Lippincott Williams & Wilkins, a Wolters Kluwer business

blood cells also become smaller than normal and their hemoglobin content decreases, as evidenced by lower mean corpuscular hemoglobin and mean corpuscular volume. Nucleated red blood cells and thrombocytosis may be evident. Serum ferritin levels also decline with iron deficiency, and levels <8 to 12 μg/L are characteristic.

If poor dietary consumption of iron continues, serum iron levels will decrease to <30 μg/dL. Total iron-binding capacity will rise as iron levels fall. Protoporphyrins, the hemoglobin precursor molecules that lack iron, accumulate and can be detected as free erythrocyte protoporphyrin. As the hemoglobin concentration falls, anemia ensues. Symptoms of anemia may include pallor, tachycardia, and fatigue, although with mild anemia, often no symptoms are present. Patients may report a desire to eat unusual substances such as ice or dirt. With hemoglobin concentrations <5 g/dL, irritability and anorexia are prominent. Tachycardia, fainting, and congestive heart failure may occur.

Children with iron-deficiency anemia may suffer long-term consequences, including poorer attention and decreased performance on motor and mental development tests. The duration and severity of anemia correlate with poorer test performance.

Treatment of anemia consists of a therapeutic trial of iron in a dosage of 3 to 6 mg/kg/day of elemental iron. If hemoglobin concentrations increase by 1 g/dL or more after 1 month of therapy, iron deficiency is confirmed. Reticulocytosis begins at 7 to 10 days after initiating therapy. Therapy should be continued for 2 to 3 months to replenish iron stores. Dietary modification includes limiting the ingestion of cow's milk to <24 oz daily.

Excessive and early consumption of cow's milk is a major risk factor for iron-deficiency anemia. The anemia can be dramatic. A detailed dietary history is essential to diagnose anemia.

SUGGESTED READINGS

Cheng TL. Iron deficiency anemia. *Pediatr Rev.* 1998;19(9):321–322.

Glader B. Iron-deficiency anemia, Chapter 447. In: Behrman RE, Kliegman RM, Jenson HB, eds. *Nelson Textbook of Pediatrics.* 17th ed. Philadelphia: Saunders; 2004:1614–1616.

168

CONSIDER CHECKING A FIBRINOGEN LEVEL IN EXCESSIVELY BLEEDING PATIENTS BECAUSE IF IT IS NOT REPLACED WITH CRYOPRECIPITATE, THEY WILL BE UNABLE TO FORM CLOTS

DOROTHY CHEN, MD

WHAT TO DO – GATHER APPROPRIATE DATA

Patients can present with bleeding after trauma, during or after a procedure, or secondary to a critical clinical state. Fortunately, the body's hemostatic processes normally respond by stopping and preventing further bleeding. Clotting requires adequate levels of both platelets and coagulation factors. Disorders of primary hemostasis indicate an abnormality in the blood vessels or platelets, whereas disorders of secondary hemostasis indicate an abnormality in the coagulation factors. The end goal of the coagulation cascade is the formation of the fibrin clot. Prothrombin is converted to thrombin, and thrombin converts fibrinogen to fibrin.

Understanding the coagulation cascade explains the rationale behind commonly ordered screening tests: complete blood count, prothrombin time, and partial thromboplastin time. When the screening tests are normal and bleeding persists, it is important to consider checking a fibrinogen level. Fibrinogen (coagulation factor I) is required to ultimately form the fibrin clot. If this factor is not adequately replaced, the patient will not be able to clot properly. Among the many available blood products used for transfusion are packed red blood cells, platelets, fresh frozen plasma (FFP), and cryoprecipitate. FFP contains the acellular components of whole blood and can be administered for volume expansion and/or the replacement of specific plasma components.

In contrast, cryoprecipitate is a concentrate containing fibrinogen, factor VIII, factor XIII, von Willebrand factor, and fibronectin. Therefore, identifying a specific coagulation factor deficiency can focus the treatment regimen. If the level of fibrinogen is low, cryoprecipitate can effectively improve hemostasis. Although FFP has the same factors as cryoprecipitate, the concentrations in FFP are much lower and inadequate to replace dramatically depleted levels. Therefore, if a patient's fibrinogen level is inadequate, FFP will not correct the problem. Only cryoprecipitate will boost the fibrinogen levels adequately.

© 2008 by Lippincott Williams & Wilkins, a Wolters Kluwer business

One of the benefits of cryoprecipitate is its concentrated nature; cryoprecipitate can effectively replace fibrinogen with a smaller volume. For a normovolemic patient, administering cryoprecipitate, rather than FFP, is extremely important because it can prevent volume overload and be timelier.

SUGGESTED READINGS

Journeycake JM, Buchanan GR. Coagulation disorders. *Pediatr Rev.* 2003;24(3):83–91.

Montgomery RR, Scott JP. Hemorrhagic and thrombotic diseases. In: Behrman RE, Kliegman RM, Jenson HB, eds. *Nelson Textbook of Pediatrics.* 17th ed. Philadelphia: Saunders; 2004:1651–1674.

Sieger L. Blood, blood components, and transfusion reactions. In: Barin R. *Pediatric Emergency Medicine.* 2nd ed. St. Louis: Mosby-Year Book, Inc.; 1997:190–195.

169

ACUTE CHEST SYNDROME (ACS) IS NOT JUST PRECIPITATED BY INFECTION

SARIKA JOSHI, MD

WHAT TO DO – GATHER APPROPRIATE DATA

There is a need to treat the multiple causes of ACS.

ACS is a common complication and reason for hospital admission in children with sickle cell disease (SCD). It is also the most common cause of death in this patient population. ACS is defined as a new pulmonary infiltrate, involving at least one complete segment, on chest radiograph and at least one of the following signs or symptoms: (a) chest pain; (b) fever; (c) increased work of breathing (i.e., use of accessory muscles, nasal flaring), tachypnea, cough, or wheeze; or (d) hypoxia.

ACS is the end result of a variety of processes that result in deoxygenation of hemoglobin S and sickling of red blood cells, leading to vaso-occlusion, local ischemia, and vascular damage. Most of the time, the trigger for ACS in an individual patient cannot be identified. However, although infection is the most common identifiable cause for ACS, other important triggers are vaso-occlusive crisis (VOC) and asthma. In fact, many patients who develop ACS have been hospitalized for a different reason, often VOC. Appropriate treatment for ACS targets these multiple etiologies, with the goal of improving oxygenation and, therefore, a reduction in sickling and lung damage.

Initial management of ACS includes antibiotics, fluids and analgesia, and respiratory support, often including bronchodilators. Transfusions are also a mainstay of therapy. Viruses (i.e., respiratory syncytial virus), bacteria (i.e., encapsulated organisms), *Mycoplasma* and *Chlamydia* are common infectious agents in acute chest syndrome. Typically, patients are treated empirically with a combination of broad-spectrum antibiotics, such as ceftriaxone (a third-generation cephalosporin) and azithromycin (a macrolide). In more severe cases of ACS, vancomycin is added to cover methicillin-resistant *Staphylococcus aureus* and penicillin-resistant *Streptococcal pneumoniae*.

Generally, fluids are administered, as dehydration increases the likelihood of sickling. Adequate analgesia for VOC, especially of the back, chest, and abdomen, prevents splinting and hypoventilation due to pain. However, oversedation from opioids can also result in hypoventilation. Hypoventilation leads to atelectasis and a mismatch of ventilation and perfusion, further

© 2008 by Lippincott Williams & Wilkins, a Wolters Kluwer business

exacerbating sickling and lung damage. Incentive spirometry should be encouraged to help prevent atelectasis.

Basic respiratory support involves oxygen supplementation to maintain an arterial oxygen saturation $\geq 92\%$. For patients with increasing oxygen requirements, or those who are unable to maintain an adequate respiratory effort, the use of positive pressure ventilation should be considered. Asthma is more common is children with SCD, and children with SCD and asthma may be at increased risk for ACS. Patients with ACS and a history of asthma should receive scheduled bronchodilator therapy, irrespective of exam findings. Bronchodilator therapy should also be considered in patients with ACS and no history of asthma.

The goal of simple transfusion in ACS is to increase hemoglobin to 11 g/dL or hematocrit to 30%, thereby improving oxygenation. Some indications include anemia (i.e., hematocrit 10%–20% below the patient's baseline), $PaO_2 < 60$ mm Hg on arterial blood gas, and disease progression. In severe cases of ACS, partial exchange transfusion may be used. In summary, common precipitants of ACS include not only infection, but also VOC and asthma. Treatment for ACS needs to address these multiple etiologies, and acute therapy includes antibiotics, fluids, analgesia, oxygen, bronchodilators, and transfusion.

SUGGESTED READINGS

Boyd JH, Moinuddin A, Strunk RC, et al. Asthma and acute chest in sickle-cell disease. *Pediatr Pulmonol.* 2004;38:229–232.
Vichinsky EP, Neumayr LD, Earles AN, et al. Causes and outcomes of the acute chest syndrome in sickle cell disease. National Acute Chest Syndrome Study Group. *N Engl J Med.* 2000; 342:1855–1865.

170

KNOW WHICH BLOOD PRODUCTS TO TRANSFUSE FOR A PATIENT'S BLEEDING

MINDY DICKERMAN, MD

WHAT TO DO – MAKE A DECISION

After the decision has been made to transfuse blood products, the most appropriate product must be chosen. Donated whole blood and other products are modified in several ways that remove varying proportions of nonred cell components. It is important to know the policies of the blood center you are working with.

Packed red blood cells (PRBCs) are the blood product of choice for replacement during surgery, red cell loss, or for transfusion therapy. PRBCs are stored with a preservative solution that enables them to be used 35 to 45 days after collection. The process of removing white blood cells (WBCs) from blood products is referred to as leukoreduction, and is done by highly efficient filters that reduce the number of WBCs by >99.9 %. There are several adverse consequences of transfused WBCs that are reduced by leukoreduction. Febrile nonhemolytic transfusion reactions are mediated by leukocyte-derived cytokines and direct donor cell leukocyte interactions.

In addition, human leukocyte antigen alloimmunization can be induced by human leukocyte antigens expressed on donor leukocytes in recipients who receive multiple transfusions. Allosensitization increases the risk of graft rejection in children who subsequently receive organ or hematopoietic cell transplantation, and increases platelet refractoriness in patients requiring multiple platelet reactions. WBCs can also transmit infectious agents that are harbored in WBCs—most notably cytomegalovirus (CMV). Leukoreduction significantly reduces, but does not completely eliminate these reactions. Many blood centers in the United States have adopted a "universal leukoreduction" policy in which all PRBCs are leukoreduced.

The few WBCs that remain after leukoreducing are capable of replicating and can cause transfusion-associated graft-versus-host disease (TA-GVHD). Gamma irradiation of PRBCs stops proliferation of foreign lymphocytes, which entirely prevents TA-GVHD. The dose of irradiation used for cellular blood products is not sufficient to kill viruses such as CMV and, therefore, does not eliminate the need for leukoreduction or CMV-negative blood products. TA-GVHD can occur from directed donor blood provided by a relative, or if the recipient has decreased cellular immunity and is unable

© 2008 by Lippincott Williams & Wilkins, a Wolters Kluwer business

to mount a response against donor lymphocytes. Directed donor blood from family members as well as PRBCs destined for immunosuppressed children should be irradiated. Irradiation can lead to reduced red cell viability and a leakage of potassium, and there is potential for hyperkalemia to occur if a patient is receiving massive transfusions of irradiated blood. To prevent this potential complication, the supernatant solution containing excess potassium can be removed by washing the red blood cells prior to transfusion.

Fresh frozen plasma (FFP) is prepared from whole blood or from plasma collected by apheresis techniques. FFP is frozen at -18°C to -30°C and is usable for 1 year from the date of collection. FFP contains all of the coagulation factors but is not a concentrate of any of the circulating plasma proteins and therefore should not be used to treat coagulation defects caused by known deficiencies. It also does not contain any platelets. FFP should be used conservatively because it serves as a source for the further manufacture of plasma derivatives such as albumin, gamma globulin, and the coagulation factors.

FFP is indicated to treat a bleeding condition caused by a deficiency of multiple coagulation factors such as is seen in warfarin overdose, vitamin K deficiency, liver failure, or dilutional coagulopathy following massive transfusion. FFP may be needed for inherited factor XI deficiency or as a source of factor V in severe cases of disseminated intravascular coagulation, when platelet and cryoprecipitate transfusions do not correct factor V, factor VIII, or fibrinogen consumption defects. There is little evidence to support the use of FFP as prophylaxis for invasive procedure in patients with a mild coagulopathy. FFP is screened for the presence of unexpected red blood cell antibodies. FFP must be ABO compatible with the patient's red blood cells. Anaphylactic reactions following transfusion of plasma may occur in patients with immunoglobulin (Ig)A deficiency and antibodies to IgA. For these patients, there is IgA-deficient plasma available. Cryoprecipitate is the precipitate that is separated out by centrifugation when FFP is thawed at 4°C. It is a concentrated preparation that contains all of the factor VIII, fibrinogen, fibronectin, factor XIII, and von Willebrand factor in FFP reduced from an initial volume of 250 mL to a final volume of 10 to 15 mL. Cryoprecipitate contains approximately 200 mg of fibrinogen and 100 units of factor VIII per bag. It is used in the treatment of congenital and acquired deficiencies of fibrinogen, factor VIII, and factor XIII, as well as for the treatment of von Willebrand disease when there is no other alternative.

SUGGESTED READINGS

Dara SI, Rana R, Afessa B, et al. Fresh frozen plasma transfusion in critically ill medical patients with coagulopathy. *Crit Care Med.* 2005;33:2667–2671.

Roseff SD, Luban NL, Manno CS. Guidelines for assessing appropriateness of pediatric transfusion. *Transfusion.* 2002;42:1398–1413.

171

ADJUST THE VACCINE SCHEDULES FOR CHILDREN WHO RECEIVE CHEMOTHERAPY, PARTICULARLY FOR LIVE VIRUS VACCINES

EMILY RIEHM MEIER, MD

WHAT TO DO – INTERPRET THE DATA, MAKE A DECISION, TAKE ACTION

Children receiving chemotherapy for treatment of malignancies are in an immune-compromised state. Immunosuppression occurs due to the underlying malignancy, the cytotoxic therapy the child is receiving, or a combination of these factors. Not only is the child at an increased risk for opportunistic infections, but any immunity associated with vaccines administered prior to chemotherapy is compromised. The loss of vaccine-associated antibody protection occurs in children with leukemia and lymphoma, as well as solid tumors, although the therapy for the former is more lymphotoxic.

Response to newly administered vaccines is also compromised in children undergoing chemotherapy. Immune reconstitution usually occurs 3 to 12 months after the cessation of chemotherapy, but younger children often take longer to recover their immune function. For these reasons, the immunization schedule for a child receiving chemotherapy needs to be altered.

Children receiving chemotherapy should not receive live vaccines because of the risk of developing an active infection from the immunization. Immunization with killed vaccines may be performed in these children. However, the degree of antibody response to vaccines administered while receiving chemotherapy has not been clearly delineated. It seems that immune response is best when vaccines are administered between cycles of chemotherapy. *Table 171.1* reviews the recommendations for administration of specific vaccines.

As mentioned earlier, reconstitution of the immune system occurs at variable times in children who have been treated with chemotherapy. The timing and degree of immune reconstitution depends on a variety of factors,

© 2008 by Lippincott Williams & Wilkins, a Wolters Kluwer business

TABLE 171.1   RECOMMENDATIONS FOR THE ADMINISTRATION OF VACCINES DURING AND AFTER CHEMOTHERAPY

VACCINE	SAFE TO ADMINISTER DURING CHEMOTHERAPY?[a]	BOOSTER NEEDED?	OTHER
DTaP	Yes, during maintenance therapy[a]	Yes, 6 months after completion of chemotherapy	—
Hepatitis B	Yes, should be given to all unimmunized patients, regardless of chemotherapy cycle	No	Titers should be checked after series is complete to verify immunity.
Hib	Yes, during maintenance therapy	Yes, 12 months after chemotherapy is complete	Hodgkin lymphoma patients should be vaccinated 7–10 days before start of chemotherapy, and should receive a booster 3–5 years after completion of chemotherapy.
Influenza	Yes, if patient >6 months old. Best response if given between cycles of chemotherapy.	N/A	The intramuscular vaccine should be given annually to all immunocompromised patients. The intranasal formulation contains a live, attenuated virus and should be avoided.
IPV	Yes, if series has been started before diagnosis.	Yes, 6 months after completion of chemotherapy	OPV should not be given to household contacts.
MMR	No	Yes, 12 months after completion of chemotherapy.	—
Pneumococcal	Yes, during maintenance therapy	Yes, 6 months after completion of chemotherapy.	Hodgkin lymphoma patients should be vaccinated 7–10 days before start of chemotherapy, and should receive a booster 3–5 years after completion of chemotherapy.
Varicella	No	Yes, 12 months after completion of chemotherapy.	In patients with ALL, initial vaccination should not be considered until at least 12 months after remission achieved and in maintenance therapy. No data for patients with solid tumors. Patients should avoid oncology clinic for at least 4 weeks after immunization. Higher rate of development of vaccine-associated rash.

[a] Maintenance therapy refers to the phase of chemotherapy that follows the initial 6 to 8 months of intensive chemotherapy. It typically lasts for 2 or 3 years.
ALL, Acute lymphoblastic leukemia; DTaP, diphtheria and tetanus toxoids and acellular pertussis, adsorbed; Hib, *Haemophilus influenza* type b; IPV, inactivated poliovirus; MMR, measles, mumps, rubella; OPV, oral poliovirus

including the type of malignancy, the age of the child, and the intensity of chemotherapy. Antibody titers can be obtained prior to vaccination to determine which series of vaccines are needed. Children should receive boosters following the completion of chemotherapy. As a general rule, immunization with killed vaccines can be resumed 6 months after the completion of chemotherapy, and live vaccines may be administered 12 months after the completion of chemotherapy.

SUGGESTED READINGS

Ek T, Mellander L, Hahn-Zoric M, et al. Intensive treatment for childhood acute lymphoblastic leukemia reduces immune responses to diphtheria, tetanus, and *Haemophilus influenzae* type b. *J Pediatr Hematol Oncol.* 2004;26:727–734.

Hastings C. Immunization. In: Altman AJ, ed. *Supportive Care of Children With Cancer: Current Therapy and Guidelines From the Children's Oncology Group.* 3rd ed. Baltimore, MD: The Johns Hopkins University Press; 2004:13–24.

Mustafa MM, Buchanan GR, Winick NJ, et al. Immune recovery in children with malignancy after chemotherapy. *J Pediatr Hematol Oncol.* 1998;20:451–457.

Zignol M, Perachhi M, Tridello G, et al. Assessment of humoral immunity to poliomyelitis, tetanus, hepatitis B, measles, rubella and mumps in children after chemotherapy. *Cancer.* 2004;101:635–641.

172

ANTICIPATE TUMOR LYSIS SYNDROME (TLS) IN CHILDREN WITH LEUKEMIA OR LYMPHOMA

EMILY RIEHM MEIER, MD

WHAT TO DO – INTERPRET THE DATA

TLS is a constellation of metabolic abnormalities that usually occur within the first 3 to 5 days of starting chemotherapy. Clinicians must be aware that hydration alone can cause cell lysis, placing patients undergoing a diagnostic oncologic work up at risk for TLS. In rare cases, TLS can occur spontaneously. Patients with non-Hodgkin lymphoma and T-cell acute lymphoblastic leukemia have the highest risk of TLS due to the bulky lymphadenopathy and leukocytosis often accompanying these diseases.

Hyperuricemia, hyperphosphatemia with associated hypocalcemia, and hyperkalemia are the laboratory abnormalities seen in patients with TLS. The intracellular ions potassium and phosphate are released when cells are lysed by chemotherapy. Hyperuricemia occurs when DNA building blocks (namely the purines, guanosine and adenosine) found within tumor cell nuclei are released and degraded to uric acid. A compensatory increase in urinary excretion of uric acid and phosphate occurs. Depending on the size of the tumor burden, the kidneys may be overwhelmed by the amount of intracellular debris that needs to be excreted. Uric acid is soluble at physiologic pH, but in the acidic conditions commonly seen with a high cell turnover rate and possible renal hypoperfusion, urate crystals can form in the renal collecting system. Calcium phosphate deposits can also precipitate in the renal tubules. These can lead to renal failure, placing the patient at risk for further hyperkalemia and life-threatening cardiac arrhythmias. The best treatment for TLS-associated renal failure is prevention. Hydration, urinary alkalinization, and inhibition of uric acid production are the standard preventative interventions for TLS. Intravenous fluids usually run at high flow rates ($3 L/m^2/day$, approximately 2 times maintenance) with sodium bicarbonate infused in a separate line, adjusting the infusion rate to maintain the urine pH between 7 and 8. Uric acid precipitates at a urine pH of <7 and calcium/phosphate stones may form in urine with a pH >8. Urine pH should be tested with each void, and adjustments to the rate of bicarbonate infusion should be made accordingly.

Allopurinol is the classic medication used to prevent uric acid formation. Allopurinol stops the conversion of xanthine (formed by purine breakdown)

© 2008 by Lippincott Williams & Wilkins, a Wolters Kluwer business

to uric acid by blocking xanthine oxidase. This leads to a build up of the byproducts xanthine and hypoxanthine. Xanthine is more likely to precipitate in the urine than uric acid, and cases of xanthine nephropathy have been reported. In patients at high risk of TLS, recombinant urate oxidase (rasburicase) can be used. Urate oxidase catalyses the conversion of uric acid to allantoin, which is up to 10 times more soluble in urine than uric acid. In high-risk patients, rasburicase dramatically drops hyperuricemia, avoiding TLS-associated renal failure and its complications.

SUGGESTED READINGS

Keaney CM, Springate JE. Cancer and the kidney. *Adolesc Med Clin.* 2005;16:121–148.
Nicolin G. Emergencies and their management. *Eur J Cancer.* 2002;38:1365–1379.
Pui CH, Mahmoud HH, Wiley JM, et al. Recombinant urate oxidase for the prophylaxis or treatment of hyperuricemia in patients with leukemia or lymphoma. *J Clin Oncol.* 2001;19: 697–704.

173

DO NOT ADMINISTER SYSTEMIC STEROIDS IN MALIGNANCY PRIOR TO CONFIRMATION OF THE DIAGNOSIS, AS THEY MAY INTERFERE WITH THE ABILITY TO DIAGNOSE AND TREAT APPROPRIATELY

EMILY RIEHM MEIER, MD

WHAT TO DO – MAKE A DECISION

Acute lymphoblastic leukemia (ALL) is the most common form of childhood cancer, with more than 2,000 children in the United States diagnosed each year. Survival rates for ALL range from 70% to 85%, depending on risk factors. Patients considered to have high-risk ALL are those with a white blood cell count >50,000/μL at diagnosis, age younger than 1 year or older than 10 years, boys with testicular disease at diagnosis, or children who have received steroids for >48 hours prior to diagnosis. These patients receive more intensive therapy because of their high-risk status.

Leukemic blasts are exquisitely sensitive to steroid therapy. In fact, in German studies in the mid-1980s to early 1990s, children with ALL were treated with prednisone plus intrathecal methotrexate alone. A peripheral blast count of $\leq$1,000/μL was achieved in 90% of these children, illustrating how effective steroids are at reducing the peripheral blast count in acute leukemia. Because initial white blood cell count is an important prognostic indicator in pediatric ALL, steroid therapy for >48 hours prior to a diagnosis of ALL automatically places the child into a higher risk category. In some cases, these children are nonrandomly assigned to receive craniospinal irradiation, depending on the length of the steroid therapy. Craniospinal irradiation can cause learning disabilities and developmental delay in children younger than 5 years. This is extremely important, because ALL is most commonly diagnosed in children aged 2 to 4 years.

Patients presenting with signs and symptoms concerning for leukemia, such as fatigue, pallor, easy bruisability, leg pain, fever, hepatosplenomegaly, lymphadenopathy, petechial rash, and with suggestive laboratory abnormalities, such as anemia, leukocytosis, and thrombocytopenia, alone or in combination, should be referred immediately to a pediatric hematologist/oncologist for further diagnosis and management. Steroids should not be given prior to evaluation.

© 2008 by Lippincott Williams & Wilkins, a Wolters Kluwer business

Many conditions can mimic ALL. One common mimicker of leukemia is Epstein-Barr virus (EBV). EBV can cause fatigue, fever, pallor, pharyngitis, hepatosplenomegaly, lymphadenopathy, and pancytopenia. Physicians are occasionally tempted to treat with steroids to decrease the uncomfortable symptoms associated with this viral illness. Although steroids may have a beneficial effect on the acute symptoms associated with EBV infection, they are not likely to change the overall course of the illness. Furthermore, even with documented positive EBV titers, leukemia cannot be definitively ruled out unless a bone marrow aspiration is performed. Thus, routine use of steroids for EBV infection should not be practiced.

Rheumatologic conditions, such as systemic lupus erythematosus and juvenile rheumatoid arthritis, can also present with symptoms similar to ALL and have associated anemia, thrombocytopenia, and leukopenia, either alone or in combination. Because steroids are the mainstay of therapy for these conditions, it is important to rule out a malignant cause of bone marrow suppression prior to initiating therapy. This can usually be done when laboratory data supports the diagnosis of a rheumatologic disorder, such as a low C3 or C4, normal uric acid and lactate dehydrogenase, and increased creatinine. In some cases, malignancy can only be excluded by a bone marrow aspiration.

SUGGESTED READINGS

Jones OY, Spencer CH, Bowyer SL, et al. A multicenter case-control study on predictive factors distinguishing childhood leukemia from juvenile rheumatoid arthritis. *Pediatrics.* 2006;117: e840–e844.

Pui CH, Evans WE. Treatment of acute lymphoblastic leukemia. *N Engl J Med.* 2006;354:166–178.

Reiter A, Schrappe M, Ludwig WD, et al. Chemotherapy in 998 unselected childhood acute lymphoblastic leukemia patients. Results and conclusions of the multicenter trial ALL-BFM 86. *Blood.* 1994;84:3122–3133.

174

BE CAREFUL CHARACTERIZING CONDITIONS AS CHILD ABUSE. THERE ARE A NUMBER OF GREAT MASQUERADERS, INCLUDING NEUROBLASTOMA

ELIZABETH WELLS, MD

WHAT DO TO – MAKE A DECISION

Although child abuse continues to be a major concern for clinicians working in emergency departments, urgent care centers, and in primary care settings, it is important for pediatricians to recognize other medical conditions of the skin, bone, brain, and retina that may mimic the appearance of child abuse.

Bruises are the most common type of injury seen in abused children, but bruising can indicate a medical disorder. For instance, it may indicate a coagulopathy, such as hemophilia (factors VIII and IX deficiencies), or a clotting disorder, such as von Willebrand disease. Bruising can also be caused by low platelets, as in idiopathic thrombocytopenic purpura or thrombocytopenia, due to leukemia. Bruising may also be a sign of a vasculitis. Henoch-Schönlein purpura should be considered, especially if the "bruising" appears in dependent parts of the body (i.e., buttocks and legs in children and back and buttocks in infants). Salicylate ingestion can cause bruising, due to decreased platelet adhesion and increased capillary permeability, and should be considered in a child presenting with vomiting and metabolic acidosis. Mongolian spots are bluish-green areas of skin discoloration caused by a dense collection of melanocytes usually on the buttocks and lower back that are often differentiated from bruising by their indistinct borders.

Several medical conditions present with burnlike lesions that may mimic child abuse. Phytodermatitis can occur when sunlight interacts with photo-sensitizing compounds found in certain fruits, vegetables, and skin products. The lesions appear as erythematous lesions and bullae, often in a pattern resembling handprints or around the hands and mouth after a child handles or ingests lime or lemon juice. Staphylococci and streptococci impetigo may be mistaken for burns; however, they usually are superficial and heal cleanly, distinguishing them from cigarette burns, which usually are deeper (full-thickness), have raised margins, and heal with scarring. Other skin conditions that can mimic burns include herpes, eczema, contact dermatitis, and chronic bullous disease. In addition, cultural practices, such as cupping, coining, and spooning, may cause skin lesions that may be mistaken for child abuse.

ⓒ 2008 by Lippincott Williams & Wilkins, a Wolters Kluwer business

Pediatricians should be able to recognize medical causes of radiologic abnormalities. The evaluation of suspected physical abuse in children younger than 2 years and in nonverbal children mandates a skeletal survey. The radiographic appearance of a fracture may be found in patients with normal variant changes in their bones, such as nutrient canals, cortical irregularities, metaphyseal beaks and spurs, distal ulnar cupping, normal symmetric peritoneal changes seen in infants, and ossification defects of the ribs. Neoplastic disease may also present with unexpected fractures. Metabolic bone disease that can lead to fractures includes rickets, a bone disease caused by vitamin D deficiency and resulting in osteopenia, metaphyseal cupping, physeal widening, and pseudofractures. Another source of multiple fractures is vitamin C deficiency (i.e., scurvy) in which children present with irritability; failure to thrive; coiled, fragmented hair; prominent hair follicles on the thighs and buttocks; and gingival hemorrhage. Other metabolic causes of pathologic fractures include McCune-Albright syndrome and Gaucher disease. Infectious etiologies of bone disease should be considered in a child who presents with a warm, swollen, and tender extremity. Proper diagnosis may require multiple radiographs, a pediatric radiologist, and, sometimes, a bone scan.

Osteogenesis imperfecta, an inherited disorder of collagen formation that increases the likelihood of repeated fractures, may present with fractures in various stages of healing. Although this condition is often considered, it is a rare disorder, occurring in only 1 in 20,000 births; self-inflicted injuries do not occur until a child is toddling or walking. Characteristic features, which may or may not be present, include blue sclera, scoliosis, hearing loss, and a positive family history. Testing for mutations in collagen types COL1A1 and COL1A2, and culture of biopsied fibroblasts should be considered if there are no other signs of abuse and if the mechanism of injury seems too minor to have caused a fracture. Taking a careful history and referring to a geneticist and pediatric orthopedic surgeon are most helpful in confirming or excluding the diagnosis of osteogenesis imperfecta.

Congenital insensitivity to pain is a rare hereditary sensory autonomic neuropathy in which the peripheral nerves fail to detect pain or temperature and may lead to multiple injuries, including fractures of varying ages. A careful neurologic examination can point a clinician to this diagnosis.

The bucket-handle fracture that occurs as a result of the indirect shearing forces generated when an extremity is pulled, pushed, twisted, or shaken, is considered specific for child abuse. However, these metaphyseal fractures may also be seen in infants undergoing serial casting for treatment of equinovarus deformity. Once again, an accurate and thorough history is essential in determining the cause of this fracture.

A subdural hemorrhage raises the clinical index of suspicion for child abuse, particularly when it coexists with retinal hemorrhages, fractures, and multiple traumatic injuries. Birth trauma and vitamin K deficiency may be the source of this hemorrhage in infants. A congenital malformation (e.g., arteriovenous malformation, aneurysm, arachnoid cyst) may cause spontaneous bleeding. Disseminated intravascular coagulation, or hemophilia or other bleeding disorders may cause subdural hemorrhages. Metabolic disorders that may cause bleeding include glutaric aciduria type 1, hemophagocytic lymphohistiocytosis, and Menkes disease. Vasculitides, including moyamoya, should also be considered. Brain tumors, cranial radiation, and chemotherapy may cause subdural hemorrhage, as well.

Any infant or child, who has intracranial hemorrhages suspicious for nonaccidental trauma, should be evaluated by a pediatric ophthalmologist to detect retinal hemorrhages (RHs). Although RHs, unilateral or bilateral, occur in 50% to 80% of abusive head injuries, they are not pathognomonic for abuse and may occur in association with other medical conditions. Although most birth-related RHs resolve within 8 days, they may persist for up to 3 months. RHs can occur in meningitis and other infectious illnesses, such as Henoch-Schönlein purpura and other vasculitides. Severe hypertension can also cause RHs in children. Iatrogenic etiologies of RHs include the use of extracorporeal membrane oxygenation. Although the issue is controversial, research indicates that RHs are not caused by cardiopulmonary resuscitation.

Child maltreatment causes significant childhood mortality and morbidity. Although steps should be taken to ensure a clinician does not miss medical conditions that mimic as child abuse, such considerations should not preclude a thorough evaluation to rule out nonaccidental trauma.

SUGGESTED READINGS

Child abuse and the eye. The Ophthalmology Child Abuse Working Party. *Eye.* 1999;13(Pt 1):3–10.

Coleman H, Shrubb VA. Chronic bullous disease of childhood–another cause for potential misdiagnosis of sexual abuse? *Br J Gen Pract.* 1997;47(421):507–508.

Diagnostic imaging of child abuse. *Pediatrics.* 2000;105(6):1345–1348.

Grayev AM, Boal DK, Wallach DM, et al. Metaphyseal fractures mimicking abuse during treatment for clubfoot. *Pediatr Radiol.* 2001;31:559–563.

Heider TR, Priolo D, Hultman CS, et al. Eczema mimicking child abuse: a case of mistaken identity. *J Burn Care Rehabil.* 2002;23(5):357–359; discussion 357.

Karmani S, Shedden R, De Sousa C. Orthopaedic manifestations of congenital insensitivity to pain. *J R Soc Med.* 2001;94:139–140.

Nimkin K, Kleinman PK. Imaging of child abuse. *Radiol Clin North Am.* 2001;39:843.

Sirotnak AP, Grigsby T, Krugman RD. Physical abuse of children. *Pediatr Rev.* 2004;25:264–277.

175

CONSIDER THE DIFFERENTIAL DIAGNOSIS OF LOW BACK PAIN IN PRE-TEENS, WHICH MAY INCLUDE ONCOLOGIC DIAGNOSES AND INFECTIONS THAT CAUSE PAIN PRIOR TO BECOMING CLINICALLY IDENTIFIABLE IN DIAGNOSTIC STUDIES

ELIZABETH WELLS, MD

WHAT TO DO – GATHER APPROPRIATE DATA

Unlike in adult medicine, low back pain is an unusual chief complaint in pediatric practice, and the majority of pediatric cases have an identifiable cause. Most cases are caused by musculoskeletal disease or trauma; however, clinicians must consider more systemic conditions, such as infection, noninfectious inflammatory disease, and neoplasm.

The most common cause of back pain is mechanical. Strains and sprains are treated with rest and simple analgesics, and typically improve in 2 to 3 days. Direct traumatic injuries are also common, and the history guides the clinician to these diagnoses.

Spinal developmental abnormalities that may cause back pain include spondylolysis and spondylolisthesis. Spondylolysis is caused by a stress or fatigue fracture or separation of the pars interarticularis, often in L5. It is more common in sports that emphasize hyperextension of the spine, such as gymnastics, tennis, and weight lifting. The defect appears as a radiolucent line around the "Scottie dog's" neck on oblique radiographs. Bilateral spondylolysis can lead to spondylolisthesis in which the proximal or cephalad vertebral body is ventrally subluxed over the next most caudal vertebral body. A patient with negative radiographs but pain on hyperextension and a classic history needs further imaging, such as with a computed tomography scan or bone scan. Treatment of spondylolisthesis includes bracing, for early lesions; and fusion surgery, for patients with progression of the subluxation or neurologic signs; followed by physical therapy with core body exercises.

A child with the sudden onset of severe back pain, fever, and an elevated erythrocyte sedimentation rate may have an infection. Discitis and vertebral osteomyelitis are two conditions to consider, with the former being more common in children older than 8 to 10 years and the latter being more common in children older than 8 to 10 years. As routine radiographs can appear normal early on in the disease, magnetic resonance imaging is the

© 2008 by Lippincott Williams & Wilkins, a Wolters Kluwer business

test of choice; a bone scan is also frequently diagnostic. Treatment of both infections includes bed rest and antibiotics.

The rheumatologic diseases juvenile rheumatoid arthritis and ankylosing spondylitis are two causes of noninfectious inflammatory back pain in children. Inflammatory diseases can present with morning stiffness that improves with activity. Sacroiliac tenderness may also be found, and joint changes may be seen on plain radiographs or magnetic resonance imaging.

Neoplastic disorders should also be included in the differential diagnosis of lower back pain in children. The benign tumors osteoid osteoma and osteoblastoma commonly present with painful scoliosis, stiffness, and night pain, and are relieved by nonsteroidal anti-inflammatory drugs or aspirin. Aneurysmal bone cysts are usually asymptomatic until a fracture, collapse, or hemorrhage occurs with the cyst as the focus. Most benign spinal tumors are cured with tumor excision and bone grafting.

Malignant neoplasms present with intractable back pain, night pain, and constitutional findings, including weight loss, fever, and elevated erythrocyte sedimentation rate. Primary malignant neoplasms of the spine are rare but include Ewing sarcoma, leukemia, and lymphoma. Metastases to the spine can be seen in lymphoma, leukemia, Wilms tumor, retinoblastoma, and teratoma-teratocarcinoma. A bone scan is usually the most appropriate imaging tool for bony neoplasm; it can detect the multiple ossification centers seen in metastatic disease.

Abdominal disease can also cause back pain in children. These conditions include retrocecal appendicitis, pleuritis, pyelonephritis or hydronephrosis, and psoas abscess. Wilms tumor, rhabdomyosarcoma, and retroperitoneal masses can also cause back pain.

It is important for clinicians to consider the broad differential diagnosis when evaluating children with low back pain. Persistent back pain in a child can have a more serious etiology, and the workup should include the appropriate diagnostic imaging and the swift referral to an orthopedic specialist. The possibility of underlying spinal cord compression should always be considered. Sickle cell disease must be ruled out. Chronic pain syndromes are a diagnosis of exclusion. If an underlying pathology, such as infection or tumor, is causing the back pain, early diagnosis may facilitate timely effective treatment.

SUGGESTED READINGS

Glancy GL. The diagnosis and treatment of back pain in children and adolescents: an update. *Adv Pediatr.* 2006;53:227–240.

Grattan-Smith PJ, Ryan MM, Procopis PG. Persistent or severe back pain and stiffness are ominous symptoms requiring prompt attention. *J Paediatr Child Health.* 2000;36(3):208–212.

McCleary MD, Congeni JA. Current concepts in the diagnosis and treatment of spondylolysis in young athletes. *Curr Sports Med Rep.* 2007;6(1):62–66.

Payne WK 3rd, Ogilvie JW. Back pain in children and adolescents. *Pediatr Clin North Am.* 1996;43(4):899–917.

Selbst SM, Lavelle JM, Soyupack SK, et al. Back pain in children who present to the emergency department. *Clin Pediatr (Phila).* 1999;38:401–406.

176

RECOGNIZE THE TRIAD OF HEADACHE, VOMITING, AND ATAXIA AS A FOCAL LESION IN THE CENTRAL NERVOUS SYSTEM (CNS)

ELIZABETH WELLS, MD

WHAT TO DO – INTERPRET THE DATA

CNS malignancies, as a group, are the most common solid tumor and the second most common malignancy of childhood, comprising about 17% of all malignancies during childhood and adolescence. National Cancer Institute (NCI) statistics show that approximately 2,200 U.S. children younger than 20 years are diagnosed annually with invasive CNS tumors. Astrocytomas account for about 50%; medulloblastomas and primitive neuroectodermal tumors account for about 25%; and other gliomas and ependymomas comprise the rest. Unlike adults and older children (older than 10 years of age), who have primarily supratentorial brain tumors, young children have an increased likelihood of malignancies in the cerebellum and brainstem. Medulloblastoma, which arises within the cerebellar vermis or within the hemispheres, is the most common malignant brain tumor in children, with about 400 new cases in U.S. children every year.

Most patients with cerebellar tumors will present with ataxia. Defined as impaired coordination of movement and balance, ataxia is associated with dysfunction of the cerebellum or of the sensory or motor pathways connecting to it. A physician must be aware of a child's developmental milestones to determine if a patient is ataxic or exhibiting age-appropriate "clumsiness." Other conditions that may be confused with ataxia include muscle weakness, myopathic or neuropathic; spasticity; or movement disorders. A careful neurologic exam is needed to distinguish these general causes. The differential diagnosis for ataxia is broad and includes head trauma, Guillain-Barré syndrome, a vascular event, hydrocephalus, labyrinthitis, certain medications, seizures, conversion disorders, and infratentorial tumors.

The occurrence of a worsening headache, nausea, or vomiting, particularly on awakening, should raise the concern for increased intracranial pressure that may be secondary to a CNS lesion or tumor. Other conditions that may present with increased intracranial pressure include traumatic brain injury, hydrocephalus, arteriovenous malformation, pseudotumor cerebri and intracranial infections. Because a lumbar puncture (LP) may result in brain herniation in patients with elevated intracranial pressure, a computed

© 2008 by Lippincott Williams & Wilkins, a Wolters Kluwer business

tomography (CT) scan must be obtained prior to the LP in a child with a headache.

The most common cause of intermittent headache and vomiting in pediatrics is migraine. Migraine headaches are usually hemicranial; throbbing or pulsating; associated with abdominal pain, nausea, or vomiting; and resolve with rest. They may be associated with an aura, and a family history of migraines is found in 80% of the patients. Other common headaches are cluster or stress-related headaches, but they are not typically accompanied by nausea. A complete neurologic exam should be performed in any child presenting with a headache, vomiting, and ataxia. In a large tertiary care center study, no patient with a normal neurologic examination had a brain tumor on neuroimaging.

Whereas headache, vomiting, and ataxia may occur in all cerebellar tumors, some features may help point clinicians toward different types. Pilocytic astrocytomas tend to have an insidious onset, whereas symptoms or signs of medulloblastomas, although similar, are more rapidly progressive. Ependymomas, arising from the floor of the fourth ventricle, often present with nausea and vomiting. Brainstem gliomas typically present with multiple cranial nerve abnormalities or upper motor neuron signs. Some patients show nonspecific signs, such as irritability, listlessness, failure to thrive, and stagnation of development or loss of developmental milestones.

Neuroimaging is an important component of the evaluation of patients with suspected brain tumors. Brain tumors are not seen on skull x-rays. CT scans of tumors typically show a hyperdense mass that markedly enhances after contrast injection; however, medulloblastomas may be missed on CT. Contrast-enhanced magnetic resonance imaging should be performed in all children suspected of having cerebellar tumors, either after or instead of a CT scan. An LP should be performed to check for neoplastic cells. The diagnosis and risk stratification will be based on neuroimaging, histology results, and genetic markers. In general, children with CNS cancer do not share the favorable prognosis of those with many other common pediatric neoplasms; however, survival is improving with new combinations of surgery, radiation therapy, and chemotherapy. Surgery remains the mainstay of treatment of most brain tumors. Risk factors for a poor prognosis include the inability to resect fully the tumor, a large tumor size, and leptomeningeal dissemination, underscoring the need for early detection and treatment. Researchers are also considering long-term sequelae from chemotherapy and radiation and examining the neurocognitive and developmental deficits of long-term survivors.

Cancer is the second most frequent cause of death, after injury, in children older than 3 months. Early detection, along with accurate diagnosis and treatment, offers families the best chance of a cure. Most brain tumors in children are infratentorial and classically present with headache, nausea and vomiting, and ataxia; therefore, pediatricians must recognize this triad. The American Academy of Pediatrics (AAP) has advised that childhood cancers are best coordinated by tertiary centers, which offer specialized, supportive care. In addition to playing a critical role in the initial detection of the lesion, the primary care physician should continue to maintain a close connection with the family and the oncologists, to provide the patient and family support and to ensure a smooth transition to routine care and surveillance following the intense treatment of the cancer.

SUGGESTED READINGS

Corrigan JJ, Feig SA. American Academy of Pediatrics. Guidelines for pediatric cancer centers. *Pediatrics.* 2004;113:1833–1835.

Davis CH, Odom GL, Woodhall B. Brain tumors in children; clinical analysis of 164 cases. *Pediatrics.* 1956;18(6):856–870.

Forsyth R, Farrell K. Headache in childhood. *Pediatr Rev.* 1999;20(2):39–45.

Goodman MR, Gurney JG, Smith MA, et al. Sympathetic nervous system tumors. In: Ries LA, Smith MA, Gurney JG, et al. (eds). *Cancer Incidence and Survival among Children and Adolescents: United States SEER Program, 1975–1995.* Bethesda, Md: National Cancer Institute; 1999:35.

Haadow MK, Winchell C, Kernohan J. Brain tumors in children. *Pediatrics.* 1949;3(6):839–844.

Medina LS, Kuntz KK, Pomeroy S. Children with headache suspected of having a brain tumor: cost-effectiveness analysis of diagnostic strategies. *Pediatrics.* 2001;108(2):255–263.

Packer RJ. Childhood tumors. *Curr Opin Pediatr.* 1997;9(6):551–557.

Reddy AT, Packer RJ. Pediatric central nervous system tumors. *Curr Opin Oncol.* 1998;10(3):186–193.

177

KNOW THE DIFFERENCES BETWEEN MELANOMA, BASAL CELL CARCINOMA, AND SQUAMOUS CELL CARCINOMA

ELIZABETH WELLS, MD

WHAT TO DO – INTERPRET THE DATA

Clinicians often have a low index of suspicion for malignant cutaneous lesions in children, which can lead to a delay in diagnosis and treatment. Below is a review of the three most common types of skin cancer, including diagnostic features, management, and important distinctions.

MELANOMA

Melanoma is a life-threatening malignant neoplasm of melanocytes, the cells that synthesize and deposit the pigment melanin. The incidence of cutaneous melanoma has been increasing more rapidly than that of any other neoplasm, and studies suggest that the rates are rising in children. Although only 2% of all cases occur in pediatric patients, melanomas account for just 5% to 10% of cutaneous malignant neoplasms in prepubescent children. Pediatricians must be aware of the potential for melanoma in children, in order to look for and recognize the lesions early in their progression, when they still may be curable by surgical resection.

The American Academy of Dermatology has adopted the ABCD criteria for morphologic characteristics of a melanoma: *a*symmetry, *b*order irregularity, *c*olor variegation, and *d*iameter >6 mm. Childhood melanoma may also appear atypically with ulceration or a lack of pigment (amelanotic). Dermatologists advise clinicians and patients to be suspicious of the "ugly duckling"—a lesion that stands out from all the others through differences in color, growth characteristics, or associated signs or symptoms. Risk factors for melanoma include a history of congenital nevi, dysplastic nevi, xeroderma pigmentosum, and immunodeficiency states. It is not clear if light skin, hair, eyes, and history of blistering sunburn confer the same increased risk in children that they do in adults.

Primary care pediatricians have the opportunity to observe the growth of benign nevi in their patients over time. Any melanocytic lesion with a substantial, unexpected change, such as rapid asymmetric growth, crusting, ulceration, and color loss, warrants a dermatologic evaluation and, possibly, removal. A skin biopsy is required for any cutaneous lesion that is suspected

© 2008 by Lippincott Williams & Wilkins, a Wolters Kluwer business

of being a melanoma. For smaller lesions, an excisional biopsy that includes a small (5 mm) margin of normal skin is recommended; incisional biopsies are performed for very large lesions. All pigmented lesions that are removed should be submitted for examination by a dermopathologist, particularly as diagnosis by histology may be more difficult in children than in adults. When a diagnosis of primary melanoma is confirmed histologically, re-excision, with margins of >1 cm, is required.

The prognosis of cutaneous melanoma depends on the Breslow depth of penetration, which is a measure of lesion thickness in millimeters. Deeper lesions have a higher risk of local and systemic recurrence. Survival rates are high for melanomas with a Breslow depth of <0.75 mm but drop precipitously with a lesion with deep invasion or metastatic spread. Staging of the lesion is based on adult recommendations and is performed by a careful palpation of the associated draining lymph nodes and the radiologic examination of the lung and liver. A sentinel lymph node biopsy is being used more often to guide management. As there are few studies of chemotherapy in children, a multidisciplinary approach to melanoma treatment is recommended with oncologists, dermatologists, surgeons, and others who specialize in pigmented lesions.

BASAL CELL CARCINOMA

Basal cell carcinoma (BCC) is the most common skin cancer in adults, and the incidence is increasing. The condition peaks in the seventh decade of life and is rare in children. When found in the pediatric age group, it is usually associated with a genetic defect, exposure to high-dose radiotherapy, or scars from a burn or trauma. Although BCC in younger people does not correspond directly with cumulative sun damage, de novo cases may be more common in areas of intense ultraviolet (UV) radiation exposure, such as the southwestern United States. BCC presents as a pink, pearly, telangiectatic smooth papule that enlarges slowly and may ulcerate. It appears most frequently on the head, neck, and upper extremities, with the majority occurring on the face. There have been a few cases of BCC on the eyelids of children. Management of BCC is usually curative and involves electrodessication and curettage (ED&C), simple excision, or Mohs microsurgery (MMS). The advantages of ED&C are that treatment requires minimal time and equipment and no suturing; however, there is no histologic examination of tissue with this method, the site takes a longer time to heal, and the procedure results in a large hypopigmented patch scar rather than the linear scar that results from excisional methods. ED&C is most commonly used on superficial BCC of the trunk or extremities. MMS is indicated when the tumor is recurrent, >2 cm in diameter, located on problematic anatomic areas, or an aggressive histopathologic type (e.g., morpheaform). The recurrence rate for BCC treated by MMS is approximately 1%, whereas that for standard excision is 5% to 10%, depending on the margins of the excision. Cryotherapy is reserved as second line for patients who cannot tolerate other procedures, and radiation therapy is no longer recommended. Imiquimod (Aldara) is a biologic response modifier that stimulates local cytokine release and T cells, which shows some promise for treating BCC, but has not yet been studied for this use in children.

In contrast to melanomas, BCCs grow slowly, invade locally, and rarely metastasize. Early recognition permits treatment of smaller tumors and can prevent extensive tissue destruction and scarring after excision. Because of the high association with a positive family history of particular syndromes, the discovery of a BCC should prompt inquiry into possible systemic associations, such as basal cell nevus syndrome, xeroderma pigmentosum, and nevus sebaceous.

SQUAMOUS CELL CARCINOMA

Squamous cell carcinoma (SCC) is the second most common skin cancer. Unlike BCC, SCC does have the potential to metastasize, especially to regional lymph nodes. Cumulative exposure to UV light appears to be more important in the pathogenesis of SCC than of BCC. Other risk factors for SCC include age, immunosuppression, ionizing radiation, environmental carcinogens, scars, chronic heat exposure or burns, genetic abnormalities (e.g., mutations in the p53 tumor-suppressor gene), and human papilloma virus (HPV).

SCC has a predilection for sun-exposed and sun-damaged regions of the body but can occur anywhere, including mucous membranes. The SCC lesion appears as a hyperkeratotic, crusted, erythematous nodule or plaque that may be friable on the surface and is often tender to palpation. Histologically, SCC may be classified into several types, including in situ, well-differentiated, poorly differentiated, keratoacanthoma, infiltrative, and verrucous carcinoma.

Treatment of SCC is fairly standardized. Cryotherapy, 5-fluorouracil creams, and ED&C are recommended only for in situ SCC. Otherwise, treatment is surgical. There are no published guidelines or randomized control studies to delineate treatment for children. For standard excisions in adults, a 4 mm margin is recommended for tumors of <1 cm in diameter and <2 mm in depth. For tumors >1 cm in diameter, >6 mm depth, or more aggressive tumors, 5-mm to 10-mm margins or Mohs microsurgery (MMS) is recommended. As with BCC, MMS is the method of choice for treatment of SCC of the head and neck; in immunosuppressed patients; and for tumors that are recurrent, perineural, >2 cm, incompletely excised, or histologically aggressive. Radiation is typically used as adjuvant treatment after the resection of aggressive tumors. SCC is usually more aggressive and prone to metastasis than BCC.

Pediatricians must be hypervigilant about skin lesions and refer patients to an experienced pediatric dermatologist, surgeon, or plastic surgeon, keeping in mind that skin cancer is often curable when recognized, diagnosed, and removed early. To gather more information about staging and therapies in children, practicing physicians are encouraged to enroll their patients in cooperative group trials. In addition, pediatricians should educate all parents and children about the deleterious effects of UV light and make recommendations for sunscreen and protective behavior to help decrease the incidence of these cutaneous malignancies.

SUGGESTED READINGS

Al-Buloushi A, Filho JP, Cassie A, et al. Basal cell carcinoma of the eyelid in children: a report of three cases. *Eye.* 2005;19:1313–1314.

Butter A, Hui T, Chapdelaine J, et al. Melanoma in children and the use of sentinel lymph node biopsy. *J Pediatr Surg.* 2005;40(5):797–800.

Ferrari A, Bono A, Baldi M, et al. Does melanoma behave differently in younger children than in adults? A retrospective study of 33 cases of childhood melanoma from a single institution. *Pediatrics.* 2005;115:649–654.

Euvrard S, Kanitakis J, Cochat P, et al. Skin cancers following pediatric organ transplantation. *Dermatol Surg.* 2004;30(4 Pt 2):616–621.

Lee PK. Common skin cancers. *Minn Med.* 2004;87(3):44–47.

Leman JA, Evans A, Mooi W, et al. Outcomes and pathological review of a cohort of children with melanoma. *Br J Dermatol.* 2005;152:1321–1323.

LeSueur BW, Silvis NG, Hansen RC. Basal cell carcinoma in children: report of 3 cases. *Arch Dermatol.* 2000;136(3):370–372.

Mancini AJ. Malignant melanoma in children not as rare as once thought. *AAP News.* 2005;26(12):14.

Orlow SJ. Melanomas in children. *Pediatr Rev.* 1995;16(10):365–369.

Pappo AS. Melanoma in children and adolescents. *Eur J Cancer.* 2003;39(18):2651–2661.

Varan A, Gököz A, Akyüz C, et al. Primary malignant skin tumors in children: etiology, treatment and prognosis. *Pediatr Int.* 2005;47(6):653–657.

178

PROVIDE SYSTEMIC ANTIMICROBIAL THERAPY FOR NEUTROPENIC PATIENTS WITH FEVER

EMILY RIEHM MEIER, MD

WHAT TO DO – TAKE ACTION

Febrile neutropenia should be considered a medical emergency in children receiving chemotherapy. Neutropenia is defined as an absolute neutrophil count (total white blood cell count in thousands multiplied by the fraction of segmented neutrophils and bands) $\leq 500/\mu L$ or an absolute neutrophil count $\leq 1,000/\mu L$ and falling. Blood counts are expected to nadir 7 to 10 days following chemotherapy. Fever is defined as an oral temperature $\geq 38.5°C$, an axillary temperature $\geq 37.5°C$ or three low-grade temperatures $(38.0°–8.4°C$ orally or $37.0°–37.4°C$ axillary) in 24 hours. Rectal temperatures should not be taken in neutropenic patients due to the increased risk of infection from gastrointestinal flora. Febrile patients who have recently received chemotherapy should be considered at high risk of infection due to their immunocompromised state and receive intravenous antibiotics within 1 hour of presenting to the emergency department.

Evaluation of a patient with fever and suspected neutropenia should include careful history and physical examination, keeping in mind that due to the lack of neutrophils, the erythema, suppuration, and edema that commonly accompany infections may be lacking. For example, a patient who has exquisite tenderness over a central line site without concomitant erythema, edema, or suppurative drainage should still be treated for cellulitis. The same can be said for patients with respiratory symptoms without infiltrate on chest x-ray or urinary symptoms without pyuria. Laboratory evaluation should include complete blood count, creatinine, and liver enzymes (to use as a baseline when monitoring for antibiotic/antifungal toxicity), and blood cultures. Some debate exists if a peripheral culture should be collected in addition to cultures from the patient's central line. Aerobic, anaerobic, and fungal cultures should be collected from all sites (including each lumen of the central line). Urinalysis and chest x-ray are not indicated unless the patient has significant symptomatology.

Treatment of febrile neutropenia should be based on the bacteria most likely to cause infection in neutropenic patients (*Table 178.1*) and susceptibility profiles at individual institutions. Although gram-positive organisms

© 2008 by Lippincott Williams & Wilkins, a Wolters Kluwer business

---

TABLE 178.1 MOST COMMON ORGANISMS CAUSING BACTEREMIA IN FEBRILE NEUTROPENIC PATIENTS

- Staphylococci
- Methicillin-resistant *Staphylococcus aureus*
- *Pseudomonas aeruginosa*
- Enterococci
- *Escherichia coli*
- *Klebsiella* species

---

cause bacteremia more frequently than gram-negative organisms, monotherapy with a third- or fourth-generation cephalosporin with antipseudomonal coverage (ceftazidime or cefepime) or a carbapenem (meropenem) is adequate coverage in most uncomplicated cases of febrile neutropenia. Bacteremia only accounts for 15% to 20% of documented infections in febrile neutropenic patients. Other sites of infection include the gastrointestinal, urinary, or respiratory tracts, where infection with gram-negative organisms is much more common. Therefore, vancomycin is not indicated for treatment of febrile neutropenia in all patients; its use should be reserved for patients considered high risk (*Table 178.2*).

Vancomycin reduces mortality from *Streptococcus viridans* when given as initial treatment (in conjunction with an anti-pseudomonal agent) in patients at high risk for *S. viridans* infections (those who have received high-dose cytarabine chemotherapy). Vancomycin may be discontinued after 48 hours of treatment if there is no evidence of *S. viridans* or other gram-positive bacteremia. Initial therapy with an antifungal is not warranted because fungal infections usually occur after prolonged neutropenia. If a patient is persistently febrile and neutropenic >5 days of broad-spectrum antibiotics, antifungal coverage should be added.

TABLE 178.2 INDICATIONS FOR INITIAL USE OF VANCOMYCIN IN FEBRILE NEUTROPENIA

- Suspected catheter infection
- Unstable clinical appearance (hypotension, etc.)
- Known colonization with organisms sensitive only to vancomycin (methicillin-resistant *Staphylococcus aureus*)
- Positive blood culture with gram-positive organism, pending identification and susceptibility testing
- Patients at high risk of *Streptococcus viridans* bacteremia, based on type of chemotherapy most recently given

SUGGESTED READINGS

Hughes WT, Armstrong D, Bodey GP, et al. 2002 guidelines for the use of antimicrobial agents in neutropenic patients with cancer. *Clin Infect Dis.* 2002;34:730–761.

Kanamaru A, Tatsumi Y. Microbiological data for patients with febrile neutropenia. *Clin Infect Dis.* 2004;39(Suppl 1):S7–S10.

179

THE PROVISION OF SEDATION IN PATIENTS WITH ANTERIOR MEDIASTINAL MASS MAY BE FATAL WITHOUT APPROPRIATE PREPARATION

RENÉE ROBERTS, MD

WHAT TO DO – MAKE A DECISION

The mediastinum is comprised of superior, anterior, middle, and posterior compartments; however, masses in the anterosuperior compartment of children can be extremely unstable and challenging for caregivers. A mass in this location may result in life-threatening airway obstruction, and can arise unexpectedly at any time and cause cardiac or pulmonary artery compression, or acute pulmonary edema from superior vena cava syndrome (SVCS), all of which represent true emergencies that mandate prompt treatment.

Compared with an adult, small decreases in a child's tracheal diameter produce larger decreases in cross-sectional area and airway resistance. The most common presentation of an anterosuperior mediastinal mass is stridor, dyspnea, and cough due to direct compression of the tracheobronchial tree. Often these children even require oxygen at presentation. Examination may demonstrate reduced breath sounds or rhonchi on auscultation, tachypnea, prolonged expiration, accessory muscle use, or cyanosis. However, patients may not be symptomatic and plain chest radiographs may not reveal the presence of airway compromise. Some studies, such as pulmonary function testing, can help to predict airway complications if they demonstrate flattened flow volume loops where expiratory flow is significantly diminished. Cardiorespiratory complications may occur abruptly in these patients and are often not related to mild preoperative symptoms and roentgenographic evidence. Extrinsic compression of the trachea or mainstem bronchi can cause significant airway obstruction and is a cause of death or morbidity with induction of or emergence from sedation or anesthesia. It is also important to understand that there is most likely some degree of SVCS in all children with anterosuperior mediastinal masses, which also can cause severe complications with any sedation.

Clinical manifestations of severe SVCS include variable degrees of face, neck, and upper thorax swelling; external jugular and superficial chest vein distension with possible cyanosis; and plethora. Cardiac or pulmonary artery compression and acute pulmonary edema can represent the initial clinical

ⓒ 2008 by Lippincott Williams & Wilkins, a Wolters Kluwer business

signs in previously healthy children. Upper body venous hypertension impedes lymphatic drainage, often leading to lymphedema or chylothorax. Although venous pressures are raised, it is not uncommon to find that edema and plethora are more impressive than large surface vein dilation. The most common cause of SVCS is surgery for congenital heart disease; the second most common cause is anterosuperior masses. Usually these masses are malignant lymphomas (usually found in adolescents) or germ cell tumors (children). Two thirds of the germ cell tumors are benign teratomas.

Because of the underlying pathophysiology of anterosuperior mediastinal masses, children may develop severe homodynamic compromise after sedation, induction of anesthesia, institution of positive pressure ventilation, or supine positioning. Compression of the right ventricular outflow tract or main pulmonary artery is probably more common than realized. In the supine position, the right ventricular outflow tract is the most superior cardiac structure. Additionally, the right ventricle is a low-pressure chamber and is more sensitive to compression than the higher-pressure ascending aorta. The right ventricle can usually compensate for moderate increases in pulmonary afterload. Adverse positioning, induction of anesthesia, hypovolemia, and reduced cardiac contractility may attenuate compensatory mechanisms. The additive effects of general anesthetics and sedation or positioning during diagnostic procedures may contribute to worsen the airway obstruction, leading to fatal cardiorespiratory failure. Sedation even for biopsy or excision of the mass is associated with a high risk for severe airway obstruction, hemodynamic compromise, and death.

Rapidly evolving symptoms of respiratory compromise from an anterior mediastinal neoplasm can occur even after the trachea has been secured through intubation. In addition, circulatory compromise becomes clinically apparent when compression of the great vessels occurs despite airway patency. As the tumor size increases, the trachea, mainstem bronchi, and major vessels may be exposed to an increasingly positive pressure. Any positive pressure ventilation can cause dynamic hyperinflation and resulting auto-positive end-expiratory pressure (auto-PEEP) because of expiratory gas flow obstruction. With sufficient elevation of intrathoracic pressure, the gradient for venous return is reduced, and right ventricular pressures are reduced, worsening the extent of vascular obstruction. Intraoperative deaths have been reported without evidence of tracheal obstruction but with cardiac compression or pulmonary artery compression or encasement demonstrated at autopsy. Once these complications occur, the death rate appears to be high.

Initial treatment efforts of a child with a symptomatic anterosuperior mediastinal mass should be toward patient stabilization. Temporary supportive measures, such as elevation of the head, oxygen, diuretics, and steroids may improve symptoms of SVCS. All children should receive cardiovascular monitoring. Spontaneous breathing should be maintained if clinically accept-able, and sedation and muscle paralysis should be avoided. For diagnosis, the least invasive procedures should be performed under local anesthesia, avoid-ing the added risks of general anesthesia. Before any procedure, a thorough evaluation and preparation needs to be done by an anesthesiologist and the operating room team from pretreatment to prevent bronchospasm, with large bore intravenous (IV) catheters and arterial catheters and special wire reinforced endotracheal tubes of different sizes as well as fiberoptic, and jet ventilation capability, if needed. Because the use of awake fiberoptic tech-niques is limited in the pediatric population, volatile agent or IV induction is usually the technique of choice. However, even under the best circumstances, adverse events occur especially in children with a tracheal area of <50%.

Ventilation after intubation is also complex, with several different ap-proaches. Handling emergence, extubation, and postoperative care must also be carefully planned. Severely symptomatic patients may require empiric pretreatment before any diagnostic procedures can be safely performed.

In a closed-claims database of the United Kingdom Medical Defense Union, eight adverse events were reported related to anterior mediastinal masses; six were younger than 8 years of age. The patients were booked for diagnostic biopsy of a mass—a trivial procedure. All eight cases suffered severe brain damage or death. A common theme was a bronchospasm or dif-ficulty with ventilation. It may be tempting to sedate patients with a "benign" appearing mediastinal mass for a simple procedure; however, the very high risk of adverse complications makes children with a mediastinal mass a sig-nificant sedation and anesthetic risk. Because sedation and general anesthesia comprise the two ends of a continuum of states ranging from minimal seda-tion (anxiolysis) through general anesthesia, it is imperative to realize that for any patient, it is not always possible to predict how an individual will respond to the administered medications. Therefore, practitioners targeting a given level of sedation should be able to rescue patients whose level of sedation becomes deeper than initially intended (i.e., rescue patients who enter a state of general anesthesia). Given the risks involved with airway obstruction and underlying SVCS in the case of a child with an anterosuperior mediastinal mass, any procedure should be carefully planned with an anesthesiologist.

SUGGESTED READINGS

American Society of Anesthesiologist Task Force on Sedation and Analgesia by Non-Anesthesiologists. Practice guidelines for sedation and analgesia by non-anesthesiologists. *Anesthesiology.* 2002;96(4):1004–1017.

Narang S, Harte BH, Body SC. Anesthesia for patients with a mediastinal mass. *Anesthesiol Clin North Am.* 2001;19(3):559–579.

Piastra M, Ruggiero A, Caresta E, et al. Life-threatening presentation of mediastinal neoplasms: report on 7 consecutive pediatric patients. *Am J Emerg Med.* 2005;23(1):76–82.

180

CONSIDER THE POSSIBILITY OF TYPHLITIS IN CANCER PATIENTS WHO PRESENT WITH SYMPTOMS SUGGESTIVE OF APPENDICITIS

CYNTHIA GIBSON, MD

WHAT TO DO – INTERPRET THE DATA

Typhlitis refers to a necrotizing colitis involving the cecum or the cecum and appendix, and is found in leukemic children. The term neutropenic enteropathy is also used to refer to these clinical findings. The vaguely defined clinical diagnosis of typhlitis is difficult, but frequent symptoms include abdominal pain, fever, tenderness on exam, and diarrhea. Typhlitis and appendicitis appear to be equally common in the young leukemic patient with right lower quadrant signs of peritoneal irritation. The classical signs of peritoneal irritation can be found in these patients despite their neutropenia and immunosuppressed condition, and have the same implications as in the nonleukemic patient. Plain radiographs are nonspecific but may demonstrate a fluid-filled mass like density in the right lower quadrant, distension of adjacent small bowel loops, and thumb printing. Free intraperitoneal air and pneumatosis coli rarely are observed. The early use of computed tomography scanning helps to facilitate the diagnosis and may provide the ability to differentiate typhlitis from other abdominal diseases for which surgery would be indicated. In typhlitis, computed tomography scan demonstrates cecal distention and circumferential thickening of the cecal wall, which may have low attenuation secondary to edema.

The greatest risk to these patients is from progressive local and systemic infection. The pathogenesis appears to be cecal distension, which may impair the blood supply, lead to mucosal ischemia and ulceration. Infection may be involved, especially cytomegalovirus. Bacterial invasion leads to transmural penetration and, ultimately, perforation then sepsis. The average mortality rate from sepsis is 40% to 45%.

Diagnosis of this disorder without pathologic examination is speculative and the differentiation from appendicitis is unclear. Operative findings range from simple edema of the cecum to a frankly necrotic and perforated cecum. The preoperative differentiation between appendicitis and typhlitis is difficult. Pediatric cancer patients with typhlitis can be treated carefully nonoperatively, with bowel rest, antibiotics, and supplemental nutrition. Usual

© 2008 by Lippincott Williams & Wilkins, a Wolters Kluwer business

indications for surgery (i.e., perforation, clinical deterioration) still should be used.

SUGGESTED READINGS

McCarville MB, Adelman CS, Li C, et al. Typhlitis in childhood cancer. *Cancer*. 2005;104(2): 380–387.

Schlatter M, Snyder K, Freyer D. Successful nonoperative management of typhlitis in pediatric oncology patients. *J Pediatr Sur*. 2002;37(8):1151–1155.

Skibber J, Matter GJ, Pizzo PA, et al. Right lower quadrant pain in young patients with leukemia. A surgical perspective. *Ann Surg*. 1987;206(6):711–716.

181

DO NOT USE CHEST PHYSIOTHERAPY (CPT) IN BRONCHIOLITIS, IT IS NOT HELPFUL

MADAN DHARMAR, MD

WHAT TO DO – MAKE A DECISION

CPT in pediatric respiratory diseases has been used to assist in the clearance of tracheobronchial secretions. The main goal is to clear the airway obstruction, open collapsed airways, reduce airway resistance, enhance gas exchange, and reduce the work of breathing. CPT can play a role in improving a patient's respiratory status and expedite recovery. CPT in pediatric patients involves various techniques such as chest percussion, vibration in postural drainage positions, chest shaking, directed coughing, and slow passive forced exhalation. CPT is useful for individuals with copious mucus or thick secretions, and those with weak respiratory mechanics or those with ineffective cough. In some situations, CPT could be harmful by causing an increase in bronchospasm, inducing pulmonary hypertension, repositioning a foreign body, or destabilizing a sick infant. CPT has been linked to adverse events such as injury (rib fracture) and long term neurologic complication. But a review of the literature shows insufficient evidence of adverse events following chest physiotherapy.

Use of Chest Physiotherapy

Cystic Fibrosis (CF) and Bronchiectasis. Removal of bronchopulmonary secretions is an integral part of the management of CF. CPT helps to remove excessive secretions, thereby improving ventilation in the short term. In patients with CF, there is evidence that CPT causes a significantly greater amount of sputum expectoration when compared to no treatment.

Primary Pneumonia With Consolidation. During the treatment of pneumonia with consolidation, CPT is found to have a beneficial effect in mobilizing and clearing secretion from the lung, especially in weakened children and children unable to participate in pulmonary exercises and deep breathing. In

ⓒ 2008 by Lippincott Williams & Wilkins, a Wolters Kluwer business

patients with consolidation, CPT helps in the repositioning of the patient for optimal ventilation and perfusion even though it may not have other direct clinical beneficial effects.

Acute Atelectasis. Acute lobar atelectasis is more commonly encountered in the intensive care unit (ICU) due to excess bronchial secretions caused by intubation, mechanical ventilation, and the inability to effectively clear sections. Airway obstruction and lung collapse can complicate the clinical course, resulting in prolonged care in the ICU. CPT is usually prescribed to assist in clearing the secretions obstructing larger airways and help in reinflation of the collapsed parts of the lung.

Selected Intubated Neonates. CPT has acquired a role in the management of low birth weight infants on prolonged ventilatory support. It is important that CPT is applied only when it is clearly indicated, because there is conflicting evidence demonstrating a beneficial effect of better oxygenation and secretion clearance and the potential deterioration of physiological parameters.

Postextubation. CPT is commonly used to prevent postextubation complications. However, it should be noted that the evidence is lacking in the utility of CPT to prevent postextubation complications.

Select Patients with Acute Asthma. CPT may have utility in expediting the recovery of ventilated children with asthma and retained secretions in the lung. CPT does not improve lung function in children with acute asthma, and when applied inappropriately in the presence of bronchoconstriction can exacerbate the asthma.

Other Indications. CPT can be used to remove secretion in children with weak respiratory mechanics such as kyphoscoliosis, cerebral palsy, and neuromuscular disorders (e.g., spinal muscular atrophy or muscular dystrophy).

Chest Physiotherapy in Bronchiolitis. Bronchiolitis is a self-limiting viral condition, which commonly affects children in the range of 6 months to 2 years old. The rationale for the use of CPT in infants with acute bronchiolitis is that it will enhance clearance of secretions and improve oxygenation parameters. The use of CPT in the treatment of acute bronchiolitis differs among institutions and countries. Although the evidence for and against the use of CPT is weak, some countries consider it unethical not to use CPT for treatment of bronchiolitis, and other countries do not use it as part of the treatment plan. A recent Cochrane review based on three trials found that there was no significant effect on the clinical scores, duration of oxygen supplementation, and length of stay when CPT using percussion and vibration technique was part of management of bronchiolitis. The studies also did not report any adverse events due to the use of CPT. It was concluded that CPT using percussion and vibration techniques could not be recommended for hospitalized infants with acute bronchiolitis.

SUGGESTED READINGS

Balachandran A, Shivbalan S, Thangavelu S. Chest physiotherapy in pediatric practice. *Indian Pediatr.* 2005;42(6):559–568.

Chalumeau M, Foix-L'Helias L, Scheinmann P, et al. Rib fractures after chest physiotherapy for bronchiolitis or pneumonia in infants. *Pediatr Radiol.* 2002;32(9):644–647.

Perrotta C, Ortiz Z, Roque M. Chest physiotherapy for acute bronchiolitis in paediatric patients between 0 and 24 months old. *Cochrane Database Syst Rev.* 2007(1):CD004873.

Wallis C, Prasad A. Who needs chest physiotherapy? Moving from anecdote to evidence. *Arch Dis Child.* 1999;80(4):393–397.

182

Assure Adequate Oxygenation for Asthmatic Patients Receiving Albuterol

Madan Dharmar, MD

What to Do – Take Action

Asthma is a condition where airway hyperresponsiveness due to a chronic inflammatory condition of the lung airways results in episodic airflow obstruction. These episodes of airflow obstruction can present with mild symptoms, such as dry coughing, expiratory wheezing, chest tightness, dyspnea; or severe symptoms, such as respiratory distress, hypoxic seizures, respiratory failure, and even death. There is no definitive cause for asthma, but an interplay of genetic and environmental causes seems likely. Nearly 80% of asthmatics report an onset of asthma before the age of 6 and not all children with recurrent wheeze develop persistent asthma in later childhood. A history of parental asthma, allergies in childhood, severe lower respiratory tract infection, wheezing apart from colds, low birth weight, male gender, and environmental tobacco smoke exposure are considered to be important risk factors for persistent asthma.

The National Asthma Education and Prevention Program classifies asthma based on four parameters: (a) frequency of daytime symptoms, (b) nighttime symptoms, (c) degree of airflow obstruction by spirometry, and/or (d) peak expiratory flow variability. According to this classification, asthmatics can be categorized in four disease severity groups, as "mild intermittent," "persistent mild," "persistent moderate," and "persistent severe." The goal of asthma management is to reduce airway inflammation by the use of daily "controller" anti-inflammatory medications, minimize exposure to proinflammatory environmental exposures, and controlling comorbid conditions that can worsen asthma.

When exacerbations do occur, early intervention using systemic glucocorticoids and β-agonist bronchodilators can reduce the severity of these episodes. The mild intermittent asthma is the only group where a daily anti-inflammatory (controller) is not used and the β-agonist bronchodilators (reliever) is used for all levels of severity groups. Pharmacotherapy in the management of asthma can be divided into quick-relief medication and long-term control medication. Quick-relief medications are used to manage acute episodes of bronchospasm, which include inhaled β_2-agonists (e.g., albuterol), inhaled anticholinergics (e.g., ipratropium), and short-course

© 2008 by Lippincott Williams & Wilkins, a Wolters Kluwer business

systemic glucocorticoids (e.g., prednisone). Long-term control medications are used to manage mild-to-moderate persistent asthma, which include non-steroidal anti-inflammatory agents (e.g., cromolyn), inhaled glucocorticoids (e.g., beclomethasone), sustained-release theophylline, long-acting inhaled β-agonists (e.g., salmeterol), and leukotriene modifiers (e.g., montelukast).

The Role of β-agonist Bronchodilators and Oxygen in Acute Severe Asthma. In acute asthma exacerbation, there is narrowing of the airway. This is caused by in airway inflammation, resulting in mucosal edema and hypersecretion, and airway obstruction due to bronchospasm. The body's homeostatic response is to decrease the blood flow to underventilated lung units. By this mechanism, the body maximizes oxygenation by matching pulmonary perfusion with alveolar ventilation. In acute severe asthma, the pattern of ventilation-perfusion is bimodal, ranging from normally perfused to areas of hypoxic pulmonary vasoconstriction.

In acute severe exacerbation of asthma, the management includes correction of hypoxemia, rapid improvement of airflow obstruction, and prevention of progression or recurrence of symptoms. Children admitted to the hospital for acute severe exacerbations of asthma are treated with supplemental oxygen, frequently administered β_2-agonists, and systemic glucocorticoids. Inhaled β_2-agonists are considered the first line of medication to treat acute asthma exacerbation. Treatment with inhaled β_2-agonists is often given to relieve bronchospasm and improve oxygenation.

In acute severe asthma, nebulization of β_2-agonists without oxygen can cause or worsen hypoxemia. The β_2-agonists can alter the homeostatic response by causing pulmonary vasodilatation and increasing perfusion to poorly ventilated lung units, resulting in ventilation perfusion mismatch and causing more hypoxemia. Hypoxia perpetuates bronchoconstriction, which further worsens the condition of the child. This mechanism was initially seen in isoproterenol, a β-agonist that was commonly used for asthma. It has also been found that salbutamol can worsen ventilation-perfusion mismatch by similar mechanism of pulmonary vasodilatation and increasing cardiac output.

SUGGESTED READINGS

Field GB. The effects of posture, oxygen, isoproterenol and atropine on ventilation-perfusion relationships in the lung in asthma. *Clin Sci.* 1967;32(2):279–288.

Harris L. Comparison of the effect on blood gases, ventilation, and perfusion of isoproterenol-phenylephrine and salbutamol aerosols in chronic bronchitis with asthma. *J Allergy Clin Immunol.* 1972;49(2):63–71.

Inwald D, Roland M, Kuitert L, et al. Oxygen treatment for acute severe asthma. *BMJ.* 2001;323(7304):98–100.

183

START EMPIRIC COVERAGE FOR RESISTANT GRAM-NEGATIVE ORGANISMS IN PATIENTS WITH CYSTIC FIBROSIS (CF) AND EXACERBATIONS OF PULMONARY DISEASE

JENNIFER MANISCALCO, MD

WHAT TO DO – TAKE ACTION

CF is an autosomal recessive disorder resulting from mutations in a single gene, located on the long arm of chromosome 7. These mutations result in the absence of a functioning cystic fibrosis transmembrane conductance regulator (CFTR), which conducts chloride across cell membranes. CFTR is expressed in exocrine glands throughout the body. In the airways, it is predominantly expressed in the submucosal glands. Abnormal or absent CFTR function clogs the glands with mucous and changes the composition and mechanical properties of the airway secretions, initiating a pathophysiologic cascade that ultimately leads to progressive and chronic lung disease. Chronic endobronchial infection and the associated intense neutrophilic inflammatory response are pathognomonic for the disease.

Individuals with CF develop pulmonary infections with a unique set of bacterial pathogens, which are acquired in an age-dependent fashion. Initial infections occur shortly after birth and are typically caused by non–type-able *Haemophilus influenzae* and *Staphylococcus aureus*. Subsequent infections are caused by *Pseudomonas aeruginosa*, the most common virulent pathogen in patients with CF. Recent investigations have confirmed that infection with *P. aeruginosa* occurs earlier than previously believed. Up to 80% of children with CF will eventually be infected, with the initial infection occurring on average by age 2. Early strains of *P. aeruginosa* remain sensitive to antibiotics and can be eradicated with aggressive antimicrobial therapy. Persistent strains become mucoid, adapting to the local environment through the formation of macrocolonies and the production of an exopolysaccharide that confers resistance to phagocytosis and penetration by antibiotics. The acquisition of *P. aeruginosa* is associated with progression of lung disease and is a limiting factor in overall survival. The mucoid strains are associated with a more significant clinical deterioration. Late in the disease process, infections are caused by other opportunistic organisms, including *Burkholderia cepacia* complex, *Stenotrophomonas maltophilia*, *Achromobacter xylosoxidans*, fungi, and nontuberculous mycobacterium. *B. cepacia* complex is a group of

© 2008 by Lippincott Williams & Wilkins, a Wolters Kluwer business

closely related species that can cause a syndrome of high fever, bacteremia, severe necrotizing pneumonia, and possibly death.

Appropriate antibiotic therapy is a critical component of both periodic exacerbations and chronic maintenance therapy in CF. Antibiotic

TABLE 183.1	ANTIBIOTIC RECOMMENDATIONS FOR THE TREATMENT OF BACTERIA ASSOCIATED WITH EXACERBATIONS OF PULMONARY DISEASE IN CYSTIC FIBROSIS
BACTERIA	ANTIBIOTIC REGIMEN
Staphylococcus aureus Methicillin-resistant *S. aureus*	Cefazolin OR Nafcillin Vancomycin
Pseudomonas aeruginosa	β-lactam (choose 1): Ceftazidime Ticarcillin Piperacillin Imipenem Meropenem Aztreonam PLUS aminoglycoside (choose 1): Tobramycin Amikacin
Burkholderia cepacia complex	Meropenem PLUS (choose 1): Minocycline Amikacin Ceftazidime Chloramphenicol Trimethoprim/sulfamethoxazole
Stenotrophomonas maltophilia	Ticarcillin/clavulanate OR Trimethoprim/sulfamethoxazole OR Ticarcillin/clavulanate PLUS Aztreonam
Achromobacter xylosoxidans	Chloramphenicol PLUS Minocycline OR Ciprofloxacin PLUS (choose 1): Imipenem Meropenem

Adapted with permission from Gibson RL, Burns JL, Ramsey BW. Pathophysiology and management of pulmonary infections in cystic fibrosis. *Am J Resp Crit Care Med.* 2003;168:918–951.

management can be divided into three phases, reflecting the progression of infection with organism as detailed above. Early in the disease process, the goal of therapy is to delay colonization with *P. aeruginosa* and prevent the decline in pulmonary function that accompanies it. Once colonization with *P. aeruginosa* has occurred, use of continuous *P. aeruginosa* coverage is recommended to stabilize lung function and reduce the likelihood of pulmonary exacerbations. This is often accomplished with inhaled antibiotics, or chronic therapy with fluoroquinolones. When periodic exacerbations do occur, intravenous antibiotics should be administered in addition to bronchodilators and anti-inflammatory agents. Typically, combination therapy with an aminoglycoside and β-lactam antibiotic is used to counteract *P. aeruginosa* and other gram-negative organisms. *Table 183.1* lists antibiotic choices for the treatment of bacteria associated with pulmonary exacerbations in CF.

Regardless of the phase of therapy, antibiotic choice should be based on the periodic isolation and identification of pathogens from respiratory secretions and a review of the susceptibility profile. If multidrug resistance is suspected, the specimen should be sent to a reference lab for synergy testing or combination bactericidal testing. Expectorated sputum has been shown to be an accurate indicator of lower airway microbiology and is the preferred source of airway secretions. Cultures collected by bronchoalveolar lavage are also very sensitive, but the procedure carries more risk and cost than simple sputum collection or hypertonic saline-induced sputum collection. In addition, specimens from bronchoalveolar lavage may miss focal or regional disease.

SUGGESTED READINGS

Gibson RL, Burns JL, Ramsey BW. Pathophysiology and management of pulmonary infections in cystic fibrosis. *Am J Resp Crit Care Med.* 2003;168:918–951.

Li Z, Kosork MR, Farrell PM, et al. Longitudinal development of mucoid *Pseudomonas aeruginosa* infection and lung disease progression in children with cystic fibrosis. *JAMA.* 2005;293:581–588.

Rowe SM, Miller S, Sorscher EJ. Cystic fibrosis. *N Engl J Med.* 2005;352:1992–2001.

184

CONSIDER THAT PATIENTS WITH SNORING MAY HAVE OBSTRUCTIVE SLEEP APNEA SYNDROME (OSAS)

SARIKA JOSHI, MD

WHAT TO DO – INTERPRET THE DATA

OSAS is an underrecognized but clinically important respiratory disorder in children. OSAS is characterized by intermittent, complete, or partial upper airway obstruction during sleep, sometimes with associated hypoxemia or carbon dioxide retention. In children, the prevalence of OSAS is 1% to 3%, with the peak incidence in preschool-aged children.

The most common symptom of OSAS in children is snoring. Snoring affects 7% to 9% of children younger than age 10. Unfortunately, there is no reliable screening test to differentiate primary snoring from OSAS. Other symptoms consistent with OSAS include restless sleep; difficulty with or irritability upon awakening; mouth breathing; and behavioral problems, such as hyperactivity and aggression. In severe cases, untreated OSAS can lead to learning difficulties, developmental delay, failure to thrive, pulmonary hypertension, cor pulmonale, and congestive heart failure. According to the American Academy of Pediatrics' practice guidelines for OSAS, pediatricians should consider the possibility of OSAS in any child presenting with snoring. If other signs or symptoms of OSAS are also present, further investigation should be undertaken.

The usual etiologies of OSAS can be divided into anatomic versus functional problems, all of which result in airway occlusion, narrowing, or collapse. Anatomic causes include both bony and soft tissue abnormalities. Many genetic syndromes are associated with craniofacial anomalies, such as micrognathia (e.g., Pierre Robin sequence, Treacher Collins syndrome), midface hypoplasia and deformities of the skull base (e.g., Down syndrome, Pfeiffer syndrome).

Adenotonsillar hypertrophy is a soft tissue abnormality, with a peak incidence in children ages 3 to 8 years old, and it is the most common anatomic cause of OSAS in children. Laryngomalacia and severe allergic rhinitis causing nasal obstruction are other soft tissue anomalies that can result in OSAS. Obesity causes increased fat deposition in the soft tissues of the upper airway. As the rates of childhood obesity in the developed world continue to climb, it is important for pediatricians to remember that obesity

---

© 2008 by Lippincott Williams & Wilkins, a Wolters Kluwer business

is a significant risk factor for OSAS. Neuromuscular diseases leading to generalized hypotonia or muscular incoordination are functional etiologies of OSAS in children. These include muscular dystrophy and cerebral palsy.

Polysomnography is the gold standard for the diagnosis of OSAS in children. The American Thoracic Society recommends obtaining a polysomnogram in the following situations: (a) to differentiate primary snoring from OSAS, (b) to evaluate a child with pathologic sleep patterns (e.g., difficulty with or irritability upon awakening), (c) to confirm suspected OSAS prior to surgical referral, (d) to evaluate the risk for respiratory complications prior to surgeries of the upper airway, (e) to evaluate children with laryngomalacia or cor pulmonale, (f) to evaluate obese children with signs or symptoms concerning for OSAS, (g) to evaluate children with sickle cell disease (due to the risk of vascular occlusion with intermittent hypoxemia during sleep), (h) to evaluate recurrent snoring postadenotonsillectomy, and (i) to titrate ongoing OSAS treatment with continuous positive airway pressure (CPAP).

Treatment for OSAS depends on the etiology. Adenotonsillectomy is curative in >75% of children with adenotonsillar hypertrophy. There are many other surgeries to treat craniofacial anomalies. In obese children, weight loss should be recommended but should not delay the initiation of other therapies. Treatment with CPAP or bilevel positive airway pressure (BiPAP) is appropriate when surgery is unsuccessful or not indicated, or when symptoms persist after surgery.

In summary, OSAS is a significant respiratory disorder of children, and failure to diagnose it can lead to considerable morbidity. At-risk groups include obese children, or children with adenotonsillar hypertrophy, craniofacial anomalies, and neuromuscular disorders. Diagnosis relies on polysomnography, and treatment options include surgery, CPAP, or BiPAP.

SUGGESTED READINGS

American Thoracic Society. Standards and indications for cardiopulmonary sleep studies in children. *Am J Respir Crit Care Med.* 1996;153:866–878.

Section on Pediatric Pulmonology, Subcommittee on Obstructive Sleep Apnea Syndrome. American Academy of Pediatrics. Clinical practice guideline: diagnosis and management of childhood obstructive sleep apnea syndrome. *Pediatrics.* 2002;109:704–712.

Sulit LG, Storfer-Isser A, Rosen CL, et al. Associations of obesity, sleep-disordered breathing and wheezing in children. *Am J Respir Crit Care Med.* 2005;171:659–664.

185

CONSIDER A DIFFERENTIAL DIAGNOSIS BEYOND EMPYEMA WHEN MANAGING A PLEURAL EFFUSION

CRAIG DeWOLFE, MD

WHAT TO DO – INTERPRET THE DATA

Although the most common etiology for a pleural effusion in the pediatric population is an empyema, its differential diagnosis is broad and the consequences of mismanaging one are significant. A practitioner should consider malignancy, congestive heart failure, autoimmune, and nephrotic processes, among others listed below, when confronted with an effusion. A careful history and physical examination, in addition to an appropriate workup and laboratory approach when considering the underlying pathophysiology, will prevent most diagnostic errors.

The work of breathing and diminished breath sounds found in pleural effusions, owing to the altered flow and absorption of pleural fluid with resultant compression of the lung, are universal. The confounding symptoms of the effusion, however, are often different because of the speed of fluid accumulation, the patient's cardiopulmonary reserve, and the associated symptoms of any underlying disease. In the case of pneumonia or other systemic inflammatory process such as a connective tissue disease, fluid accumulates because of the increased capillary permeability of vessels and oncotic pressure of proteins in the pleural space. These patients present with systemic symptoms of inflammation, such as fever and myalgia, in addition to cough or arthritis. In congestive heart failure, the capillary hydrostatic pressure is increased and results in bilateral effusions. Neonates with congenital heart disease commonly present as afebrile, cyanotic, with poor perfusion, and have a murmur. In older patients with congestive heart failure caused by a previously compensated and/or undiscovered congenital disorder, myopathy, myocarditis, pericarditis, or pericardial effusion, the associated symptoms include fatigue, failure to thrive, tachycardia, hepatosplenomegaly, and poor perfusion. Malignancies that result in mediastinal lymphadenopathy or obstruction of the lymphatic ducts, such as in lymphoma or superior vena cava syndrome, prevent lymphatic drainage from the pleural space and often manifest with more indolent fever, weight loss, night sweats, or facial edema. Patients with effusions resulting from nephrotic syndrome with its associated hypoalbuminemia and low plasma oncotic pressure present with

© 2008 by Lippincott Williams & Wilkins, a Wolters Kluwer business

dependent edema—commonly of the extremities, perioral or scrotal areas. Finally, patients who present with trauma, pancreatitis, or Down's or Noonan syndrome should be considered at risk for evolving effusions.

Radiographs are crucial in the diagnosis and management of pleural effusions. The practitioner should first use posteroanterior and lateral plain film radiographs in order to measure the effusion and identify associated parenchymal or cardiac disease. Lateral decubitus films should then be obtained to assess for mobile fluid. In the case of nonloculated effusions, placing the unaffected side inferior may also help the practitioner visualize the underlying parenchyma. Practitioners should avoid obtaining a supine film—common in portable x-rays when the patient is considered too sick to transfer—as effusions may manifest as diffuse haziness and be overlooked. Ultrasounds and computed tomography are second line studies for the practitioner concerned with managing a significant effusion. Ultrasounds differentiate solid versus liquid lesions with 92% accuracy and can often facilitate a thoracentesis so that fluid is obtained with the least amount of radiation exposure and risk to the patient. Chest computed tomographic scans are invaluable to surgeons when the predominance of evidence suggests an empyema and the extent of loculations and presence of an abscess will help them determine their surgical approach.

When pleural effusions are not clearly related to pneumonia, a thoracentesis will allow the clinician to evaluate the pleural fluid and either make the diagnosis or limit the differential. Gross visualization of the fluid may identify pus (suggestive of a bacterial process), chyle, blood, or fluid that can be further characterized as an exudate or transudate. An exudate suggests an inflammatory process that disrupts the integrity of the pleural lining and allows the movement of inflammatory cells and other proteins across the pleura. Alternatively, a transudate results from a pressure gradient across an intact lining and is characterized by a relative paucity of cells with chemistries similar to serum. The clinician should order a protein level, glucose, lactase dehydrogenase (LDH), cell count, and culture when differentiating a transudate from an exudate, whereas cytology, pH, amylase, triglyceride, or antinuclear antibody may be helpful for further classification. The Light's criteria for diagnosing an exudate include any one of the following: (a) the ratio of pleural protein to serum protein is >0.5, (b) the ratio of pleural LDH to serum LDH is >0.6, or (c) the ratio of pleural LDH to the upper limit of normal for serum is 2/3. If the fluid is an exudate, the clinician should consider bacteria, tuberculosis, virus, neoplasm, connective tissue, pancreatitis, esophageal perforation, or pulmonary infarction high on the differential. If the fluid is a transudate, the differential diagnosis includes congestive heart failure, nephrotic syndrome, cirrhosis, peritoneal fluid, or hypothyroidism. A milky fluid suggests a chylothorax from an injury to the lymphatic channel from a neoplasm, surgery, tuberculosis, or congenital chylothorax. A bloody fluid in the absence of trauma suggests malignancy, lung infarction, or postpericardiotomy syndrome.

The degree of symptoms and pathology will determine the extent of intervention, which includes close monitoring without further drainage, intermittent therapeutic thoracentesis, or placement of a tube with or without surgical thoracotomy. Any patient with respiratory compromise attributed to the effusion should have the fluid drained. In addition, a grossly purulent fluid suggestive of an empyema should be drained with a chest tube because of the high likelihood of developing loculations, pleural peel, or other tissue injury. Further use of antibiotics, diuretics, anti-inflammatory drugs, or other therapeutic measures is dictated by the ultimate diagnosis.

In summary, not all pleural effusions are empyemas, but with the appropriate clinical suspicion, thorough history, exam, and logical diagnostic approach, the clinician will avoid most therapeutic mishaps or delays.

SUGGESTED READINGS

Boyer DM. Evaluation and management of a child with a pleural effusion. *Pediatr Emerg Care.* 2005;21:63–68.

Montgomery M, Sigalet D. Air and liquid in the pleural space. In: Chernick V, Boat TR, Willmont RW, et al., eds. *Kendig's Disorders of the Respiratory Tract in Children.* 7th ed. Philadelphia: Saunders; 2006, chapter 21.

186

DO NOT USE STEROIDS IN PATIENTS WITH RESPIRATORY SYNCYTIAL VIRUS (RSV) BECAUSE IT MAY LEAD TO SUPERINFECTION WITH BACTERIA

DOROTHY CHEN, MD

WHAT TO DO – MAKE A DECISION

RSV is the major cause of lower respiratory tract infections in young children. It is a paramyxovirus that is found in ocular or nasal secretions and on fomites. It is also a nosocomial pathogen, so it is crucial to take precautions and prevent the spread of disease. The incubation period varies from 2 to 8 days. RSV may localize to the upper airway, but 50% or more of infections in infants spread to the lower respiratory tract. Therefore, bronchiolitis and pneumonia are often a result of RSV infection.

In bronchiolitis, viruses induce necrosis of bronchiolar epithelium, increased mucus secretion, and edema of the submucosa. Mucus obstructs the bronchioles and this leads to hyperinflation and collapse of lung tissue. Patients initially experience fever, rhinorrhea, pharyngitis, and cough; after the initial few days, they can develop tachypnea and wheezing. Each year, as many as 90,000 infants are hospitalized in the United States for bronchiolitis.

The treatment for RSV is largely supportive care. Children often require close observation, intravenous fluids, and supplemental oxygen. Bronchodilators and steroids are often used, but have limited efficacy. Steroids are postulated to have an impact on bronchiolitis by decreasing bronchiolar inflammation and hyperactivity. However, treatment with intravenous steroids has not demonstrated clinical improvements. The American Academy of Pediatrics' 2006 clinical practice guidelines, Diagnosis and Management of Bronchiolitis, does not recommend corticosteroids or bronchodilators in the management of bronchiolitis.

In a randomized controlled trial of 147 infants hospitalized with documented RSV infection, prednisolone was not shown to have a significant effect on the course of hospitalization or the duration of hospital stay. At the 1-month and the 1-year follow-up, variables, such as the number of admissions for respiratory tract infection, the number of children coughing at night, and the number of children with otitis media, were examined. There were no significant differences between the two groups.

© 2008 by Lippincott Williams & Wilkins, a Wolters Kluwer business

Other studies have studied the effect of steroids on bronchiolitis, but the patients did not all have RSV. A meta-analysis of six studies showed that corticosteroids decreased the clinical symptom scores and length of stay in children with bronchiolitis. However, only two of the studies included only children with positive RSV tests.

The Cochrane Database of Systemic Reviews completed a meta-analysis of 13 studies to review the use of glucocorticoids for acute viral bronchiolitis in infants and young children. The analysis included 1,198 children, ages 0 to 30 months, and only randomized controlled studies. The length of stay was lower in children treated with glucocorticoids, but the findings were not statistically significant. Similarly, there were no differences between the treatment and placebo groups in regards to clinical outcome scores (respiratory rate, hemoglobin oxygen saturation or readmission rates).

SUGGESTED READINGS

American Academy of Pediatrics Subcommittee on Diagnosis and Management of Bronchiolitis. Diagnosis and management of bronchiolitis. *Pediatrics.* 2006;118(4): 1774–1793.

Bülow SM, Nir M, Levin E, et al. Prednisolone treatment of respiratory syncytial virus infection: a randomized controlled trial of 147 infants. *Pediatrics.* 1999;104:e77.

Garrison MM, Christakis DA, Harvey E, et al. Systemic corticosteroids in infant bronchiolitis: a meta-analysis. *Pediatrics.* 2000;105(4):E44.

McCarthy CA, Hall CB. Respiratory syncytial virus: concerns and control. *Pediatr Rev.* 2003;24(9):301–309.

McIntosh K. Respiratory Syncytial Virus. In: Behrman RE, Kliegman RM, Jenson HB, eds. *Nelson Textbook of Pediatrics.* 17th ed. Philadelphia: Saunders; 2004:1076–1079.

Patel H, Platt R, Lozano JM, et al. Glucocorticoids for acute viral bronchiolitis in infants and young children. *Cochrane Database Syst Rev.* 2004;(3):CD004878.

187

DO NOT USE NEBULIZED DEXAMETHASONE IN CROUP BECAUSE IT IS INFERIOR TO INTRAVASCULAR, INTRAMUSCULAR, OR ENTERAL DEXAMETHASONE

CAROLINE RASSBACH, MD

WHAT TO DO – MAKE A DECISION

Viral croup is the most common form of airway obstruction in children 6 months to 6 years of age. When symptoms are severe enough to seek medical attention, oral dexamethasone is the preferred therapy because of cost, ease of administration, and efficacy. Intravascular and intramuscular dexamethasone are reasonable alternatives. Nebulized steroids are more expensive and less efficacious than oral dexamethasone for the treatment of croup. Croup is a viral illness caused most commonly by parainfluenza viruses (types 1, 2, and 3). Croup can also be caused by influenza A and B, adenovirus, respiratory syncytial virus, rhinovirus, and enteroviruses. Croup can affect the larynx, trachea, bronchi, and lungs, causing inflammation and swelling. The subglottic area is particularly affected, resulting in a narrowed airway. Classic symptoms of croup include a barking cough, hoarse voice, inspiratory stridor, and varying degrees of respiratory distress. Croup most commonly affects children between 6 months and 6 years of age, with a peak incidence at 2 years. The incidence in children younger than 6 years of age is approximately 6 per 100 annually. The illness predominates in the fall and winter.

When a child presents with stridor, other diagnoses such as foreign body aspiration, angioedema, epiglottitis, and bacterial tracheitis must be considered in the differential. Croup is diagnosed clinically based on its characteristic history. It begins with 12 to 72 hours of nasal congestion and low-grade fevers, followed by hoarseness and a barky cough. Patients may also have inspiratory stridor and respiratory distress. Symptoms of croup are worse at night, when in the supine position, and with agitation and crying. Symptoms peak between 24 and 48 hours, and usually resolve within 1 week.

Patients with croup usually have normal oxygen saturation. Neck radiographs may be performed if the diagnosis is uncertain; however, the classic "steeple sign" is present in only about 50% of cases. Laryngoscopy should be performed in children with suspected croup if they have a long-standing history of stridor, were previously intubated, or are younger than 4 months

ⓒ 2008 by Lippincott Williams & Wilkins, a Wolters Kluwer business

of age. Croup is usually managed in the outpatient setting with mist therapy, steroids, and close follow-up. Mist is thought to work by moistening secretions, decreasing airway inflammation, and decreasing the viscosity of secretions. Any child with croup and respiratory distress is a candidate for steroid treatment. Steroids have been shown to improve symptoms within 6 hours. For hospitalized children, steroids also result in shorter hospital stays and less use of epinephrine. One study to determine the efficacy of oral dexamethasone compared with nebulized budesonide showed that both are equally effective, although oral dexamethasone is cheaper and easier to administer than nebulized budesonide. Another study comparing oral versus nebulized dexamethasone showed greater improvement in symptoms and less need for subsequent medical intervention in patients treated with oral dexamethasone. As a result, oral dexamethasone in a single dosage of 0.15 mg/kg is used for the treatment of mild-to-moderate croup. Intravenous and intramuscular routes are equally effective when oral administration is not feasible.

For patients with moderate respiratory distress, nebulized racemic epinephrine may also be used. Racemic epinephrine reduces bronchial and tracheal secretions as well as mucosal edema through its α- and β-adrenergic properties. This usually results in decreased inspiratory stridor and intercostals retractions within 30 minutes of administration. The benefits of racemic epinephrine last approximately 2 hours.

Only a small number of patients with croup will require hospitalization. Patients should be hospitalized for croup if they have hypoxemia or cyanosis, altered mental status, worsening stridor or respiratory distress, stridor at rest, restlessness, or toxic appearance. Patients who have received steroids and racemic epinephrine in the outpatient setting can safely be discharged home if they do not show signs of respiratory distress at least 3 hours after racemic epinephrine.

Croup is a self-limited viral illness resulting from inflammation and swelling of the upper airway. When respiratory distress is present, patients should receive oral dexamethasone to decrease airway swelling. Intravenous and intramuscular dexamethasone are alternatives. Patients may also receive racemic epinephrine and mist therapy to alleviate symptoms.

SUGGESTED READINGS

Klassen TP, Craig WR, Moher D, et al. Nebulized budesonide and oral dexamethasone for treatment of croup: a randomized controlled trial. *JAMA.* 1998;279(20):1629–1632.

Knutson D, Aring A. Viral croup. *Am Fam Physician.* 2004;69(3):535–540.

Luria JW, Gonzalez-del-Rey JA, DiGiulio GA, et al. Effectiveness of oral or nebulized dexamethasone for children with mild croup. *Arch Pediatr Adolesc Med.* 2001;(155):1340–1345.

188

CONSIDER THE REASONS FOR HYPOVENTILATION AFTER ANESTHESIA. IT MAY REPRESENT RESIDUAL ANESTHESIA, BUT NOT ALWAYS

RENÉE ROBERTS, MD

WHAT TO DO – GATHER APPROPRIATE DATA

Mild hypoxemia, airway obstruction, hypercapnia, atelectasis, and bronchospasm are so common during emergence from anesthesia that anesthesiologists and postanesthetic nurses routinely provide good prophylactic therapy in the modern surgical setting. These problems are often considered a natural consequence of giving drugs that depress central respiratory drive, temporarily decrease lung volume, impair protective airway reflexes, depress secretion mobilization, and eliminate sighing (auto-positive end-expiratory pressure [auto-PEEP], preventing atelectasis). Adverse pulmonary outcomes are often attributed to anesthesia care, but a significant component of perioperative risk derives from the surgical site, postoperative pain, and effects of pharmacologic pain management. These risks must be recognized by the perioperative staff so that more serious perioperative pulmonary complications, such as bronchitis, pneumonia, pulmonary edema, aspiration, and respiratory failure, do not evolve.

Problems with oxygenation, ventilation, and airway maintenance are cardinal signs of perioperative pulmonary complications and can be discussed within the context of hypoxia. Hypoxia is defined as decreased oxygen tension with concomitant decreased oxygen supply in the blood delivered to the tissues. The common postoperative causes of hypoxia fall into two categories: anemic hypoxia and hypoxemic hypoxia. Anemic hypoxia results from a reduction in hemoglobin concentration, either from diseases such as sickle cell disease, or from unreplaced surgical losses. Anemic hypoxia can also be due to the conditions that shift the oxyhemoglobin dissociation curve (acid base balance, temperature) and or change the binding capacity of hemoglobin such as HbF found in infants. Postoperative hypoxemic hypoxia results when oxygen exchange in the lungs is problematic and can be divided into two categories: ventilation/perfusion mismatch and hypoventilation.

When the ratio of ventilation ($\dot{V}$) and perfusion ($\dot{Q}$) of the lungs is not normal, the resulting hypoxemia is from $\dot{V}/\dot{Q}$ mismatch. Acute changes in $\dot{V}$ and $\dot{Q}$ take place as a function of changes in chest wall configuration,

ⓒ 2008 by Lippincott Williams & Wilkins, a Wolters Kluwer business

surgical positioning, intraoperative ventilation modes, and anesthetic effects on pulmonary blood flow. Acute anesthetic effects are largely reversed at the end of surgery; however, certain surgeries have postoperative implications for lung function. For instance, after upper abdominal and thoracic surgery, lung capacities are reduced by approximately 40% for the first few days following surgery, and measurable decrement in respiratory mechanics persists for up to 2 weeks. Other causes of $\dot{V}/\dot{Q}$ mismatch include partial airway obstruction (postextubation stridor, laryngospasm or bronchospasm); inadequate tidal volumes and cough (from recurarization or residual sedation); and atelectasis (from sustained reduction of peak air flows and total lung volume during and after anesthesia).

Moderate V/Q mismatch may evolve to severe mismatch otherwise known as shunt (there is no oxygen exchange (V) with the circulating blood (Q). Pneumonia, bronchitis, and pulmonary edema are examples of shunt. Pulmonary aspiration and the ensuing pneumonia is widely viewed as the most common serious complication of anesthesia that can be avoided by adherence to fasting and preventative measures. An increased risk for aspiration includes emergency surgery, obesity, reflux, neuromuscular disease, a full stomach, and sedation. Another preoperative risk factor for a PPC that can lead to shunt is sleep apnea (from congenital syndromes, craniofacial abnormalities, obesity, cardiac dysfunction). If not managed carefully, dramatic hypoxic episodes in the postoperative period can cause cardiovascular decompensation, postobstructive pulmonary edema, or pulmonary aspiration syndrome. And finally, negative pressure pulmonary edema caused by inspiration against closed vocal cords after extubation should also be in the differential for hypoxemic hypoxia from shunt.

The other etiology of hypoxemic hypoxia is hypoventilation: inadequate minute ventilation (respiratory rate × tidal volume) to remove the carbon dioxide produced. Whenever alveolar ventilation is inadequate, carbon dioxide increases in the blood and alveolus and there is little remaining for other gases (including oxygen); when hypoventilation occurs in a patient breathing room air, hypoxia inevitably occurs. Causes of postoperative hypoventilation in spontaneously ventilating patients are airway obstruction, acute depression of the brainstem respiratory center by drugs (opiates, barbiturates, inhaled agents), pain (after thoracotomy, chest trauma, high upper abdominal incision), pneumothorax, neuromuscular blocking drugs, abnormalities of spinal conducting pathways (C3–5) as in high cervical surgery, phrenic nerve injury via cold injury (cardiopulmonary bypass) or ablation. Postoperative hypoventilation may also result from respiratory muscle weakness from unrecognized dystrophy, malnutrition, prolonged mechanical ventilation, and problems with the respiratory drive from the medullary center due to surgery for trauma, neoplasm, or hemorrhage.

The neurologic symptoms of hypoxemia (anxiety, confusion, restlessness, somnolence, and coma) may be masked in the postanesthetized patient. Because anesthetics attenuate, many of the normal cardiorespiratory responses to hypoxia, other subtle warning signs, such as tachycardia and tachypnea, are blunted. Furthermore, oxygen consumption in the newborn is two to three times that of older children and adults and the newborn responds to hypercarbia and hypoxia paradoxically with apnea rather than hyperventilation. This paradoxic response is even more prominent in premature infants.

Anesthesia and postanesthetic care unit nursing staff routinely manage partial airway obstruction, hypoventilation, and hypoxemia associated with the residual effects of muscle relaxants, sedatives, narcotics, and anesthetic agents. It is imperative that postoperative patients have their saturation monitored with pulse oximetry and their ventilation carefully monitored. If hypoxemia persists or worsens despite supplemental oxygen, bronchodilators, airway management, techniques to expand atelectatic lungs, or reversal of sedative/narcotic and relaxant drugs, the patient should undergo new clinical assessment directed toward the most likely problems and supportive maneuvers such as continuous positive airway pressure or ventilation. Evolving respiratory distress should be worked up with studies to rule out pulmonary edema, pneumothorax, pulmonary embolism, or obstruction of upper or lower airway. In the case of hypoxemia after thoracic and upper abdominal surgery, postoperative care should recognize the need for multimodal pain control without excessive narcotic, sedative, mobilize patient and secretions, preserve lung volume, and ambulate (if appropriate) as soon as possible.

SUGGESTED READINGS

Watson CB. Respiratory complications associated with anesthesia. *Anesthesiol Clin North Am.* 2002;20(3):513–537.
Wilson WC, Shapiro B. Perioperative hypoxia. The clinical spectrum and current oxygen monitoring methodology. *Anesthesiol Clin North Am.* 2001;19(4):1271–1282.

189

Use appropriate oxygen delivery devices to achieve the necessary fraction of inspired oxygen (FiO_2)

Renée Roberts, MD

What to Do – Make a Decision

When assessing a patient who is hypoxic, monitors to measure pulse oximetry, electrocardiogram, and blood pressure should be placed while providing supplemental oxygen. The mental status should be observed and the chest should be auscultated to ensure that the airway is patent, that the lungs are clear, and that spontaneous respiratory efforts are adequate. Quickly check areas to rule out include obstruction either via collapse of the soft tissues or via a foreign object (such as a mucous plug or vomitus), stridor, and bronchospasm. These reasons for hypoxia should be ruled out and addressed before significant improvement is seen with supplemental oxygen.

In certain patient populations, the benefits of supplemental oxygen must be weighed with the potential risks. Neonates, especially expremature infants younger than 44 weeks' postconceptual age, are at risk of developing retrolental fibroplasia (otherwise known as retinopathy of prematurity). It is suggested that PaO_2 does not rise above 80 torr in this population. Supplemental oxygen in patients with certain congenital heart lesions (hypoplastic left heart syndrome, single ventricle physiologies, ventricular septal defect, patent ductus arteriosus) will cause an increase in alveolar oxygen tension and may compromise the balance between pulmonary and systemic flow. Patients taking certain chemotherapeutic drugs, such as bleomycin, may be prone to oxygen toxicity and pulmonary fibrosis.

Nasal cannulae fall under the category of low-flow systems. They are used to provide a low concentration of oxygen to the patient. The actual FiO_2 delivered depends on oxygen flow, nasopharyngeal volume, and inspiratory flow. FiO_2 roughly increases 1% to 2% above 21% per liter of oxygen flow in a normally breathing adult. So, at oxygen flows of 3 to 4 L/min, nasal cannulas can deliver an FiO_2 of 30% to 35%. An FiO_2 of 40% to 50% can be attained with flows of >10 L/min. In infants, FiO_2 of 0.35, 0.45, 0.6, and 0.68, with flows of 0.25, 0.5, 0.75, and 1 L/min, respectively, can be attained.

Although nasal cannulae have the advantage of allowing feeding and increased mobility while delivering supplemental oxygen, they do dry out

© 2008 by Lippincott Williams & Wilkins, a Wolters Kluwer business

mucous membranes and are poorly tolerated by patients at high flows. In fact, if higher flows are needed to achieve a higher FIO_2, alternative methods of oxygen delivery should be considered. "Simple" or oxygen masks without a reservoir bag are suited for patients who require higher levels of oxygen for short periods. The body of the mask serves as the reservoir or both the inspired oxygen and expired carbon dioxide (CO_2). The required minimum flow needs to be checked with the manufacturer so that rebreathing of CO_2 is prevented. The FIO_2 delivered is variable; it may range from 0.3 to 0.6 at 5 to 10 L/min.

When higher levels of FIO_2 are needed, the partial rebreather mask and the nonrebreathing mask can be used. Both have a reservoir bag at the end of the mask but the nonrebreather uses valves between the bag and mask and at least one of the mask's exhalation ports. Typical minimum flows range from 10 to 15 L/min. Partial rebreathers can attain an FIO_2 between 0.4 and 0.6, whereas nonrebreathers are used to deliver $FIO_2 > 0.6$. Both masks are useful for patients with normal spontaneous minute ventilation, such as trauma patients and victims of mild carbon monoxide poisoning. As with all the mask methods of supplemental oxygen delivery, the maximum FIO_2 attainable has not been well established in infants and children.

Do not leave dyspneic patients on nonrebreather masks. These patients are candidates for fixed-performance, high-flow oxygen systems. These include anesthesia bags or bag-mask-valve systems and air entrapment "Venturi" masks. For practical purposes, bag-mask-valve systems are often used in resuscitation situations. The "Venturi" mask system comes in fixed and adjustable FIO_2 models, with minimum flow instructions. An FIO_2 of 1.0 is attainable depending on flow.

Many infants and children cannot tolerate nasal cannulae or masks. Oxygen hoods are an alternative. FIO_2 can vary from 0.21 to 1.0 and cannot be easily controlled because a constant flow of gas is needed through and out of the system to remove CO_2. Flows of >7 L/min are required to wash out expired CO_2. The hood is useful for short-term oxygen therapy for relatively inactive infants.

Supplemental oxygen will improve oxygenation. However, it will not improve hypercarbia. If the patient is hypoventilating, dyspneic, or shows an altered mental status that does not improve with oxygen, obtain an arterial blood gas if time permits. Use your clinical judgment instead of waiting for lab results if additional measures are needed. More supportive measures, such as the insertion of a nasal or oral airway, continuous positive airway pressure, bilevel positive airway pressure, positive pressure ventilation, or intubation may be required.

Suggested Reading

Myers TR, American Association for Respiratory Care (AARC). AARC Clinical Practice Guideline: selection of an oxygen delivery device for neonatal and pediatric patients—2002 revision & update. *Respir Care.* 2002;47(6):707–716.

190

ABSENT BREATH SOUNDS IN AN INTUBATED PATIENT SHOULD MAKE YOU ENSURE THAT THE PATIENT IS POSITIVELY INTUBATED

RENÉE ROBERTS, MD

WHAT TO DO – INTERPRET THE DATA

Also consider *major* bronchospasm, right mainstem intubation, or tension pneumothorax—these conditions happen often more than you think.

The sudden onset of peak inspiratory pressures and reduced or absent sounds after intubation can have many causes. In cases where intubation was confirmed by direct vision or by prior knowledge of ventilation, mechanical factors should be considered first. Mechanical factors (e.g., kinked endotracheal tube [ETT] or circuit), endobronchial intubation, mucous plug, or leaning on the ETT neck or chest can be resolved easily. If there is no reason to believe there is a pneumothorax (i.e., there is not hyperresonance on percussion on one side of the chest, shift in the mediastinum, or unilateral breath sounds), then bronchospasm should be considered.

Etiologies of bronchospasm include the patient's intrinsic disease, chemical, or neurogenic causes. Bronchospasm is a common sequelae for those patients having intrinsic disease, such as reactive airway disease (RAD) and asthma. These patients are more sensitive to airway manipulation, which may result in severe bronchospasm with intubation. Furthermore, patients with a recent upper respiratory tract infection are more prone to bronchospasm because of the increased airway "irritability."

The second most common reason for severe bronchospasm is drugs. Histamine-releasing drugs, such as muscle relaxants, morphine, antibiotics (vancomycin), and gastrointestinal drugs (omeprazole), are usual culprits. Even nonsteroidal anti-inflammatory drugs have been related to an acute attack of asthma developing within minutes of the drug given. Other concomitant reactions to the histamine include profuse rhinorrhea, conjunctival injection, and scarlet flushing. However, any drug can be a suspect. If no other reasons for a change in pulmonary status are identified and the symptoms occurred just after a drug had been given, one should consider drug-induced bronchospasm as a cause. These reactions usually occur within a short period of time after the administration of drug and usually in patients with history of RAD or asthma.

© 2008 by Lippincott Williams & Wilkins, a Wolters Kluwer business

Chemical factors that cause bronchospasm include aspiration, either of secretions or of aerosolized irritants such as latex. Lastly, bronchospasm also can result from direct activation of receptors in the pulmonary system or from neurogenic activation. There have been cases of vagally induced bronchospasm (vagal tumor resection, vagal nerve stimulators).

Bronchospasm can be a severe, life-threatening occurrence that must be considered after intubation if no breath sounds are auscultated. When a patient is in severe bronchospasm, even after removing the tube to check for mucous plug, often one will see that mask ventilation is also impossible. When the tube is reinserted and reintubating is accurate, no breath sounds, chest movement, ETT fogging, end-tidal carbon dioxide, nor gastric sounds are detected. The use of albuterol, diphenhydramine (Benadryl), and small doses of epinephrine may be required to treat severe episodes of bronchospasm. Remember, epinephrine can be administered via the endotracheal tube or intravenously.

SUGGESTED READINGS

Carroll CL, Goodman DM. Endotracheal albuterol treatment of acute bronchospasms. *Am J Emerg Med.* 2004;22(6):506–507.

Kron SS. Severe bronchospasm and desaturation in a child associated with rapacuronium. *Anesthesiology.* 2001;94(5):923–924.

Liu M, Schellenberg A, Patterson T, et al. Intraoperative bronchospasm induced by stimulation of the vagus nerve. *Anesthesiology.* 1998;88(6):1655–1677.

Looney Y, O'Shea A, O'Dwyer R. Severe bronchospasm after parenteral parecoxib: cyclooxygenase-2 inhibitors: not the answer yet. *Anesthesiology.* 2005;102(2):473–474.

191

CONSIDER THE BROAD-DIFFERENTIAL DIAGNOSIS FOR WHEEZING IN CHILDREN

SARIKA JOSHI, MD

WHAT TO DO – GATHER APPROPRIATE DATA

Wheezing is a continuous musical sound produced by airflow through a narrowed or compressed airway. Wheezing can originate from both small and large airways. Ten to 15% of infants wheeze during the first year of life, and as many as one fourth of children younger than 5 years of age present to a physician with wheezing. Although asthma is the most common cause of recurrent wheezing, the differential diagnosis of wheezing in children includes foreign body aspiration, infections, vascular rings and slings, tracheobronchomalacia, tracheoesophageal fistula (TEF), mediastinal masses, gastroesophageal reflux (GER), dysfunctional swallow, immunodeficiency syndromes, cystic fibrosis (CF), and vocal cord dysfunction (VCD).

Conceptually, it is helpful to distinguish between acute-onset wheezing versus chronic or recurrent wheezing. Common causes of acute-onset wheezing in children are foreign body aspiration and infections. Foreign body aspiration occurs more in children younger than 3 years of age but less in infants. Classically, patients present with the history of a choking episode, but acute-onset wheezing alone warrants suspicion for foreign body aspiration. Exam may reveal unilateral wheezing or unequal breath sounds. Chest radiograph (CXR) may show unilateral hyperinflation or atelectasis or may be normal. Patients are usually unresponsive to bronchodilators. Definitive diagnosis is made by bronchoscopy. Common infectious agents that cause wheezing in children include respiratory syncytial virus, parainfluenza virus, metapneumovirus, rhinovirus, and *Mycoplasma pneumoniae*. Patients typically present with other signs of infection such as nasal congestion, rhinorrhea, cough, and fever. CXR findings and response to bronchodilator are variable.

Etiologies for recurrent wheezing can be categorized as anatomic or structural versus functional. Vascular rings and slings, tracheobronchomalacia, TEF, and mediastinal masses are some anatomic or structural causes of recurrent wheezing in children. Vascular rings and slings (i.e., double aortic arch, right-sided aortic arch, pulmonary artery sling) can compress large airways, such as the trachea and mainstem bronchi, thereby leading to stridor or wheezing. Patients generally present early in life, and CXR is almost always abnormal. Bronchodilator may actually exacerbate wheezing

© 2008 by Lippincott Williams & Wilkins, a Wolters Kluwer business

due to associated tracheobronchomalacia. Further workup involves barium esophagram, echocardiogram, and cardiac magnetic resonance imaging. In addition to vascular rings and slings, cardiac lesions that lead to pulmonary artery dilation, left atrial enlargement, left ventricular failure, or pulmonary venous outflow obstruction can lead to wheezing. Tracheobronchomalacia also presents early in life with stridor or wheezing but generally becomes more pronounced at 2 to 3 months of age. Stridor and wheezing worsen with infections and activity. CXR is often nondiagnostic, and bronchodilator may exacerbate wheezing due to the increasing airway obstruction caused by smooth muscle relaxation. Definitive diagnosis is made by bronchoscopy.

TEF generally presents in the immediate postnatal period. Patients present with coughing, choking, and wheezing from aspiration with feeds; older infants may also have a history of recurrent pneumonias. CXR may be consistent with recurrent pneumonias, and response to bronchodilator is variable. Further workup involves barium esophagram, esophagoscopy, and bronchoscopy. Mediastinal masses (i.e., tumors, bronchogenic cysts, enlarged lymph nodes) can compress the trachea or bronchi, thereby leading to stridor or wheezing. Patients may also have associated lymphadenopathy. CXR is usually abnormal, and patients are generally unresponsive to bronchodilator.

GER, dysfunctional swallow, immunodeficiency syndromes, CF, VCD, and asthma are some functional causes of recurrent wheezing in children. When GER is associated with chronic microaspiration, it leads to inflammation and edema, which results in airway narrowing and wheezing. Patients usually have other signs and symptoms of GER such as vomiting, arching and nighttime cough. CXR is usually normal, and response to bronchodilator is variable. Further workup involves pH probe or milk scan. Dysfunctional swallow should be suspected in children with neurologic or muscular disease. Classically, patients present with coughing from aspiration with feeds, but aspiration may be silent, and older children may have a history of recurrent pneumonias. Definitive diagnosis is made by barium swallow. Immunodeficiency syndromes, especially those with immunoglobulin(Ig)A or IgG deficiency, can result in recurrent pneumonias with wheezing. Patients may also present with recurrent otitis or pharyngitis. Preliminary immune workup includes complete blood count, quantitative immunoglobulins, and total hemolytic complement levels. CF is the most common autosomal recessive disease in whites, and patients may present with recurrent wheezing. CF should be suspected in children with concomitant respiratory and gastrointestinal symptoms, including failure to thrive. Definitive diagnosis is made by sweat or genetic testing. For dysfunctional swallow, immunodeficiency syndromes, and CF, CXR may be consistent with recurrent pneumonias, and response to bronchodilator is variable.

VCD is classically diagnosed in adolescent females. In patients with VCD, the true vocal cords adduct on inspiration and abduct on expiration, thereby causing recurrent stridor or wheezing. The etiology of VCD appears to be psychogenic, and symptoms may resolve when the patient is not being observed or is sleeping. CXR is usually normal, and response to bronchodilator is variable. Definitive diagnosis is made by bronchoscopy. Asthma is the most common cause of recurrent wheezing in children. Most patients with asthma present before 5 years of age, and cough is another common symptom. Usual triggers are infections, exercise, weather changes, and allergen exposure. CXR may show hyperinflation, peribronchial thickening, or atelectasis due to mucus plugging, and patients should respond to bronchodilator. Definitive diagnosis is made by pre- and postbronchodilator spirometry in children old enough to perform pulmonary function testing (typically older than 5 years of age).

In summary, the differential diagnosis for wheezing in children is broad. CXR findings and response to bronchodilator may help to narrow this differential. Remember the medical cliché: "all that wheezes is not asthma."

SUGGESTED READINGS

Finder JD. Understanding airway disease in infants. *Curr Probl Pediatr.* 1999;29:65–81.
Fireman P. The wheezing infant. *Pediatr Rev.* 1986;7:247–254.
Marinati LC, Boner AL. Clinical diagnosis of wheezing in early childhood. *Allergy.* 1995;50: 701–710.

192

CONSIDER THE DIAGNOSIS OF INTUSSUSCEPTION IN A CHILD WITH PAROXYSMAL BOUTS OF ABDOMINAL PAIN OR EMESIS

MICHAEL CLEMMENS, MD

WHAT TO DO – INTERPRET THE DATA

Intussusception is the most common cause of bowel obstruction in children after the newborn period. The incidence peaks in late infancy but may be seen at any age. Intussusception occurs when a part of the bowel collapses into the segment immediately distal to it, much in the way that a telescope collapses upon itself. The immediate consequence is restriction of venous flow, resulting in engorgement of the involved section and subsequent bowel obstruction. Arterial flow may eventually be compromised, leading to necrotic bowel and perforation. Untreated intussusception may lead to peritonitis, sepsis, and death. However, an early diagnosis minimizes the occurrences of these complications.

In children younger than 5 years, approximately 75% of classic ileocolic intussusceptions are idiopathic. After that age, the presence of a lead point is more common. The lead point may be a Meckel diverticulum, lymphoma, duplication, hypertrophied lymphoid tissue, or associated with a bowel wall lesion from Henoch-Schönlein purpura.

The initial history may be suggestive of gastroenteritis, with vomiting and abdominal pain as the presenting symptoms. However, in cases of intussusception, the vomiting may be clear initially, but it often becomes bilious with time. Bilious emesis in any child implies the presence of a bowel obstruction until proven otherwise. Also, in intussusception, the pain is more severe and classically occurs in waves every 10 to 20 minutes. The stool may be normal, have the appearance of currant jelly, or be grossly bloody. A history of lethargy is common, especially between bouts of pain. A viral syndrome frequently precedes intussusception.

© 2008 by Lippincott Williams & Wilkins, a Wolters Kluwer business

The physical examination may be normal in children with intussusception. The child's general appearance may be lethargic and suggestive of central nervous system disease. The abdomen may be flat, soft, and nontender. However, the classic finding is a right-sided, sausage-shaped mass, which is the intussusception. A more nondescript mass may be present or there may be no mass at all. Peritoneal signs are only present late in the course of the disease. A rectal exam may be helpful by confirming the presence of blood in the stool.

The majority of children with intussusception have some of these findings. The clinical triad of bilious emesis, an abdominal mass, and currant jelly stools is the exception rather than the rule. The clinician should consider the diagnosis of intussusception in any child with altered sensorium, bilious emesis, severe abdominal pain, abdominal mass, or blood in the stool.

Plain abdominal radiographs may demonstrate a bowel obstruction with dilated loops and the presence of air-fluid levels. However, early in the course, the plain films may be normal. The diagnostic test of choice is the contrast enema. This study may also be therapeutic, reducing the intussusception in more than 80% of cases. Barium is most commonly used, although air or saline may also suffice. When the contrast meets the obstruction, the diagnosis is established. The contrast is then instilled with slightly more pressure until the intussusception is reduced and there is free flow beyond the blockage. Failure to obtain reduction increases the likelihood that a lead point is present.

Prior to obtaining contrast studies, the patient should be stabilized. Most patients require intravenous hydration, bowel decompression with a nasogastric tube, and pain control. Antibiotics are administered when peritonitis is suspected. In addition, a contrast enema should not be attempted without the immediate availability of a pediatric surgeon because of the risk of perforation. When contrast enema does not reduce the intussusception, the next step is surgery. Manual reduction at laparotomy can usually be accomplished. Resection is required if nonviable bowel or a pathological lead point are found.

SUGGESTED READINGS

Davis CF, McCabe AJ, Raine PA. The ins and outs of intussusception: history and management over the past 50 years. *J Pediatr Surg.* 2003;38(7 Suppl):60–64.

del-Pozo G, Albillos JC, Tejedor D, et al. Intussusception in children: current concepts in diagnosis and enema reduction. *Radiographics.* 1999;19:299–319.

West KW, Grosfeld JL. Intussusception. In: Wyllie R, Hyams JS. *Pediatric Gastrointestinal Disease: Pathophysiology, Diagnosis, Management.* Philadelphia: WB Saunders; 1999:427.

193

HAVE A HIGH INDEX OF SUSPICION FOR PYLORIC STENOSIS IN A NEONATE WITH PERSISTENT, PROGRESSIVE, OR FORCEFUL EMESIS

BRIAN KIT, MD

WHAT TO DO – INTERPRET THE DATA

Infantile hypertrophic pyloric stenosis (IHPS) results in marked hypertrophy of both the circular and longitudinal muscular layers. The effect of the muscular hypertrophy is a lengthening of the canal and thickening of the pylorus, causing the classic "olive" shape. Hypertrophy of the pyloric muscle occurs during the postnatal period, which becomes clinically apparent between 3 and 6 weeks of age.

In their report, Applegate et al., described the incidence of IHPS to be approximately 2 in 1,000. Boys have a four- to fivefold higher risk of developing IHPS compared to girls, and there appears to be a predilection for the first-born child. The development of IHPS is believed to be multifactorial, with both genetic and environmental factors playing a role.

The classic presentation is an afebrile, first-born male child who develops nonbilious, projectile vomiting immediately following feeding, and who is interested in feeding after episodes of emesis. The diagnosis should be considered in any child when there is emesis worsening over days to weeks, becoming more frequent and increasingly forceful. It is extremely important for the clinician to observe the baby feeding, noting the amount of the feed, onset of emesis following feeding, and the quality and quantity of emesis. Depending on the duration of symptoms, there may be physical exam findings associated with dehydration. Classically, infants with pyloric stenosis have hyponatremia, hypochloremia, hypokalemia, and metabolic alkalosis, resulting from chronic loss of gastric secretions.

The abdominal exam is generally benign, although with advanced gastric obstruction there may be gastric distension. The examiner may note peristaltic waves progressing from left to right prior to the episode of emesis. In the past, there has been emphasis placed on palpation of the "olive" sign to accurately diagnose pyloric stenosis, which is done by palpating the right upper quadrant while raising the infant's feet and flexing the legs. The "olive" is approximately 1 cm. When palpated, a pyloric mass is pathognomonic for IHPS. However, palpation of the "olive" sign is often difficult, and practitioners

ⓒ 2008 by Lippincott Williams & Wilkins, a Wolters Kluwer business

often rely on radiographic evidence of pyloric stenosis to confirm the diagnosis.

In the past, the radiographic imaging test of choice was an upper gastrointestinal (GI) series and it remains the most common test for the diagnosis of IHPS in some centers. In the upper GI series, the diagnosis of IHPS demonstrates obstruction of contrast beyond the stomach. There is a relatively high rate of error with the upper GI series. Additionally, because this is a fluoroscopic study, it carries the additional risks of radiation. Ultrasound is now the test of choice. Ultrasound can be performed without the risks of radiation but is often said to be "operator-dependent," limiting its implementation into universal practice. A common ultrasound criterion for pyloric stenosis is 3 to 4 mm transpyloric muscle thickness or pyloric muscle length of >17 mL.

The first step in the treatment of pyloric stenosis involves repletion of fluid losses and correction of electrolyte abnormalities. Surgical repair should be deferred until the electrolytes have been corrected. Failure to correct the metabolic alkalosis is associated with an increased risk of postoperative apnea. Generally, correction begins with normal saline, followed by fluids containing dextrose, sodium chloride, and potassium chloride. After fluid and electrolyte correction, surgery is performed, which is curative and involves incision and division of the pyloric muscle. The procedure of choice is called the Ramstedt pyloromyotomy.

SUGGESTED READINGS

Applegate MS, Druschel CM. The epidemiology of infantile hypertrophic pyloric stenosis in New York State, 1983 to 1990. *Arch Pediatr Adolesc Med*. 1995;149:1123–1129.

Hernanz-Schulman M, Sells LL, Ambrosino MM, et al. Hypertrophic pyloric stenosis in the infant without a palpable olive: accuracy of sonographic diagnosis. *Radiology*. 1994;193:771–776.

Stunden RJ, LeQuesne GW, Little KE. The improved ultrasound diagnosis of hypertrophic pyloric stenosis. *Pediatr Radiol*. 1986;16:200–205.

194

CONSIDER THE DIAGNOSIS OF TESTICULAR TORSION IN CHILDREN WITH ACUTE SCROTAL PAIN OR SWELLING

MICHAEL CLEMMENS, MD

WHAT TO DO – GATHER APPROPRIATE DATA, INTERPRET THE DATA, MAKE A DECISION, TAKE ACTION

Consult a urologist early and obtain an emergent color Doppler ultrasound in cases of suspected torsion, as delay in diagnosis increases the likelihood of a poor outcome.

Torsion of the testicle occurs when the testicle twists on its vascular pedicle, compromising blood flow to and from the testes. Torsion may occur prenatally, during the newborn period, or anytime throughout childhood. The peak incidence is during adolescence, but a smaller peak occurs late in gestation and in the first months of life. Swelling from vascular engorgement occurs when venous drainage is impaired by torsion of the spermatic veins. Arterial compromise occurs when the testicle twists more severely or after longer-standing venous occlusion. The likelihood of testicular viability is directly related to the length of time between the event and surgical detorsion. When corrected within 6 hours of the event, testicular viability approaches 100%; beyond 24 hours, the viability nears 0%. Therefore, a high index of suspicion and immediate surgical consultation are mandatory.

Scrotal pain and swelling are the most common symptoms of testicular torsion. The pain is usually sudden in onset, unilateral, and severe. Irritability may be the presenting symptom in infants. Older children may complain of groin, thigh, or abdominal pain. Vomiting and nausea are sometimes seen. Scrotal swelling may be noted by the parents or the patient.

The physical exam reveals a child in severe discomfort. The hemiscrotum is swollen and may be erythematous. The testicle is large and tender compared to the uninvolved side. It may be high in the scrotum or oriented horizontally. The cremasteric reflex is almost always absent. Its presence points away from the diagnosis of torsion. Its absence, however, does not rule out other scrotal conditions, such as epididymitis.

Color Doppler ultrasonography is most commonly used to evaluate testicular size, adnexal structures, and blood flow. The testicle is usually enlarged compared to the unaffected side. Compromise of blood flow is almost

© 2008 by Lippincott Williams & Wilkins, a Wolters Kluwer business

always seen in torsion; however, some arterial flow may still be present. Complete absence of arterial flow is highly suggestive of the diagnosis. Nuclear scanning is also reliable but may take more time than sonography.

When testicular torsion is suspected on clinical grounds, surgical consultation should be requested immediately. Consultation should not be delayed to obtain diagnostic studies. When the diagnosis is unclear, the clinician should obtain imaging studies in an effort to rule out torsion.

There are several pitfalls to be avoided when evaluating the child with an acute scrotum. The provider must obtain a detailed history, especially regarding pain and swelling, and perform a complete examination. Always evaluate the cremasteric reflex. The diagnosis of torsion must be considered in any child with a swollen or painful hemiscrotum. Imaging studies and surgical consultation must be obtained in a timely fashion.

SUGGESTED READINGS

Kadish HA, Bolte RG. A retrospective review of pediatric patients with epididymitis, testicular torsion, and torsion of the testicular appendages. *Pediatrics.* 1998;102(1 Pt 1):73–76.

Karmazyn B, Steinberg R, Kornreish L, et al. Clinical and sonographic criteria of the acute scrotum in children: a retrospective study of 172 boys. *Pediatr Radiol.* 2005;35:302–310.

Kass EJ, Lundak B. The acute scrotum. *Pediatr Clin North Am.* 1997;44:1251–1266.

195

DO NOT CONSIDER PAINLESS VAGINAL BLEEDING IN ADOLESCENT FEMALES AS DUE TO MENARCHE ALONE

ESTHER FORRESTER, MD

WHAT TO DO – INTERPRET THE DATA

The evaluation of gynecologic problems in prepubertal girls is often a complex, challenging process. This is partly due to the pediatricians' lack of training in gynecologic examination techniques and the inability to differentiate normal variants from abnormal findings. The rise in concern and incidence of sexual abuse has placed the pediatrician as a central provider in this social, physical, and psychological issue, therefore, mandating an increased knowledge, skills, and comfort in evaluating gynecologic conditions in children. Most girls presenting with genital symptoms have normal findings or a nontraumatic disorder.

When a patient presents with (or her parent describes) a complaint of vaginal bleeding, many questions should come to mind. What is the age of the patient? Is it really blood? What is the sexual maturity rating (SMR) of the patient? A red or brown discoloration present in the diaper or underpants may represent stool, bloody stool, bloody urine, or color-stained urine. The bleeding cannot be due to normal menarche if the patient is only SMR 1 or 2 for breast development because menarche typically occurs at SMR 3 or 4 breast development. It is extremely common to have vaginal bleeding during the first weeks of life (small amounts). This is due to withdrawal bleeding secondary to decreasing maternal estrogen. The differential diagnosis of vaginal bleeding in children is included in *Table 195.1*.

It is important to note that vaginal bleeding occurs in >90% of cases of vaginal foreign body, as compared to a foul-smelling discharge, which is far less common. The most common foreign body encountered is wadded toilet paper. Also, accidental trauma must be differentiated from abusive trauma. Vaginal trauma, resulting in bleeding that is due to a straddle injury, rarely results in hymenal trauma. Trauma caused by inserted objects or sexual

ⓒ 2008 by Lippincott Williams & Wilkins, a Wolters Kluwer business

TABLE 195.1	DIFFERENTIAL DIAGNOSIS OF VAGINAL BLEEDING	
VISIBLE LESION	**NO VISIBLE LESION**
Lichen sclerosis et atrophicus	Neonatal withdrawal bleeding
Urethral prolapse	Hematuria
Straddle injury	Rectal bleeding
Penetrating injury	Infectious vaginitis
Genital warts	Vaginal foreign body
External hemangioma	Blood dyscrasia
Precocious puberty	Exogenous hormone withdrawal
Pseudoprecocious puberty	Isolated premature menarche
Neoplasm–vulva or lower vagina	Neoplasm–upper vagina or uterus

abuse often results in laceration of the hymen. Urethral prolapse is caused by a weakness in the tissues supporting the urethra. It may present during the toddler years or as late as adolescence; it often presents as painless vaginal bleeding. It is more common in African American girls than white girls. On examination, a bulging, dark red to black mass is seen at the introitus.

This mass is a vascular ring of congested edematous tissue. Treatment includes the application of a small amount of estrogen cream to the affected area daily for 1 week, then every other day for an additional week. Warm sitz baths may also be helpful. Stool softeners may need to be included in the treatment regimen, as straining exacerbates the prolapse. If the aforementioned treatments are ineffective, or if the patient is unable to urinate at presentation, surgical intervention is necessary.

Lichen sclerosis et atrophicus is an additional cause of painless vaginal bleeding. It is autoimmune in nature and usually affects postmenopausal women. The most common complaint in the pediatric patient is genital itching. Examination reveals a figure-of-eight pattern of pale, atrophic skin around the anus and vulva. The introitus is spared. Treatment involves the use of 1% hydrocortisone cream as needed. This conservative method is associated with episodic exacerbation at least until puberty. Topical tacrolimus and pimecrolimus are being studied as to their efficacy in treating this condition in pediatrics.

Vaginal bleeding is concerning for both parents and children. Common causes and treatments need to be kept in mind to provide the family with reassurance and treatment.

SUGGESTED READINGS

Bernard D, Peters M, Makoroff K. The evaluation of suspected pediatric sexual abuse. *Clin Pediatr Emerg Med.* 2006;7:161–169.
Index of suspicion. *Pediatr Rev.* 2002;23:25–33.
Sugar NF, Graham EA. Common gynecologic problems in prepubertal girls. *Pediatr Rev.* 2006; 27:213–223.

196

DO NOT FORGET TO ADD IRON (FE) TO THE TREATMENT REGIMEN OF DYSFUNCTIONAL UTERINE BLEEDING (DUB)

ANJALI SUBBASWAMY, MD

WHAT TO DO – TAKE ACTION

DUB is defined as abnormal vaginal bleeding without an identifiable pathologic condition. This is in contrast to abnormal uterine bleeding (AUB), which results from a broad spectrum of conditions. In adolescents, DUB is most often due to the anovulatory cycles that result from an immature hypothalamic-pituitary-ovarian axis. Etiologies of AUB, which must be excluded, are numerous and include genital tract abnormalities (ovarian, fallopian tube, uterine, cervical, vaginal, and vulval), trauma, drugs (oral contraceptives, corticosteroids, chemotherapy, phenytoin [Dilantin], antipsychotics) and systemic diseases (*Table 196.1*). Optimal management of DUB requires a systematic diagnostic and therapeutic approach.

By definition, other causes of irregular menses must be excluded before a diagnosis of DUB can be made. In girls in whom a diagnosis of DUB is considered, additional evaluation may include follicle-stimulating hormone, luteinizing hormone, thyroid-stimulating hormone, and prolactin on day 3 of the menstrual cycle (by convention, the first day of menses is day 1 of the cycle, even in girls with irregular cycles). A complete blood count and coagulation tests are standard.

It is important to first exclude pregnancy, and next, to distinguish between ovulatory (cyclic) and anovulatory (acyclic) DUB. The differential diagnosis varies accordingly. For example, DUB is the most common cause of excessive menstrual flow in adolescents with anovulatory bleeding, whereas blood dyscrasias and structural anomalies (e.g., polyps, fibroids) are more common in those with ovulatory bleeding.

Ovulatory AUB is typically cyclic, but heavy or prolonged. Bleeding in these women is usually due to an anatomic lesion (polyp, fibroid, adenomyosis, neoplasm, foreign body), hemostatic defect, infection, trauma, or local disturbances in prostaglandins. Gonadotropin and sex steroid levels, if checked, are normal. Anovulatory uterine bleeding, the most common cause of DUB, refers to unpredictable endometrial bleeding of variable flow and duration. In these patients, sex steroids are produced, but not cyclically, so bleeding is irregular. Anovulation is most common at menarche or

ⓒ 2008 by Lippincott Williams & Wilkins, a Wolters Kluwer business

TABLE 196.1   THE CAUSES OF ABNORMAL UTERINE
              BLEEDING IN CHILDREN VARY WITH AGE

Neonates
Estrogen withdrawal

Premenarchal
Foreign body
Trauma, including sexual abuse
Infection
Urethral prolapse
Sarcoma botryoides
Ovarian tumor
Precocious puberty

Early postmenarche
Anovulation (hypothalamic immaturity)
Bleeding diathesis
Stress (psychogenic, exercise-induced)
Pregnancy
Infection

menopause but can occur at any time. Polycystic ovary syndrome is the most common endocrine disorder associated with anovulation, affecting 6% of reproductive-aged women. Signs include obesity, hirsutism, acanthosis nigricans, and irregular menstrual cycles. Thyroid dysfunction and elevated prolactin levels are other common endocrine disorders related to anovulation.

Treatment of mild DUB (slightly prolonged cycles) may be limited to iron supplementation. Moderate DUB (menses every 1–3 weeks) requires iron and folate supplementation and hormonal therapy. Estrogen is the treatment of choice and 90% of adolescents respond well. Combination estrogen/progesterone therapy is also an option; the estrogen promotes hemostasis, whereas the progesterone promotes endometrial proliferation and stability. Actively bleeding patients require hemodynamic stabilization (hospital admission and blood transfusion may be necessary) and aggressive combination hormonal therapy. Some suggest oral contraceptives three times a day until bleeding stops and then a 1-week taper to daily dosing. In recurrent or debilitating cases, a dilation and curettage may be considered.

Potential sequelae of AUB include anemia and endometrial cancer. Timely evaluation and treatment can prevent these problems.

SUGGESTED READINGS

Lavin C. Dysfunctional uterine bleeding in adolescents. *Curr Opin Pediatr.* 1996;8(4):328–332.
Matytsina LA, Zoloto EV, Sinenko LV, et al. Dysfunctional uterine bleeding in adolescents: concepts of pathophysiology and management. *Prim Care.* 2006;33(2):503–515.
Minjarez D. Abnormal bleeding in adolescents. *Semin Reprod Med.* 2003;21(4):363–373.

197

Do not prescribe oral contraceptive pills (OCPs) to females with undiagnosed vaginal bleeding

Anjali Subbaswamy, MD

What to do – Make a Decision

OCPs are widely available and advocated for use in the adolescent population. They work via several mechanisms of action, but the most important for providing contraception is estrogen-induced inhibition of the midcycle surge of gonadotropin secretion so that ovulation does not occur. Combination OCPs are potent in this regard, but progestin-only pills are not. Although, OCPs are widely available and used, they do carry some inherent risks. Contraindications include previous thromboembolic event, history of an estrogen-dependent tumor, liver disease, pregnancy, undiagnosed abnormal uterine bleeding, cerebral vascular or coronary artery disease, women older than 35 years who smoke heavily (>15 cigarettes/day).

It is imperative that one does not prescribe OCPs to females with undiagnosed vaginal bleeding. The patient may be pregnant in which case the hormonal therapy may induce bleeding or result in birth anomalies. Also, breakthrough bleeding is one of the best known side effects of OCPs. This occurs because the endometrial lining thins, becomes less stable on hormonal therapy (particularly combination estrogen-progesterone therapy), and becomes more prone to breakdown, with resultant bleeding. A systematic workup for abnormal uterine bleeding should be initiated on presentation. The first two steps of this include a pregnancy test and determining through history whether the bleeding is ovulatory or anovulatory in nature. Follicle-stimulating hormone and leuteinizing hormone levels may assist with this determination.

Some relative contraindications to hormonal contraception include inherited thrombophilias, uncontrolled hypertension, anticonvulsant medications, and migraine headaches (because they may carry an additional risk of stroke).

Patients must be well apprised of the side effects of oral contraceptive therapy. These include breakthrough bleeding, amenorrhea (5%–10%), drug interactions (phenobarbital, phenytoin, rifampin), increased cardiovascular morbidity and mortality from stroke and myocardial infarction, venous thromboembolic disease, hypertension, weight gain, nausea, and mood

© 2008 by Lippincott Williams & Wilkins, a Wolters Kluwer business

swings. Over the years, there has been controversy regarding an increased risk of breast and cervical cancer. There are no data implying a concrete relationship. Most of these side effects were more prevalent with the older, high-dose estrogen OCPs. The past 20 years have seen a reduction in both the estrogen and progestin component of oral contraception. This has led to a reduction in both side effects and cardiovascular complications. These preparations can be given cyclically (21 or 24 active, followed by 7 or 4 inactive pills) or by an extended cycle regimen (e.g., 84 active, followed by 7 inactive pills).

SUGGESTED READINGS

Brinton LA, Daling JR, Liff JM, et al. Oral contraceptives and breast cancer risk among younger women. *J Natl Cancer Inst.* 1995;87(11):827–835.

Cerel-Suhl SL, Yeager BF. Update on oral contraceptive pills. *Am Fam Physician.* 1999;60:2073–2084.

Felice ME, Feinstein RA, Fisher M, et al. American Academy of Pediatrics, Committee on Adolescence. Contraception in adolescents. *Pediatrics.* 1999;104(5 Pt 1):1161–1166.

198

OBTAIN A COMPUTED TOMOGRAPHY (CT) SCAN OF THE ORBIT TO RULE OUT ORBITAL INVOLVEMENT IN CASES OF PERIORBITAL CELLULITIS

BRIAN KIT, MD

WHAT TO DO – GATHER APPROPRIATE DATA

The orbital septum is connective tissue from the periosteum of the bony rim that inserts into the tarsal plate, which forms the connective tissue structures of the eyelid. The septum serves as a barrier to the spread of infection, preventing microbes anterior to the septum from spreading posteriorly. Infections posterior to the septum are called orbital cellulitis (or postseptal cellulitis) and those anterior to the septum are called periorbital cellulitis (or preseptal cellulitis).

The most typical presentation of orbital cellulitis is lid swelling. Patients may complain of eye pain or visual disturbances, including blurry vision. The physical examination may be significant for proptosis, poor lid closure, conjunctival injection, restricted ocular movements (ophthalmoplegia), altered pupillary reactivity, pain on movement of the eye, or decreased visual acuity. There may be associated erythema to the bony rim of the orbit where the septum originates. Younger children are less likely to present with ophthalmoplegia or proptosis. The presence of fever, systemic signs, and toxicity is variable.

Orbital cellulitis is secondary to sinusitis in >90% of cases. The ethmoid sinuses are the most commonly involved sinuses, but frontal sinus disease may be present in adolescents. The pathogenesis of orbital cellulitis usually involves the development of subperiosteal abscess and spread of infection from the involved paranasal sinus. Organisms commonly found in orbital cellulitis reflect those found in sinus disease, including *Streptococcus pneumoniae*, *Haemophilus influenzae*, *Moraxella catarrhalis*, *Streptococcus pyogenes*, *Staphylococcus aureus*, both alpha- and nonhemolytic streptococci,

© 2008 by Lippincott Williams & Wilkins, a Wolters Kluwer business

and anaerobes. Many patients, particularly those older than 9 years, have polymicrobial infections.

An orbital CT scan with coronal and axial images, with and without contrast, should be obtained in patients with signs and symptoms of orbital cellulitis. Findings on CT that would indicate orbital cellulitis include subperiosteal abscess, orbital abscess, proptosis, and inflammation of ocular muscles along with ipsilateral or bilateral sinusitis. Orbital cellulitis requires prompt systemic antibiotics. Occasionally, surgical intervention to drain the infected sinuses or the abscess may be needed.

The presentation of periorbital cellulitis is also most commonly eyelid swelling. Eye pain is not a feature of the disease, especially early in the clinical course before significant edema. Examination of the affected skin may reveal an erythematous or violaceous discoloration and swelling. Vision, pupillary response, and eye motility are normal and there is no proptosis. Fever and signs of systemic illness may be present, particularly in children whose disease is the result of bacteremia.

Periorbital cellulitis often results from either bacteremia or eyelid trauma with subsequent infection. In the immunized child, *S. pneumoniae* is the most common bacteria that causes periorbital cellulitis. *H. influenza* must be considered in the nonimmunized child. *S. aureus* or Group A streptococcus are the most common bacterial etiologies of periorbital cellulitis in those who sustained eyelid trauma, such as an insect bite or mild abrasion, with subsequent infection. Mild cases of preseptal cellulitis in children older than 1 year can be managed on an outpatient basis with oral antibiotics if there are no signs of systemic illness and the child is appropriately vaccinated.

If the eye exam reveals normal orbital motility and there are no other signs or symptoms suggestive of orbital cellulites, imaging is generally not required. However, if the eye exam is limited secondary to swelling or if there are other factors limiting the assessment of the eye, radiologic evaluation with orbital CT is indicated. Any child with signs or symptoms consistent with orbital cellulitis should also undergo CT evaluation.

SUGGESTED READINGS

Givner LB. Periorbital versus orbital cellulitis. *Pediatr Infect Dis J*. 2002;21(12):1157–1158.
Periorbital and Orbital Infections. http://www.emedicine.com/oph/topic205.htm and http://www.emedicine.com/oph/topic206.htm
Nageswaran S, Woods CR, Benjamin DK Jr, et al. Orbital cellulitis in children. *Pediatr Infect Dis J*. 2006;25(8):695–699.
Uzcátegui N, Warman R, Smith A, et al. Clinical practice guidelines for the management of orbital cellulitis. *J Pediatr Ophthalmol Strabismus*. 1998;35(2):73–79; quiz 110–111.

199

OBTAIN AN EMERGENT OPHTHALMOLOGY CONSULT FOR SERIOUS EYE DISORDERS SUCH AS HYPHEMA, RUPTURED GLOBE, CORNEAL ULCER, FOREIGN BODY, AND HERPETIC KERATITIS

NICKIE NIFORATOS, MD

WHAT TO DO – MAKE A DECISION, TAKE ACTION

The role of the pediatrician in managing health concerns of the eye is to recognize early pathology and ophthalmic emergencies. Abnormalities can be detected before the child becomes symptomatic, and emergencies referred for early intervention can greatly improve morbidity and preserve visual acuity and health.

Eye screenings are often age dependent and focus on both anatomy and function. For example, preterm infants should be referred to ophthalmology regardless of their physical exam by the fourth to sixth week of life to allow for a detailed funduscopic examination and evaluation for retinopathy of prematurity. At birth, all infants should be evaluated for the presence and symmetry of the red reflex. A defect in the light reflex may be the result of a congenital cataract. Without appropriate and early intervention, a congenital cataract may lead to deprivational amblyopia and limit visual potential during a critical period of visual development. The red reflex should also be monitored at all routine well-child physicals, as an asymmetry of color or brightness of the reflex can occur at any age. Such variations in the color or brightness of the reflex, such as a "white reflex," may reflect a refractive error or a retinoblastoma. At ages 6 months to 1 year, the physician should be able to test for strabismus in a cooperative infant through the corneal light reflex. If there is any asymmetry in the reflection, the child should be referred to ophthalmology. Similarly, infants should also be able to fix and follow by 6 months of age; any such failures in a cooperative infant should again be referred to a specialist.

Visual acuity may be difficult to measure in infancy and early childhood, but a number of tests can detect gross anomalies and alert the physician to potential deficits. In alert infants, a light stimulus should elicit wincing behavior. By age 6 months, the infant should object equally when either eye is occluded; if there is decreased fussing or "objection" when one eye is occluded, the physician should suspect decreased acuity in the occluded eye.

© 2008 by Lippincott Williams & Wilkins, a Wolters Kluwer business

Preverbal children can be tested by observing their ability to reach an object (toy), when either eye is occluded. By age 3 years, charts using pictures of cartoons, shapes, or symbols can be used to measure acuity. By age 5 years, most children should be able to cooperate with the Snellen letter chart or number chart. Whenever visual acuity is <20/40 in either eye or there is a difference of two lines of acuity between the eyes, the child should be referred for further testing.

The techniques used in routine screens are also used to evaluate the eye in case of trauma. In addition, a full funduscopic exam should be performed on all patients to evaluate the clarity of the media and the appearance of the optic nerve head and vessels, as well as the presence of retinal hematomas. The pupils can be dilated to allow for full examination, as the risk of precipitating acute angle closure glaucoma is minimal and greatly outweighed by the benefit of detecting intraocular pathology.

A child that presents with a chemical injury to the eye should be treated immediately with copious irrigation; families should be instructed to irrigate the eye at home first with tap water prior to coming to the emergency department. In the medical setting, clinicians should continue irrigation with saline or sterile water. In most instances, 20 to 30 minutes of irrigation is adequate. Severe burns may require débridement of necrotic tissue and must be followed by ophthalmology.

A child who presents with intense pain and photophobia should be evaluated for a corneal abrasion. Many will require an initial application of a topical anesthetic to allow for a complete examination and a fluorescein dye test. Patients should be treated with topical cycloplegic drops, antibiotics, and a semipressure patch. To prevent infection, corneal abrasions must be re-examined every 24 hours. If an infection develops, the eye should be patched.

If there is a suspicion of an open or ruptured globe, the examination should not continue, as further inspection or palpation may lead to extrusion of ocular contents and loss of the eye. A protective shield should be applied. Intravenous antibiotics should be ordered, and ophthalmology should be emergently consulted. If there were blunt trauma to the eye, the patient may require computed tomography scans to determine the extent of the injury and look for fractures of the orbital bones. Fracture of the superior orbit or frontal sinus may track into the intracranial space and lead to infection and, in severe cases, cerebrospinal fluid leaks. If the trauma leads to hyphema, the patient will often be hospitalized. Treatment consists of bed rest, with elevation of the head of the bed; eye protection; and topical steroids with or without systemic antifibrinolytic medications. Patients with hyphemas are at risk for rebleeding, and the secondary hyphema can induce glaucoma or hemophthalmitis and vision loss.

Patients who report a shower of "floaters" with progressive visual loss may be showing signs of a posterior segment hemorrhage. If there is a report of a curtain or cloud moving across the visual field, the patient may be experiencing signs of retinal detachment. A sudden loss of vision, partial or complete, with pain may reflect optic neuritis. These patients require immediate referral to ophthalmology.

Fever, swelling, redness, and warmth of the skin surround the eye may be a sign of preorbital cellulitis. These children require imaging studies (computed tomography scan) to determine the extent of the infection and to evaluate for orbital cellulitis, an ophthalmologic emergency. Complications include meningitis, intracranial abscess, or cavernous sinus thrombosis.

SUGGESTED READINGS

Klein BR, Sears ML. Pediatric ocular injuries. *Pediatr Rev.* 1992;13(11):422–428.
Tingley DH. Vision screening essentials: screening today for eye disorders in the pediatric patient. *Pediatr Rev.* 2007;28(2):54–61.

200

PERFORM A SLIT LAMP EXAMINATION FOR PATIENTS WITH ZOSTER ON THE FACE TO IDENTIFY DENDRITIC CORNEAL LESIONS OF HERPETIC KERATITIS

CAROLINE RASSBACH, MD

WHAT TO DO – TAKE ACTION

Herpes zoster is an unusual condition in pediatrics caused by reactivation of latent varicella virus. It presents most often in children who are immune suppressed, who had chickenpox when younger than age 1 year, or who contracted the virus transplacentally. When zoster appears in the distribution of cranial nerve V1, herpes zoster ophthalmicus often occurs. Practitioners should know how to diagnose and treat this condition.

Clinically, the physician should be alerted to zoster in the region of the face extending from the level of the eye to the vertex of the skull. This is the region innervated by cranial nerve V1, the ophthalmic nerve. Zoster lesions on the tip or side of the nose are called the Hutchinson sign and are highly associated with herpetic eye involvement. This is because the same branch of the ophthalmic nerve that innervates the eye, the nasociliary nerve, also innervates the nose.

To review the anatomy, cranial nerve V, the trigeminal nerve, provides sensory and motor innervation to the face. The trigeminal nerve branches into the ophthalmic, maxillary, and mandibular nerves (V1, V2, and V3, respectively). The ophthalmic nerve is then divided into the frontal, lacrimal, and nasociliary nerves. Involvement of any of the divisions of the ophthalmic nerve can result in herpes zoster ophthalmicus; however, the nasociliary nerve correlates with severe disease. The eye is spared when zoster affects other branches of the trigeminal nerve.

Herpes zoster ophthalmicus may involve the conjunctiva, cornea, or sclera. An affected eye appears red and painful, and the lid may be swollen. A slit lamp examination is urgently required and may reveal herpetic dendritic lesions on the cornea. Prompt referral to an ophthalmologist is essential to treating herpetic eye disease and preventing long-term complications. The most common ocular problems are anterior uveitis and corneal keratitis. Long-term complications include decreased visual acuity, decreased corneal sensitivity, and corneal clouding. Early initiation of antiviral drugs has been shown to reduce the severity of the skin eruption and the incidence and severity of late eye complications.

© 2008 by Lippincott Williams & Wilkins, a Wolters Kluwer business

It is important to be aware of other symptoms that accompany herpes zoster ophthalmicus, as well. Prior to presentation with rash, there may be a prodrome of headache, nausea, vomiting, as well as lymphadenopathy of the ipsilateral preauricular and submaxillary nodes. Meningeal signs and third and sixth nerve palsies may be present because the ophthalmic nerve extends to the tentorium and to the third and sixth cranial nerves.

SUGGESTED READINGS

De Freitas D, Martins EN, Adan C, et al. Herpes zoster ophthalmicus in otherwise healthy children. *Am J Ophthalmol.* 2006;142(3):393–399.

Habif T. Warts, herpes simplex, and other viral infections. *Clinical Dermatology*, 4th ed. New York: Mosby, 2004, pages 381–388.

201

OBTAIN AN EAR, NOSE, AND THROAT (ENT) CONSULT FOR INFANTS AND TODDLERS WITH INCREASING HOARSENESS (OR SOFT VOICE) TO RULE OUT JUVENILE LARYNGEAL PAPILLOMATOSIS (JLP)

JOHANN PETERSON, MD

WHAT TO DO – TAKE ACTION

Laryngeal papillomatosis is infection of the airway with human papilloma virus (usually strains 6 and 11), leading to papillomas on the vocal cords. The juvenile form is thought to be caused by vertical transmission of human papilloma virus at birth. It has a peak incidence between 2 and 4 years, but has been diagnosed in neonates. Most juvenile cases are diagnosed before age 5 years. Risk factors include a vaginal birth, a young or primiparous mother, and a mother with genital warts during pregnancy.

The typical course is one of frequent relapses, requiring multiple surgeries over many years, usually every few months but for rapidly growing papillomas as often as every 1 to 2 weeks. Ultimately, spontaneous remission is common, but spread into the tracheobronchial tree, causing cystic lung lesions and even malignant transformation, is possible. Laryngeal papillomas have caused fatal airway obstruction even after diagnosis. JLP is a relatively rare disease, affecting 3 to 4/100,000 children, but the burden of disease for affected children is huge, with some requiring >40 surgeries during their lives. Stridor in infants and toddlers is common, is most often acute and in such cases is usually related to infection (e.g., croup) or aspiration. Chronic stridor has an extensive differential, including laryngomalacia, tracheoesophageal fistula, vocal cord paralysis, subglottic stenosis, hemangioma of the airway, and extrinsic compression from a tumor or vascular anomaly ("rings and slings"). The clinical clues in laryngeal papillomatosis are first, that the stridor is progressive, whereas that of laryngomalacia, the most common cause of chronic stridor in infants, should slowly improve; and second, the changes in the voice quality, which suggest insolvent of the

ⓒ 2008 by Lippincott Williams & Wilkins, a Wolters Kluwer business

vocal cords. Children with fixed or progressive laryngeal obstructions often present with recurrent croup, because they are more prone to significant airway obstruction during viral illnesses; therefore, a child with hoarseness plus recurrent croup or episodes of stridor should always prompt a referral for laryngoscopy. Evaluation in a child with chronic or recurrent stridor should include plain films of the neck to visualize the upper airway, and an esophagram, which may offer clues to extrinsic compression (e.g., anomalous vasculature) or tracheoesophageal fistula.

SUGGESTED READINGS

Derkay CS. Recurrent respiratory papillomatosis. *Laryngoscope.* 2001;111(1):57–69.

Mancuso RF. Stridor in neonates. *Pediatr Clin North Am.* 1996;43(6):1339–1356.

Shah KV, Stern WF, Shah FK, et al. Risk factors for juvenile onset recurrent respiratory papillomatosis. *Pediatr Infect Dis J.* 1998;17(5):372–376.

Silverberg MJ, Thorsen P, Lindeberg H, et al. Condyloma in pregnancy is strongly predictive of juvenile-onset recurrent respiratory papillomatosis. *Obstet Gynecol.* 2003;101(4):645–652.

202

DO NOT IGNORE DELAYS IN SPEECH, WHICH ARE OFTEN ATTRIBUTABLE TO HEARING LOSS OR DEFICITS

ELIZABETH WELLS, MD

WHAT TO DO – GATHER APPROPRIATE DATA

Hearing deficits contribute to or cause speech delay in children. The incidence of profound-to-severe hearing loss is estimated to be 1 in 1,000 live births, and twice that in infancy and childhood. Hearing loss or deficits may be classified as conductive, due to dysfunction of the external or middle ear, or sensorineural, due to a malfunction of the cochlea or auditory nerve. Most sensorineural hearing loss appears to be present at birth and is, therefore, termed congenital.

Hearing loss can have numerous etiologies. Most inherited hearing loss is autosomal recessive and the child's sole disability. There are also many genetic disorders associated with hearing loss, including Treacher Collins syndrome (deformed auricles), Waardenburg syndrome (white forelock, irises of different colors), CHARGE association (eye, gastrointestinal, and other malformations), Down Syndrome (small auricles, frequent otitis media), trisomy 13 and trisomy 18 (central nervous system malformations), Usher syndrome (retinitis pigmentosa, central nervous system effects, loss of smell, associated psychosis), and cleft palate. Nongenetic causes of hearing loss include prenatal and postnatal infections, exposure to ototoxic agents (e.g., aminoglycosides), anoxia, prematurity, and trauma.

Universal hearing screening is recommended before postpartum hospital discharge and for any infant born outside of a hospital. Audiological and medical evaluation of children who failed their screen and 1-month rescreen should be performed to confirm hearing loss before 3 months of age, and intervention must occur before 6 months of age. As infant screening can miss children with mild-to-moderate, progressive, or acquired hearing loss, a hearing assessment should be repeated in any child with a language or speech delay. Published guidelines for receptive and expressive skills exist to help delineate a language delay. After infancy, a rough estimate of a child's expressive language skills can be used as follows: speech should be 50% intelligible by age 2, 75% intelligible by age 3, and 100% intelligible by age 4. A delay of 25% or greater is considered significant.

© 2008 by Lippincott Williams & Wilkins, a Wolters Kluwer business

Once a child is diagnosed with hearing impairment, management depends on the degree of loss and the preference of families. Amplification devices (e.g., hearing aids, assistive listening devices) are the mainstay of management for moderate-to-profound hearing loss and require a pediatric audiologist for proper prescription and fit. Cochlear implantation should be considered for children with bilateral severe-to-profound sensorineural hearing loss who do not benefit from amplification. Research has shown large, unpredictable individual differences, but significant overall improvement in language development and speech production. The mode of communication (primarily aural-oral vs. manual sign language) is an important decision for the family. Early identification and intervention for hearing loss is crucial, because it enables children to stimulate brain pathways, promote brain maturation, and acquire language skills during critical stages of development.

The most common cause of mild-to-moderate hearing loss in children is chronic otitis media with effusion. Most otitis media-associated hearing loss is transient, but a persistent (1–2 weeks) or recurrent infection may add a sensorineural component to the typical conductive hearing loss, because bacterial toxins can damage the organ of Corti. There is considerable controversy surrounding whether a history of otitis media with effusion in early childhood causes later speech and language problems. Early studies suggested that chronic infection and hearing loss may affect speech and language development in a preschooler and scholastic achievement in a school-aged child, a recent meta-analysis published in Pediatrics (2004) found little to no association. A recent Cochrane Review found no benefit on language development and behavior from screening the general population of asymptomatic children for otitis media effusion.

As otitis media treatment outcomes and their effects on speech and language development are variable, the need for prevention and treatment of chronic otitis media is under debate. For many years, tympanostomy tubes were inserted for bilateral effusions persisting 3 to 4 months. A recent large, randomized clinical trial of tympanostomy tube insertion in otherwise healthy children did not find an advantage for the early tympanostomy group and found that tympanostomy increases the rates of abnormal tympanic membrane findings, when compared with children managed medically. Several other studies have agreed that the high rate of complications of tympanostomy tube insertion outweighs the beneficial effect on hearing loss in patients with persistent, asymptomatic middle ear effusion that is not complicated by sensorineural or severe conductive hearing loss, balance dysfunction, or severe tympanic membrane retraction. Watchful waiting, with medical management for each symptomatic episode, is currently recommended for children with chronic otitis media unless other developmental risk factors exist.

The association between hearing and language development in infancy has been well established, and it is important for pediatricians to screen for hearing loss when they encounter signs of language delay. Although otitis media has been shown to cause hearing loss, the impact of otitis media effusion on language development is still under investigation. Children with a history of chronic middle-ear problems may need their hearing checked after a course of treatment. Currently, treatment is left to the discretion of the pediatrician, the otolaryngologist and the family.

SUGGESTED READINGS

Briggs RJ, Luxford WM. Correction of conductive hearing loss in children. *Otolaryngol Clin North Am.* 1994;27:607–620.

Feldman HM. Evaluation and management of language and speech disorders in preschool children. *Pediatr Rev.* 2005;26(4):131–142.

Herer GR, Knightly AC, Steinberg AG. Hearing: sounds and silences. In: Batshaw ML. *Children with Disabilities.* 5th ed. Baltimore: Paul H. Brookes; 2002:193–227.

Johnstrom LC, Feldman HM, Paradise JL, et al. Tympanic membrane abnormalities and hearing levels at the ages of 5 and 6 years in relation to persistent otitis media and tympanostomy tube insertion in the first 3 years of life: a prospective study incorporating a randomized clinical trial. *Pediatrics.* 2004;114(1):e58–e67.

Paradise JL, Campbell TF, Dollaghan CA, et al. Developmental outcomes after early or delayed insertion of tympanostomy tubes. *N Engl J Med.* 2005;353(6):576–586.

Pisoni DB. Cognitive factors and cochlear implants: some thoughts on perception, learning, and memory in speech perception. *Ear Hear.* 2000;21:70–78.

Simpson SA, Thomas CL, van der Linden MK, et al. Identification of children in the first four years of life for early treatment for otitis media with effusion. *Cochrane Database Syst Rev.* 2007;24(1):CD004163.

Stenstrom R, Pless IB, Bernard P. Hearing thresholds and tympanic membrane sequelae in children managed medically or surgically for otitis media with effusion. *Arch Pediatr Adolesc Med.* 2005;159(12):1151–1156.

Winskel H. The effects of an early history of otitis media on children's language and literacy skill development. *Br J Educ Psychol.* 2006;76(Pt 4):727–744.

203

REMEMBER THAT CHILDREN WHO PRESENT WITH A NECK MASS HAVE A NUMBER OF CONSIDERATIONS THAT CAN ASSIST WITH THE DIAGNOSIS, INCLUDING LOCATION AND ASSOCIATED FINDINGS

MICHAEL S. POTTER AND ANTHONY SLONIM, MD

WHAT TO DO – GATHER APPROPRIATE DATA

Several considerations need to be taken into account when a pediatric patient presents with a neck mass. Most neck masses in children are benign and due to either inflammation or congenital abnormalities, with 2% to 15% of persistent masses exhibiting malignancy. *Figure 203.1* provides the three major categories for neck masses based upon age grouping.

In children, inflammation is the number one cause of neck masses. Lymphadenopathy is very common in children. However, 50% of children presenting with palpable lymph nodes of an appreciable size (1–1.5 cm) are not obviously infected or systematically ill. Children with cervical lymphadenopathy should be examined to determine a source for the adenopathy. Other variations of lymphadenopathy include lymphadenitis (acute and chronic) and suppurative lymphadenitis. Acute cervical lymphadenitis is usually caused by regional viral infections such as rhinovirus or adenovirus. Similarly, chronic cervical lymphadenitis is also usually due to viral infections. When lymph nodes are unilateral or fluctuant, suppurative lymphadenitis caused by bacterial infections or common granulomatous diseases should be considered. The differential diagnosis includes *Mycobacteria,* cat-scratch disease, toxoplasmosis, actinomyces, but group A β-hemolytic streptococci and *Staphylococcus aureus* are often the primary causes. Salivary glands can also be the origin of neck masses: sialolithiasis, acute suppurative sialoadenitis, acute nonsuppurative sialoadenitis, or human immunodeficiency virus can all affect the salivary glands and cause neck masses.

Neck masses due to congenital conditions occur next in frequency after inflammation (*Table 203.1*). They are most easily classified by location either in the midline or lateral neck. Branchial cleft cysts and thyroglossal duct cysts are the most common congenital neck masses. Branchial cleft cysts, which occur in the lateral neck regions, typically present in childhood or early adulthood as nontender masses that become inflamed in the

© 2008 by Lippincott Williams & Wilkins, a Wolters Kluwer business

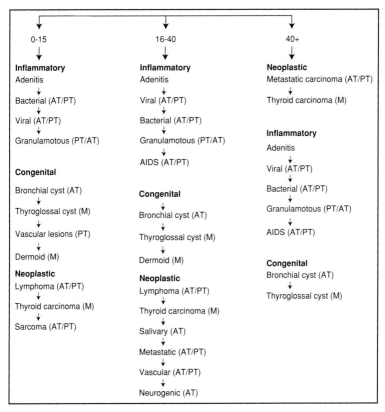

FIGURE 203.1. Relative frequency of specific neck masses within causative groups by age. AIDS, acquired immunodeficiency syndrome. Fedok FG, Burnett M. Evaluation of Neck Masses. In: Nobel J. *Textbook of Primary Care Medicine.* 3rd ed. St. Louis: Mosby, Inc.; 2001.

presence of an upper respiratory tract infection. Lymphangiomas are also common lateral neck masses that typically present during a child's first year of life. Thyroglossal duct cysts, occurring in the midline neck area, typically present as a midline neck mass that is asymptomatic. As with branchial cleft cysts, thyroglossal duct cysts can become infected. Other congenital neck masses include vascular anomalies, teratomas, and dermoid cysts. Vascular anomalies are typically noted at birth and can result in disfiguring and local compressive symptoms. Teratomas and dermoid cysts are usually painless masses that always occur in the neck's midline.

Though infrequent in younger children, neoplastic neck masses can present in older children as painless, cervical masses that are fixed to the

TABLE 203.1	NONINFECTIOUS CAUSES OF NECK MASSES
CONDITION	**COMMENTS**
Congenital anomalies	
Thyroglossal duct cyst	Most common congenital neck mass; discrete 1-cm midline nodule that may elevate with tongue protrusion; elective excision best; may contain only existing thyroid tissue
Second pharyngeal (branchial) cleft anomaly	Second most common congenital neck mass; anterior to upper or middle one third of sternomastoid muscle; external sinus opens anterior to sternal head of muscle; tract needs to be excised; cyst associated with lymphatic tissue
Cystic hygroma	Third most common congenital neck mass; occurs along jugular lymphatic chain in posterior supraclavicular fossa; failure of mesenchymal clefts to fuse; varies from few cm to massive collarlike lesions; may extend into mediastinum
Dermoid or epidermoid cysts	Midline, deep to mylohyoid muscle; soft, fluid-filled midline mass; may elevate with tongue protrusion; contain caseous material or epithelial debris
Nonlymphomatous malignancies	
Neuroblastoma	Second most common malignant neck mass in children (first in younger children)
Thyroid cancer	Third most common neck malignancy; high incidence of malignancy in thyroid nodules; prompt biopsy required
Rhabdomyosarcoma	Most common nasopharyngeal malignancy in children
Nasopharyngeal carcinoma	Cervical adenopathy often initial and only symptom; arises most often in fossa of Rosenmüller
Parotid tumors	Vascular anomalies most common; asymptomatic node may be malignant and should be excised
Miscellaneous	
Sternocleidomastoid tumor	Fibrous mass within muscle; detected at 2–4 weeks of age in 0.4% of infants; head turned away from mass; ipsilateral facial hypoplasia
Sinus histiocytosis with massive lymphadenopathy (Rosai-Dorfman disease)	Bilateral, painless cervical nodes; generalized lymphadenopathy may develop; systemic manifestations include fever and hypergammaglobulinemia; self-limited
Giant lymph node hyperplasia (Castleman disease)	Asymptomatic lymphadenopathy in mediastinum or neck; systemic symptoms include fever and hypergammaglobulinemia; surgical removal curative
Histiocytic necrotizing lymphadenitis (Kikuchi-Fujimoto disease)	Asymptomatic cervical or generalized adenopathy; skin lesions, fever, and leukopenia; spontaneous resolution; recurrences possible
Kimura disease	Benign, chronic, unilateral lymphadenopathy; adjacent subcutaneous nodules, peripheral eosinophilia and increased serum immunoglobulin E

(Used with permission from Long S. *Principles and Practice of Pediatric Infectious Diseases.* Philadelphia: Saunders; 2007).

deep cervical tissue, have grown quickly, or are located in the supraclavicular or posterior triangle areas of the neck (Table 203.1). Half of masses located in the posterior triangle area are malignant with half of those being Hodgkin lymphoma or non-Hodgkin lymphoma. Approximately 15% of these malignancies are due to neuroblastoma. Finally, thyroid tumors make up a significant percentage of malignant neck masses in children. Children who are younger than 6 years are most susceptible to neuroblastoma, non-Hodgkin lymphoma, rhabdomyosarcoma, and Hodgkin lymphoma, in that order of frequency. Children between the ages of 7 and 15 are equally likely to develop Hodgkin lymphoma or lymphosarcoma, followed by thyroid carcinoma, rhabdomyosarcoma, and parotid adenocarcinoma.

The diagnostic tests that may be helpful to differentiate the etiology of neck masses are contained in *Table 203.2*. In general, excisional biopsy and

---

TABLE 203.2   DIAGNOSTIC EXAMINATION AND TESTS FOR HEAD AND NECK MASSES

Physical examination: Repeated; most important

Radionucleotide scanning: Obtain in lesions of anterior neck compartment; helpful in thyroid lesions and in localizing a lesion to be within a salivary gland. PET scan may be helpful in differentiating tumor from postirradiation changes, equivocal adenopathy by CT scan or MRI exam, and identifying distant metastasis.

Ultrasonography: To differentiate solid from cystic masses; especially useful in congenital and developmental cysts; also useful noninvasive technique for vascular lesions

Arteriography: For vascular lesions and tumors fixed to the carotid artery

Sialography: To diagnose diffuse sialadenopathies or to locate mass within or outside a salivary gland

CT and MRI imaging: Single most informative test; differentiates cysts from solid lesions; locates mass within or outside a gland or within a nodal chain; mucosal disease enhancement; provides anatomic relationships

X-ray, plain: Rarely of help in differentiating neck masses

Antibiotic course: Clinical test for suspected inflammatory bacterial lymphadenopathy; must pursue workup if unresolved after course of antibiotics.

Culture with sensitivities: Inflammatory tissue at open biopsy

Skin tests: Used when chronic or granulomatous inflammatory lesion is suspected

Needle biopsy: Gold standard in diagnosis of a neck mass; use small-gauge needle; obtain flow cytometry of lymphoid population

Endoscopy and biopsy: To identify primary tumor as source of metastatic node; use in all patients suspected of having neoplasia

Open biopsy: Use only after workup is complete and if diagnosis is not evident; specimen for histologic frozen section; be prepared to do simultaneous neck dissection

---

CT, computed tomography; MRI, magnetic resonance imaging; PET, positron emission tomography

(Used with permission from Bailey BJ. *Otolaryngology: Head & Neck Surgery*. Philadelphia: Lippincott Williams & Wilkins; 2006:)

antibiotic therapy are appropriate for inflammatory neck masses. However, inflammation due to viral (rather than bacterial) infection may require a different approach. If an inflamed lymph node develops an abscess, incision and drainage is usually appropriate. The treatment for most congenital neck masses is surgical excision, and in general, surgery is a logical treatment for masses that do not exhibit malignancy. Malignant neck masses are uncommon in children. When present, the child and family will benefit from the collaboration of a team of pediatric specialists, including surgeons, oncologists, and radiation oncologists to strategize the best course of action for the patient.

SUGGESTED READINGS

Chesney PJ. Cervical lymphadenitis and neck infections. In: Long SS, Pickering LK, MD, Prober CG. *Principles and Practice of Pediatric Infectious Diseases.* 2nd ed. Philadelphia: Churchill Livingstone; 2003.

Fedok FG, Burnett M. Evaluation of neck masses. In: Nobel J. *Textbook of Primary Care Medicine.* 3rd ed. St. Louis: Mosby, Inc.; 2001.

McGuirt WF Sr. Differential diagnosis of neck masses. In: Cummings CW, Flint PW, Haughey BH, et al. *Otolaryngology: Head & Neck Surgery.* 4th ed. Philadelphia: Mosby, Inc.; 2005.

O'Handley JG, Tobin E, Tagge B. Otolaryngology. In: Rakel RE. *Textbook of Family Practice.* 6th ed. Philadelphia: W.B. Saunders Company; 2002.

204

ASSURE THAT YOUR PATIENT WHO HAS A PRESUMED PERFORATED OTITIS MEDIA (OM) OR OTITIS EXTERNA DOES NOT HAVE A CHOLESTEATOMA

DOROTHY CHEN, MD

WHAT TO DO – INTERPRET THE DATA

Concern for otitis infections is a common reason for pediatric outpatient visits. Untreated ear infections can have serious consequences. Diagnosing and differentiating between the different types of otitis infections is vital. OM includes suppurative acute OM and nonsuppurative or secretory OM. Perforation, spontaneous rupture of the tympanic membrane, can occur during acute OM. Otitis externa includes bacterial infection or inflammation of the external ear canal. Similar to OM, there is acute ear pain, decreased hearing acuity, and visible debris and secretions in the ear canal. When either OM with perforation or otitis externa is suspected, a cholesteatoma should be considered.

Cholesteatomas are benign skin tumors, usually located in the middle ear and mastoid spaces. The cysts are lined with keratinized and stratified squamous epithelium with deposits of desquamated epithelium and keratin. Cholesteatomas grow progressively over time. There are both congenital and acquired cholesteatomas.

A congenital cholesteatoma is a cystlike structure of epithelial tissue in the ear, usually medial to an intact tympanic membrane. Children with acquired cholesteatomas do not typically have a history of infection or tympanic perforation. The etiology of the collection of epithelial tissue is unclear. On physical exam, cholesteatomas appear as a small white ball behind the tympanic membrane, next to the eustachian tube. Retraction pockets, chronic drainage, and keratin debris can also be present.

Acquired cholesteatomas are often a complication of chronic OM. However, they can also arise from retraction pockets or cell migration. They will appear as white debris or drainage in the ear canal, after having broken through the tympanic membrane. Retraction pockets develop when there is prolonged damage to the eustachian tube. The pars flaccid, the weakest part of the tympanic membrane, will enter the middle ear and become a collection of squamous epithelial tissue. Chronic infection allows metaplasia of the cuboidal mucosa into squamous epithelium. Lastly, epithelial cells can

---

ⓒ 2008 by Lippincott Williams & Wilkins, a Wolters Kluwer business

migrate to the middle ear when there is tympanic membrane perforation or insertion of tympanostomy tubes.

The negative impact of cholesteatomas is due to their location and their activity. Because cholesteatomas are found in the middle ear, mastoid spaces, tympanic membrane or the ear canal wall, they grow and can erode bone with easy access to the brain. The lysozymes within the matrix of cells can dissolve both soft tissue and bone. Infection is another common complication, resulting in serious meningitis; thrombi; and epidural, subdural, and brain abscesses. A computed tomography scan of the temporal bone should be performed to evaluate the disease extent. Surgical intervention is usually required to treat cholesteatomas.

SUGGESTED READINGS

Haddad J. Congenital malformations. In: Behrman RE, Kliegman RM, Jenson HB, eds. *Nelson Textbook of Pediatrics*. 17th ed. Philadelphia: Saunders; 2004:2136.

Hughes W, Lee JH. Otitis externa. *Pediatr Rev.* 2001;22(6):191–197.

Paradise JL. Otitis media. In: Behrman RE, Kliegman RM, Jenson HB, eds. *Nelson Textbook of Pediatrics*. 17th ed. Philadelphia: Saunders; 2004:2138–2148.

Stone KE. Otitis externa. *Pediatr Rev.* 2007;28(2):77–78.

Thompson JW. Cholesteatomas. *Pediat Rev.* 1999;20(4):134–136.

205

PRESCRIBE AN ANTIBIOTIC FOR PATIENTS TREATED AS OUTPATIENTS WITH NASAL PACKING DUE TO THE RISK OF TOXIC SHOCK SYNDROME AND SINUSITIS

WILLIAM GIASI, JR., MD

WHAT TO DO – TAKE ACTION

The rich vascular network of the nose makes it vulnerable to either spontaneous bleeds or bleeds secondary to trauma. In the majority of cases, epistaxis is mild and self-limiting. Epistaxis can result from local or systemic causes. Common etiologies of epistaxis include upper respiratory infection, sinusitis, local trauma, foreign bodies, irritants, and medications. Less common etiologies include vascular malformations, leukemia, thrombocytopenia, coagulopathies, or hepatic disease.

Anterior bleeds arise from the rich venous vascular network on the anterior nasal septum, the Kiesselbach plexus, and account for the majority of episodes. The thin and adherent nature of the anterior venous plexus makes it especially susceptible to trauma. The venous source of anterior bleeds results in a slow and oozing quality. In contrast, posterior bleeds occur less often and arise from branches of the sphenopalatine artery. The arterial source results in more profuse bleeds that may drain into the nasopharynx, thus carrying a higher risk of airway compromise.

Epistaxis generally requires minimal intervention. Those patients who are not actively bleeding should be given anticipatory guidance to avoid local trauma as well as to keep the mucosa moist. If a patient is actively bleeding, there are several management options that lie along a continuum ranging from conservative to invasive surgical interventions.

Patients should be instructed hold keep their head elevated and to pinch the nose without interruption for at least 5 minutes and up to 20 to 30 minutes. Hyperextension should be avoided to prevent aspiration of blood. In the event that a bleed doesn't resolve with simple pressure, the clinician can place a piece of gauze soaked in either nasal decongestant in the anterior nasal cavity, followed by direct pressure. If bleeding remains active, chemical cautery using silver nitrate or thermal cautery may be helpful. Epistaxis that is unresponsive to cautery may require anterior nasal packing with petroleum jelly gauze strips or commercial packing that are used to tamponade the

© 2008 by Lippincott Williams & Wilkins, a Wolters Kluwer business

vessels. Posterior bleeds are less responsive to cautery and often require the use of either nasal packing or balloons.

The presence of nasal packing may serve as a medium for bacteria growth. Application of antibiotic ointment to the packing as well as an oral course of prophylactic antibiotics, with *Staphylococcus* coverage, may decrease infection. Patients with nasal packing should be closely monitored for complications such as sinusitis or toxic shock syndrome. Although it is uncommon, toxic shock can result in multiple organ failure and ultimately death. Early recognition of complications, removal of the packing, and initiation of appropriate management is important.

SUGGESTED READINGS

Bernius M, Perlin D. Pediatric ear, nose, and throat emergencies. *Pediatr Clin North Am.* 2006;53(2):195–214.

Kucik CJ, Clenney T. Management of epistaxis. *Am Fam Physician.* 2005;71(2):305–311.

Epistaxis. In: Cummings CW, Flint PW, Haughey BH, et al. eds. *Otolaryngology: Head & Neck Surgery.* 4th ed. Philadelphia: Mosby Inc., 2000, pages 942–960.

Kucik CJ, Clenney T. Management of epistaxis. *Am Fam Physician.* 2005;71(2):305–311.

206

Do not use aminoglycoside antibiotic eardrops in the presence of a perforation or ventilation tube, because they may be ototoxic if they enter the middle ear

William Giasi, Jr., MD

What to Do – Make a Decision

Acute otitis externa (AOE) is the acute onset of inflammation of the external auditory canal, which may involve the pinna and tympanic membrane. AOE classically has a rapid onset, symptoms of ear canal inflammation, and findings of ear canal inflammation. Symptoms of otitis externa include otalgia, itching, fullness, or ear canal pain with chewing. The hallmark physical finding of AOE is intense tenderness and pain of the tragus and/or pinna with movement. Otitis externa is common with an incidence of 1:100 to 250 in the general population and peaks between 7 and 12 years of age. Otitis externa is a cellulitis of the external ear with acute inflammation and edema, and bacterial organisms account for 98% of cases. The most common pathogens are *Pseudomonas aeruginosa, Staphylococcus aureus,* and polymicrobial infections. Gram-negative organisms (excluding *Pseudomonas*) account for no more than 2% to 3% of cases and fungal infections are a rare cause of primary AOE.

The treatment objective in otitis externa is to eradicate the pathogens responsible for the infection and reduce ear pain. Topical antibiotics are the most beneficial and efficacious for the treatment of AOE. Topical antibiotics are recommended for the initial treatment of diffuse uncomplicated AOE. Oral antibiotics are often prescribed in addition to topical antibiotics but have limited efficacy against *P. aeruginosa* and *S. aureus.* Topical therapy allows for a high concentration of antimicrobial that exceeds the minimal inhibitory concentration needed for pathogen eradication and has little systemic absorption, thus limiting systemic side effects. Furthermore, there are lower persistence and recurrence rates with topical antimicrobials.

There are many different types of antimicrobial treatments that are efficacious and available for treatment of otitis externa. Special consideration must be given to the patient with a nonintact tympanic membrane, whether it is perforated or has tympanostomy tubes. Visual assessment of the tympanic membrane may be difficult and impeded by pain, edema, drainage, or debris. If the tympanic membrane is not intact, topical medications may enter the

© 2008 by Lippincott Williams & Wilkins, a Wolters Kluwer business

middle, and ultimately, the inner ear. Topical drops that contain alcohol, have a low pH, or both should be avoided with nonintact membranes because they cause pain and have an ototoxic potential. Ototoxic medications, such as aminoglycosides, have in experimental animals caused severe hearing loss and injury to the inner ear. Clinical experience has shown that ototoxicity does result in cases of excessive administration or prolonged courses. Medications that are ototoxic or potentially ototoxic should not be used with a perforated tympanic membrane because the risk of ototoxicity outweighs the benefits of nonototoxic antimicrobials that are equally efficacious. The only U.S. Food and Drug Administration-approved topical antimicrobials approved for middle ear use are otic ofloxacin and ciprofloxacin/dexamethasone.

SUGGESTED READINGS

Beers SL, Abramo TJ. Otitis externa review. *Pediatr Emerg Care.* 2004;20(4):250–256.

Dohar JE. Evolution of management approaches for otitis externa. *Pediatr Infect Dis J.* 2003;22:299–308.

McCoy SIZell ER, Besser RE. Antimicrobial prescribing for otitis externa in children. *Pediatr Infect Dis J.* 2004;23(2):181–183.

Rosenfeld RM, Brown L, Cannon CR, et al. American Academy of Otolaryngology–Head and Neck Surgery Foundation. Clinical practice guideline: acute otitis externa. *Otolaryngol Head Neck Surg.* 2006;134(4 Suppl):S4–S23.

Rosenfeld RM, Singer M, Wasserman JM, et al. Systemic review of topical antimicrobial therapy for acute otitis externa. *Otolaryngol Head Neck Surg.* 2006;134(4 Suppl):S24–S48.

207

Perform Prompt Evaluation to Exclude Complications of Chronic Sinusitis When a Patient Presents with Ocular or Central Nervous System Signs and Symptoms

William Giasi, Jr., MD

What to Do – Gather Appropriate Data

Sinusitis is a common infection that affects children each year. On average, children will experience 5 to 8 viral upper respiratory infections per year, of which 5% to 13% may be complicated by a secondary bacterial infection of the paranasal sinuses. When a sinus infection goes unrecognized or untreated, complications may result. Complications of sinusitis include preseptal, periorbital cellulitis; orbital cellulitis; subperiosteal abscess; and intracranial complications.

Intracranial complications of sinusitis in order of frequency are epidural abscess, subdural empyema, meningitis, encephalitis, intracerebral brain abscess, dural sinus thrombophlebitis, and middle cerebral artery ischemia. Intracranial complications can arise from the spread of septic thrombi or emboli from the sinus via the valveless diploic veins of the skull base that penetrate the dura, osteomyelitis of the sinus wall that extends posteriorly, or an infection that penetrates an existing bony defect in the sinus cavity.

Clinicians should suspect intracranial complications of sinusitis in any children with sinusitis and any neurologic finding, other signs of complicated sinusitis, persistent headache, persistent fever, or nausea/vomiting after antibiotic therapy.

Children with intracranial complications of sinusitis often present with nonspecific symptoms such as fever, headache, facial mass, or swelling. The physical exam may be significant for fever, facial mass or edema, abnormal vision, abnormal extraocular muscle movements, proptosis, or an abnormal neurologic exam. It is important to recognize that more than half of patients with intracranial complications of sinusitis may have a normal exam, so the clinician should maintain a high suspicion.

Several organisms have been identified in the pathogenesis of intracranial complications from sinusitis. They include *Streptococcus* species (*S. anginosus, S. constellatus, S. intermedius*), *Staphylococcus aureus*, facultative anaerobes, and gram-negative rods.

© 2008 by Lippincott Williams & Wilkins, a Wolters Kluwer business

The radiological evaluation of a patient for intracranial complications of sinusitis should either be conducted via a computed tomography scan of the sinuses with contrast, including coronal cuts or a magnetic resonance imaging scan of the brain with contrast. Noncontrast computed tomography scans lack sensitivity and may be falsely reassuring, leading to a delay in diagnosis.

The treatment of intracranial complications of sinusitis requires a sustained multidisciplinary team approach, including broad antibiotic therapy and prompt surgical drainage.

SUGGESTED READINGS

Adame N, Hedlund G, Byington CL. et al. Sinogenic intracranial empyema in children. *Pediatrics.* 2005;116:e461–e467.

American Academy of Pediatrics. Subcommittee on Management of Sinusitis and Committee on Quality Improvement. Clinical practice guidelines: management of sinusitis. *Pediatrics.* 2001;108:798–808.

Brook I, Friedman EM, Rodriguez WJ, et al. Complications of sinusitis in children. *Pediatrics.* 1980;66:568–572.

Bussey MF, Moon RY. Acute sinusitis. *Pediatr Rev.* 1999;20(4):142.

Germiller JA, Monin DL, Sparano AM, et al. Intracranial complications of sinusitis in children and adolescents and their outcomes. *Arch Otolaryngol Head Neck Surg.* 2006;132:969–976.

Nash D, Wald E. Sinusitis. *Pediatr Rev.* 2001;22(4):111–117.

208

STEROIDS ARE NOT OFTEN USED TO TREAT INFECTIONS. HOWEVER, FOR OTITIS EXTERNA (OE), CONSIDER USING OTIC STEROIDS AS PART OF THE TREATMENT REGIMEN TO REDUCE THE PAIN AND INFLAMMATION OF OTITIS ETERNA

DOROTHY CHEN, MD

WHAT TO DO – MAKE A DECISION

Diseases of the ear, nose, and throat (ENT) are common in pediatrics. Infections are often viral or bacterial in origin, so antibiotics are prescribed when appropriate. Steroids, however, are not routinely prescribed for ENT infections. In OE, there is both inflammation and infection of the external ear canal. Because of the inflammatory nature of OE, steroids can be considered in the management.

Acute or diffuse OE is the most common infection of the external ear canal. It is often referred to as "swimmer's ear" or "tropical ear." Patients can present with a range of symptoms including pain, pruritus, erythema, otorrhea, hearing loss, and a feeling of fullness. The most common pathogens in otitis externa are *Staphylococcus aureus* and *Pseudomonas aeruginosa*. When treating OE, it is important to eliminate the micro-organisms, while also limiting the patient's otalgia.

Treatment regimens include cleansing of the canal, avoidance of moisture, ototopical medications, and systemic analgesics, when necessary. The topical otic preparations should focus on eliminating microorganisms, decreasing the pH of the ear canal, and decreasing inflammation of the ear canal. The most commonly used agents are antibiotics, acidifying agents, and steroids. Neomycin is active against gram-positive and some gram-negative organisms; polymyxin is active against gram-negative organisms, including *Pseudomonas;* and fluoroquinolones provide coverage against both staphylococci and *Pseudomonas.* Acetic acid is the most commonly prescribed acidifying agent; many bacteria grow best in alkaline environments, so acidifying the ear canal prevents further bacterial growth. Many of the topical otic medications are a combination of steroids with either antimicrobials or acetic acid. Although some patients experience pain that requires oral nonsteroidal anti-inflammatory medications, steroid drops have also been shown to decrease the duration of otalgia.

ⓒ 2008 by Lippincott Williams & Wilkins, a Wolters Kluwer business

In one randomized controlled trial, patients were given acetic acid drops, a combination of acetic acid and steroid drops, or a combination of antimicrobial and steroid drops (van Balen et al.). Patients who used the combination drops with steroids self-reported a shorter duration of symptoms such as ear pain. The addition of steroids to acetic acid also decreased the rate of OE recurrence, in comparison to the use of acetic acid alone.

SUGGESTED READINGS

Haddad J. Disease of the external ear. In: Behrman RE, Kliegman RM, Jenson HB, eds. *Nelson Textbook of Pediatrics*. 17th ed. Philadelphia: Saunders; 2004:2136–2137.

Hughes E, Lee JH. Otitis externa. *Pediatr Rev.* 2001;22(6):191–197.

Rosenfeld RM, Brown L, Cannon CR, et al. American Academy of Otolaryngology–Head and Neck Surgery Foundation. Clinical practice guideline: acute otitis externa. *Otolaryngol Head Neck Surg.* 2006;134(4 Suppl):S4–S23.

Sander R. Otitis externa: a practical guide to treatment and prevention. *Am Fam Physician.* 2001;63(5):927–935.

van Balen FA, Smit WM, Zuithoff NP, et al. Clinical efficacy of three common treatments in acute otitis externa in primary care: randomised controlled trial. *BMJ.* 2003;327:1201–1205.

209

IDENTIFY THE ETIOLOGY BEHIND LONG BONE FRACTURES

LAURA HUFFORD, MD

WHAT TO DO – GATHER APPROPRIATE DATA

Preverbal children presenting with acute fractures should bring about the suspicion of child abuse for the clinician. Thus, one must evaluate the child to determine if the true cause of the injury. The key in distinguishing between accidental and inflicted trauma involves a close look at the type of fracture, mechanism of injury, and history given by the parent.

The history must seem plausible for the child's stage of development. For example, you see a 2-month-old infant who reportedly rolled off a bed presents with a femur fracture. This history raises suspicion of abuse because a 2-month-old child cannot typically roll at this stage of development. Other concerning clues in the history involve a relative lack of information, such as histories that seem vague or change over time. If the parents state a child fell down the stairs, they should be able to say how many stairs, where exactly it occurred, and at what time. These details should remain consistent throughout the interview.

Additionally, the history of the injury should be consistent with the type of fracture found on x-ray. Asking how the patient was initially standing, how he or she fell, and how they landed can give the clinician clues to the types of forces exerted on a bone and the likely fractures that should result. For example, spiral fractures tend result from torsional loading. A toddler who was running, twisted, and fell may have a nondisplaced oblique, spiral fracture of the distal tibia (toddler's fracture). However, the same fracture in a nonambulatory 8-month-old infant would be highly suspicious of abuse.

Certain fracture types are suggestive of abuse. Multiple fractures of the hands and feet are unlikely to occur unless the child is involved in a car accident, crush injury, or from deliberate abuse. Rib fractures in a young child are also suspicious signs of abuse and the child should be evaluated for concomitant head and abdominal injuries. Femur fractures, which result

© 2008 by Lippincott Williams & Wilkins, a Wolters Kluwer business

from large forces, can be both accidental and inflicted in origin, but are a marker for serious trauma. Infants presenting with metaphyseal fractures are likely to have been shaken. Rapid acceleration and deceleration applies alternating forces to the metaphysis, resulting in fracture. Finally, any child presenting with multiple fractures in the absence of a validated large force trauma should be evaluated for abuse.

Suspicion of abuse prompts the clinician to obtain additional studies to screen for further injury. A skeletal survey should be ordered in children younger than 2 years of age to look for occult or healing fractures. Liver transaminases and urine analysis and a lipase should be ordered to screen for abdominal trauma. Complete blood count, prothrombin time, and partial prothrombin time may provide clues to ongoing bleeding or a bleeding disorder. An inconsolable infant, lethargic child, or abnormal neurologic exam should be evaluated with a head computed tomography scan to check for skull fractures, and intracranial bleeds. Finally, Child Protective Services should be notified of any child in whom an abuse workup is being initiated.

SUGGESTED READINGS

Nimkin K, Spevak MR, Kleinman PK. Fractures of the hands and feet in child abuse: imaging and pathologic features. *Radiology.* 1997;203:233–236.

Pierce MC, Bertocci GE, Janosky JE, et al. Femur fractures resulting from stair falls among children: an injury plausibility model. *Pediatrics.* 2005;115:1712–1722.

Rewers A, Hedegaard H, Lezotte D, et al. Childhood femur fractures, associated injuries, and sociodemographic risk factors: a population-based study. *Pediatrics.* 2005;115:e543–e552.

210

DO NOT ASSUME THAT PATIENTS HAVE FRACTURES WITHOUT OBTAINING COMPARISON VIEWS OF THE CONTRALATERAL BODY PART

MADAN DHARMAR, MD

WHAT TO DO – GATHER APPROPRIATE DATA

Fractures account for nearly 15% of all pediatric injuries. The anatomical, physiologic, and biomechanical differences in the bones make fractures in children different from adult fractures. Hence, children have some unique types of fractures that can be problematic to diagnose, and at the same time, their bones typically heal faster, so it is important that pediatric fractures be managed in a timely manner.

The difference in children's bones are:

1. The bones are more porous and, hence, can absorb more energy before they are fractured or deformed. They have greater plasticity.
2. The bones have a thicker periosteum, which can help in stabilizing the fracture and can also result in faster healing. In some instances, this makes it difficult to diagnose a fracture.
3. In children, the long bones have growth plates or physis, which are present between the epiphysis and the metaphysis of the bone.
4. The bones have more cartilage than adult's bone, which changes as children grow older. The bones are composed of perosseous cartilage, physes, and an osteogenic periosteum.
5. Variation in the appearance of ossification centers in the growing bone can make it difficult to diagnose fractures in children.
6. Children also heal differently due to their high propensity for remodeling. The factors that could affect remodeling are the age of the child, proximity to a joint, and relation of residual deformity to the plane of the joint axis of movement.

Types of fracture in children:

1. **Complete fracture:** This is the most common type of fracture, where the bone is broken on both the sides. Comminuted fractures are rare in children.
2. **Buckle or torus fracture:** They commonly occur in the metaphysic of the long bones. This fracture occurs when the bone buckles due to a

© 2008 by Lippincott Williams & Wilkins, a Wolters Kluwer business

longitudinal force applied along the long axis of the bone (e.g., a fall onto an outstretched hand).

3. **Bowing of bone:** Occurs when the bone is angulated beyond its limits of plastic deformation, resulting in bending of the bone, but is not fractured.

4. **Greenstick fracture:** When the bone is angulated beyond its limits of plastic deformation, resulting in a fracture, but the force is insufficient to cause a complete fracture.

5. **Growth plate (physeal) fractures:** Growth plates are unique to children; they are present in growing long bones. A growth plate is a cartilaginous disc present between metaphysic (widened area of the shaft) and the epiphysis (end of the bone). The Salter-Harris classification is most commonly used to classify growth plate fractures. The five classification of growth plate fractures are:

   a. Type 1: Fracture through the physis separating the epiphysis from the metaphysis.

   b. Type 2: Fracture through the physis extending through metaphysis.

   c. Type 3: Fracture through physis extending through epiphysis.

   d. Type 4: Fracture through epiphysis and metaphysis crossing the physis.

   e. Type 5: Compression fracture through the physis not extending to epiphysis or metaphysis.

   Growth plate fractures need immediate management, as they could result in progressive angular deformity, progressive limb length discrepancy, and joint incongruity.

Assessment of fractures in children. Evaluation of the fracture involves a detailed history to determine the mechanisms of injury, examination of the affected region, and imaging studies. When a child presents with deformity, swelling, or localized bony tenderness following trauma, a fracture must be suspected. If a younger child does not move a limb or refuses to bear weight on a limb, a fracture must be suspected. The suspected region must be examined for deformity, swelling, point tenderness, skin wound around the injured region (open fracture), peripheral pulse, and signs of neurologic impairment distal to the injury. The child must also be examined for signs of compartment syndrome such as tense compartment, excessive pain, and pain on movement of fingers or toes.

X-rays are used to determine the type of fracture and decide on a treatment plan. X-ray of the suspected injured region, including the joints on either side of the injured region, must be obtained. X-rays should include both anteroposterior and lateral views for diagnosis of fracture. Growth plate are seen in x-rays as either spaces or sometimes they are difficult to see, and as children are in different stages of development, the presence of primary and secondary ossification center can make a diagnosis from an initial x-ray difficult. Hence in many circumstances, when a fracture is suspected based on the mechanisms of injury and/or based on examination, it is important to take a comparison x-ray of the uninjured side to make a diagnosis of fracture. This is particularly true if a fracture involving the growth plate is suspected. In growth plate fractures, magnetic resonance imaging can provide useful information on the appearance of the growth plate. Other diagnostic tests, such as computed tomography scan or ultrasound, can also be used.

SUGGESTED READINGS

Beaty JH, Kasser JR. *Rockwood and Wilkins' Fractures in Children.* 6th ed. Philadelphia: Lippincott Williams & Wilkins; 2006.

Bernier J. Fractures. *Pediatr Rev.* 1999;20(5):179.

Macewen GD, Kasser JR, Heinrich SD. *Pediatric Fractures: A Practical Approach to Assessment and Treatment.* Baltimore: Williams & Wilkins; 1993.

Wenger DR, Pring ME, Rang M. *Rang's Children's Fractures.* 3rd ed. Philadelphia: Lippincott Williams & Wilkins; 2006.

Young SJ, Barnett PL, Oakley EA. II. Fractures and minor head injuries: minor injuries in children II.*Med J Aust.* 2005;182(12):644–648.

211

CONSIDER THAT BLUNT TRAUMA IN PEDIATRIC PATIENTS MAY RESULT IN SOLID ORGAN (MOST NOTABLY, THE LIVER AND SPLEEN) TRAUMA

MICHAEL S. POTTER AND ANTHONY SLONIM, MD

WHAT TO DO – INTERPRET THE DATA

In industrialized countries, injury is the primary cause of death in children, although most trauma does not result in death. Trauma is classified by the number of significantly injured body parts, the severity of the injuries, and the mechanism of injury: penetrating or blunt (*Table 211.1*). Firearm injuries are the most significant cause of penetrating trauma. Penetrating trauma is far less common in pediatric patients than adults, but when it does occur in children, it is likely to be in the adolescent age group. Blunt trauma, or blunt abdominal trauma (BAT), is usually caused by motor vehicle accidents (the most significant contributor), falls, impairments resulting from recreation, and assault. Coincidentally, the most affected organs of BAT are the liver and the spleen. Due to their retroperitoneal location, the kidney, pancreas, and duodenum are frequently spared significant injury after blunt trauma. In contrast to penetrating trauma, BAT accounts for 80% to 90% of all pediatric trauma.

Pediatric blunt trauma patients should be initially evaluated according to the advanced-trauma life support (ATLS) standards. First, as a part of the primary survey, evaluating the airways, breathing, and circulation (ABCs) is essential. An abbreviated neurologic assessment and a thorough injury search via complete patient exposure are appropriate during the primary survey as well. A secondary survey should focus on a complete, head-to-toe, physical examination to determine all traumatic injuries. About 24 hours after admission, a tertiary survey should also be conducted to once again perform a full, physical examination to assure that no injuries were previously missed.

Because blunt trauma most often results in abdominal injury, detection of intra-abdominal wounds is critical; however, this can be difficult when dealing with very young children. Gastric distention as a result of a crying or an uncooperative child can result in misleading physical examination findings. During examination, one should focus on distention, bruising, tenderness detected by palpitating, and rectal bleeding. The use of an abdominal

ⓒ 2008 by Lippincott Williams & Wilkins, a Wolters Kluwer business

TABLE 211.1 PATTERNS OF ABDOMINAL ORGAN INJURY BY MECHANISM OF INJURY

FREQUENCY OF ORGAN INJURY	BLUNT (%)	PENETRATING (%)
Liver	15	22
Spleen	27	9
Pancreas	2	6
Kidney	27	9
Stomach	1	10
Duodenum	3	4
Small bowel	6	18
Colon	2	16
Other	17	6

(Source: Saxena AK, Nance ML, Lutz N, et al. Abdominal Trauma. eMedicine. Available at: www.emedicine.com/ped/topic3045.htm. Accessed July 3, 2007.)

computed tomography (CT) scan with intravenous contrast enhancement can quickly locate structural abnormalities. The advantage of CT scans is that their sensitivity for identifying splenic, hepatic, and renal injuries is very high. On the other hand, pancreatic and intestinal injuries are not so clearly identified by an abdominal CT scan. The use of ultrasonography may also be beneficial in identifying acute abdominal traumatic injuries and following their progression.

After careful surveys have been performed and the extent of the child's injuries are clear, the appropriate treatment should be administered. It is worth noting that nonoperative treatment strategies have become the standard for hemodynamically stable children with splenic, hepatic, and renal injuries resulting from blunt trauma. Such treatment can avoid perioperative complications, decrease the need for blood transfusions, and reduce length of stay.

SUGGESTED READINGS

Kristoffersen KW, Mooney DP. Long-term outcome of nonoperative pediatric splenic injury management. *J Pediatr Surg.* 2007;42:1038–1041; discussion 1041–1042.
Saxena AK, Nance ML, Lutz N, et al. Abdominal Trauma. eMedicine. Available at: www.emedicine.com/ped/topic3045.htm. Accessed July 3, 2007.

212

PAY IMMEDIATE ATTENTION TO THE AIRWAY FOR VICTIMS SUSTAINING BURNS THAT ARE CIRCUMORAL, INTRA-AORAL, OR WHO DEMONSTRATE HOARSENESS, STRIDOR, WHEEZING, CYANOSIS, OR PULMONARY EDEMA

MINDY DICKERMAN, MD

WHAT TO DO – TAKE ACTION

One third of all burn unit admissions and deaths involve children. Flame and scald burns are the major mechanisms of injury in the pediatric burn population. Children younger than 4 years of age are at greatest risk. Despite improvement in burn care, burn injury remains the fifth leading cause of unintentional child injury-related death. Approximately 10% to 20% of pediatric burns are a result of child abuse. The majority of all deaths related to burns are due to smoke inhalation rather than surface burns or their sequelae.

As with any patient, the priority during the assessment of a child with a burn is the adequacy of the *a*irway, *b*reathing, and *c*irculation (ABCs). Early identification and treatment of life-threatening injuries are critical. It is crucial to evaluate for the possibility of inhalation injury early on. It is equally important to understand the mechanism of injury and the circumstances surrounding the burn so that other life-threatening injuries, such as a closed head injury, can be identified.

Smoke inhalation injury can cause respiratory decompensation by several mechanisms. Direct thermal injury to the airway can cause airway obstruction and require immediate intubation. Clinical markers to suspect upper airway compromise include respiratory distress, hypoxemia, hoarseness, stridor, deep burns to the face or neck, blistering on the oropharynx, tongue swelling, carbonaceous sputum, and singed eyebrows and nasal hairs.

The physician must maintain a high index of suspicion for airway involvement. The presence or absence of surface burns does not reliably predict the extent of inhalation injury. Respiratory distress may not develop in a patient with inhalation injury for several hours. Chest x-ray at presentation is also a poor predictor of inhalation injury. If there is any doubt about potential for airway deterioration, an early decision to intubate is always justified. Delayed intubation can be more difficult, especially in a pediatric airway

© 2008 by Lippincott Williams & Wilkins, a Wolters Kluwer business

because it is smaller and, therefore, more at risk to be occluded by progressive edema.

A child who sustains a flame injury in an enclosed space is at risk for carbon monoxide intoxication and acute lung injury from smoke inhalation. If a child presents obtunded with a history of an isolated flame injury, it should be presumed that the child is hypoxic from carbon monoxide intoxication. This child may have a normal oxygenation by pulse oximetry reading. Pulse oximetry is not accurate for assessing carbon monoxide poisoning because it does not differentiate between oxyhemoglobin and carboxyhemoglobin. Treatment is with high concentrations of inspired oxygen, which displaces carbon monoxide from hemoglobin, reduces the half life of carboxyhemoglobin, and allows for oxyhemoglobin formation. It is recommended to intubate children with carboxyhemoglobin levels >25% because delivery of 100% oxygen is most effective endotracheally. If a patient appears obtunded, has profound metabolic acidosis, and does not respond to oxygen, one needs to consider cyanide poisoning.

Smoke injury in this setting can also lead to acute lung injury. Acute lung injury is a result of toxin-induced injury to the lung parenchyma that impairs alveolar function. Symptoms of acute lung injury may not manifest until 24 to 48 hours after the initial burn. Treatment is supportive and includes intubation, ventilation, oxygen, and pulmonary toilet. The clinical course is similar to that of adults with acute respiratory distress syndrome and is associated with significant morbidity, prolonged intubation, and mortality.

SUGGESTED READINGS

Duffy BJ, McLaughlin PM, Eichelberger MR. Assessment, triage, and early management of burns in children. *Clin Ped Emerg Med.* 2006;7:82–93.

Lee AS, Mellins RB. Lung injury from smoke inhalation. *Pediatr Resp Rev.* 2006;7:123–128.

213

KNOW HOW TO TREAT THE DIFFERENT TYPES OF DROWNING

MINDY DICKERMAN, MD

WHAT TO DO – INTERPRET THE DATA

In 2002, the World Congress on Drowning published expert consensus recommendations regarding the terminology, evaluation, and management of drowning. For decades, lack of uniformity in terminology has resulted in confusion among clinicians, leading to difficulty in comparing and interpreting data. "Drowning" was defined by the 2002 World Congress as the process resulting in primary respiratory impairment from submersion/immersion in a liquid medium regardless of whether the ultimate outcome is survival or death. Previously used descriptive terminology, such as "near-drowning," leads to confusion and should be abandoned. In the past, there has also been an attempt to distinguish drowning with aspiration from drowning without aspiration. It is also the consensus that drowning without aspiration does not occur.

The literature formerly emphasized the distinction between salt water and fresh water drowning, believing that the effects from the hypertonicity of salt water were very different than the effects from the hypotonicity of fresh water. It is thought now that rarely enough water is aspirated to cause these varying effects. After voluntary breath-holding takes place, small amounts of water initially are aspirated from the oropharynx, which triggers involuntary laryngospasm, resulting in hypoxia. Larger amounts of water are subsequently swallowed as laryngospasm abates from prolonged hypoxia. Aspiration of water leads to destruction of surfactant, impaired alveolar capillary gas exchange, intrapulmonary shunting, and pulmonary edema. These events lead to progressive hypoxia, hypercarbia, and acidosis. Vomiting and aspiration of gastric contents can contribute to acute lung injury. Prolonged hypoxia leads to intense peripheral vasoconstriction, and decreased cardiac output and arterial blood pressure. If the hypoxic drowning process is not reversed, the brain and the heart can become permanently injured. Ultimately, profound bradycardia and circulatory arrest can occur. The extent of hypoxic insult will ultimately determine outcome.

Unfortunately, no single variable or combination of variables has proven to be reliably predictive of outcome. The first priority for managing drowning victims at the scene as well as in the emergency room is to reverse hypoxemia

ⓒ 2008 by Lippincott Williams & Wilkins, a Wolters Kluwer business

by restoring adequate oxygenation and ventilation. Initial care is directed to the ABCs, including consideration of the need for cervical spine immobilization. Many patients will need tracheal intubation. Both fresh water and salt water drowning victims need aggressive fluid resuscitation with crystalloid solution.

Submersion in cold water can produce physiologic changes that can be beneficial or disastrous. Potential benefits of cold water are decreasing the metabolic demands of the body and helping to delay the effects of hypoxia. The adverse effects of cold water causing arrhythmias are seen more often. It is important when managing hypothermia that goal body temperature is clear, and appropriate rewarming techniques are used depending on severity of hypothermia and the patient's cardiovascular status. The degree of hypothermia can be classified as mild, moderate, or severe. The priority in managing hypothermia is to establish a safe and steady rewarming rate while also maintaining cardiovascular stability. The goal should be to rewarm a patient $1°C$ to $2°C$ per hour to a range of $33°C$ to $36°C$. If a patient is hemodynamically stable, aggressive rewarming and hyperthermia should be avoided due to evidence that hyperthermia can worsen cerebral injury.

If a patient has mild hypothermia, defined as $32°C$ to $35°C$, passive rewarming by removing wet, cold clothing or applying warm blankets is sufficient. It is reasonable to maintain a temperature of $34°C$ to $35°C$ in a child who remains comatose and is stable cardiovascularly for 24 hours. Active rewarming should be used if a patient has moderate hypothermia, defined as $28°C$ to $32°C$, or severe hypothermia, defined as $<28°C$. Arrhythmias, extreme bradycardia, and asystole may occur at these temperatures. When a core temperature is $<30°C$, cardioactive medications and defibrillation attempts are ineffective. Active external rewarming involves applying hot packs and heat lamps, both of which need to be done cautiously to avoid iatrogenic burns. Active internal rewarming includes applying warmed humidified oxygen, giving warmed intravenous fluid, or performing warm saline lavages, via peritoneal dialysis. Extracorporal rewarming is the most efficient warming method (able to increase body temperature $1°C$ to $2°C$ per 5 minutes) and is the preferred treatment for victims in cardiac arrest, those with persistent cardiac instability, and those who have core temperatures of $<24°C$.

SUGGESTED READINGS

Olshaker JS. Submersion. *Emerg Med Clin North Am.* 2004;22:357–367.
Zucherbraun NS, Saladino RA. Pediatric drowning: current management strategies for immediate care. *Clin Ped Emerg Med.* 2005;6:49–56.

214

REMEMBER THAT THE LOSS OF ABDOMINAL ELASTANCE DUE TO A REDUCTION IN MUSCLE TONE MAY SIGNIFY A HIGH SPINAL CORD LESION

MEGHA SHAH FITZPATRICK, MD

WHAT TO DO – INTERPRET THE DATA

The primary function of the lung is gas exchange. The mechanics of respiration are as important to adequate gas exchange as the properties inherent to the lung itself. The muscles that aid in inspiration and expiration play an important role in the mechanics of respiration. Often, an injury to these muscles or the nerves that control them can result into altered respiratory mechanics and an impairment of gas exchange.

The diaphragm is the primary muscle used during inspiration. It consists of a thin dome-shaped muscle that inserts into the lower ribs. It is innervated by the phrenic nerves arising from cervical segments 3, 4, and 5. During inspiration, the dome of the diaphragm contracts downward and forward, expanding the vertical dimension of the chest. In addition, there is an elevation of the lower ribs where the diaphragm inserts and the ribcage moves outward, resulting in an increase in the transverse diameter of the chest. Other accessory muscles of inspiration, not necessarily used during quiet respiration, include the sternocleidomastoid, scalenes, internal intercostal, and external intercostal muscles.

In contrast, expiration is passive during quiet breathing. After being expanded during inspiration, the elastic properties of the lung and chest wall allow them to return to their positions of equilibrium. Once expiration becomes active, as it does during hyperventilation, the muscles of the abdominal wall become the most important. When these muscles contract, the diaphragm is pushed upward. This return to the equilibrium position is further assisted by the internal intercostal muscles, which pull the ribs down and inward.

Because the respiratory mechanics of the lung rely on the diaphragm innervated high up in the cervical spinal cord and the abdominal musculature innervated from the midthoracic to the lumbar spine, an injury to the cervical spinal cord could potentially impair the mechanics of respiration. A cervical spinal cord injury can be classified into two categories: complete or incomplete. With a complete cervical spinal cord injury, there is an absence

---

© 2008 by Lippincott Williams & Wilkins, a Wolters Kluwer business

of sensory and motor function in the lowest sacral segments (i.e., the absence of anal sensation on rectal examination and of voluntary external anal sphincter contraction). Incomplete cervical spinal cord injury is defined as the presence of sensory or motor function below the neurologic level of spinal cord injury, and must include the lowest sacral segments. Patients with incomplete cervical spinal cord injury have a better prognosis for recovery in comparison to patients with complete cervical spinal cord injury.

Generally, the signs and symptoms of cervical spinal cord injury include new weakness, paralysis, spasticity, pain, cough, shortness of breath, bladder or bowel incontinence, and skin breakdown, but will depend on the level of the lesion. The physical exam may provide overt or subtle clues as to the level of the cervical spinal cord lesion.

With a high cervical spinal cord lesion—complete or incomplete—the tone and contraction of the abdominal musculature can be affected. As a result, the diaphragm is unable to contract across what should be incompressible abdominal contents, and instead the abdominal contents are forced outward during inspiration. The physiologic consequence of this loss of abdominal muscle tone is a loss in functional residual capacity, defined as the volume of gas in the lung after normal expiration. This lung volume relies on the ability of the lung and chest wall to return back to their equilibrium position. Furthermore, with very high cervical spinal cord injury, the movement of the diaphragm itself could be affected, causing severe respiratory compromise. Consequently, when evaluating patients with cervical spinal cord lesions it is important to obtain pulmonary function testing and observe their mechanics of respiration to detect changes, whether subtle or obvious.

SUGGESTED READING

Wratney A, and Chiefetz IM. Chapter 41, Disorders of the chest wall and respiratory muscle. In: Slonim AD and Pollack MM. *Pediatric Critical Care Medicine*. Lippincott Williams & Wilkins, Philadelphia: 2006, pages 705–716.

215

DO NOT DRAMATICALLY LOWER THE BLOOD PRESSURE IN PATIENTS WITH INCREASED INTRACRANIAL PRESSURE (ICP)

EMILY RIEHM MEIER, MD

WHAT TO DO – MAKE A DECISION

Brain parenchyma, cerebrospinal fluid (CSF), and blood are the three components of the intracranial cavity (*Table 215.1*). The durability of the skull protects the brain from outside insults, but cannot accommodate an increase in the amount of intracranial contents. Increased ICP is, therefore, a medical emergency that requires careful diagnosis, monitoring, and management.

The Cushing triad is classically associated with increased ICP but is a relatively late finding. It consists of hypertension, bradycardia, and hypopnea. Hypertension occurs as the body attempts to maintain cerebral perfusion pressure (CPP). CPP can be calculated by subtracting the mean arterial pressure (MAP) from ICP (CPP = MAP – ICP). Because CPP is interdependent on MAP, an acute fall in blood pressure in patients with increased ICP places them at risk for cerebral hypoperfusion and long-term neurologic damage. Hypertension associated with increased ICP causes a compensatory bradycardia. Decreased respiratory rate is a late finding, signaling impending herniation and is secondary to compression of brainstem respiratory centers from the increased pressure. Ideally, increased ICP should be identified and treatment started before these findings arise (*Table 215.2*).

Evacuation of a fluid (CSF or blood) collection or mass removal are the surgical interventions for increased ICP. Medical management of increased ICP includes elevation of the head of the bed, osmotic diuretics, hypertonic saline, hyperventilation, sedation, and hypothermia. Varying amounts of evidence exist for the effectiveness of these interventions in decreasing ICP. Elevating the head of the bed to 30 degrees is one of the simplest interventions for patients with suspected increased ICP. It improves venous outflow from the brain and can be an effective measure at preventing increased ICP from escalating.

© 2008 by Lippincott Williams & Wilkins, a Wolters Kluwer business

TABLE 215.1   CAUSES OF INCREASED INTRACRANIAL PRESSURE

Brain parenchyma
Space-occupying lesion
- Epidural or subdural hematoma
- Mass
- Abscess
Cerebral edema
- Infection (meningitis/encephalitis)
- Toxin induced encephalopathy (lead, liver failure, Reye syndrome)
- Hypertensive encephalopathy

CSF
Hydrocephalus
- CSF Overproduction
- Decreased CSF absorption
- Blockage of CSF flow (aqueductal stenosis)

Blood
Head trauma
Subarachnoid hemorrhage
Venous sinus thrombosis
Miscellaneous
Pseudotumor cerebri

CSF, cerebrospinal fluid.

Mannitol is the most thoroughly studied medication used to induce an osmotic diuresis in patients with increased ICP. Doses range from 0.25 to 1 g/kg and should be given as a bolus infusion. Mannitol is a large sugar that does not cross the blood–brain barrier. This allows it to exert an osmotic effect on brain parenchyma, effectively decreasing the volume of the intracranial

TABLE 215.2   MANAGEMENT GUIDELINES FOR INCREASED INTRACRANIAL PRESSURE

First-Line Therapy
- Sedation, analgesia, paralytics
- CSF drainage if ventriculostomy present
- Hyperosmotic therapy (mannitol of hypertonic saline)
- Mild hyperventilation (P_aCO_2 30–35 mm Hg)

Second-Line Therapy
- Barbiturate coma
- Hypothermia
- Aggressive hyperventilation (P_aCO_2 <30 mm Hg)

CSF, cerebrospinal fluid; P_aCO_2, partial pressure of arterial carbon dioxide.

space, which lowers ICP. Mannitol also increases intravascular volume, which improves cerebral blood flow and perfusion. If autoregulation is maintained within the brain, the improved oxygenation can lead to vasoconstriction in certain areas, which would also decrease ICP. One side effect of mannitol therapy is renal failure when serum osmolarity is >320 mOsm/L. If this problem arises, hypertonic (3%) saline can provide similar effects and can increase serum osmolarity to 360 mOsm/L without a concomitant risk of renal failure.

Hyperventilation is a controversial intervention for increased ICP. Cerebral blood flow (CBF) is exquisitely sensitive to changes in oxygenation and ventilation, with hypoxia and hypercapnia causing increased CBF and hypocapnia decreasing CBF. Intentionally inducing hypocapnia by hyperventilating a patient with increased ICP can lead to cerebral hypoperfusion. Even mild hypocapnia (partial pressure of arterial carbon dioxide [P_aCO_2] of 32–35 mm Hg) leads to hypoxia and generation of lactic acid, leading to possible neurologic damage. CBF decreases in the first 24 hours following head trauma and gradually improves over the next 3 to 4 days. Therefore, aggressive hyperventilation is not generally used in the treatment course to minimize additional risk of neurologic damage, but mild-to-moderate hyperventilation may be effective particularly for refractory ICP problems.

Two other therapeutic options may be tried if ICP is not lowered by hyperosmolarity and hyperventilation: barbiturate coma and hypothermia. Because of decreased cerebral metabolism, cerebral oxygenation requirements are lower for patients when they are in barbiturate coma. Pentobarbital is the most frequently used barbiturate used to induce coma. These patients should have continuous electroencephalograph monitoring to ensure adequate suppression of brain activity. Mechanical ventilation and pressor support will likely be needed in these patients. Hypothermia is another strategy aimed at decreasing cerebral metabolism and subsequently decreasing CBF.

Steroids are commonly used to treat cerebral edema in patients with brain tumors. However, there is no evidence to support the use of steroids in increased ICP, unless patients have a documented decreased cortisol level.

SUGGESTED READINGS

Allen CH, Ward JD. An evidence-based approach to management of increased intracranial pressure. *Crit Care Clin.* 1998;14:485–495.

Jankowitz BT, Adelson PD. Pediatric traumatic brain injury: past, present and future. *Dev Neurosci.* 2006;28(4-5):264–275.

Soustiel JF, Mahamid E, Chistyakov A, et al. Comparison of moderate hyperventilation and mannitol for control of intracranial pressure control in patients with severe traumatic brain injury–a study of cerebral blood flow and metabolism. *Acta Neurochir (Wien).* 2006;148:845–851.

Tasker RC. Neurological critical care. *Curr Opin Pediatr.* 2000;12:222–226.

216

LIMIT THE ACTIVITY OF A CHILD WHO SUFFERS A CONCUSSION TO AVOID CUMULATIVE BRAIN INJURY AND TO PREVENT SECOND IMPACT SYNDROME

MICHAEL CLEMMENS, MD

WHAT TO DO – TAKE ACTION

Concussion is defined as a closed head injury associated with transient alteration in mental status or neurologic function, which may or may not involve loss of consciousness (LOC). In the pediatric population, the etiology of concussion is variable and is influenced by age. Young infants and children commonly suffer concussion after a fall from a height. Older children and adolescents may suffer concussion as a result of sports activity. Child abuse should always be considered in the differential diagnosis of head injury, especially in children younger than 2 years of age who are at risk for both shaken baby syndrome and blunt head trauma.

A complete and detailed history, with emphasis on the mechanism of injury and the presence and duration of LOC, is an important part of the head injury and concussion evaluation. For fall injuries, the height of the fall and the composition of the surface that the head strikes are two major factors in determining the degree of force generated by a fall. The degree of force is an important factor in assessing risk for serious injury. For example, a 4-foot fall onto concrete may generate more force than an 8-foot fall onto wood chips. An inconsistent or implausible history should raise the suspicion of inflicted injury.

The most common immediate symptoms of concussion are confusion and amnesia, although a variety of other neurologic deficits may be seen. These include, but are not limited to, headache, dizziness, vomiting, slowing, poor coordination, LOC, and emotional lability. Following the injury, children may develop postconcussive symptoms (PCS), which may persist for days, weeks, or even months. These symptoms may manifest as somatic complaints, emotional or behavioral changes, or cognitive problems. A thorough history and age-appropriate neurologic exam, with emphasis on mental status, should elicit any evidence of ongoing central nervous system dysfunction. If the exam is normal, the diagnosis of concussion or PCS can be made on the basis of the history. Several tools exist for the assessment of both immediate, on-site symptoms, and PCS, and these are reviewed in the references.

ⓒ 2008 by Lippincott Williams & Wilkins, a Wolters Kluwer business

Computed tomography (CT) scan is useful in ruling out intracranial injuries that may require neurosurgical intervention. Historical factors that suggest the need for CT include severe mechanism of injury, LOC, seizure, persistent vomiting, and suspicion of child abuse. Persistence or worsening of PCS may also warrant an imaging study. Physical exam findings that may indicate the need for imaging include abnormal mental status, focal neurologic findings, skull fracture, scalp hematoma, and a full or bulging fontanel. Low-risk patients are those who do not have a severe mechanism of injury and do not have any of the signs and symptoms listed above. These low-risk patients likely do not need a CT scan.

Sports participants who sustain a concussion and wish to return to play should be advised carefully. Cumulative brain injury from recurrent concussions can occur. In rare circumstances, a child may develop second impact syndrome. This syndrome occurs when a child receives a second concussion before having fully recovered from the first, and subsequently develops malignant cerebral edema. This syndrome is thought to occur as a result of disruption to the autoregulation of the brain's blood supply, leading to vascular engorgement, cerebral edema, increased intracranial pressure, herniation, and possibly death. Even though the exact relationship between a second impact and the resultant pathophysiologic response is unclear, immaturity of the brain is a documented risk factor.

To prevent these complications, several guidelines have been published that propose a grading system for concussions and detail when return to play is safe, and these are reviewed in the references. Among these guidelines, there is consensus that athletes should refrain from play until all signs and symptoms have resolved, including somatic, emotional or behavioral, and cognitive symptoms. Although there are some minor differences among the guidelines regarding other recommendations, the more severe the concussion, the longer the child should refrain from play. Severity is gauged by the presence or absence of LOC and the duration of symptoms. If there has been any LOC, return to play should be delayed for approximately 1 to 2 weeks. If there is no LOC, but initial symptoms persist beyond 15 minutes, then the wait time is 1 week. Any ongoing symptoms preclude return to play until resolution is complete and a waiting period has been observed. Furthermore, in all cases, special consideration should be given to a gradual and step-wise increase in activity level.

SUGGESTED READINGS

Duhaime AC, Alario AJ, Lewander WJ. Head injuries in very young children: mechanisms, injury types, and ophthalmologic findings in 100 hospitalized patients younger than 2 years of age. *Pediatrics.* 1992;90(2 Pt 1):179–185.

Kirkwood MW, Yeates KO, Wilson PE. Pediatric sport-related concussion: a review of the clinical management of an oft-neglected population. *Pediatrics.* 2006;117:1359–1371.

The management of minor closed head injury in children. Committee on Quality Improvement, American Academy of Pediatrics. Commission on Clinical Policies and Research, American Academy of Family Physicians. The management of minor closed head injury in children. *Pediatrics.* 1999;104:1407–1415

Wojtys EM, Hovda D, Landry G, et al. Current concepts. Concussion in sports. *Am J Sports Med.* 1999;27:676–687.

217

WHEN THERE ARE CONCERNS FOR VENTRICULOPERITONEAL SHUNT (VPS) MALFUNCTION, RELYING ENTIRELY ON THE HEAD COMPUTED TOMOGRAPHY (CT) SCAN AND SHUNT SERIES FOR VENTRICULOPERITONEAL SHUNT MALFUNCTION WILL MISS 30% OF SHUNT FAILURE

DAVID STOCKWELL, MD

WHAT TO DO – GATHER APPROPRIATE DATA

Perform a complete history and physical examination, evaluate the radiographic studies and their comparisons, and combine all of this information to make an accurate diagnosis.

VPSs are a relatively common device in pediatrics. As with any artificial device placed internally, the possibility of malfunctioning exists. Missing the diagnosis of shunt malfunction may lead to permanent neurologic injury or death. Unfortunately the diagnosis of shunt failure is not a simple task. Commonly used techniques to diagnose shunt malfunction are a combination of the patient's history, clinical exam, and radiographic studies. Often, however, the ultimate decision is based on the head CT and "shunt series." This chapter will explain how relying solely on those results will result in approximately one third of cases of shunt failure being missed.

Noninfectious shunt failure occurs due to obstruction, mechanical failure of the shunt (e.g., disconnection, fractured tubing, misplacement, or migration of the shunt), overdrainage, cerebrospinal fluid drainage other than from the shunt, loculations within the ventricular system, and abdominal causes. Timing of the malfunction may assist in diagnosing the type of shunt failure. Obstruction of the shunt system can occur at any time after shunt placement and at any point along the shunt. Early shunt malfunctions are usually due to misplacement, disconnection, or migration of the shunt components. Common causes for late shunt failure include tubing fractures, shunt overdrainage, ventricular loculations, and erosion of the distal tubing into a hollow viscus in the abdomen.

Radiographic evidence of shunt malfunction is typically observed either on plain radiographs or by CT scan. Plain radiographic images of the entire shunt tract, the so-called shunt series, help identify a mechanical

ⓒ 2008 by Lippincott Williams & Wilkins, a Wolters Kluwer business

disruption of the shunt. It will typically show broken tubing or disconnections. Common locations for fractures are near the clavicle or lower ribs.

Computed tomographic studies present evidence of increased ventricular size and reveal intraventricular catheter location. Shunt failure is manifest on head CT scan by increasing ventricular size. It is imperative to compare current studies against a baseline study obtained after successful shunt placement. Several studies note that current head CTs have been incorrectly read as normal when compared to earlier head CTs because the comparison was taken at another point of shunt failure.

When evaluating a head CT scan, it is important to realize that normal ventricular size or even small ventricles does not rule out shunt dysfunction. For this reason, CT and magnetic resonance imaging scans should not be used as the definitive diagnostic modality. Some of the causes of small ventricles other than shunt failure include poor compliance, overdrainage, slit ventricle syndrome, intermittent shunt malfunction.

When a scan shows large ventricles, an effort should be made to find out whether the ventricles have ever been smaller in size, thus usually implying that the current shunt has failed. All previous scans should be reviewed and compared with the current scan. Furthermore, it is crucial to know which of the comparison scan represents normal shunt functioning. Finally, even if the ventricles had never changed in size, the presence of large ventricles still should raise the suspicion for shunt failure.

In patients with high clinical suspicion for shunt failure but nonconfirmatory radiographic studies, further studies could include shunt taps, intracranial pressure monitoring, shunt patency studies, long periods of observation in the hospital, and even an occasional surgical exploration.

Evaluating a shunt malfunction is difficult; certainly neurosurgical input should be requested early in the patient's evaluation. Unfortunately, the radiographic studies that are the mainstay of evaluation are not infallible.

SUGGESTED READINGS

Browd SR, Ragel BT, Gottfried ON, et al. Failure of cerebrospinal fluid shunts: part I: obstruction and mechanical failure. *Pediatr Neurol.* 2006;34(2):83–92.

Iskandar BJ, McLaughlin C, Mapstone TB, et al. Pitfalls in the diagnosis of ventricular shunt dysfunction: radiology reports and ventricular size. *Pediatrics.* 1998;101(6):1031–1036.

218

Perform a Stat Sodium and Glucose Level in Patients with Refractory Seizures

Caroline Rassbach, MD

What to Do – Interpret the Data

Seizures are one of the most common neurologic conditions affecting children. The majority are short, self-limited seizures that occur secondary to disorders originating outside the brain. Examples include high fever, infection, head trauma, hypoxia, and toxins. Less than one third of seizures in children occur as a result of epilepsy. When a child presents with a first-time seizure, or when a child with a known seizure disorder presents with prolonged seizure, metabolic causes should be considered. Obtaining stat serum glucose and sodium levels are essential in these children.

Initial assessment of any child with a seizure should include evaluation of the *a*irway, *b*reathing, and *c*irculation (ABCs). The provider should perform vital signs and place the patient on a cardiac monitor and on supplemental oxygen. The provider should then obtain a detailed history and perform a quick physical examination, including a neurologic examination, searching for clues to the etiology of the seizure. Life-threatening conditions, such as meningitis, sepsis, head trauma, and toxin ingestion, should be considered in the differential diagnosis.

When a seizure lasts >5 minutes, intravenous access should be attained and stat serum glucose and sodium levels drawn. Serum calcium, phosphorus, magnesium, blood urea nitrogen, and a complete blood count may also be indicated. Urine for toxicology and serum anticonvulsant levels may be helpful. A benzodiazepine such as lorazepam or a barbiturate should be administered as a first-line drug to stop the seizure. Lorazepam administration can be repeated every 10 to 15 minutes if needed.

If the seizure continues for >10 minutes, a second anticonvulsant, such as phenobarbital or phenytoin, should be administered. Metabolic derangements, such as hypoglycemia and hyponatremia, should be treated as soon as they are diagnosed.

When the seizure activity persists >30 minutes, it is referred to as status epilepticus. Administration of a second long-acting anticonvulsant is indicated for status epilepticus. In addition, the practitioner should prepare for intubation and general anesthesia as the seizure approaches 45 minutes.

© 2008 by Lippincott Williams & Wilkins, a Wolters Kluwer business

Complications of status epilepticus include hypoxia, lactic acidosis, hyperkalemia, hypoglycemia, shock, hyperpyrexia, renal and respiratory failure, and death.

Hypoglycemia and hyponatremia are the most frequent metabolic derangements that cause seizure. Hypoglycemia occurs most commonly in neonates in the setting of hypoxia, toxemia, gestational diabetes, or a normal delivery. In older children, it occurs because of prolonged fasting, malabsorption and malnutrition, systemic disease, and hyperinsulinemia. Hypoglycemia in infants presents as cyanosis, apnea, hypothermia, hypotonia, poor feeding, lethargy, or seizures. In older children, signs of hypoglycemia include anxiety, tachycardia, sweating, tremulousness, weakness, hunger, and seizures. At any age, hypoglycemia should be considered as a cause of a seizure. Seizures secondary to hypoglycemia should be treated with 2 mL/kg of 50% glucose intravenously.

Hyponatremia, another metabolic cause for seizure, is one of the most common electrolyte disturbances occurring in hospitals. It usually results from excess free water intake in the presence of impaired free water excretion. Examples include syndrome of inappropriate secretion of antidiuretic hormone (SIADH), postoperative hyponatremia, water intoxication, overdilution of infant formula, and diuretic use. When hyponatremia occurs, water shifts into the intracellular space, resulting in cellular swelling. This may present clinically as cerebral edema and encephalopathy with headache, nausea, vomiting, emesis, and weakness. It may progress to altered mental status, seizures, respiratory arrest, and cerebral herniation.

Symptomatic hyponatremia is a medical emergency and should be treated with hypertonic 3% saline intravenously. For seizing patients or for those with increased intracranial pressure, the hypertonic saline should be infused rapidly enough to raise the serum sodium level by 4 to 8 mEq/L during the first hour or until seizure activity ceases. For less severe symptoms, hypertonic saline should be infused with a goal of raising the serum sodium by 1 mEq/L/hr. In general, 1 mL/kg of hypertonic saline will raise the serum sodium level by 1 mEq/L. Practitioners should be aware that overly fast correction of hyponatremia can result in devastating cerebral demyelination.

Practitioners should remember to consider metabolic derangements in patients with seizures. Stat serum glucose and sodium levels should be checked for all patients with prolonged or refractory seizures.

SUGGESTED READINGS

Johnston MV. Seizures in childhood. In: Behrman RE, Kliegman RM, Jenson HB, eds. *Nelson Textbook of Pediatrics.* 17th ed. Philadelphia: Saunders; 2004: chapter 586, pages 1993–2009.

Moritz ML, Ayus JC. Disorders of water metabolism in children: hyponatremia and hypernatremia. *Pediatr Rev.* 2002;23(11):371–380.

Sabo-Graham T, Seay AR. Management of status epilepticus in children. *Pediatr Rev.*
1998;19(9)306–310.

Sperling MA. Hypoglycemia. In: Behrman RE, Kliegman RM, Jenson HB, eds. *Nelson Textbook
of Pediatrics.* 17th ed. Philadelphia: Saunders; 2004: – .

219

AGGRESSIVELY TREAT ACUTE PAIN: FOR ANYONE IN ACUTE PAIN THE MANAGEMENT SHOULD INCLUDE A BASAL MEDICATION IN ADDITION TO A PRN FOR BREAKTHROUGH PAIN

DAVID STOCKWELL, MD

WHAT TO DO – MAKE A DECISION

An important responsibility of physicians who care for children is treating pain and suffering when possible. Several studies have documented that a large percentage of patients do not have their pain adequately addressed. The most common type of pain experienced by children is acute pain resulting from injury, illness, or necessary medical procedures. It is the responsibility of the physician to understand and practice the basic tenets of pain control including the anticipation of pain, identification of pain and treatment of pain.

Prior to discussing tenets of pain control, several barriers to the adequate treatment of pain in children should be recognized. These barriers identified by the American Association of Pediatrics include the following: (a) the myth that children, especially infants, do not feel pain the way adults do, or if they do, there is no untoward consequence; (b) lack of assessment and reassessment for the presence of pain; (c) misunderstanding of how to conceptualize and quantify a subjective experience; (d) lack of knowledge of pain treatment; (e) the notion that addressing pain in children takes too much time and effort; and (f) fears of adverse effects of analgesic medications, including respiratory depression and addiction.

Health care professionals should *anticipate* predictable painful experiences and monitor the condition of patients accordingly. Additionally, it should be discussed with the patient and family that pain may be present. One of the large misconceptions is that all pain can be nullified. However, having a discussion with the family and the patient, if appropriate, allows them to understand that some discomfort may occur but that the pain will be anticipated and treated adequately.

To treat pain adequately, ongoing *identification* of the presence and the severity of pain is essential. Several reliable, valid, and clinically sensitive assessment tools are available for neonates through adolescents. In a hospital setting, pain and response to treatment, including adverse effects, should be monitored routinely and documented clearly and in a visible place.

© 2008 by Lippincott Williams & Wilkins, a Wolters Kluwer business

Identification of pain in the preterm infant can be particularly difficult. When pain is prolonged, striking changes occur in the infant's physiologic and behavioral indicators. During episodes of prolonged pain, neonates enter a state of passivity with few, if any, body movements; an expressionless face; decreased heart rate and respiratory variability; and decreased oxygen consumption—all suggestive of a marked conservation of energy. Prolonged or repeated pain also increases the response elicited by future painful stimuli and even by usually nonpainful stimuli.

Early effective *treatment* of pain is safer and more efficacious than delayed treatment and results in improved patient comfort and possibly less total analgesic administered. For moderate to severe pain expected to persist, continuous dosing or around-the-clock dosing at fixed intervals is recommended; there are few indications for an as-needed regimen used alone. Dosages and the dosing interval should be adjusted based on the patient's response.

Therefore, the recommendations of many pain experts are to have an ongoing medication. For example this is the reason for the basal infusion in a patient-controlled analgesia system. The use of an around-the-clock regimen of a nonsteroidal anti-inflammatory drug is also an alternative to the ongoing continuous medication.

In both scenarios, if there is an exacerbation of pain that exceeds the efficacy of the continuous medication, then an intermittent analgesic can be administered. In the patient-controlled analgesia system, the patient will trigger the system to deliver a bolus dose of medication. In the oral regimen, the patient is given another dose of medication (as a prn) or a dose of medication from another class of analgesics.

SUGGESTED READINGS

American Academy of Pediatrics Committee on Fetus and Newborn; American Academy of Pediatrics Section on Surgery; Canadian Paediatric Society Fetus and Newborn Committee; Batton DG, Barrington KJ, Wallman C. Prevention and management of pain in the neonate: an update. *Pediatrics.* 2006;118(5):2231–2241.

American Academy of Pediatrics. Committee on Psychosocial Aspects of Child and Family Health; Task Force on Pain in Infants, Children, and Adolescent. The assessment and management of acute pain in infants, children, and adolescents. *Pediatrics.* 2001;108(3):793–797.

BE SURE TO APPROPRIATELY POSITION AND CUSHION INTENSIVE CARE UNIT AND ANESTHETIZED PATIENTS BECAUSE THEY ARE PRONE TO THE DEVELOPMENT OF FOCAL NEUROPATHIES AT COMPRESSION SITES

RENÉE ROBERTS, MD

WHAT TO DO – TAKE ACTION

Be sure to appropriately position and cushion intensive care unit and anesthetized patients because they are prone to the development of focal neuropathies at compression sites (e.g., ulnar nerve at elbow, peroneal nerve at fibular head, and radial nerve in spiral groove), due to positioning and weight loss.

Be aware of pressure points when the patient is under anesthesia or medically unable to sense or respond to pressure points or extremities in limb position. Pre-existing conditions to note during a preoperative history and physical include body habitus, diabetes mellitus, pre-existing neurologic conditions, peripheral vascular disease, alcohol dependence, and arthritis.

Especially in patients with a limited range of motion, assess if the patient can tolerate the anticipated operative position before administering anesthesia. The most common sites of injury under anesthesia as analyzed by closed claim analysis are the ulnar nerve, followed by the brachial plexus. Arm abduction should not exceed 90 degrees in supine patients but may do so in prone patients. Arms should be positioned to decrease pressure on the postcondylar groove of the humerus so as to protect the ulnar nerve. For instance, when the patient is supine with the arms abducted, the forearm should be supinated or in a neutral position.

Pressure on the radial nerve in the spiral groove of the humerus should be avoided. Make sure that the armrest is properly padded. Check that the blood pressure cuff is the correct size for the patient and rests on the arm rather than the forearm. There have been case reports of radial and ulnar nerve injuries hypothesized to be have been induced by blood pressure cuffs. However, the Task Force on Prevention of Peripheral Neuropathies (supported by the American Society of Anesthesiologists) agrees that the use of a blood pressure cuff placed above the antecubital fossa does not change the risk of peripheral neuropathy. Avoid prolonged extension of the elbow. This may result in median nerve injury. Limit extension of the elbow to

© 2008 by Lippincott Williams & Wilkins, a Wolters Kluwer business

≤90 degrees. Remember, safe positioning takes precedence over optimum surgical exposure. To avoid sciatic nerve injury, avoid stretching the biceps femoris muscle (hamstring) beyond a comfortable range. Limit hip flexion to <120 degrees when the patient is supine or in lateral position. To prevent femoral neuropathy, limit hip flexion to ≤90 degrees for supine patients. To protect the peroneal nerve, be sure that there is adequate padding and no direct pressure on the fibular head and lateral tibia. In other words, be sure there is pad between the outside of the leg below the knee in order the prevent contact of the peroneal nerve with a hard surface, that is, during procedures in the lithotomy position. Protective padding does reduce the incidence of perioperative peripheral neuropathies. Other examples include padded arm boards, foam or gel pads at the elbow, and a chest roll placed under the chest (rather than the axilla) for patients in the lateral position to protect the brachial plexus.

Postoperative physical assessment improves detection and results in early treatment of peripheral neuropathies. Recording of specific positioning actions on the anesthesia record is important not only for documentation purposes but also to determine the possible etiology of a postoperative peripheral neuropathy.

SUGGESTED READINGS

Cheney FW, Domino KB, Caplan RA, et al. Nerve injury associated with anesthesia: a closed claims analysis. *Anesthesiology.* 1999;90(4):1062–1069.

Lin CC, Jawan B, de Villa MV, et al. Blood pressure cuff compression injury of the radial nerve. *J Clin Anesth.* 2001;13(4):306–308.

Practice advisory for the prevention of perioperative peripheral neuropathies: a report by the American Society of Anesthesiologists Task Force on Prevention of Perioperative Peripheral Neuropathies. *Anesthesiology.* 2000;92:1168–1182.

221

MONITOR GLUCOSE LEVELS IN PATIENTS PRESENTING WITH AN ALTERED MENTAL STATUS

SOPHIA SMITH, MD

WHAT TO DO – GATHER APPROPRIATE DATA

Children with altered mental status show a change in personality, behavior, or responsiveness. They may appear somnolent, difficult to rouse, or completely unresponsive. This can be life-threatening if it is not recognized and treated promptly. It often results in hypotonia, which may lead to airway obstruction and interfere with respiration, resulting in hypoxemia and eventual respiratory failure.

Infants and young children may present with altered mental status from causes including hypoxemia, shock, seizures, sepsis, meningitis, hyperthermia, hypothermia, and hypoglycemia. The focus here is on hypoglycemia as a common cause that requires immediate treatment. Transient hyperinsulinemic neonatal hypoglycemia is seen in neonates of diabetic or pre-eclamptic mothers, premature infants, small-for-gestational age infants, or infants with fetal distress. Infants of mothers taking hypoglycemia-inducing drugs may be predisposed to hypoglycemic conditions. There are cases of persistent hyperinsulinism in infants that may be due to familial and nonfamilial hyperinsulinism, beta-cell adenoma (insulinoma), or beta-cell hyperplasia. Other causes of newborn hypoglycemia include endocrine deficiencies and congenital inborn errors of metabolism.

A high degree of suspicion is required to identify children who have metabolic disorders. The presentation of inborn errors of metabolism is usually nonspecific and can mimic many other conditions. Metabolic diseases individually are rare, but collectively constitute a full range of disorders. Each disorder is due either to an absence or reduced activity of a specific enzyme. The patient may have a nonfunctional form of an enzyme or be missing a cofactor that is necessary for the metabolism of an amino acid, carbohydrate, fatty acid, or more complex compound. The clinical presentation results from the accumulation of toxic metabolites, lack of production of the necessary intermediates or byproducts, or both.

The organic acidemias comprise a group of metabolic disorders in which the defect produces an accumulation of organic acids. The central emergency features of the organic acid disorders are profound metabolic ketoacidosis

© 2008 by Lippincott Williams & Wilkins, a Wolters Kluwer business

and hypoglycemia. The ketoacidosis, hyperammonemia, and hypoglycemia can explain the lethargy and obtundation. The increased organic acids overwhelm the body's acid–base balance, resulting in metabolic acidosis. This metabolic stress produces an increased need for cellular energy, which is provided by enhanced degradation of glucose, resulting in hypoglycemia. The hypoglycemia is exacerbated by the inhibition of gluconeogenesis induced by one or more of the accumulated organic acids. The hypoglycemia causes hormonal changes with the release of free fatty acids from adipose tissue.

It is important to make a diagnosis quickly to prevent permanent neurologic damage. Organic acids and ammonia are toxic to the brain and accumulations of these products may result in cerebral edema. Metabolic decompensation is treated with intravenous glucose and bicarbonate. Early decompensation or persistent ketonuria are treated by eliminating protein in the diet and encouraging a high-carbohydrate diet. The treatment for acute metabolic decompensation in these disorders includes hydration, correction of the biochemical abnormalities (metabolic acidosis, hyperammonemia, hypoglycemia), the reversal of catabolism/promotion of anabolism, elimination of toxic metabolites, treatment of the precipitating factor when possible (e.g., infection, excess protein ingestion), and cofactor supplementation.

It is important that clinical parameters are utilized to monitor the patient's clinical condition but also the biochemical parameters are needed to monitor closely the acid–base status and glucose control as recovery begins.

SUGGESTED READINGS

Hale D. Endocrine emergencies: hypoglycemia. In: Fleisher G, Ludwig S, eds. *Textbook of Pediatric Emergency Medicine.* 4th ed. Baltimore: Lippincott Williams & Wilkins; 2000.

222

KNOW THE EARLY SIGNS OF BRAIN HERNIATION

MEGHA SHAH FITZPATRICK, MD

WHAT TO DO – INTERPRET THE DATA

Herniation occurs when the brain shifts across structures within the skull, from one intracranial compartment to another, as a result of pressure gradients created by high intracranial pressure (ICP). Although the brain has considerable elasticity, the arteries and veins responsible for its blood supply are relatively fixed in space, leading to the risk that a shifting brain will cause moving portions to lose their blood supply. It is essential to be able to recognize the early clinical manifestations of herniation syndromes and to rapidly institute therapies to decrease ICP in order to reverse the process and maintain viability of the patient. Herniation syndromes of the brain can be classified as follows: central, uncal, cerebellar tonsillar, subfalcine, and transcalvarial.

CENTRAL HERNIATION SYNDROME

Central (transtentorial) herniation syndrome occurs as a result of diffuse brain swelling due to trauma or a centrally located mass. This causes the diencephalon (thalamus, hypothalamus, epithalamus, subthalamus, and pretectum) to move caudally through the tentorial notch. The resulting alteration of consciousness is thought to be caused by cerebral hypoperfusion secondary to increased ICP as well as dysfunction of the reticular formation. The reticular formation is involved in stereotypical actions such as walking, sleeping, and lying down. It is absolutely essential for the basic functions of life and is evolutionarily one of the oldest portions of the brain. Consequently, an initial presenting sign of potential central herniation is a decreased level of alertness, which later progresses to stupor and coma.

Other key early features of the central herniation syndrome include meiotic but reactive pupils secondary to loss of sympathetic output from the hypothalamus; decorticate or flexor posturing that can be elicited spontaneously or via noxious stimuli; and Cheyne-Stokes respiration, an abnormal pattern of breathing characterized by periods of breathing with gradually increasing and decreasing tidal volumes scattered with periods of apnea. It is crucial to recognize this constellation of symptoms in the face of severe traumatic brain injury or a known central intracranial mass, because at this stage, herniation is potentially reversible.

© 2008 by Lippincott Williams & Wilkins, a Wolters Kluwer business

In addition to these early signs of central herniation, it is crucial to be able to recognize signs and symptoms of Parinaud syndrome. Children with midbrain or pineal tumors, as well as direct or compressive trauma to the midbrain often present with Parinaud syndrome, also known as dorsal midbrain syndrome or pretectal syndrome. This syndrome consists of paralysis of up gaze, Pseudo-Argyll Robertson pupils (light–near dissociation), convergence-retraction nystagmus, and eyelid retraction (Collier sign). If this group of symptoms is present or even just a limitation of upward gaze is present, it behooves the physician to obtain neuroimaging to rule out an intracranial process.

With progression of the central herniation syndrome, there is a marked decrease in the likelihood of reversibility. As the failure progresses to the midbrain from the diencephalon, the pupils enlarge to midposition and posturing becomes decerebrate or extensor. Attempts to elicit horizontal eye movements via the cerebro-ocular reflex (commonly known as doll's eyes) or the cerebrovestibular reflex (also known as the cold calorics test) fail, respiratory patterns continue to become more irregular, and the patient becomes overtly comatose. At this point, the patient will also display signs of Cushing triad (hypertension, bradycardia, and alteration in respiratory pattern) and will likely continue to complete loss of all brainstem reflexes and death.

UNCAL HERNIATION SYNDROME

Uncal herniation (or lateral mass herniation) syndrome occurs when a lateral expanding cerebral mass pushes the uncus and the hippocampal gyrus over the lateral edges of the tentorium. Initially, prior to the herniation syndrome developing, signs and symptoms are often due to the mass itself (i.e., contralateral hemiparesis). With shifting of the diencephalon away from the mass, the initial two signs of impending herniation are alteration in consciousness and an ipsilateral third nerve palsy, which is present in about 85% of patients. As the third cranial nerve is compressed against the tentorial notch, the papillary fibers—which are located most peripherally within the nerve—are damaged and cause a dilated pupil. This unilateral dilated pupil, along with contralateral hemiparesis with or without significant impairment in consciousness, are the hallmarks of the uncal herniation syndrome.

As the lateral displacement of the midbrain continues, an ipsilateral hemiplegia is produced secondary to compression of the contralateral corticospinal tract within the cerebral peduncle against the edge of the tentorium. This hemiplegia is also referred to as Kernohan notch phenomenon. Patients may also have bilateral papillary dilatation secondary to distorted cranial nerve three anatomy and midbrain ischemia. After the initial triad of symptoms, uncal herniation begins to affect the midbrain and pons, producing bilateral fixed pupils and decerebrate posturing. Symptoms are often rapidly progressive, and at this point, the signs and symptoms of uncal herniation are no longer distinguishable from central herniation.

CEREBELLAR TONSILLAR HERNIATION SYNDROME

Cerebellar tonsillar herniation is seen in patients with posterior fossa masses, causing brainstem compression, cranial nerve dysfunction, and obstructive hydrocephalus. The cerebellar tonsils are pushed into and eventually through the foramen magnum as the pressure gradient across the foramen increases. Patients can initially present with neck pain prior to losing consciousness. In addition, compression of the medulla affects respiratory centers within this structure and results in apnea.

Conversely, patients undergoing ventriculostomy for relief of obstructive hydrocephalus can have a caudal or upward transtentorial herniation of the posterior fossa into the diencephalic region. Consequently, neurosurgeons performing a ventriculostomy also prepare the patient for an emergent posterior fossa decompression before beginning the procedure, given the risk of caudal herniation of the posterior fossa.

As discussed earlier, it is crucial as a physician to be able to identify the signs and symptoms of brain herniation syndromes. Often, patients are asymptomatic in their presentation of an intracranial mass until increased ICP is above a threshold necessary to cause pressure gradients that lead to shifting of parts of the brain between compartments and ischemia secondary to compression of the vasculature. Once this cascade of symptoms has begun, there is often very limited time to initiate treatment to decrease intracranial pressure and eliminate the pressure gradients preventing complete herniation and death.

SUGGESTED READINGS

Furhman BP, Zimmerman J, eds. *Pediatric Critical Care.* 3rd ed. Philadelphia: Mosby Elsevier; 2006.

Goetz CG, Pappert EJ, eds. *Textbook of Clinical Neurology.* 2nd Ed. Philadelphia: WB Saunders Company; 2003.

223

KNOW HOW TO CORRECT FOR A LEUKOCYTOSIS IN THE FACE OF A BLOODY CEREBROSPINAL FLUID (CSF) TAP

MEGHA SHAH FITZPATRICK, MD

WHAT TO DO – INTERPRET THE DATA

CSF is comprised of >99% water. Other components of CSF include the major ions, oxygen, sugars, lactate, proteins (e.g., albumin, globulins), amino acids, urea, ammonia, creatinine, lipids, neurotransmitters and their metabolites, hormones, and vitamins. The blood–CSF barrier protects the brain and CSF from potentially harmful or toxic substances in the blood. Only lipophilic substances can diffuse unrestricted across the blood–CSF barrier. In addition, substances such as glucose that are lipophobic are transported across the blood–CSF barrier into the CSF space via facilitated diffusion using a proteolipid carrier. If the integrity of the blood–CSF barrier is compromised, abnormal amounts of protein, cells, and glucose may be present in the CSF.

The composition of CSF and the mechanism of transport across this barrier are important when evaluating CSF fluid samples obtained by lumbar puncture (LP) in an attempt to diagnose and treat central nervous system (CNS) disease. The most common CSF studies obtained include gram stain and culture, cell count and differential, as well as glucose and protein concentrations. Abnormal results of these studies help to determine whether CNS disease is present and also help indicate what type of disease is present. CSF for analysis is obtained via a LP and should be clear and colorless secondary to the large water content of the fluid if no CNS disease is present. The CSF typically contains no red blood cells (RBCs) and 0 to 1 white blood cells (WBCs). Often, the LP can be a technically challenging procedure and not uncommonly may result in minor trauma to the blood–CSF barrier, leading to bleeding within the CSF space. As a result, some of the lab values, such as the protein count and WBC count, may be elevated secondary to the increased RBC count of the CSF, but not necessarily secondary to the presence of CNS disease, such as an infection or an inflammatory process.

It is important to account for the presence of blood when ruling in or out different types of CNS disease. This is achieved using a correction factor in the form of a ratio. For every 700 RBCs per microliter present, 1 WBC per microliter is present. If the WBC count exceeds this ratio, another cause

ⓒ 2008 by Lippincott Williams & Wilkins, a Wolters Kluwer business

of CSF leukocytosis must be investigated. For example, in the evaluation of fever, especially in infants younger than 6 months of age, a LP is a common diagnostic tool used to look for the presence of meningitis. Although blood in the CSF secondary to subarachnoid hemorrhage may not be common in this population, blood as a result of a traumatic LP sometimes occurs. Using the ratio of 700 RBC to every 1 WBC per microliter of CSF helps differentiate the cause of the CSF leukocytosis prior to committing an infant to a course of antibiotics and a hospitalization secondary to a diagnosis of meningitis for a traumatic LP.

A second laboratory test used to look for CNS disease is CSF glucose. CSF glucose is normally 60% of the plasma glucose concentration. Although an elevated CSF glucose level (hyperglycorrhachia) is the result of elevated plasma glucose, a low CSF glucose level (hypoglycorrhachia) can be due to many causes, including low peripheral blood sugar (hypoglycemia). If the hypoglycorrhachia is not caused by hypoglycemia, it could indicate a deficiency of glucose transport or increased utilization of glucose by the brain because of infection or another CNS disease process.

Together, the CSF glucose and WBC count are useful diagnostic tests for abnormal CNS processes, such as an infection. In addition to the clinical presentation and the results of other common CSF studies, such as protein level, Gram stain, and culture, the ability to accurately interpret abnormal CSF laboratory values is extremely useful for diagnosing CNS disease.

SUGGESTED READINGS

Haslam RHA. Neurologic Evaluation, chapter 584. In: Behrman RE, Kleigman RM, Jenson HB, eds. *Nelson Textbook of Pediatrics.* 17th ed. Philadelphia: Saunders; 2004:1980–1981.

224

KNOW HOW TO APPROPRIATELY CORRECT FOR THE CEREBROSPINAL FLUID (CSF) GLUCOSE CONCENTRATION

MEGHA SHAH FITZPATRICK, MD

WHAT TO DO – INTERPRET THE DATA

The lowered CSF glucose concentration is the result of defective glucose transport into the CSF and the increased utilization of glucose in the brain. The CSF glucose depends on the blood glucose concentration. A CSF glucose of <40% of the blood glucose is considered abnormally low.

Glucose is an essential substrate for the metabolism of most cells. Because glucose is a polar molecule, transport through biological membranes requires specific transport proteins. GLUT-1 was one of the first glucose transporters reported. It is widely distributed in the endothelial tissues of the blood–brain barrier, making it responsible for the glucose uptake required by the tissues to sustain normal respiration in all cells.

Glucose is usually present in the CSF; the level is usually 60% that of the peripheral circulation. To appropriately judge the relative normality of the glucose concentrations, a simultaneous measurement of serum glucose (especially if the CSF glucose level is likely to be low) is recommended. Reduced CSF glucose levels can indicate fungal, tuberculous, or pyogenic infections; lymphomas; leukemia spreading to the meninges; meningoencephalitic mumps; or hypoglycemia. This low CSF glucose level associated with bacterial infection is probably due to enzymatic inhibition rather than actual bacterial consumption of the glucose. A decreased CSF glucose concentration is usually present in purulent meningitis. It has little value beyond supporting a diagnosis because the important information is derived from the CSF culture results.

The reduced CSF glucose appears to be the result of decreased glucose transport across the blood–CSF barrier and conversion of the brain's metabolism to a less efficient glycogenolysis mechanism. Thus, a lowered glucose suggests more severe brain involvement.

A deficiency in glucose transport (glucose transporter type 1 deficiency syndrome) has also been linked with epileptic encephalopathy. It is also well characterized in children and should be considered in intractable epilepsy. Thus, glucose transporter 1 deficiency syndrome is an important condition for the general pediatrician's differential armamentarium.

© 2008 by Lippincott Williams & Wilkins, a Wolters Kluwer business

SUGGESTED READINGS

Deane R, Segal MB. The transport of sugars across the perfused choroid plexus of the sheep. *J Physiol.* 1985:362:245–260.

Klepper J. Impaired glucose transport into the brain: the expanding spectrum of glucose transporter type 1 deficiency syndrome. *Curr Opin Neurol.* 2004;17(2):193–196.

225

RECOGNIZE THE REASONS FOR AN ELEVATED CEREBROSPINAL FLUID (CSF) PROTEIN LEVEL

MEGHA SHAH FITZPATRICK, MD

WHAT TO DO – INTERPRET THE DATA

The majority of CSF is produced by the choroid plexus, which is present throughout the ventricular system and the subarachnoid space that surround the brain and spinal cord. The choroid plexus is formed by the choroidal epithelium, a bilayered structure, and its accompanying blood vessels and interstitial connective tissue. The brain and its surrounding fluid are protected from substances in the blood by the blood–CSF barrier. Only substances that can cross biological membranes because of their lipophilic nature may diffuse unrestricted across the blood-brain barrier. Proteins are not included in this subset of substances.

CSF is clear and colorless because it is comprised of 99% water. The majority of protein in CSF is derived from the serum. When the integrity of the blood–CSF barrier is intact, the CSF to serum albumin ratio is 1:200, implying that normal entry rate of protein from the serum to the CSF space is 200 times less than its rate of exit. Any compromise to the integrity of this barrier results in a higher rate of entry and thus a higher protein level in the CSF. The normal CSF protein ranges from 10 to 40 mg/dL in a child, to as high as 120 mg/dL in a neonate.

The CSF protein may be elevated in many processes, including infectious; immunologic, vascular, and degenerative diseases; as well as tumors of the brain and spinal cord. Hemorrhage within the CSF space, such as a subarachnoid hemorrhage or secondary to a traumatic lumbar puncture, can also cause an increase in the protein level of the CSF. This differs from other causes of elevated CSF protein in that the integrity of the blood–CSF barrier is not necessarily compromised. It is important to consider the amount of blood present and determine if it alone accounts for the elevation of CSF protein or if there is compromise to the blood–CSF barrier. For every 1,000 red blood cells in the CSF, the protein level increases by 1 mg/dL.

An elevation of CSF protein is a nonspecific indicator of central nervous system disease. Although it may provide an indication that the blood–brain barrier is compromised, the presence of blood in the CSF must be first ruled out as a cause of the elevated protein.

© 2008 by Lippincott Williams & Wilkins, a Wolters Kluwer business

SUGGESTED READINGS

Fishman RA, ed. *Cerebrospinal Fluid in Diseases of the Nervous System.* 2nd ed. Philadelphia: WB Saunders; 1992:431.

Haslam RHA. Neurologic Evaluation, chapter 584. In: Behrman RE, Kleigman RM, Jenson HB, eds. *Nelson Textbook of Pediatrics.* 17th ed. Philadelphia: Saunders; 2004:1980–1981.

226

ALWAYS CONSIDER THE DIAGNOSIS OF SEPTIC ARTHRITIS AND OSTEOMYELITIS IN ANY CHILD PRESENTING WITH FEVER AND LIMB PAIN

ANJALI SUBBASWAMY, MD

WHAT TO DO – INTERPRET THE DATA

In septic arthritis, the knee is most commonly infected, followed by the hip. An early peak in incidence appears to occur in the first months of infancy, with an overall average age of 3 to 6 years. Males and females seem to be at equivalent risk. Bacteria can reach the joint by hematogenous or direct spread from an adjacent focus. The hip joint is particularly susceptible, as it is intracapsular and shares blood supply with adjacent femoral metaphysis. *Staphylococcus aureus* and streptococcal species are the most common offending agents. Joint and growth plate destruction result from bacterial enzymes, inflammation, and pressure from purulent fluid collection in a confined space. Reduced leg length and decreased joint mobility are common sequelae. Symptoms include fever, ill appearance, joint or limb pain, leukocytosis, and elevated erythrocyte sedimentation rate. Diagnosis is confirmed by joint aspiration and culture. It is not uncommon to obtain culture-negative purulent exudate, in which case antibiotic therapy is targeted towards the most common organisms.

Osteomyelitis evolves and presents in much the same fashion. Etiologies include hematogenous, direct inoculation by trauma or surgery, and local infection spread. The incidence of hematogenous osteomyelitis is highest in the first two decades of life, more common in immunodeficiency, minor trauma coincident with bacteremia, and indwelling vascular catheters. Diagnostic workup includes plain radiographs, magnetic resonance and/or radionuclide bone scan imaging of affected limb. Subacute and chronic infection may subsequently develop, necessitating long-term antibiotic therapy, up to 6 weeks. The most common bacterial pathogens are *S. aureus*, streptococcal species, and *Kingella kingae* (mostly in children younger than the age of 5 years).

© 2008 by Lippincott Williams & Wilkins, a Wolters Kluwer business

Both septic arthritis and osteomyelitis constitute medical emergencies and any child who presents with fever and joint or limb pain should be evaluated and treated expeditiously.

SUGGESTED READINGS

Kiang KM, Ogunmodede F, Juni BA, et al. Outbreak of osteomyelitis/septic arthritis caused by *Kingella kingae* among child care center attendees. *Pediatrics.* 2005;116(2):e206–e213.

Offiah AC. Acute osteomyelitis, septic arthritis and discitis: differences between neonates and older children. *Eur J Radiol.* 2006;60(2):221–232.

Yuan HC, Wu KG, Chen CJ, et al. Characteristics and outcome of septic arthritis in children. *J Microbiol Immunol Infect.* 2006;39(4):342–347.

227

OBTAIN A MAGNETIC RESONANCE IMAGING (MRI) SCAN IN PATIENTS WITH LEGG-CALVÉ-PERTHES DISEASE (LCPD) BECAUSE IT IS MORE SENSITIVE FOR DETECTING EARLY CHANGES THAN RADIOGRAPHS

YOLANDA LEWIS-RAGLAND, MD

WHAT TO DO – GATHER APPROPRIATE DATA

LCPD is estimated to affect approximately 1 in 1,200 children, mostly male. LCPD is also referred to as ischemic necrosis of the hip, coxa plana, osteochondritis, and avascular necrosis of the femoral head.

SIGNS AND SYMPTOMS OF LEGG-CALVÉ-PERTHES DISEASE

The first symptoms characterized of LCPD are usually a limp, and pain in one hip, groin, or knee, with decreased abduction and internal rotation of the hip. Often the parent will first notice limping during the child's active play. The child usually cannot remember an injury, nor can he or she accurately specify the location of the pain.

ETIOLOGY

LCPD is of unknown origin; however, a hypothesis of clotting abnormalities with vascular thrombosis has been entertained. This vascular thrombosis leads to bone death that occurs in the head of the femur due to an interruption in blood flow. As bone death occurs, the femoral head develops a fracture, which signals the beginning of bone reabsorption by the body. As bone is slowly absorbed, it is replaced by new tissue and bone. LCPD appears to take place in four distinct phases:

1. The femoral head becomes dense with possible fracture of supporting bone
2. Fragmentation and reabsorption of bone
3. Reossification when new bone has been laid down
4. Healing, when new bone remodels.

© 2008 by Lippincott Williams & Wilkins, a Wolters Kluwer business

RISK FACTORS FOR LEGG-CALVÉ-PERTHES DISEASE

Some of the risk factors for LCPD include children who are small for their age and are extremely active; ethnic predominance in Asians, Eskimos, and whites; and an exposure to secondhand smoke.

DIAGNOSIS

Initial diagnosis will require an x-ray, MRI scan, or bone scan. Other diagnostic measures may include tests for limitation of abduction, a measurement of the thigh to determine muscle atrophy, and tests to determine the child's range of motion. Several studies have focused on MRI's sensitivity for early diagnosis. Several studies of early LCPD demonstrated the superiority of MRI to radiography and nuclear scans. MRI demonstrated avascular necrosis of the affected hip when radiography and scintigraphy were normal. Weeks to months later, the repeat roentgenograms subsequently also became positive for LCPD.

SUGGESTED READINGS

Khan AL, Seriki D, Hutchinson CE, et al. Legg-Calvé-Perthes-Disease. Available at: www.emedicine.com/radio/topic387.htm. Accessed January 3, 2008.

MedlinePlus Medical Encyclopedia. Legg-Calvé-Perthes Disease. Available at: www.nlm.nih.gov/medlineplus/ency/article/001264.htm. Accessed January 3, 2008.

National Osteonecrosis Foundation. Legg-Calvé-Perthes Disease Brochure. Baltimore: National Osteonecrosis Foundation. 2000. Available at: www.nonf.org/perthesbrochure/perthes-brochure.htm. Accessed January 3, 2008.

228

KNOW THAT HIP PAIN IN CHILDREN CAN BE A DIAGNOSTIC DILEMMA FOR HEALTH CARE PROVIDERS

LAURA HUFFORD, MD

WHAT TO DO – GATHER APPROPRIATE DATA

Although most conditions that cause hip pain are benign and self-limiting, evaluation for pathology and rapid treatment is often very important and needed to prevent significant morbidity and mortality.

Patients presenting with a limp and impaired internal rotation of the hip may have a slipped capital femoral epiphysis. In this condition, the femoral epiphysis is shifted in a posterior position. Importantly, hip pain may be referred to the knee. The mean age of presentation is 12 years old, and risk factors include obesity, hypothyroidism, and growth hormone deficiency. Once the diagnosis is confirmed with plain radiographs, the patient should be placed on crutches, in non–weight-bearing status and referred to orthopedics for possible operative management.

Idiopathic necrosis of the capital femoral epiphysis of the femoral head is known as Legg-Calvé-Perthes disease (LCPD). Peak ages of presentation are between 5 and 7 years of age, and it is more common in boys than girls. Patients may initially present with a limp, as the necrosis progresses they develop hip, thigh, or knee pain. On exam, they have pain during internal rotation and abduction, and typically, plain x-rays (including frog leg views) are sufficient for diagnosis. Therapy for LCPD remains controversial. Indeed, 70% to 90% of patients have good range of motion and are without pain at 20-year follow-up regardless of initial treatment. Thus, if LCPD is suspected, the patient should be placed on non–weight-bearing status and referred to orthopedics for further evaluation and management.

Transient synovitis is a self-limiting inflammation of the synovial lining in hip joint. It occurs in boys twice as often as in girls and is most commonly found in children between 3 and 8 years old. The patient is usually afebrile and presents with a limp and unilateral hip pain. However, a small percentage of children with transient synovitis present with bilateral pain. One study found that 25% of children with transient synovitis had a joint effusion or synovial swelling on the contralateral side. The pain usually lasts for 3 to 10 days and is treated with anti-inflammatory medications and rest.

© 2008 by Lippincott Williams & Wilkins, a Wolters Kluwer business

Septic arthritis is a bacterial infection of the joint space and can lead to permanent disability and death if not treated promptly. The patient is usually ill-appearing with fever and irritability or lethargy. The hip is usually held in a flexed, externally rotated and abducted position, and has impaired mobility. The gold standard for diagnosis of septic arthritis involves aspiration of the synovial fluid. The fluid is generally turbid, with the white blood cell count $>50,000/\mu L$ and a neutrophilic predominance. Culture of the fluid yields the offending organism in 70% of patients. This condition is a medical emergency because any delay in surgical washing of the infected hip is associated with joint necrosis and osteomyelitis.

Differentiating the causes of hip pain is a difficult but important task. Plain film radiographs can help rule out such musculoskeletal disease such as LCPD and slipped capital femoral epiphysis. However, discriminating between transient synovitis and septic hip can be difficult. A study by Kocher et al. recommends using four predictors to determine the patient's probability of septic arthritis. Predictors include a history of fever $>38.5°C$, refusal to bear weight, erythrocyte sedimentation rate of ≥ 40, and a serum white blood cell count $\geq 12,000$ cell/mL^3. Kocher's study suggests that if three or four predictors are present, there is a $>93\%$ chance that the patient has septic arthritis and should be taken for joint aspiration and likely therapeutic arthrotomy. If a patient has two predictors, Kocher recommends ultrasound guided aspiration of joint fluid and then treatment as indicated by fluid analysis.

SUGGESTED READINGS

Burrow SR, Alman B, Wright JG. Short stature as a screening test for endocrinopathy in slipped capital femoral epiphysis. *J Bone Joint Surg Br*. 2001;83(2):263–268.

Ehrendorfer S, LeQuesne G, Penta M, et al. Bilateral synovitis in symptomatic unilateral transient synovitis of the hip: an ultrasonographic study in 56 children. *Acta Orthop Scand*. 1996;67:149–152.

Frick SL. Evaluation of the child who has hip pain. *Orthop Clin North Am*. 2006;37(2):133–140.

Hart JJ. Transient synovitis of the hip in children. *Am Fam Physician*. 1996;54:1587–1591.

Kocher MS, Zurakowski D, Kasser JR. Differentiating between septic arthritis and transient synovitis of the hip in children: an evidence-based clinical prediction algorithm. *J Bone Joint Surg Am*. 1999;81(12):1662–1670.

Luhmann SJ, Jones A, Schootman M, et al. Differentiating between septic arthritis and transient synovitis of the hip in children: an evidence-based clinical prediction algorithm. *J Bone Joint Surg Am*. 2004;86-A(5):956–962.

229

REMEMBER TO CHECK A CREATININE PHOSPHOKINASE (CPK) IN PATIENTS WHO PRESENT WITH SIGNIFICANT "MUSCLE ACHES"

LINDSEY ALBRECHT, MD

WHAT TO DO – GATHER APPROPRIATE DATA, INTERPRET THE DATA

Rhabdomyolysis is often misdiagnosed and not worked up in children and adolescents with systemic viral illnesses, extreme heat, or who have over-exercised.

Complaints of muscle aches are common in pediatrics. In most instances, the aches are transient and benign; occasionally, though, a more significant underlying problem may exist. Rhabdomyolysis is a potentially serious cause of myalgia in childhood and is characterized by the breakdown of striated muscle tissue. Muscle breakdown results in the leakage of muscle cell constituents, including creatine kinase (CK) and myoglobin, into the circulation. Myoglobinuria may result in acute renal failure, the most severe consequence of rhabdomyolysis. Rhabdomyolysis in the pediatric population differs from rhabdomyolysis in the adult population with respect to etiology, clinical presentation, and prognosis.

In children, rhabdomyolysis is frequently the result of viral myositis, trauma, connective tissue disease, and drug overdose. In early childhood, viral infection is the leading cause, accounting for almost 40% of all childhood rhabdomyolysis. Trauma, resulting in muscle compression or muscle injury, is the leading cause of rhabdomyolysis in children older than 9 years of age. Trauma accounts for approximately 26% of all pediatric cases of rhabdomyolysis. Vigorous exercise is well known to occasionally induce rhabdomyolysis in children and adults and accounts for approximately 4% of pediatric cases. In one case report, 119 students developed myalgia and elevation in CK after being instructed to perform 120 pushups in 5 minutes by their gymnastics teacher. Exercise-induced rhabdomyolysis is especially likely if the temperature and humidity are high. Metabolic disorders, such as diabetic ketoacidosis, McArdle disease, and aldolase A deficiency, may additionally result in rhabdomyolysis in the pediatric patient.

The classic presentation consists of a triad of muscle pain, weakness, and dark urine, but occurs infrequently in the pediatric patient. In the largest

© 2008 by Lippincott Williams & Wilkins, a Wolters Kluwer business

pediatric study to date, only 1 out of 191 patients had all three symptoms. Myalgia was noted in 45% of patients, weakness in 38%, and dark urine in approximately 4% of children in this study. Common additional presenting features included fever in 40%, muscle tenderness in 39%, and viral symptoms in 39%.

Laboratory evaluation of rhabdomyolysis should include serum CK, basic chemistry panel, and urinalysis. Definitive diagnosis of rhabdomyolysis is usually made when serum CK is >5 times normal without evidence of significant elevation of cardiac or brain fractions (CK-MB or CK-BB). Urine dipstick analysis may be positive for hemoglobin but have a microscopic examination that does not demonstrate erythrocytes. This represents myoglobinuria rather than *hematuria*. Acute renal failure (ARF) is rarely seen in pediatric patients with urinary heme dipstick results of <2+. ARF is more frequent with higher heme dipstick results (>2+), but still only occurs in 5% of all pediatric cases. The serum CK is correlated with the degree of renal dysfunction, because higher CK values are associated with higher serum creatinine levels. In addition to the much lower incidence of ARF versus that in adults, children also tend to not develop chronic renal failure as frequently.

Treatment of rhabdomyolysis in childhood should include early initiation of fluid therapy. Most clinicians tend to treat with 1.5 to 2 times maintenance fluid needs. The need for bicarbonate administration to alkalinize the urine, although effective in adults, has not been shown to prevent ARF in children. Significant electrolyte abnormalities, such as hyperkalemia, are rare but need to be managed appropriately and aggressively.

Prompt diagnosis of rhabdomyolysis in the pediatric population is often hampered by a lack of classical symptoms. Patients with myalgia, weakness, or muscle tenderness should be evaluated for rhabdomyolysis, because serious sequelae such as ARF may occur if early aggressive intravenous fluid administration is not initiated. Because viral illness and trauma are the leading causes of rhabdomyolysis in childhood, these conditions should raise suspicion for the diagnosis.

SUGGESTED READINGS

Lin AC, Lin CM, Wang TL, et al. Rhabdomyolysis in 119 students after repetitive exercise. *Br J Sports Med.* 2005;39(1):e3.

Mannix R, Tan ML, Wright R, et al. Acute pediatric rhabdomyolysis: causes and rates of renal failure. *Pediatrics.* 2006;118(5):2119–2125.

Melli G, Chaudhry V, Cornblath DR. Rhabdomyolysis: an evaluation of 475 hospitalized patients. *Medicine (Baltimore).* 2005;84(6):377–385.

230

REMEMBER THAT JOINT OR LIMB PAIN, PARTICULARLY IN THE LOWER EXTREMITIES, MAY BE REFERRED PAIN FROM ANOTHER LOCATION

MICHAEL CLEMMENS, MD

WHAT TO DO – INTERPRET THE DATA

Perform a thorough physical exam and consider radiographs of both the area in question, as well as those areas proximal and distal.

Lower extremity pain may be a sign of significant pathology in children. In toddlers, it often presents as a limp or refusal to bear weight. Infants may present with discomfort during diaper changes or refusal to move one extremity. Localizing the pathology may be difficult because young children are often unable to communicate the site of pain. Also, disease in one area may present as referred pain to another area. This happens most commonly with the hip, which may present as referred pain to the thigh or knee. However, limp and referred pain may also be secondary to spinal pathology or gastrointestinal disease, such as appendicitis. The clinician may be misled if the entire lower extremity and the adjacent body parts are not evaluated.

The differential diagnosis of lower extremity pain, or limp, is broad and depends on the age of the child. *Table 230.1* lists some of the common etiologies of lower extremity pain for different age groups. A selection of diagnoses that require urgent recognition, evaluation, and treatment will be reviewed here. A more expanded differential diagnosis can be found in the references provided or in separate chapters on developmental dysplasia of the hip and fracture patterns in nonaccidental trauma. Generally, specific causes of limp fall into one of three categories: pain, weakness, or structural abnormality. A thorough history, a meticulous exam, and the judicious use of lab studies and x-rays will usually lead to the correct diagnosis.

Legg-Calvé-Perthes disease (LCPD) and slipped capital femoral epiphysis are diseases of the hip, that if diagnosed early lead to improved outcomes. LCPD is a syndrome of avascular necrosis of the femoral head. Pain in LCPD is generally not severe and may be referred to the anteromedial thigh or knee. Some cases present with limp only. On exam, range of motion may be limited. Slipped capital femoral epiphysis occurs from acute or repetitive trauma to a presumably abnormal femoral growth plate. It occurs most commonly in the early teenage years, just prior to the adolescent growth spurt, and it is

TABLE 230.1	COMMON CAUSES OF LOWER EXTREMITY PAIN BY AGE GROUP
AGE	**CAUSES**
Birth to 2 years	Septic arthritis
	Osteomyelitis
	Developmental dysplasia of the hip
	Nonaccidental trauma
2 to 10 years	Septic arthritis
	Osteomyelitis
	Legg-Calvé-Perthes disease
	Juvenile rheumatoid arthritis
	Transient synovitis of the hip
	Leukemia
	Fractures
10 to 18 years	Fractures
	Slipped capital femoral epiphysis
	Transient synovitis of the hip
	Tumors
	Osteomyelitis

associated with obesity. Along with external rotation of the affected limb, the presenting complaint is often limp with pain in the hip, thigh, or knee.

The early diagnosis and treatment of septic arthritis, a bacterial infection of the joint, is also critical to prevent morbidity from joint destruction. Although it can occur in any joint, it commonly affects the hip and knee. Fever is usually present, and the exam is most significant for severe pain upon passive range of motion of the joint. Serum inflammatory markers are elevated, and bacteria may be present in the synovial fluid of the affects joint or in the bloodstream. The most common mimicker of septic arthritis is transient synovitis of the hip, a self-limited, temporary inflammatory process of unclear etiology. Children with transient synovitis are not systemically ill and usually have normal laboratory values.

Childhood accidental spiral tibial (CAST) fractures, formerly called toddler's fractures, result from minor trauma such as twisting the ankle, tripping, or jumping from a low height. CAST fractures present with leg or foot pain, limp, or refusal to bear weight in children younger than 7 years. Swelling and deformity are often absent. The diagnosis is made by eliciting point tenderness over the fracture site, which is usually the lower third of the tibia. Pain may also be elicited by gently twisting the foot and the upper foreleg in opposite directions. CAST fractures are best seen radiographically with an anterior oblique view. In many instances, however, the x-ray will be normal and the diagnosis made on clinical grounds alone.

Acute lymphoblastic leukemia is the most common childhood malignancy and frequently presents with long bone pain or limp. The diagnosis of acute lymphoblastic leukemia should be entertained in any child with lower extremity pain at night or persistent leg pain. A thorough history, physical examination, peripheral blood smear, and plain x-rays may lead to the diagnosis. Malignant tumors of the bone that arise in the distal femur or proximal tibia may also present with knee pain.

SUGGESTED READINGS

Fischer SU, Beattie TF. The limping child: epidemiology, assessment and outcome. *J Bone Joint Surg Br.* 1999;81:1029–1034.

Frick SL. Evaluation of the child who has hip pain. *Orthop Clin North Am.* 2006;37:133–140.

Mellick LB, Milker L, Egsieker E. Childhood accidental spiral tibial (CAST) fractures. *Pediatr Emerg Care.* 1999;15:307–309.

Singer JI. The cause of gait disturbance in 425 pediatric patients. *Pediatr Emerg Care.* 1985;1: 7–10.

231

DO NOT MISS THE DIAGNOSIS OF NONACCIDENTAL TRAUMA IN CHILDREN WITH SKELETAL TRAUMA

MICHAEL CLEMMENS, MD

WHAT TO DO – INTERPRET THE DATA

Know the common patterns or features of fractures associated with inflicted injury. Child abuse is a common cause of skeletal fractures in young children, especially in those younger than 2 years. Children who are not independent walkers rarely have accidental fractures of their long bones. When such fractures do occur in this age group, there is usually a clear-cut history of a fall or other plausible injury. Any fracture in a nonambulatory child should raise the clinician's index of suspicion for abuse.

Several factors in the clinical history should alert the clinician to the possibility of nonaccidental trauma. Unexplained or unwitnessed injuries leading to fractures, especially in small children, are suspect for abuse. When the reported mechanism of injury is inconsistent with the child's developmental stage or with the injuries noted on exam or x-ray, the likelihood of inflicted injury is significantly higher. Also of concern is a changing or implausible history, a history that suggests the child was injured by a sibling or another caregiver, or contradictory histories obtained from separate caregivers.

Many nonaccidental fractures are solitary. However, some children will have a history of repeated injuries, with visits to a variety of health care providers in search of treatment. Multiple fractures, especially those in various stages of healing, or fractures associated with other injuries, such as burns or bruises, should make the examiner suspicious of child abuse.

The classic metaphyseal lesion occurs as a result of a shearing injury and represents a series of microfractures across the metaphysis. A classic metaphyseal lesion, also called the corner or bucket handle fracture based on its radiographic appearance, is pathognomonic for inflicted injury. Furthermore, in the absence of a history of trauma, rib fractures in young children are highly suspicious for inflicted injury. These fractures are often sustained along the posterior and lateral aspects of the ribs, and result from the compression forces exerted while being tightly held around the thorax. Finally, scapular fractures or fractures of different ages are highly correlated with inflicted injury.

© 2008 by Lippincott Williams & Wilkins, a Wolters Kluwer business

Several other fractures can be seen in abuse but are not as specific as those mentioned above. These include skull fractures, especially if they are complex or associated with an implausible history and spinous process or spinal compression fractures. Epiphyseal separations and phalangeal, metacarpal, and metatarsal fractures are also associated with inflicted injury.

The most common site for an inflicted fracture is the mid-shaft of a long bone. A broken humerus or femur in a nonambulatory child is suggestive of inflicted injury. Forearm and foreleg fractures are also frequently seen in abuse, but in ambulatory children these injuries may also be accidental. Clavicle fractures and linear skull fractures commonly occur as a result of abuse but can happen in a variety of other settings as well.

In cases of nonaccidental trauma diagnostic imaging begins with plain radiographs. Anteroposterior and lateral radiographs of the affected body part should be obtained in all instances of reported or suspected injury. A complete skeletal survey is indicated in children younger than 2 years when child abuse is suspected. In some cases, skeletal surveys may be helpful in older children. The skeletal survey consists of an anteroposterior view of all bones, lateral views of the spine and skull, and bilateral posterior oblique views of the ribs. Cone down views of suspicious or involved areas should also be performed. When additional information is needed about the presenting or associated injuries, secondary modalities include bone scan, computed tomography scan, or magnetic resonance imaging scan.

The diagnosis of child abuse is not always obvious. The physician or other health care provider must maintain a high level of alertness for the potential of inflicted injury. A thorough history and physical exam and judicious use of imaging studies can lead to the recognition of nonaccidental trauma. The provider is responsible for reporting not only straightforward cases of abuse to the proper authorities, but also cases of *suspected* abuse. This allows for a thorough investigation by a multidisciplinary team of professionals and assists the provider in making a more informed diagnosis.

SUGGESTED READINGS

Diagnostic imaging in child abuse. *Pediatrics.* 2000;105:1345–1348.
Loder RT, Bookout C. Fracture patterns in battered children. *J Orthop Trauma.* 1991;5:428–433.
Vandeven AM, Newton AW. Update on child physical abuse, sexual abuse and prevention. *Curr Opin Pediatr.* 2006;18:201–205.

232

PERFORM A THOROUGH HIP EXAMINATION ON INFANTS AND CHILDREN AT EVERY WELL VISIT UNTIL THEY ARE WELL-ESTABLISHED WALKERS

MICHAEL CLEMMENS, MD

WHAT TO DO – GATHER APPROPRIATE DATA

Developmental dysplasia of the hip (DDH) refers to an abnormal anatomic relationship between the head of the femur and the acetabulum. Without the usual ball-in-socket configuration, the joint will not develop normally, resulting in lifelong morbidity. The hip may be dislocated at birth or merely dislocatable, with dislocation occurring in the first months of life. DDH may present at any time during childhood, but is most commonly diagnosed at birth or in infancy. Early recognition leads to more rapid and less invasive treatment. Young infants usually can be treated without surgery, whereas most children diagnosed after the age of 2 require open surgical reduction.

Risk factors for DDH include female sex, breech presentation, and a positive family history. Girls who are breech are at particularly high risk. The presence of torticollis, metatarsus adductus, or an underlying neuromuscular disorder also increases the risk for DDH. Parents of older children may report a limp, a waddling gait, or a leg length discrepancy.

DDH is primarily diagnosed by the physical exam. The Ortolani and Barlow maneuvers detect most but not all DDH in the newborn period and during the first 4 months of life. The examiner must take care to examine the infant while she or he is calm, and to examine one hip at a time. A palpable clunk with either maneuver indicates a positive test. Ligamentous clicks generally do not indicate pathology. Asymmetry of femur length or skin folds also suggests the diagnosis. Limited abduction of the hip is a cardinal sign of DDH after 3 months of age. It is imperative that the clinician carefully perform and document the hip examination at each well visit because hip dysplasia may develop after a normal newborn exam. Ultrasound is the imaging study of choice in children younger than 4 months because it can determine mobility of the hip and the anatomy. After that age, plain radiographs are useful because the femoral heads are beginning to ossify.

When DDH is suspected, the child should be immediately referred to an orthopedic surgeon skilled in the diagnosis and treatment of this condition. Treatment is age-dependent. The Pavlik harness is used in early infancy to

© 2008 by Lippincott Williams & Wilkins, a Wolters Kluwer business

maintain flexion and abduction. Triple diapering is not an effective treatment for DDH. Older infants and young toddlers most often undergo closed reduction. The diagnosis after approximately 18 months of age commonly requires open reduction and fixation.

Pitfalls to be avoided in evaluating children for DDH include failure to consider risk factors, failure to evaluate the hips at every well visit in the first 2 years of life, and performing an inadequate or incorrect hip exam. In questionable cases, the clinician should not hesitate to seek a second opinion from a more experienced pediatrician or an orthopedic surgeon. Plain radiographs are not helpful in children under the age of 4 months. When the diagnosis is clear, there should not be a delay in making the appropriate referral.

SUGGESTED READINGS

Clinical practice guideline: early detection of developmental dysplasia of the hip. Committee on Quality Improvement, Subcommittee on Developmental Dysplasia of the Hip. American Academy of Pediatrics. *Pediatrics.* 2000;105(4 Pt 1):896–905.

Harcke HT. Developmental dysplasia of the hip: a spectrum of abnormality. *Pediatrics.* 1999; 103:152.

Novacheck TF. Developmental dysplasia of the hip. *Pediatr Clin North Am.* 1996;43:829–848.

233

KNOW HOW TO RECOGNIZE AND MANAGE SCOLIOSIS BECAUSE AN EARLY DIAGNOSIS AND TREATMENT ARE ESPECIALLY IMPORTANT TO PREVENT SERIOUS CONSEQUENCES

ELIZABETH WELLS, MD

WHAT TO DO – INTERPRET THE DATA, MAKE A DECISION

WHEN TO SCREEN

Scoliosis may be congenital, neuromuscular, degenerative, or idiopathic. The spine should be examined in all pediatric patients as part of routine newborn and annual exams. Idiopathic scoliosis is seen in otherwise healthy, rapidly growing preadolescent and adolescent children (typically grades 5–9). Females require treatment five to eight times more frequently than males. It is important to ask about scoliosis when obtaining a family history, as there is a 20 times more frequent occurrence of scoliosis in patients with an immediate family member affected.

HOW TO SCREEN

During the examination, the child's back should be fully exposed. The pediatrician should instruct older children to stand up straight with feet together, shoulders back, and hands hanging at their sides, head up and looking straight ahead. Signs of scoliosis include asymmetry of shoulder height, scapulae, or flanks (sometimes seen as a bony prominence) or misalignment of spinous processes. After inspecting the back in an upright position, the examiner should ask the child to bend forward at the waist (with feet and palms together) and check again for asymmetry. This forward-bending test to check for thoracic asymmetry is the single most important screening technique.

TREATMENT

The American Academy of Pediatrics recommends that infants, children, and adolescents with severe scoliosis be referred to a pediatric orthopedic surgeon. The orthopedist will conduct a standing anteroposterior roentgenogram of the spine to confirm the diagnosis. Treatment recommendations will depend on the degree, flexibility, and location of the curve. Current guidelines are to follow closely every 3 to 6 months with spinal radiographs and photographs for <15- to 20-degree curvature; to use a

© 2008 by Lippincott Williams & Wilkins, a Wolters Kluwer business

Milwaukee brace for between 20 and 40 degrees; bracing or surgery between 40 and 50 degrees; and spinal fusion for >50 degrees.

CONSEQUENCES OF MISSING SCOLIOSIS

As severe scoliosis (>50–60 degrees) requires treatment with surgical spinal fusion, pediatricians must recognize scoliosis at earlier stages in order to avoid major surgery. Nonsurgical treatment is preferred, because back surgery, in addition to the general risks associated with surgery and anesthesia, can be associated with problems, such as nerve and spinal cord damage. Left untreated, the lateral curve will continue to grow until skeletal maturity is reached, usually between ages 13 and 16 for girls and 14 and 17 years for boys. Without surgery, severe scoliosis may irreversibly limit vital capacity and impair cardiopulmonary function, leading to pulmonary hypertension and congestive heart failure.

DO NOT MISS OTHER CONDITIONS PRESENTING WITH SCOLIOSIS

Although most children with scoliosis are otherwise structurally normal, it is important not to miss a broader developmental problem of which lateral spinal curvature represents one feature. Infants with scoliosis should be evaluated, usually with radiographs, to determine whether it is due to in utero compression or malformation of vertebral bodies. A patient with malformed vertebral bodies should be carefully examined for other malformations. Older children with scoliosis should be evaluated to determine if the scoliosis is acquired or the result of a programming deficit. A child who is short, disproportionate, or has altered structures of long bones should receive a skeletal survey to rule out a skeletal dysplasia or metabolic bone disease. Skin should be thoroughly inspected to rule out a neurocutaneous syndrome, such as neurofibromatosis or incontinentia pigmentosa. If severe mental retardation is present in an adolescent boy with scoliosis, short stature, and coarse facies, Coffin-Lowry syndrome should be considered. Primary neuromuscular disease may be the cause in older children with scoliosis, if the neurologic exam reveals weakness, altered deep tendon reflexes, poor coordination, or gait disturbances. Finally, connective tissue differences should be considered, and ophthalmic and cardiac evaluation should be pursued when other abnormalities in support structures (e.g., marfanoid body habitus, generalized joint laxity, subluxed eye lenses) are recognized.

All children should be examined for scoliosis. Classification of the scoliosis and evaluation for underlying causes will depend on the age at presentation and associated abnormalities. Pediatricians must give particular focus to the spine during the adolescent growth spurt to prevent the consequences of surgery or untreated disease.

SUGGESTED READINGS

Berwick DM. Scoliosis screening. *Pediatr Rev*. 1984;5(8):238–247.
Dunn BH, Hakala MW, McGee ME. Scoliosis screening. *Pediatrics*. 1978;61:794–797.
Jones MC. Clinical approach to the child with scoliosis. *Pediatr Rev*. 1985;6(7):219–222.
Surgical Advisory Panel. American Academy of Pediatrics. Guidelines for referral to pediatric surgical specialists. *Pediatrics*. 2002;110(1 Pt 1):187–191.

234

DO NOT OVERLOOK COMMON MUSCULOSKELETAL PROBLEMS THAT HAVE BAD CONSEQUENCES SUCH AS OVERUSE INJURIES, GROWTH PLATE FRACTURES, AND SCAPHOID FRACTURES

NAILAH COLEMAN, MD

WHAT TO DO – INTERPRET THE DATA

Athletic competition, be it Little League, Junior Varsity, Varsity, or collegiate sports, can often result in athletic injury. Some injuries are easy to recognize; however, there may be a few that are difficult to recognize and, if left untreated, can have potentially devastating consequences. Overuse injuries, scaphoid fractures, and growth plate fractures represent injuries that should be diagnosed and treated in a timely manner.

Overuse injuries, which include tendonitis, apophysitis, and stress fractures, can occur with excessive sports participation. While still growing and developing, young athletes can be particularly predisposed to injuries from repetitive use sports (e.g., running, pitching). These injuries can include traction apophysitis (e.g., Osgood-Schlatter disease, a tibial tubercle apophysitis), medial epicondylitis (e.g., Little League elbow, caused by the traction and compression forces from repetitive and forceful throwing on the medial and lateral parts of the elbow), injuries to developing joint surfaces (e.g., osteochondritis dissecans, collapse and deformity of part of the joint, also seen in Little League elbow), and injuries of the immature spine (e.g., spondylolysis, a defect in the pars interarticularis, caused by repetitive hyperextension of the spine, often seen in gymnasts). Early recognition of an overuse injury can help to avoid future chronic joint disease and disability. Depending on when they are diagnosed, the management of overuse injuries ranges from rest and bracing to surgical correction.

The scaphoid bone, also called the carpal navicular bone, is a frequent site of fracture in adolescents and adults, and should be considered in someone who falls on an outstretched hand and has pain over the anatomic snuffbox. An untreated fracture through the waist of the scaphoid bone, due to its unique blood supply, could result in nonunion, wrist arthrosis, and avascular necrosis of the proximal fragment. Fortunately, most pediatric fractures of the scaphoid bone occur through the distal third of the bone. Once suspected, and even without radiographic confirmation, a scaphoid fracture should

ⓒ 2008 by Lippincott Williams & Wilkins, a Wolters Kluwer business

be treated with a thumb spica or cast. Once confirmed via scaphoid view radiographs (anteroposterior view of the wrist held at 30 degrees supination and ulnar deviation), a scaphoid fracture should be treated with 8 to 12 weeks of immobilization for waist fractures and with 6 to 8 weeks of immobilization for distal pole fractures. Due to the seriousness of the consequences of delayed treatment, an orthopedic consult is warranted for all suspected or confirmed scaphoid fractures.

Physeal injuries, also known as growth plate fractures, occur only in people with developing skeletal systems, in which the growth plate is still open and functioning. Physeal injuries have most notably been classified into five groups, known as Salter-Harris (SH) classification system of fractures.

- **SH I fractures** pass completely through the physis cartilage without disruption of the epiphysis and metaphysis. These injuries are diagnosed by the presence of pain over the physis without any radiographic signs of injury and usually heal well without an adverse affect on growth.
- **SH II fractures,** the most common physeal injury, pass through the physis and part of the metaphysis but do not involve the epiphysis. They also generally heal well.
- **SH III fractures** pass through the epiphysis and physis but do not involve the metaphysis. As these fractures involve the articulating joint surface, they require reduction to restore joint alignment and to reduce the likelihood of growth disruption on that side of the joint.
- **SH IV fractures** cut through the epiphysis and cross the physis to cut through the metaphysis. They also require reduction to restore joint alignment and to reduce the likelihood of growth disruption or growth deformity in that area.
- **SH V fractures,** also known as crush injuries and often mistaken as SH I fractures, have a high incidence of growth disruption. The early recognition and treatment of these injuries can help avoid potentially long-term morbidity.

SUGGESTED READINGS

Agvepong M. Index of Suspicion, Case 3. Kawasaki disease. *Pediatr Rev.* 1999;20:199, 202–203.

Cantu S Jr, Connors GP. Index of suspicion. Case 2. Fracture of the scaphoid bone. *Pediatr Rev.* 1999;20(6):199, 201–202.

Children Committee on Sports Medicine and Fitness. American Academy of Pediatrics: risk of injury from baseball and softball in children. *Pediatrics.* 2001;107:782–784.

DeWolfe C. Back pain. *Pediatr Rev.* 2002;23:221.

Ganley TJ, Gaugles RL, Moroz LA. Consultation with the specialist: patellofemoral conditions in childhood. *Pediatr Rev.* 2006;27:264–269; quiz 270.

Intensive training and sports specialization in young athletes. American Academy of Pediatrics. Committee on Sports Medicine and Fitness. *Pediatrics.* 2000;106(1 Pt 1):154–157.

Metzl JD. Preparticipation examination of the adolescent athlete: part 1. *Pediatr Rev.* 2001;22: 199–204.

235

REMEMBER THAT COMMON SKIN LESIONS MAY BE PASSED FROM FAMILY MEMBER TO FAMILY MEMBER

JOHANN PETERSON, MD

WHAT TO DO – GATHER APPROPRIATE DATA

Tinea capitis is a fungal infection of the hair follicles of the scalp and is more common in prepubertal children than in adolescents or adults. It is typically caused by fungal species of the genera *Trichophyton* and *Microsporum*. Infection can be passed between members of a family, especially on fomites such as hairbrushes and pillows, and some species can be acquired from household pets. Clinically, tinea capitis takes both inflammatory and noninflammatory forms. The noninflammatory form consists of patches of localized scaly alopecia, which are often itchy, with an annular appearance. Ringworm may also be present on the body. The inflammatory form manifests as scattered pustules, abscesses, or a kerion (a boggy, inflamed swelling of the scalp, often painful or pruritic). Lymphadenopathy, especially occipital, is common. Tinea capitis is sometimes accompanied by an id (dermatophytid) reaction, especially after trauma to the affected skin or after the initiation of treatment. An id reaction is a systemic immune-mediated response to a localized dermatitis, and presents as a symmetric, pruritic, fine papulovesicular rash, although it can sometimes mimic a drug eruption. Fungal studies of the id lesions will be negative, and the rash resolves with effective treatment of the primary infection.

Diagnosis of tinea capitis can be made clinically in obvious cases, by fungal culture of hair or scrapings, or by identification of fungal elements on light microscopy of a potassium hydroxide preparation. Some dermatophytes fluoresce under Wood's light, but this depends on the species and is unreliable. Treatment consists of systemic antifungals for an extended period, until signs of infection have resolved or culture is negative. Griseofulvin is the agent of choice and is typically prescribed for a minimum of 8 weeks. Other choices include fluconazole or terbinafine. Other family members should be

ⓒ 2008 by Lippincott Williams & Wilkins, a Wolters Kluwer business

examined and treated if necessary. Some recommend that infected patients use a topical treatment (e.g., selenium sulfide shampoo every other day for 1 to 2 weeks) initially to reduce the risk of spreading the infection.

Some patients with inflamed tinea can appear to have cellulitis. Their lesions are sometimes treated as such, with incision and drainage plus intravenous antibiotics. A fluctuant, inflamed lesion on the scalp without fever should make you doubt the diagnosis of cellulitis. Also look for tinea elsewhere on the patient and his or her family. If your patient is not ill–appearing, consider diagnostic studies before you treat.

SUGGESTED READINGS

Elewski BE. Clinical diagnosis of common scalp disorders. *J Investig Dermatol Symp Proc.* 2005;10(3):190–193.

Elewski BE. Tinea capitis: a current perspective. *J Am Acad Dermatol.* 2000;42(1 Pt 1):1–20.

Martin ES, Elewski BE. Tinea capitis in adult women masquerading as bacterial pyoderma. *J Am Acad Dermatol.* 2003;49(2 Suppl):S177–S179.

236

RASHES ARE NOT ALL BENIGN. BE ALERT FOR RASHES THAT MAY BE SIGNALING A SYSTEMIC CONDITION

LAURA HUFFORD, MD

WHAT TO DO – INTERPRET THE DATA

Specific types of rashes provide important clues to many systemic illnesses in pediatrics. One must become expert at inspecting, describing, and identifying rashes so appropriate treatment can be initiated. Some rashes can be suggestive of cancer; immunologic disorders; systemic infection; or even impending cardiovascular collapse and signal the need for rapid, intensive management to avoid significant morbidity and mortality.

Mottling of the skin is described as a lacy, reticular rash. Mottling is seen in many conditions including shock, however if the child is otherwise well-appearing, shock is unlikely to be the cause. Infants tend to develop mottling when they are cold or when they have been exposed for a long period of time. This is often seen when an infant has been undressed and waiting in an exam room for an extended period of time for the doctor. However, mottling of the skin should raise concern for shock if it is coupled with other physical exam signs such as lethargy, tachycardia, and hypotension. For example, mottling can be a sign of decreased perfusion as in the case of coarctation of the aorta, with accompanying unilateral cutaneous mottling of the arm.

Other rashes can be signs of serious underlying illnesses. Petechiae are small red, macular, nonblanching lesions. These are frequently seen in viral illnesses and streptococcal infections. However, petechiae, especially when coupled with fever, may be a sign of bacterial infection and disseminated intravascular coagulation. Thus, a clinician must raise suspicion for serious infection when petechiae are present.

Purpura are raised violaceous, nonblanchable lesions that are always a sign of underlying disease. Generalized vasculitides, such as Henoch-Schönlein purpura, and diseases involving thrombocytopenia, such as idiopathic thrombocytopenia purpura, can present with petechiae and purpura. However, patients with fever and petechiae or purpura may have an invasive infection, requiring immediate attention.

Neisseria meningitides is a gram-negative diplococcus that is spread by respiratory droplets and can cause meningitis and meningococcemia. Patients with fulminant meningococcemia initially have weakness, fever, and

ⓒ 2008 by Lippincott Williams & Wilkins, a Wolters Kluwer business

malaise but rapidly develop shock, disseminated intravascular coagulopathy, and multiorgan system failure. Purpura develops when fibrin clots occur in small vessels and produce hemorrhage and necrosis of the skin. Thus in any patient with fever and purpura meningococcal infection must be considered and antibiotic therapy initiated.

Rocky Mountain spotted fever should also be considered in a patient with fever and purpura. The disease, caused by *Rickettsiae rickettsii*, is transmitted by ticks primarily in the southeastern area of the United States. Rash initially presents on the ankles and wrists and then spreads throughout the rest of the body. In Rocky Mountain spotted fever, the rickettsiae flourish within the endothelial cytoplasm, and produce a vasculitis of the venules and capillaries within the skin, producing petechiae and purpura. Vasculitis also commonly involves other internal organs. Rapid recognition and treatment with doxycycline is imperative to prevent poor outcomes.

SUGGESTED READING

Pearson IC, Holden CA. Delayed presentation of persistent unilateral cutaneous mottling of the arm following coarctation of the aorta. *Br J Dermatol.* 2003;148(5):1066–1068.

237

PETECHIAE ARE COMMON IN BENIGN VIRAL ILLNESSES BUT CAN BE A SIGN OF MORE SERIOUS CONDITIONS, SUCH AS MENINGOCOCCEMIA AND THROMBOCYTOPENIA

JOHANN PETERSON, MD

WHAT TO DO – INTERPRET THE DATA

Petechiae are nonblanching, usually red, macules <1 mm in diameter. They are a form of purpura, which as a general term refers to rashes caused by the extravasation of red blood cells into the skin. Other purpuric lesions are ecchymoses (nonblanching macules >1 cm), and purpura (macules from 1 mm to 1 cm in diameter). Thus, the term *purpura* (somewhat confusingly) can be used either to refer to all of these purpuric rashes as a group, or specifically to mean purpura per se. Purpura fulminans refers to large, confluent "lakes" of ecchymoses, which become necrotic. Broadly, purpuric rashes are caused by disorders of coagulation, platelet disorders, or disorders affecting the walls of blood vessels. Thus, the process leading to purpura may be thrombocytopenia (immune-mediated, infectious, malignant, Kasabach-Merritt syndrome) or platelet dysfunction, coagulopathy (inherited [e.g., protein C or S deficiency or other factor deficiency] or acquired [e.g., hemorrhagic disease of the newborn, disseminated intravascular coagulation]), vasculitis, or connective tissue disease (scurvy, Ehlers-Danlos). Petechiae are most often the result of platelet dysfunction or thrombocytopenia. The differential diagnosis of purpura is enormous and includes everyone's favorite suspect, meningococcemia, as well as many other infections, noninfectious acquired diseases, congenital disorders, and trauma.

In neonates, a common cause of petechia is immune-mediated thrombocytopenia, due either to maternal alloimmunization against fetal platelets or to transplacental passage of maternal autoantibodies (e.g., idiopathic thrombocytopenic purpura, lupus, or drug reactions). Kasabach-Merritt syndrome refers to thrombocytopenia from the sequestration or coagulative consumption of platelets within a hemangioma or similar vascular anomaly. Other causes of thrombocytopenia in infants are congenital disorders of platelet number (Wiskott-Aldrich, Fanconi, thrombocytopenia-absent radii syndromes) or function (Bernard-Soulier, Glanzmann thrombasthenia), and heparin-induced thrombocytopenia. Infectious possibilities

© 2008 by Lippincott Williams & Wilkins, a Wolters Kluwer business

include TORCH (*t*oxoplasmosis, *o*ther infections, *r*ubella, *c*ytomegalovirus, *h*erpes simplex virus) infections, human immunodeficiency virus, parvovirus B19, and bacterial sepsis.

For children, the most worrisome (but uncommon) cause of petechia and fever is bacteremia, and most children with these signs typically undergo sepsis "rule-out," including culture of at least blood and urine plus empiric antibiotics for 48 hours. However, in several published series, other causes are far more common, including presumed viral urinary tract infection, Group A streptococcal pharyngitis, respiratory syncytial virus, and otitis media. In these series, only 8% to 20% of children with fever and petechiae had documented invasive bacterial disease. *Neisseria meningitidis* was the most common organism causing bacteremia among children with fever and petechiae, but *Streptococcus pneumoniae*, group-B *Streptococcus, Haemophilus influenzae, Staphylococcus aureus,* and *Escherichia coli* were also identified in blood cultures. Other ostensible causes were urinary tract infections, aseptic meningitis; Henoch-Schönlein purpura; acute leukemia Rocky Mountain spotted fever; idiopathic thrombocytopenic purpura; roseola; *Mycoplasma pneumonia;* rotavirus; and reaction to the measles, mumps, rubella (MMR) vaccine.

In some of these series, several criteria were found to completely exclude serious bacterial infection: well-appearance (although this was variably defined), absence of petechiae below the nipples, and a normal C-reactive protein. However, there does not seem to be consensus regarding safe criteria, which, in the presence of fever and petechiae, will identify seriously ill children with acceptable sensitivity. The list of possible infections in a child with fever and a purpuric rash is long, and in fact it is common for no agent to be identified.

A number of features may provide clues to the diagnosis. Meningococcemia is classically associated with generalized petechiae that are often stellate, and that progress rapidly, eventually into ecchymoses and necrosis. A petechial rash is a common presenting symptom, but some children will have a nonspecific maculopapular rash, or none at all. The rash of Rocky Mountain spotted fever begins with petechiae on the palms and soles and spreads centrally, and the child will typically appear quite ill. Epidemic typhus causes petechiae or purpura beginning on the trunk. Both are caused by *Rickettsiae*, which directly invade endothelial cells. A number of viruses, especially parvovirus B19, have been associated with "papular purpuric gloves and socks syndrome," which consists of symmetric erythema and edema of the hands and feet, which is sharply demarcated and usually painful, or pruritic. An associated petechial body rash, fever, and oral erosions are common. Henoch-Schönlein purpura is an immunoglobulin (Ig)A-mediated vasculitis that is common in children and classically presents with a symmetric palpable purpuric rash on the legs and buttocks, but petechiae and/or ecchymoses may coexist or be the only rash. Other common features include fever, abdominal pain, arthralgias, and hematuria with or without proteinuria. Localized petechiae, or petechiae in an unusual distribution, may be due to minor trauma (e.g., from a blood pressure cuff) and should also alert to the possibility of child abuse. Vigorous coughing may cause petechiae in the distribution of the superior vena cava, including scleral hemorrhage.

SUGGESTED READINGS

Baker RC, Seguin JH, Leslie N, et al. Fever and petechiae in children. *Pediatrics.* 1989;84(6): 1051–1055.

Baselga E, Drolet BA, Esterly NB. Purpura in infants and children. *J Am Acad Dermatol.* 1997;37(5 Pt 1):673–705.

Brogan PA, Raffles A. The management of fever and petechiae: making sense of rash decisions. *Arch Dis Child.* 2000;83(6):506–507.

Mandl KD, Stack AM, Fleisher GR. Incidence of bacteremia in infants and children with fever and petechiae. *J Pediatr.* 1997;131(3):398–404.

Van Nguyen Q, Nguyen EA, Weiner LB. Incidence of invasive bacterial disease in children with fever and petechiae. *Pediatrics.* 1984;74(1):77–80.

238

SEARCH FOR A GENETIC DISORDER IN PATIENTS WITH MULTIPLE CAFÉ AU LAIT (CAL) SPOTS

DOROTHY CHEN, MD

WHAT TO DO – GATHER APPROPRIATE DATA, MAKE A DECISION

Dermatological findings are often a concern of parents. CAL spots are uniformly hyperpigmented discrete round or oval skin lesions. They are brown in color, with both smooth and irregular borders. The lesions are small in a newborn, increasing in size during childhood, and then become less prominent in adulthood. Histologically, CAL spots have increased melanocytes and melanin in the epidermis.

Children commonly have solitary spots. In the general population, the number and frequency of CAL spots depends on ethnicity and age. In children younger than 10 years of age, the frequency of ≥ 1 CAL spot has been reported as 13% in white children versus 27% in African American children. When multiple lesions are noted on physical exam, they should raise concern for underlying genetic disorders. Although an evaluation of the child is ongoing, the presence of multiple CAL spots should also prompt investigations of family members.

Neurofibromatosis type 1 (NF1) (Von Recklinghausen disease) is an autosomal dominant disorder (NF1 gene on chromosome 17) and is the genetic disorder most commonly associated with CAL spots. In the general population, NF1 occurs in approximately 1 in 3,500. The CAL spots in NF1 are usually oval-shaped, uniform in color, 1 to 3 cm in diameter, with well-defined borders. The diagnostic criteria for NF1 require two or more physical findings listed in *Table 238.1*.

In infants, the presence of axillary or groin freckling with CAL spots is diagnostic of NF-1. By age 10, approximately 80% of children with NF1 have axillary/groin freckling. In addition to the impact of the physical findings listed in the diagnostic criteria, it is necessary to identify NF1 to address its comorbidities. The frequency of learning disabilities ranges from 30% to 60% of patients. Patients with NF1 have also been noted to have short stature, macrocephaly, renal artery stenosis, and hypertension.

CAL spots have also been reported in other genetic disorders, so these should be considered as well. The NF type 2 (NF2) gene is found on

© 2008 by Lippincott Williams & Wilkins, a Wolters Kluwer business

TABLE 238.1	**DIAGNOSTIC CRITERIA FOR NEUROFIBROMATOSIS (NF)-1**

Two or more of the following:
1. Six or more Café au lait spots
   a. ≥1.5 cm in postpubertal persons
   b. ≥0.5 cm in prepubertal persons
2. Two or more neurofibromas of any type or one or more plexiform neurofibromas
3. Freckling in the axillary or inguinal region
4. Optic glioma
5. Two or more Lisch nodules
6. Distinctive osseous lesion
   a. Dysplasia of the sphenoid bone
   b. Dysplasia or thinning of long bone cortex
7. First-degree relative with NF-1, based on the preceding criteria

chromosome 22 and is less common than NF-1. CAL spots can be present in this disease but are not required for diagnosis. Similarly, CAL spots have been found on patients with tuberous sclerosis, but hypopigmented macules are the more commonly noted skin finding.

McCune-Albright syndrome is a sporadic genetic disease and CAL spots are a typical skin finding. However, the spots usually have more irregular borders and occur over the upper spine, sacrum, and buttocks. McCune-Albright also has very different clinical manifestations from NF1. The mutation in McCune Albright results in an overproduction of cyclic adenosine monophosphate, and thus an increase in the growth and function of the osteoblasts, melanocytes, gonads and adrenal cortex.

CAL spots have also been reported in Fanconi anemia, Bloom syndrome, ataxia telangiectasia, and Russell-Silver syndrome. However, CAL spots are not diagnostic for these disorders. The presence of multiple CAL spots should prompt an evaluation for an underlying genetic disorder, particularly NF1.

SUGGESTED READINGS

Darmstadt GL, Sidbury R. The skin. In: Behrman RE, Kliegman RM, Jenson HB, eds. *Nelson Textbook of Pediatrics.* 17th ed. Philadelphia: Saunders; 2004:2153–2250.
Halsam RH. Neurocutaneous syndromes. In: Behrman RE, Kliegman RM, Jenson HB, eds. *Nelson Textbook of Pediatrics.* 17th ed. Philadelphia: Saunders; 2004:2015–2019.
Tekin M, Bodurtha JN, Riccardi VM. Café au lait spots: the pediatrician's perspective. *Pediatr Rev.* 2001;22(3):82–89.

239

DO NOT GIVE TOPICAL STEROIDS FOR A TINEA INFECTION, IT WILL WORSEN THE INFECTION

WILLIAM GIASI, JR., MD

WHAT TO DO – MAKE A DECISION

The dermatophytes, or ringworm fungi, include a group of fungi that have the ability to infect and survive only on dead keratin, the top layer, of skin, hair, and nails. The dermatophytes are ubiquitous in the environment and tinea infections are among the most common dermatologic disorders in the world. Dermatophytes are classified into three genera: *Microsporum, Trichophyton,* and *Epidermophyton.* The prevalent species of dermatophytes change with time and geographic location. The organisms may invade both the stratum corneum and the terminal hair shaft. Transfer of the organism may occur through the shedding of scales, autoinoculation, or transfer of spores. *Microsporum canis* is a frequent cause of tinea infections in children and is transferred from affected cats, dogs, horses, or cattle. Clinically, infections caused by dermatophytes are classified by the affected body region.

The history and physical exam will often establish the diagnosis of a dermatophyte infection. The use of laboratory resources, such as direct visualization of branching hyphae under a microscope, culture, or Wood's light examination, increases diagnostic accuracy.

In many cases of tinea infections, topical antifungal treatment is efficacious. Oral antifungal therapy is needed to efficaciously treat tinea capitis and tinea barbae when large portions of the body are involved or if the patient is immunocompromised. Combination antifungal and corticosteroid preparations are widely used by physicians for the treatment of superficial tinea infections. These preparations include an antifungal agent in combination with a mid- to high-potency steroid. The proposed mechanism of these agents is to treat the symptoms in addition to the dermatophyte infection. Physicians are often unaware of the potency of the steroid component of these preparations and, thus, their potential for local and systemic complications. Furthermore, the use of topical steroids for tinea infections may prolong the course of treatment.

Topical corticosteroid therapy suppresses inflammation and gives the patient and physician the false impression that the lesion is improving, whereas the fungal infection continues to flourish in the face of an altered

© 2008 by Lippincott Williams & Wilkins, a Wolters Kluwer business

immunologic defense. Following cessation of steroid treatment, the rash will return and may be transformed into an unrecognizable skin eruption, referred to as tinea incognito. The lesion may be characterized by the absence of scaling or a well defined border, diffuse erythema, scattered papules or pustules, and brown hyperpigmentation. Hyphae are easily demonstrated and can be seen a few days after discontinuing the use of a topical steroid.

SUGGESTED READINGS

Alston SJ, Cohen BA, Braun M. Persistent and recurrent tinea corporis in children treated with combination antifungal/corticosteroid agents. *Pediatrics.* 2003;111:201–203.

Drake LA, Dinehart SM, Farmer ER, et al. Guidelines of care for superficial mycotic infections of the skin: tinea capitis and tinea barbae. Guidelines/Outcomes Committee. American Academy of Dermatology. *J Am Acad Dermatol.* 116;34(2 Pt 1):290–294.

Stein DH. Tineas–superficial dermatophyte infections. *Pediatr Rev.*1998;19(11):368–372.

Weinstein A, Berman B. Topical treatment of common superficial tinea infections. *Am Fam Physician.* 2002;65(10):2095–2102.

240

WHEN A MISTAKE IS MADE, IT IS BEST TO DISCLOSE

LINDSEY ALBRECHT, MD

WHAT TO DO – MAKE A DECISION

Despite efforts by individual physicians and health care systems, medical errors inevitably occur. Errors may range from minor (as in the case of medication dosing errors with no adverse outcome) to severe (as in wrong-site surgery). Estimates of the frequency of such mistakes are high, with a significant proportion of errors resulting in increased hospital stay or producing measurable disability. It is estimated that up to 98,000 people die in the United States per year secondary to medical errors. Disclosure of mistakes is not routine; just 30% of respondents in one national survey who experienced an error in their care reported that they were informed of the error by the involved medical professional. Physicians cite fear of litigation, fear of losing their patient's trust, fear of having their reputation damaged, and desire to avoid the awkwardness of such a discussion among their reasons for withholding information about medical errors from their patients.

Errors in the field of pediatrics pose unique challenges, as caregivers and not the patients themselves are typically the ones involved in discussions with the health care provider. Attitudes of pediatricians with respect to mistake disclosure have recently been assessed. Although the vast majority of survey respondents supported reporting errors to patients' families, many identified factors that would deter them. Failure of the patient's family to understand what they were being told was the most frequently cited of these factors. Most pediatricians feel they would benefit from disclosure training, particularly those still in residency.

Patient attitudes with respect to disclosure of error differ markedly from physician attitudes. Patients define errors much more broadly than physicians do; examples of "medical error" cited by patients included poor service quality and physician rudeness. Physicians, in contrast, defined error solely as deviations from standard of care. Patients unanimously desired that

© 2008 by Lippincott Williams & Wilkins, a Wolters Kluwer business

all errors leading to harm be disclosed and would like to be told everything about the error. Many would additionally prefer to be told about events that nearly led to error, but did not actually result in a mistake. In contrast, physicians felt that all errors causing harm should be disclosed, except if the harm was trivial in nature, if the patient was unable to understand the error, or if the patient did not want to know about the error. Patients also desire compassionate disclosure and an apology from the physician.

In contrast to what many physicians assume, the likelihood of litigation has been shown to decrease when mistakes are fully disclosed; this decrease exists for all ranges of severity of medical mistakes. Additionally, patients are more likely to keep seeing their physician and less likely to report the physician to a supervising body if they are informed of a mistake. An apology in and of itself may actually decrease the likelihood of legal action being taken. Failure to disclose error leads to higher damage awards if litigation does occur and may, in some cases, be considered fraudulent behavior.

The best method for disclosing error to patients is unclear and depends to large extent on the details of the particular event. Although guidelines have been proposed and are implemented in many institutions, many questions remain. What is clear is that disclosure of error is strongly desired by patients, can be considered an ethical obligation, and is required by many hospital policies and some state laws. Honest disclosure results in higher patient satisfaction and decreased likelihood of litigation.

SUGGESTED READINGS

Blendon RJ, DesRoches CM, Brodie M, et al. Views of practicing physicians and the public on medical errors. *N Eng J Med.* 2002;347(24):1933–1940.

Gallagher TH, Waterman AD, Ebers AG, et al. Patients' and physicians' attitudes regarding the disclosure of medical errors. *JAMA.* 2003;289(8):1001–1007.

Garbutt J, Brownstein DR, Klein EJ, et al. Reporting and disclosing medical errors: pediatricians' attitudes and behaviors. *Arch Pediatr Adolesc Med.* 2007;161(2):179–185.

Kohn LT, Corrigan JM, Donaldson MS, eds. *To Err Is Human: Building a Safer Health System.* Washington, DC: Committee on Quality of Health Care in America, Institute of Medicine. National Academy Press; 2000.

Leape LL, Brennan TA, Laird N, et al. The nature of adverse events in hospitalized patients. Results of the Harvard Medical Practice Study II. *N Engl J Med.* 1991;324(6):377–384.

Witman AB, Park DM, Hardin SB. How do patients want physicians to handle mistakes? A survey of internal medicine patients in an academic setting. *Arch Int Med.* 1996;156(22):2565–2569.

241

ASSURE APPROPRIATE ASSENT AND CONSENT IN PEDIATRIC CLINICAL RESEARCH

SARIKA JOSHI, MD

WHAT TO DO – GATHER APPROPRIATE DATA, TAKE ACTION

The values of autonomy, beneficence, nonmaleficence, and justice guide bioethics and clinical research in the United States and around the world today. The Nuremberg code established the requirement of informed consent and limited research involving children, in order to protect this vulnerable population from exploitation; however, this ruling resulted in a lack of research targeting this special population. Federal guidelines in the United States now encourage the inclusion of children in clinical research so that this population can benefit from new studies and technology. The issue of consent in pediatric research aims to reconcile the competing ideas of informed consent and research application to all, requiring both informed consent from parents and assent from children.

Informed consent necessitates disclosure by the researcher, discussion between the researcher and potential subject, and a subject's full understanding of the proposed research. Once these requirements are fulfilled, a subject may then voluntarily wish to participate in the research protocol. By law, informed consent must be given by an autonomous individual who is younger than 18 years of age and makes independent decisions and is responsible for them. In pediatric research, parental consent permits the researcher to ask the child if he or she wants to participate in the protocol. The researcher must then ask for assent from the child. Assent should be obtained using developmentally appropriate tools.

There are both internal and external factors that affect a child's ability to give assent. Internal factors include age and developmental maturity. Younger children have more difficulty understanding research protocols. Individual Institutional Review Boards (IRBs) are responsible for determining age requirements for children's assent to participate in research. A specific child's developmental maturity must also be taken into account, because children advance through developmental stages at varying rates. External factors that affect a child's ability to give assent include the effects of role constraints, of family, and of the consent seeker on the child. Role constraints are created by social and institutional customs. In addition, both

© 2008 by Lippincott Williams & Wilkins, a Wolters Kluwer business

family and the consent seeker may directly affect a child's ability to give assent.

There are three levels of protection for children who participate in research. The first is the IRB. The second is the family, who must give informed consent. The third is the requirement for voluntary assent from the child. Some approaches to ensuring voluntary assent from a child include using a variety of developmentally appropriate media and obtaining consent in an environment that minimizes family influences. Pediatric research must strike a balance between protecting children from the burdens of research and allowing them to participate so that they may benefit from it.

SUGGESTED READINGS

Barfield RC, Church C. Informed consent in pediatric clinical trials. *Curr Opin Pediatr.* 2005; 17(1):20–24.

Meaux JB, Bell PL. Balancing recruitment and protection: children as research subjects. *Issues Compr Pediatr Nurs.* 2001;24(4):241–251.

242

DO NOT IGNORE A PARENT'S CONCERNS

NICKIE NIFORATOS, MD

WHAT TO DO – GATHER APPROPRIATE DATA

Parents are often well accommodated to their children and know the subtle signs of change, especially for children with chronic or complex conditions.

Psychosocial stressors and the personal perceptions of health and disease that lead patients to seek medical care are not unique to pediatrics. However, what is unique in pediatrics is that fear, anxiety, and stress come from the patients' parents or caregivers and not the patients themselves.

Personal and past experiences have an interesting and complex role in how, when, and why parents seek care. On one end of the spectrum are children who experienced serious illness in the recent or distant past. Though the child may have made a complete recovery, with no long-term sequelae, the stress of the initial illness has a long-term impact on the parents. This leads parents to be concerned about disease susceptibility. For example, a mother might bring her 8-month-old infant to a clinic with a chief complaint of "runny nose and congestion." The recent history might be benign, as the mother describes a happy, playful infant, who eats and voids well without fevers, cough, or respiratory distress. The physical exam also might be benign, without significant rhinorrhea or congestion. On further discussion with the mother, she might report that, several months earlier, her child was hospitalized with respiratory syncytial virus (RSV) bronchiolitis, and she had been concerned the infection would recur. Without the knowledge of the previous infection, the provider might offer reassurance that the child does not have a concerning condition. However, without eliciting the mother's underlying concerns, such as "Will the RSV infection recur?" or "Will my child be hospitalized again?," the clinician might not address the mother's fears.

The child with a complex medical history and multiple medical problems represents another important challenge. Many of these children have unique medical needs and a considerable variation in baseline developmental achievements and physical exam findings. In these situations, parents can be helpful to the clinician, who is unfamiliar with the patient. Parents can assist in identifying new and concerning signs and symptoms of disease. For example, the family could help with the delineation of symptoms in a 4-year-old girl with an inherited mitochondrial disorder, severe developmental delay, cerebral palsy, epilepsy, tracheomalacia, and chronic lung disease. If this

© 2008 by Lippincott Williams & Wilkins, a Wolters Kluwer business

patient does not respond to verbal commands but withdraws from painful stimuli, a determination needs to be made if this represents a significant change in mental status or her level of functioning.

Regardless of why a child is brought to the doctor's office, whether it is an acute illness or parental anxiety, it is important for the clinician to remember the parent is often the child's greatest advocate. Parents spend more time with their children than physicians do in a relatively brief office visit, and it is the parent who can alert physicians to subtle changes in behavior or clinical signs. Providing a comfortable, open environment that enables parents to speak freely and share their concerns, lead to improved patient care and satisfaction.

SUGGESTED READINGS

Levy JC. Vulnerable children: parent's perspectives and the use of medical care. *Pediatrics.* 1980;65(5):956–963.

Wasserman RC, Inui TS, Barriatua RD, et al. Pediatric clinician's support for parents makes a difference: an outcome-based analysis of clinician-parent interaction. *Pediatrics.* 1984;74(6): 1047–1053.

243

WORK UP THE POTENTIAL CAUSES OF MENTAL RETARDATION (MR) TO ASSIST FAMILIES IN IDENTIFYING POTENTIALLY MODIFIABLE CONDITIONS OR CONDITIONS THAT ARE GENETIC IN ORIGIN SO THAT THEY CAN RECEIVE APPROPRIATE COUNSELING FOR THEIR NEXT CHILD OR OTHER FAMILY RELATIVES

SONYA BURROUGHS, MD

WHAT TO DO – GATHER APPROPRIATE DATA

MR is common, affecting approximately 1% to 3% of the general population and defined as an intelligence quotient (IQ) of <70, coupled with limitations in adaptive abilities.

The differentiation between mild and severe MR is clinically important because this helps to determine which educational programs are most beneficial for patients.

MR results from genetic and environmental factors. Genetics provide the cognitive potential, which is molded by environmental factors. Fragile X syndrome (FXS), fetal alcohol syndrome (FAS), and Down's syndrome have been identified as the three most common identifiable causes of MR.

FXS is the leading cause of inherited MR. The prevalence of FXS is 1 in 4,000 males; 1:6,000 females. Approximately, 4% to 8% of the cases of MR in males are due to this syndrome. The primary mutation is an increase in the number of CGG trinucleotide repeats in the promoter region of the fragile X mental retardation gene (FMR1) on the X chromosome. Individuals with >230 CGG repeats have a "full mutation." Those with a modest increase in repeats (55–230) are considered to have a "premutation." Based on the mutation leading to this syndrome, it makes sense that the diagnosis of FXS is via molecular testing of the FMR1 gene to detect a CGG repeat expansion. Chromosome analysis to detect the fragile site of the X-chromosome is *no* longer used as a stand alone test because of its low sensitivity.

© 2008 by Lippincott Williams & Wilkins, a Wolters Kluwer business

FXS is inherited in an X-linked dominant fashion. Remember, pre-mutations may be carried by males. These males are usually phenotypically normal until late adulthood. The premutation is passed to all of their daughters, but none of their sons. Women with the premutation or full mutation have a 50% chance of passing the mutation to each offspring. Sons, who inherit the full mutation, develop FXS. Half of daughters who inherit a full mutation manifest mild-to-moderate symptoms, and the other half are asymptomatic carriers.

Physical features associated with FXS usually become apparent after puberty. Large ears and macro-orchidism are the two most commonly described physical features. Developmental delay (especially speech) and MR are the most common prepubertal findings.

FAS is the most common preventable cause of MR. IQ scores range from 20 to 120 in affected children. Those with normal IQ scores may have significant neurobehavioral deficits. Children with FAS have a higher likelihood of psychiatric and behavioral disorders than those with other identifiable causes of MR. Diagnosis of FAS is easier between ages 2 and 11 years when the physical features (short palpebral fissures, smooth philtrum, thin upper lip) are still present and central nervous system dysfunction emerges (memory deficits, slow information processing, hearing deficits, etc).

Down's syndrome is the most common genetic disorder causing mild-to-moderate MR. It is usually identified based on physical features, including hypotonia, flat facial profile, hyperflexibility of joints, poor Moro reflex, excess skin on back of neck, single palmar crease, and abnormal ears. Chromosome analysis confirms the diagnosis.

These three syndromes are the most common identifiable causes of MR, but other causes such as Prader-Willi, Angelman, Sotos, Autism, Rett, and cri-du-chat (5p-) exist and should be considered in the differential diagnosis when appropriate.

Identifying a cause of MR is extremely important because it relates to treatment, prognosis, and genetic counseling. The initial evaluation should focus on a detailed history and physical exam. This will help make some diagnoses more likely than others. Inquire about family members with learning disabilities, stillbirths, miscarriages, and consanguinity. Routine chromosome studies may be the next step in the evaluation, or high-resolution chromosome analysis may be needed for more subtle chromosomal abnormalities. Fluorescent in situ hybridization may be helpful when considering a particular syndrome. Newborn screening tests are also effective in identifying metabolic disorders associated with MR. Because most of these disorders are amenable to early treatment, newborn screening can also be seen as preventative.

SUGGESTED READINGS

Walker WO Jr, Johnson CP. Mental retardation: overview and diagnosis. *Pediatr Rev.* 2006; 27:204–212.

Weisner GL, Cassidy SB, Grimes SJ, et al. Clinical consult: developmental delay/fragile X syndrome. *Prim Care.* 2004;31:621–625.

244

CONSIDER THE DIAGNOSIS OF INBORN ERRORS OF METABOLISM IN AN INFANT OR CHILD WITH "SHOCK," ALTERED MENTAL STATUS, CYCLIC VOMITING, OR AN EXAGGERATED RESPONSE TO TYPICALLY ROUTINE INFECTIONS

JOHANN PETERSON, MD

WHAT TO DO – INTERPRET THE DATA

Infants have a typical response to stress and illness (e.g., lethargy, poor feeding, seizures, temperature derangements, or hypotonia), and these findings are nonspecific. Most acutely ill infants will be treated empirically for sepsis or other serious bacterial infections, and cultures of urine, blood, and possibly cerebrospinal fluid will be sent. The possibility of occult trauma (intracranial hemorrhage, blunt abdominal injury) is also a consideration. Inborn errors of metabolism also need to be considered because it is often said that, in some form, these disorders are "individually rare but collectively not so rare." Although it is beyond the scope of this chapter to consider even the most common of the hundreds of individual diseases or their diagnosis and management, there are general clues that may provide clues for screening for a metabolic defect.

Broadly, children who are "puzzles," that is, who do not respond as expected to specific therapy, who do not have a clear etiology for their presentation despite a thorough search, who become excessively ill in response to what should be a mild infection, who have repeated episodes (of shock, vomiting, altered mental status, seizures, etc.), or an inexorable deterioration (e.g., progressive encephalopathy or myopathy) deserve a workup for a metabolic abnormality. Other clues include dysmorphology, chronically ill siblings or parents, and siblings who have died or been miscarried. Children who have acidosis without poor perfusion may have a defect in cellular energy consumption or in the production of substrates, such as glucose or ketones, or may have a defect that results in the buildup of an amino acid or another organic acid.

Altered mental status or seizures may be due to poor perfusion, toxic ingestion, infection or other causes of inflammation, intracranial blood or a mass lesion, hypoglycemia or electrolyte abnormalities, or a focal lesion acting as a seizure focus or causing hydrocephalus. However, if the initial evaluation

ⓒ 2008 by Lippincott Williams & Wilkins, a Wolters Kluwer business

for these entities is negative, the consideration of metabolic encephalopathies such as hyperammonemia needs to be entertained. Saudubray and Charpentier (2007) provide a thorough approach to diagnostic testing.

The initial management of a child suspected of having a metabolic disorder should focus on clearing toxic metabolites and minimizing their production, and provide adequate calories to prevent catabolism. In children where a suspected protein metabolism disorder (amino acidopathy, organic acidopathy, urea cycle defects) is suspected, usually glucose (10% dextrose) with electrolytes, and without protein, lipids, or other carbohydrates, is the first choice. Manage hyperglycemia with insulin to ensure adequate intracellular glucose. Protein can be withheld for 2 to 3 days while awaiting diagnosis. Ammonia encephalopathy can cause permanent neurologic damage in infants, so patients with hyperammonemia and encephalopathy should receive urgent hemodialysis. Some forms of empiric therapy directed at specific disorders may be attempted. For example, intravenous arginine hydrochloride may be effective in reducing ammonia levels in citrullinemia or ureidosuccinic aciduria, and vitamin B_{12} and biotin are sometime effective in methylmalonic acidemia and multiple carboxylase deficiency, respectively. Severe metabolic acidosis should be corrected with intravenous bicarbonate or dialysis if necessary.

In children with a suspected metabolic defect, an initial screening evaluation should include blood electrolytes and a hepatic panel (including transaminases, prothrombin time/partial prothrombin time, and bilirubin), peripheral blood count and smear, glucose, lactate, pyruvate, ammonia, uric acid, blood gasses, and a urinalysis, including reducing substances and ketones. In a hypoglycemic patient, serum ketones, insulin, cortisol, growth hormone, and C peptide levels should be submitted to the laboratory at the time of hypoglycemia if possible. In patients with metabolic acidosis, plasma ketones and amino acids may also be helpful. Additional specific testing includes urine organic and amino acid panels, plasma carnitine levels, acylcarnitine panel, and plasma amino acid panel. It is best to discuss this testing with a metabolic specialist so that the important tests are obtained early.

For patients who die or are critically ill, samples should be taken and saved, if possible, for later testing. Genetic testing can help the family even if the patient does not survive. Frozen blood, urine and cerebrospinal fluid, and blood spots on filter paper (Guthrie card) should be taken as soon as possible after death with biopsies of skin, liver, and muscle.

SUGGESTED READINGS

Burton BK. Inborn errors of metabolism in infancy: a guide to diagnosis. *Pediatrics.* 1998; 102(6):E69.

Leonard JV, Morris AA. Diagnosis and early management of inborn errors of metabolism presenting around the time of birth. *Acta Paediatr.* 2006;95(1):6–14.

Saudubray JM, Charpentier C. Clinical phenotypes: diagnosis/algorithms. In: Scriver, et al., eds. *Online Metabolic and Molecular Bases of Inherited Disease.* McGraw-Hill; 2007.

Saudubray JM, Sedel F, Walter JH. Clinical approach to treatable inborn metabolic diseases: an introduction. *J Inherit Metab Dis.* 2006;29(2–3):261–274.

245

OBTAIN A CARDIOLOGY CONSULT FOR THOSE PATIENTS PRESENTING WITH A GENETIC SYNDROME

RUSSELL CROSS, MD

WHAT TO DO – GATHER APPROPRIATE DATA, MAKE A DECISION, TAKE ACTION

The complex relationship between genetic composition and environmental influences leading to congenital heart disease (CHD) is just beginning to be understood. From a clinical standpoint, however, there are several well-described genetic syndromes and nongenetic associations involving CHD, of which the pediatric clinician should be aware. *Table 245.1* outlines the most commonly encountered genetic syndromes and nongenetic associations that are commonly seen with CHD.

TABLE 245.1	GENETIC SYNDROMES AND NONGENETIC ASSOCIATIONS INVOLVING CONGENITAL HEART DISEASE	
SYNDROME	**GENETIC ASSOCIATION**	**RELATED CONGENITAL HEART DISEASE**
Down's syndrome	Trisomy chromosome 21	• Atrioventricular septal defect (35%) • Ventricular septal defect ± other lesions (8%) • Patent ductus arteriosus (7%) • Tetralogy of Fallot (4%) • Some studies suggest adults with Down's syndrome have increased risk of mitral and aortic valve disease, like mitral valve prolapse and aortic insufficiency
Trisomy 18	Trisomy chromosome 18	• Congenital heart disease in >50% • Most commonly ventricular septal defect and patent ductus arteriosus
• DiGeorge syndrome • Velocardiofacial syndrome	Deletion in chromosome 22q11	• Congenital heart disease in approximately 75% • Tetralogy of Fallot • Interrupted aortic arch • Other conotruncal abnormalities • Ventricular septal defect

(continued)

© 2008 by Lippincott Williams & Wilkins, a Wolters Kluwer business

TABLE 245.1   (*CONTINUED*)

SYNDROME	GENETIC ASSOCIATION	RELATED CONGENITAL HEART DISEASE
Williams-Beuren syndrome	Deletion in chromosome 7q11.23, resulting in involving elastin	• Supravalvar aortic stenosis • Supravalvar pulmonic stenosis • Stenosis of peripheral vessels, such as renal arteries
Turner syndrome	45, X	• Left-sided heart disease • Coarctation of the aorta (10%) • Aortic valve disease—stenosis, insufficiency, bicuspid aortic valve (18%)
Marfan syndrome	FBN1 mutation causing abnormalities in fibrillin-1	• Aortic root dilation • Mitral valve prolapse
Holt-Oram syndrome	Related to TBX5 gene	• Atrial septal defect • Ventricular septal defect • Tetralogy of Fallot
Noonan syndrome	PTPN11 mutation in 50%	• Valvar pulmonic stenosis • Hypertrophic cardiomyopathy
VACTERL Association		• Atrial septal defect • Ventricular septal defect
CHARGE Association		• Conotruncal abnormalities—Tetralogy of Fallot, Truncus arteriosus • Aortic arch abnormalities—Interrupted aortic arch, vascular rings

CHARGE, Coloboma, *h*eart defect, *c*hoanal atresia, *r*etarded growth and development, *g*enital hypoplasia, *e*ar abnormality; VACTERL, *V*ertebral anomaly, *i*mperforate anus, *c*ardiac abnormality, *t*racheo*e*sophageal fistula, *r*enal abnormalities, *l*imb abnormalities.

A thorough cardiac evaluation and, in many cases, consultation with a pediatric cardiologist, is appropriate when patients are identified with one of these syndromes. Likewise, the practitioner should also consider the possibility of one of these syndromes or associations when these particular forms of CHD are identified. It is also important to be aware of progressive forms of CHD that may develop, as individuals with specific genetic syndromes age, such as hypertrophic cardiomyopathy in Noonan syndrome or mitral and aortic valve disease in Trisomy 21.

SUGGESTED READINGS

Bernier FP, Spaetgens R. The geneticist's role in adult congenital heart disease. *Cardiology Clin.* 2006;24:557–569.

Freeman SB, Taft LF, Dooley KJ, et al. Population-based study of congenital heart defects in Down syndrome. *Am J Medl Genet.* 1998;80(3):213–217.

Goldmuntz E. The genetic contribution to congenital heart disease. *Pediatr Clin North Am.* 2004;51:1721–1737.

Gøtzsche CO, Krag-Olsen B, Nielsen J, et al. Prevalence of cardiovascular malformations and association with karyotypes in Turner's syndrome. *Arch Dis Child.* 1994;71(5):433–436.

246

PERFORM ANNUAL C SPINE FILMS IN CHILDREN WITH DOWN'S SYNDROME BEFORE CLEARING THEM FOR PARTICIPATION IN EXERCISE

WILLIAM GIASI, JR., MD

WHAT TO DO – GATHER APPROPRIATE DATA

Children with Down's syndrome have multiple malformations due to presence of extra genetic material from chromosome 21. An ongoing assessment and management should be performed throughout childhood for specific morbidities. Early identification of these potential risks may maintain or even improve their level of functioning as well as to facilitate transition to adulthood.

Atlantoaxial instability is one of these areas of concerns. The incidence of instability ranges from 10% to 25%. Screening for atlantoaxial instability requires regular assessment for those individuals participating in sports.

Atlantoaxial instability, also called atlantoaxial subluxation, refers to increased mobility at the atlantoaxial joint between the first and second cervical vertebrae. The etiology of atlantoaxial instability is not well understood nor is it unique to Down's syndrome. Atlantoaxial instability may include abnormalities of the ligaments or bony structures of C1 and C2.

Almost all of the patients are affected by atlantoaxial instability are asymptomatic. Patients who are symptomatic may exhibit neurologic signs and symptoms associated with upper motor or posterior column lesions such as easy fatigability, difficulty walking, abnormal gait, neck pain, limited neck mobility, incontinence, torticollis, incoordination, sensory deficits, spasticity, hyperreflexia, and clonus.

Instability can be detected radiographs of the lateral cervical spine. It is recommended to obtain lateral cervical spine radiographs in flexion, neutral, and extension. Radiographic findings of instability are significant for an increased distance between the odontoid process of the axis (C2) and the anterior arch of the atlas (C1). Asymptomatic individuals are thought to be at risk of symptomatic atlantoaxial instability. Studies have found that 7% to 20% of patients with Down's syndrome who have normal neck radiographs initially will have abnormal radiographs later.

ⓒ 2008 by Lippincott Williams & Wilkins, a Wolters Kluwer business

Screening of patients with Down's syndrome includes the possibility of preventing catastrophic spinal cord injury amongst individuals with asymptomatic atlantoaxial instability. Furthermore, screening may identify previously unrecognized patients with symptomatic atlantoaxial instability.

Individuals with asymptomatic atlantoaxial instability should be restricted from participating in activities that have a high risk of spinal cord injury and require further evaluation and periodic assessments.

SUGGESTED READINGS

American Academy of Pediatrics: Committee on Sports Medicine and Fitness. Atlantoaxial instability in Down syndrome: subject review. *Pediatrics.* 1995;96(1 Pt 1):151–154.

American Academy of Pediatrics: Committee on Genetics. American Academy of Pediatrics: supervision for children with Down syndrome. *Pediatrics.* 2001;107:442–449.

Haslam RAH. Spinal Cord Disorders. In: Behrman RE, Kleigman RM, Jenson HB, eds. *Nelson Textbook of Pediatrics.* 17th ed. Philadelphia: Saunders, 2004:2050.

Thompson GH. Atlantoaxial instability. In: Behrman RE, Kliegman RM, Jenson HB, eds. *Nelson Textbook of Pediatrics.* 17th ed. Philadelphia: Saunders; 2004:2289–2290.

247

KNOW WHICH CHILD WITH A GENETIC SYNDROME MAY BE A DIFFICULT INTUBATION

RENÉE ROBERTS, MD

WHAT TO DO – INTERPRET THE DATA

It is generally agreed upon that a difficult airway is a situation when problems exist in establishing adequate ventilation via mask or artificial airway. This situation can be both unanticipated and anticipated. The scope of this discussion will consist of the anticipated difficult airway caused from genetic syndromes with craniofacial disorders. Early recognition of these syndromes increases the likelihood of a possible difficult airway being identified and proper preparation occurring. This includes both proper equipment and additional skilled personnel.

There are multiple challenges involved in managing the airway of a patient with craniofacial disorders. A thorough understanding is needed of the normal anatomy, including both bony structures and soft tissue, and how these are affected by various disorders. The resulting abnormalities can affect airway management: ventilation, intubation, or both. Well-known congenital disorders that can affect the anatomy of the airway include Pierre Robin syndrome, Treacher Collins syndrome, Klippel-Feil syndrome, Beckwith-Wiedemann syndrome, Trisomy 21, Freeman–Sheldon syndrome, Goldenhar syndrome, craniofacial dysostosis (Apert syndrome), as well as mucopolysaccharidosis syndromes that include Hunter and Hurler syndromes. Following is a brief discussion of these disorders and their associated anatomic abnormalities.

Pierre Robin Syndrome. This disorder is characterized by severe micrognathia, glossoptosis, and cleft soft palate, or cleft lip. Relaxation of the soft tissue in the oropharynx can lead to total airway obstruction as the tongue falls posteriorly. Ventilation by mask can be difficult; therefore, airway management often requires additional planning and the availability of alternate methods and skilled providers to establish the airway. This can include the laryngeal mask airway and a fiberoptic scope.

Treacher Collins Syndrome. This disorder is characterized by maxillary, zygomatic, and mandibular hypoplasia. Additional features that can affect airway include a small mouth and high arched palate. Secondary issues

ⓒ 2008 by Lippincott Williams & Wilkins, a Wolters Kluwer business

can consist of cleft palate and velopharyngeal incompetence. If temporo-mandibular joint abnormalities are present, mask ventilation and intubation can be very difficult, if not impossible. As patients age, airway issues become more difficult. Severe airway obstruction can occur and may necessitate a tracheostomy.

Klippel-Feil Syndrome. Characterized by atlanto-occipital abnormalities, fusion of cervical vertebrae, scoliosis, and stenosis of the spinal cord. Although bag–mask ventilation is often not difficult, the limitation in movement of the cervical vertebrae make intubation very difficult. Often a fiberoptic scope or laryngeal mask airway are needed to intubate the patient, as aggressive manipulation of the cervical spine can result in injury.

Beckwith-Wiedemann Syndrome. Large protuberant tongue, exomphalos, and giantism are key characteristics. The large tongue can cause airway obstruction severe enough to result in cor pulmonale over time. Bag–mask ventilation is difficult, as the tongue remains in the mouth and can cause obstruction; this should be avoided. However, intubation can be achieved because the tongue can be moved out of the way with a laryngoscope.

Trisomy 21. This is the most common chromosomal disorder affecting the airway. Abnormal characteristics that may be present and affect the airway in these patients include large fissured tongue, atlanto-occipital and atlantoaxial instability, and hypoplastic nasal bone and subglottic stenosis. Due to the possible presence of subglottic stenosis, an endotracheal tube smaller than expected for age may be needed for intubation. These patients obstruct easily and an oral airway is often needed to mask ventilate.

Freeman-Sheldon Syndrome. This is a rare myopathic dysplastic disorder. Patients with this disorder are at higher risk for malignant hyperthermia. Therefore, rapid sequence induction for establishing an airway using succinylcholine is not recommended. Patients have masklike facies due to contraction of the soft tissue and musculature of the face, with microstomia and circumoral fibrosis. Additionally, some patients will have contractures that limit neck movement, resulting in difficult intubation.

Goldenhar Syndrome. This syndrome is variant of hemifacial microsomia. Mandibular hypoplasia, auricular abnormalities, overlying soft-tissue loss, and facial nerve involvement are key features in hemifacial microsomia, and are often asymmetric in nature. As the severity of the mandibular deformity increases, the level of difficulty in intubation increases. The additional features of vertebral abnormalities and macrostomia characterize Goldenhar syndrome. The vertebral abnormalities may be total fusion or hemivertebrae that result in decreased flexion and extension, resulting in a more difficult intubation.

Apert Syndrome. This syndrome is also known as craniofacial dysostosis. Midface hypoplasia, craniosynostosis, high arched palate, proptosis, and some degree of choanal stenosis characterize this disorder. Due to the abnormalities, mask ventilation can be difficult, as the tongue can fill the small oral cavity. This can be overcome by holding the mouth open slightly during mask ventilation. Unless an issue with cervical spine mobility is present, intubation is generally not very difficult; however, a smaller tube may be needed for patients with tracheal ring abnormalities.

Hunter and Hurler Syndromes. Both variants in the mucopolysaccharidoses group of genetic disorders are characterized by varying enzyme production that affects mucopolysaccharides in the body. Mucopolysaccharides accumulate in the body secondary to enzyme deficiencies. This affects the airway, as deposits cause tongue enlargement, soft tissue in the oropharynx becomes thickened, and redundant tissue is present and nasal passages become blocked. All of these issues result in worsening airway obstruction over time and increased difficulty in mask ventilation and intubation.

SUGGESTED READINGS

Gregory GA, Riazi J. Classification and assessment of the difficult pediatric airway. *Anesthesiol Clin North Am.* 1998;16(4):739–741.

Nargozian C. The Airway in patients with craniofacial abnormalities. *Paediatr Anaesth.* 2004; 14:53–59.

Steward DJ. Anesthesia considerations in children with Down syndrome. *Sem. Anesth Periop Med Pain* 2006;25:136–141.

248

USE MEDICAL TESTS JUDICIOUSLY

MADAN DHARMAR, MD

WHAT TO DO – GATHER APPROPRIATE DATA, INTERPRET THE DATA, MAKE A DECISION

Using the appropriate test or study for a particular disease helps to optimize the risk-benefit profile of the diagnostic testing and improve the diagnostic capabilities of the test.

Medical tests can be classified into two types: screening tests and diagnostic tests. Screening tests are usually applied in the community to identify a disease early and thus able to appropriately intervene as a measure of secondary prevention; and they are also used as a basis for primary prevention. Diagnostic tests are applied to an individual in the clinical setting to identify and provide effective health care to that individual. The results of the tests could fall into one of the four groups:

- **True positive** (TP): when the patient's test is *positive* and *is* diseased
- **False positive** (FP): when the patient's test is positive but *not* diseased
- **True negative** (TN): when the patient's test is *negative* and is *not* diseased
- **False negative** (FN): when the patient's test is negative but *is* diseased.

An ideal test is one that, when applied to an individual or a population, can separate patients into two groups (TP and TN). In reality, the majority of tests are far from ideal and are influenced by many factors, which affects the way they separate the population into groups. Hence, it is important to know how the test performs before interpreting the test's results.

The first step in understanding a test is to assess the ability of the test to correctly diagnose the diseased and nondiseased. Sensitivity and specificity are test characteristics that help to access the ability of the test to make that distinction in an individual.

- The sensitivity of a test is the ability of the test to correctly identify the diseased. It could also be defined as the proportion of TP among the diseased [TP/(TP+FN)].

© 2008 by Lippincott Williams & Wilkins, a Wolters Kluwer business

■ The specificity of a test is the ability of the test to correctly identify the individual as not diseased. It could also be define as the proportion of TN among the not diseased [TN/(TN+FP)].

To illustrate with an example, let us consider a population of 100 people, of whom 20 are diseased and 80 are not diseased. Let us say that when each of the individuals was tested using Test A, we found that 18 were correctly identified as diseased (TP) and that 64 were correctly identified as not diseased (TN).

Disease Status

		+	−	
Test	+	18 (TP)	16 (FP)	24
Status	−	2 (FN)	64 (TN)	64
		20	80	100

Sensitivity of the test $= \text{TP}/(\text{TP} + \text{FN}) = 18/20 = 0.90\,(90\%)$

Specificity of the test $= \text{TN}/(\text{TN} + \text{FP}) = 64/80 = 0.80\,(80\%)$

It is important to understand that tests may be chosen based on the situation it is being applied to the individual. It is essential to understand the impact of false positive and false negative before choosing a test. A positive result in a screening test may need to be followed with more tests to confirm the disease, which could be burdensome to the health system; and it could cause anxiety and worry in the person who had been told that the test was positive when he or she was, in fact, not diseased. A person who has been diagnosed as positive based on false-positive results from a screening test may never be able to remove that label, even when it was later found to be negative on subsequent evaluation. Similarly, consider the impact of a false-negative test result in a diseased individual, especially with a serious disease, which, when diagnosed in a timely manner, could affect management of that disease (e.g., early stages of cancer).

Sensitivity and specificity of a test provides the probability of the test results in the presence or absence of disease, but a physician is more interested in knowing the probability of disease in the presence of positive or negative results from the test. That is, if the test is positive for an individual, then what is the probability that the individual is truly positive? And similarly, if a test is negative for an individual, then what is the probability that the individual is truly negative?

Predictive Value and Prevalence. Positive predictive value (PPV) is defined as the proportion of TP among the test-positive individuals [TP/(TP+FP)]. Negative predictive value (NPV) is the proportion of TN among the test negative individuals [TN/(TN+FN)]. Using the sample example above,

$$PPV = TP/(TP + FP) = 18/24 = 0.53$$

$$NPV = TN/(TN + FN) = 64/66 = 0.97$$

Prevalence of a disease is defined as the number of cases of a disease present in a population at that specific time divided by the number of persons in the population at that time. It is the probability of disease in the population. The predictive value of a test is dependant on the prevalence of the disease in that population. To illustrate this let us go back to the example above. The prevalence of disease in the population is 0.20 (20/100) and we know that the predictive values are 0.53 and 0.97 (positive and negative, respectively). Using the same test, (sensitivity = 90% and specificity = 80%) let us calculate the predictive values for population with prevalence of 0.4 (40/100).

Disease Status

		+	−	
Test	+	54 (TP)	8 (FP)	62
Status	−	6 (FN)	32 (TN)	38
		60	40	100

$$PPV = TP/(TP + FP) = 54/62 = 0.87$$

$$NPV = TN/(TN + FN) = 32/38 = 0.84$$

The PPV increased from 0.53 to 0.87 when the same test was applied to a population with greater prevalence of the disease. When the prevalence of a disease is very low, then the PPV of the test will not be even close to 1, even when the test is highly sensitive and specific. When the test is used to screen a population with low prevalence, it is inevitable that many people will have false positive results. This shows that test results must be interpreted only after taking into consideration the prevalence of the disease in that population.

Most of the tests during development are evaluated under ideal conditions (experimental condition): sensitivity being determined by testing on diseased individuals, and the specificity determined by testing on individuals who do not have the disease. Therefore, test specifications may vary when the test is used in real-world conditions and applied to a different population with different prevalence of disease. Prevalence affects the positive and negative predictive value of the test. Prevalence can be considered the pretest probability that the individual could have the disease, and the positive and negative predictive values (PPV and NPV) of the test are the revised estimate for the individuals who are positive or negative on the test, and are post-test probabilities or posterior probabilities. The positive (PPV) and negative (NPV) predictive value can be calculated for different population prevalence for a test by,

$$PPV = \frac{sensitivity \times prevalence}{(((sensitivity \times prevalence) + ((1 - specificity) \times (1 - prevalence)))}$$

$$NPV = \frac{specificity \times (1 - prevalence)}{(((1 - sensitivity) \times prevalence) + (specificity \times (1 - prevalence)))}$$

The usefulness of the test can be assessed by the difference between the pre- and posttest probabilities.

In a clinical setting, the physician, following his or her initial evaluation, arrives at a probability (pretest probability or prevalence) of that individual being diseased. Based on the initial assessment, the physician could either decide the individual is not diseased, or test the individual further for the disease, or treat the individual for the disease. This approach was described by Pauker and Kassirer in their article about clinical decision making. The pretest probability for any individual can fall into the category of: (a) no disease, (b) may have the disease but need to test, and (c) has the disease. The medical test is used to enable the physician to arrive at a diagnosis. If a test is used in an individual with a low pretest probability, there is greater chance for a false positive result, that could in turn result in a misdiagnosis for the individual. It is essential to avoid testing an individual when there is a greater likelihood that one or more of the results could be a false positive. The judicious use of medical testing based on the sensitivity, specificity, and predictive values of the test in important.

In conclusion, when choosing or interpreting a test result in an individual we need to consider:

- The pretest probability of the disease in the individual.
- Sensitivity and specificity are specific characteristics of a test, which could help to assess quality of the test.

■ Predictive values of a test could help us to assess how good the test is at identifying diseased patients correctly.

■ Impact of false-positive and false-negative results of a test.

SUGGESTED READINGS

Altman DG, Bland JM. Diagnostic tests 2: predictive values. *BMJ*. 1994;309(6947):102.

Gordis L. *Epidemiology*. 3rd ed. Philadelphia: Saunders; 2004.

Pauker SG, Kassirer JP. The threshold approach to clinical decision making. *N Engl J Med*. 1980;302(20):1109–1117.

249

UNDERSTAND HOW YOUR PATIENT'S CONDITION MAY BE RELATED TO THE CONDITIONS IN THE COMMUNITY OR POPULATION WITHIN WHICH YOU PRACTICE

MADAN DHARMAR, MD

WHAT TO DO – GATHER APPROPRIATE DATA

Disease in an individual is an interaction between the individual (host), the disease-causing agent, and the environment. Each disease is unique in its causation and its effect on the individual. For example, the genetic make-up of an individual plays an important role in determining susceptibility and immunity of the individual when interacting with the disease agent and the environment. Exposure to a causative agent is a necessary step in the causation of disease in an individual. Disease could be caused by direct contact with another individual who has the disease or by contact with a common vehicle or vector (e.g., contaminated food or mosquito). For an individual, the risk of exposure to an agent could be related the distribution of the disease and the causative agent in community or population. Therefore, to understand the causation of a disease in a community, frequency of the disease and their determinants in the community or population need to be measured. By knowing the conditions in the community, health care providers can plan to deliver appropriate services. The disease burden in a community, and the evolution of that disease, helps to estimate the risk of disease development in the people in the community.

Incidence and prevalence are measures that help us to better understand the trend and patterns of disease occurrence. The most important step in determining these measures is to define the disease or what differentiates the individual as diseased or nondiseased.

Incidence. Incidence is the measure of the frequency of new cases of a disease in a population. Incidence is represented as the "number of new cases of a disease occurring in the population during a specified period of time" divided by the "number of persons at risk of developing the disease during the same period of time."

If the disease is uncommon, for example, incidence can be expressed as incidence per 1,000 persons by multiplying it by 1,000. For an incidence to be a measure of risk, a period of time must be specified and all the individuals

© 2008 by Lippincott Williams & Wilkins, a Wolters Kluwer business

in the groups represented in the denominator must have been followed up for the entire period.

Prevalence. Prevalence is the measure of the frequency of all cases of a disease in a population. Prevalence is represented as the "number of cases of a disease present in the population at a specific time" divided by the "number of persons in the population at that specified time." Prevalence can also be expressed per number population such as per 1,000 population.

There are two types of prevalence: point prevalence, which is the prevalence of a particular disease at one point in time, and period prevalence, which is the prevalence of a particular disease at any time during a certain period. For period prevalence, the numerator would include individuals who had the disease at some point during this time period and they could either still have the disease, recovered from the disease, or died from the disease.

Here is an example to illustrate the above concepts:

1. In January 2001, a community of 5,000 people underwent a free evaluation for diabetes mellitus. During this evaluation, 40 people were noted to have diabetes: 15 were newly diagnosed and 25 were already-known cases undergoing treatment.
2. The same 5,000 people had a repeat evaluation in January 2003: 30 people were noted to have diabetes; 10 of them were previously diagnosed with diabetes by their personal physician in last 12 months. Five of the people diagnosed in the 2001 screening had died of various causes in 2002.

$$\text{Point prevalence in January 2001} = (40/5{,}000) \times 1{,}000$$
$$= 8 \text{ cases per } 1{,}000 \text{ people.}$$

$$\text{Point prevalence in January 2003} = [(40 - 5 + 30)/(5000 - 5)] \times 1000$$
$$= 13.01 \text{ cases per } 1{,}000 \text{ people}$$

$$\text{Period prevalence (January 2001 to January 2003)}$$
$$= [(40 + 30)/5{,}000)] \times 1{,}000 = 14 \text{ cases per } 1{,}000$$

$$\text{Incidence during January 2001 to January 2003}$$
$$= [(30)/(5000 - 40)] \times 1000 = 6.04 \text{ cases per } 1{,}000$$

Relationship Between Prevalence and Incidence. Prevalence of a disease at a particular time point is dependant on the incidence of the disease and the duration of the disease. An increase in the incidence of disease results in an increase of the prevalence of the disease, and a decrease in duration of disease (cured or died) will result in a decreased prevalence.

SUGGESTED READINGS

Altman DG, Bland JM. Diagnostic tests 2: predictive values. *BMJ*. 1994;309(6947):102.

Gordis L. *Epidemiology*. 3rd ed. Philadelphia: Saunders; 2004.

Pauker SG, Kassirer JP. The threshold approach to clinical decision making. *N Engl J Med*. 1980;302(20):1109–1117.

KNOW THE CATEGORIES OF MEDICAL EVIDENCE AND THE EVIDENCE-BASED MEDICINE APPROACH

SARIKA JOSHI, MD

WHAT TO DO – GATHER APPROPRIATE DATA

Know the categories of medical evidence and the evidence-based medicine (EBM) approach.

Physicians are charged with the task of keeping up-to-date with the latest medical research and innovations. The practice of EBM enables clinicians to synthesize this ever-growing body of knowledge, as well as helps them to apply this information to individual patients. Physicians also need to be familiar with the classes of research reports and the conclusion grades for evidence.

EBM is practiced when clinicians integrate the best available evidence and their clinical expertise in making decisions about their patients' care. There are five necessary steps in the practice of EBM.

First, the need for information must be converted into answerable questions. Research can only answer specific questions. For instance, "How effective are inhaled corticosteroids in the prevention of asthma symptoms?" is an answerable question, whereas "What is the best way to treat asthma?" is not. An appropriate question has four components: (a) a patient or a problem, (b) an intervention, (c) an intervention for comparison, if applicable, and (d) a clinical outcome.

Second, the best evidence must be found in the most efficient manner. The *ACP Journal Club* and *Evidence-Based Medicine* are two journals that screen, analytically appraise, and compile articles from other publications. The Cochrane Database is a growing collection of comprehensive reviews of clinical interventions based on meta-analyses of rigorously chosen articles. These sources of information give physicians quick access to the best evidence.

Third, the evidence must be critically appraised for its internal validity and generalizability. Internal validity examines whether the results for the patients in the study are true, and it is threatened by bias and chance. Bias is a systematic error that could falsify the results. Chance effects, which are depicted with P values, power, and confidence intervals, can be minimized by studying a large population. Generalizability requires the judgment of the

© 2008 by Lippincott Williams & Wilkins, a Wolters Kluwer business

clinician and refers to whether the study results are applicable to a particular population of patients.

Knowing the classes of research reports and the conclusion grades for evidence is useful when trying to sort through the literature. The classes of research reports are as follows:

- Class A reports come from a randomized, controlled trial.
- Class B reports are generated from a cohort study.
- Class C reports follow a nonrandomized trial with current or historical controls, a case-control study, a study about the sensitivity or specificity of a diagnostic test, or a descriptive, population-based study.
- Class D reports come from a cross-sectional study, a case series, or a case report.
- Class M reports are generated from a meta-analysis, a systematic review, or a decision or cost-effectiveness analysis.
- Class R reports follow a consensus statement or report or a narrative review.
- Class X reports demonstrate a medical opinion.

The conclusion grades for evidence are as follows:

- Grade I evidence draws from the conclusions of well-designed studies with consistent results. The results are internally valid, generalizable, and have adequate statistical power.
- Grade II evidence draws from the conclusions of well-designed studies, but there is some uncertainty about the results, due to minor concerns about internal validity, generalizability or statistical power. Alternatively, grade II evidence may come from study designs that are weaker but have consistent results.
- Grade III evidence draws from the conclusions of well-designed studies, but there is a lot of uncertainty about the results, due to major concerns about internal validity, generalizability or statistical power. Alternatively, grade III evidence may come from study designs that are weak and few in number.

The fourth step in EBM is putting together the appraised evidence with clinical expertise and applying it to an individual patient.

The fifth step in EBM is self-evaluation. Physicians should ask themselves if they formulated an answerable question, if they efficiently found the best evidence, if they critically appraised the evidence they found, and if they integrated this evidence with their clinical experience. By taking the time to go through this assessment, clinicians continually improve their EBM skills.

In summary, EBM is the process by which physicians find and evaluate evidence to incorporate into their clinical practice, combine it with their own experience and knowledge, and ultimately help take better care of their patients.

SUGGESTED READINGS

Sackett DL, Rosenberg WM. The need for evidence-based medicine. *J R Soc Med.* 1995;88(11):620–624.

Straus SE, Sackett DL. Using research findings in clinical practice. *BMJ.* 1998;317(7154):339–342.

Note: Page numbers followed by *f* indicate figures; page numbers followed by *t* indicate tables.

Alcohol (*contd.*)
 smell of, 183
 toxicity, 174–175
Aldara. *See* Imiquimod
Aldolase A deficiency, 580
Algorithms
 for acne, 100–101
 for hyperbilirubinemia, 27
Alkaline phosphatase (AP), 397
Alkalosis. *See* Metabolic alkalosis
ALL. *See* Acute lymphoblastic
  leukemia
Allergies
 iodine, 240–241
 milk, 31, 429–430
 penicillin, 243–244, 250–251
 seafood, 240–241
Allopurinol, 440–441
Alpha blockers, 340
ALT. *See* Alanine aminotransferase
ALTE. *See* Apparent life threatening
  events
Altered mental status, 563–564, 616
Alveoli, 408
Ambiguous genitalia, 45–47
American Academy of Dermatology, 453
American Academy of Pediatrics, 36,
  97, 98, 100, 102, 120, 125, 245,
  429, 452
American Academy of Rheumatology,
  289
American College of Cardiology, 303
American Dietetic Association, 120
American Heart Association, 303
American Liver Foundation, 121
Amino acids, 140, 154, 563
Aminoglycoside, 472, 527–528
Ammonia, 220, 398–399, 564
Ammonium chloride, 365
Amoxicillin, 162, 303
Amphetamines, 194, 195*t*
Ampicillin, 303
ANA. *See* Antinuclear antibody
Anal fissures, 83
Anal tags, 83
Anaphylactoid reactions, 240–241
Anaphylaxis, 230–232
Ancylostoma duodenale, 252
Androgen receptors, 46
Androstenedione, 154

Anemia, 141, 429–430. *See also* Sickle
  cell anemia
 aplastic, 424–425
 hemolytic, 142
Anesthesia, hypoventilation, 482–484
Angelman syndrome, 614
Angiotensin-converting enzyme (ACE),
  158
Anhedonia, 115
Anion gap, 358–360, 382
 formulas related to, 359*t*
Ankylosing spondylitis, 448
Anomalous left coronary artery (ALCA),
  148
Anorectal fissures, 31, 411
Anorexia, 150
Anterior mediastinal masses, 460–462
Anterolateral hymenal flaps, 82
Anteromedial surface, 203–204
Antibiotic therapy, 72, 250–251, 525–526
 for puncture wounds, 264–265
Antibodies to double-stranded DNA
  (anti-dsDNA), 289
Anticipatory guidance, 102–104
 family discord in, 107–109
 in infants, 102–103
 in older adolescents, 103–104
 in school age children, 103
 in toddlers, 103
 in younger adolescents, 103
Antideoxyribonuclease B (anti-DNAse
  B), 356
Antidiuretic hormone (ADH), 349*f*, 351,
  377
anti-DNAse B. *See*
  Antideoxyribonuclease B
anti-dsDNA. *See* Antibodies to
  double-stranded DNA
Antifungals, 605
Antihistamines, 90, 241
Anti-inflammatory agents, 290
Anti-Müllerian hormone, 45
Antinuclear antibody (ANA), 288, 289,
  293
Antioxidants, 154
Antipyretics, 90
Anti-Smith antibody, 288–290
Antithrombin (AT), 418
Anxiety, 68–70
AOE. *See* Acute otitis externa